Review for
Textbook of Pediatric Emergency Medicine

Fourth Edition

Review for
Textbook of Pediatric Emergency Medicine

Fourth Edition

Editors

Sujit Sharma, MD
Clinical Fellow in Pediatrics
Harvard Medical School
Fellow in Pediatric Emergency Medicine
Division of Emergency Medicine
Children's Hospital
Boston, Massachusetts

Vincent J. Wang, MD
Assistant Professor of Clinical Pediatrics
Keck School of Medicine of
the University of Southern California
Attending Physician
Division of Emergency Medicine
Childrens Hospital Los Angeles
Los Angeles, California

Assistant Editors

Robert L. Cloutier, MD
Instructor in Pediatrics
University of Pennsylvania School of Medicine
Fellow in Pediatric Emergency Medicine
Children's Hospital of Philadelphia
Philadelphia, Pennsylvania

Barbara M. Garcia Peña, MD, MPH
Clinical Fellow in Pediatrics
Harvard Medical School
Fellow in Pediatric Emergency Medicine
Division of Emergency Medicine
Children's Hospital
Boston, Massachusetts

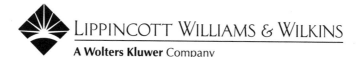

LIPPINCOTT WILLIAMS & WILKINS
A Wolters Kluwer Company
Philadelphia • Baltimore • New York • London
Buenos Aires • Hong Kong • Sydney • Tokyo

Acquisitions Editor: Anne M. Sydor
Developmental Editor: Tanya Lazar
Supervising Editor: Mary Ann McLaughlin
Production Editor: Janet Domingo, Compset, Inc.
Manufacturing Manager: Kevin Watt
Cover Designer: David Levy
Compositor: Compset, Inc.
Printer: Maple Press

© 2000 by LIPPINCOTT WILLIAMS & WILKINS
530 Walnut Street
Philadelphia, PA 19106 USA
LWW.com

Printed in the USA

ISBN: 0-7817-2467-8

Care has been taken to confirm the accuracy of the information presented and to describe generally accepted practices. However, the authors, editors, and publisher are not responsible for errors or omissions or for any consequences from application of the information in this book and make no warranty, expressed or implied, with respect to the currency, completeness, or accuracy of the contents of the publication. Application of the information in a particular situation remains the professional responsibility of the practitioner.

The authors, editors, and publisher have exerted every effort to ensure that drug selection and dosage set forth in this text are in accordance with current recommendations and practice at the time of publication. However, in view of ongoing research, changes in government regulations, and the constant flow of information relating to drug therapy and drug reactions, the reader is urged to check the package insert for each drug for any change in indications and dosage and for added warnings and precautions. This is particularly important when the recommended agent is a new or infrequently employed drug.

Some drugs and medical devices presented in this publication have Food and Drug Administration (FDA) clearance for limited use in restricted research settings. It is the responsibility of the health care provider to ascertain the FDA status of each drug or device planned for use in their clinical practice.

10 9 8 7 6 5 4 3 2 1

Dedication

To our parents:

Visho and Kamlesh Sharma

Jaw and Jean Wang

Contents

Contributing Authors . . . . **xiii**
Foreword . . . . **xvii**
Preface . . . . **xix**
Acknowledgments . . . . **xxi**
Pre-test . . . . **xxiii**
Abbreviations . . . . **xxxviii**

SECTION I   Life-Threatening Emergencies

1 Resuscitation—Pediatric Basic and Advanced Life Support   3
   Vincent J. Wang, M.D.
2 Neonatal Resuscitation   8
   Jacqueline Bryngil, M.D.
3 Shock   10
   Karen Dull, M.D.
4 Sedation and Analgesia   13
   Atima Chumpa, M.D.
5 Emergency Airway Management—Rapid-Sequence Intubation   16
   Atima Chumpa, M.D.
6 Prehospital Care   19
   Sujit Sharma, M.D.
7 Transport   21
   Jeffrey P. Louie, M.D.
8 Myocardial Infarction   24
   Neil Schamban, M.D.

SECTION II   Signs and Symptoms

9 Abdominal Distension   29
   Barbara M. Garcia Peña, M.D., M.P.H.
10 Apnea   32
   Jill C. Posner, M.D.
11 Ataxia   35
   Joyce Soprano, M.D.
12 Breast Lesions   37
   Mark Waltzman, M.D.
13 Coma and Altered Level of Consciousness   39
   Joyce Soprano, M.D.
14 Constipation   41
   Vincent J. Wang, M.D.
15 Cough   44
   Bema K. Bonsu, MBChB, M.D.
16 Cyanosis   47
   Sujit Sharma, M.D.
17 Crying and Colic in Early Infancy   49
   Vincent J. Wang, M.D.
18 Dehydration   51
   Ron L. Kaplan, M.D.

19 Diarrhea 53
Mark Waltzman, M.D.

20 Disturbed Child 55
Thomas H. Chun, M.D.

21 Dizziness 57
Joyce Soprano, M.D.

22 Edema 59
Vincent J. Wang, M.D.

23 Epistaxis 61
Dominic Chalut, M.D.

24 Eye—Red 63
Andrea Stracciolini, M.D.

25 Eye—Strabismus 66
Mark E. Ralston, M.D., M.P.H.

26 Eye—Unequal Pupils 69
Mark E. Ralston, M.D., M.P.H.

27 Eye—Visual Disturbances 71
Mark E. Ralston, M.D., M.P.H.

28 Fever 74
Bema K. Bonsu, MBChB, M.D.

29 Foreign Body—Ingestion/Aspiration 85
Andrea Stracciolini, M.D.

30 Gastrointestinal Bleeding 87
Ron L. Kaplan, M.D.

31 Groin Masses 90
Vincent J. Wang, M.D.

32 Hearing Loss 92
Mark E. Ralston, M.D., M.P.H.

33 Heart Murmurs 95
Sujit Sharma, M.D.

34 Hematuria 97
Vincent J. Wang, M.D.

35 Hypertension 100
Vincent J. Wang, M.D.

36 Immobile Arm 102
Vincent J. Wang, M.D.

37 Injury—Ankle 104
Vincent J. Wang, M.D.

38 Injury—Head 106
David Greenes, M.D.

39 Injury—Knee 109
Andrea Stracciolini, M.D.

40 Injury—Shoulder 112
Vincent J. Wang, M.D.

41 Jaundice—Unconjugated Hyperbilirubinemia 114
Jacqueline Bryngil, M.D.

42 Jaundice—Conjugated Hyperbilirubinemia 116
Jacqueline Bryngil, M.D.

43 Limp 118
Robert G. Flood, M.D.

44 Lymphadenopathy 121
Ben Willwerth, M.D.

CONTENTS

45 Neck Mass 124
Ben Willwerth, M.D.

46 Neck Stiffness 126
Jill C. Posner, M.D.

47 Odor—Unusual 129
Michele M. Burns, M.D.

48 Oligomenorrhea 132
Jeffrey P. Louie, M.D.

49 Oral Lesions 134
Vincent J. Wang, M.D.

50 Pain—Abdomen 136
Barbara M. Garcia Peña, M.D., M.P.H.

51 Pain—Back 139
John J. Reeves, M.D.

52 Pain—Chest 141
John J. Reeves, M.D.

53 Pain—Dysphagia 144
Vincent J. Wang, M.D.

54 Pain—Dysuria 146
Vincent J. Wang, M.D.

55 Pain—Earache 148
Vincent J. Wang, M.D.

56 Headaches 150
Mark Waltzman, M.D.

57 Joint Pain 152
Vincent J. Wang, M.D.

58 Pain—Scrotal 155
Vincent J. Wang, M.D.

59 Pallor 158
Robert L. Cloutier, M.D.

60 Polydipsia 161
Dominic Chalut, M.D.

61 Rash—Eczematous 163
Karen Dale Gruskin, M.D.

62 Rash—Maculopapular 167
Karen Dale Gruskin, M.D.

63 Rash—Papular Lesions 170
Karen Dale Gruskin, M.D.

64 Rash—Papulosquamous Lesions 172
Karen Dale Gruskin, M.D.

65 Rash—Purpura 174
Vincent J. Wang, M.D.

66 Rash—Urticaria 176
Karen Dale Gruskin, M.D.

67 Rash—Vesicobullous 178
Karen Dale Gruskin, M.D.

68 Respiratory Distress 180
Vincent J. Wang, M.D.

69 The Septic-Appearing Infant 183
Robert L. Cloutier, M.D.

70 Seizures 186
Vincent W. Chiang, M.D.

71 Sore Throat 188
    Cynthia R. Jacobstein, M.D.

72 Stridor 190
    Sujit Sharma, M.D.

73 Syncope 192
    Vincent J. Wang, M.D.

74 Tachycardia/Palpitations 195
    Sujit Sharma, M.D.

75 Urinary Frequency in Childhood 198
    Vincent J. Wang, M.D.

76 Vaginal Bleeding 201
    Jacqueline Bryngil, M.D.

77 Vaginal Discharge 203
    Jacqueline Bryngil, M.D.

78 Vomiting 205
    Ron L. Kaplan, M.D.

79 Weakness/Flaccid Paralysis 207
    Karen Dull, M.D.

80 Wheezing 210
    Vincent J. Wang, M.D.

81 Weight Loss 212
    Vincent J. Wang, M.D.

SECTION III   Medical Emergencies

82 Cardiac Emergencies 217
    Sujit Sharma, M.D.

83 Neurologic Emergencies 222
    Joyce Soprano, M.D.

84 Infectious Diseases 227
    Stephen Porter, M.D.

85 Human Immunodeficiency Virus Infection 240
    Cynthia R. Jacobstein, M.D.

86 Renal and Electrolyte Emergencies 243
    Sujit Sharma, M.D.

87 Hematologic Emergencies 248
    Robert L. Cloutier, M.D.

88 Toxicology Emergencies 254
    Michele M. Burns, M.D

89 Environmental Emergencies 264
    Vincent J. Wang, M.D.

90 Radiation Accidents 269
    Thomas H. Chun, M.D.

91 Bites and Stings 274
    Vincent J. Wang, M.D.

92 Allergic Emergencies 280
    Cynthia Johnson Mollen, M.D.

93 Gastrointestinal Emergencies 285
    Vincent J. Wang, M.D.

94 Pediatric and Adolescent Gynecology 291
    Jacqueline Bryngil, M.D.

95 Pulmonary Emergencies 297
    John J. Reeves, M.D.

96 Cystic Fibrosis 303
Andrea Stracciolini, M.D.

97 Endocrine Emergencies 306
Karen Dull, M.D.

98 Metabolic Emergencies (Inborn Errors of Metabolism) 310
Ron L. Kaplan, M.D.

99 Dermatology 312
Michele M. Burns, M.D.

100 Oncologic Emergencies 318
Ben Willwerth, M.D.

101 Rheumatologic Emergencies 323
Barbara Walsh, M.D.

102 Problems of the Very Early Neonate 328
Jacqueline Bryngil, M.D.

SECTION IV Trauma

103 An Approach to the Injured Child 335
Atima Chumpa, M.D.

104 Major Trauma 337
Atima Chumpa, M.D.

105 Neurotrauma 341
David Greenes, M.D.

106 Neck Trauma 346
Neil Schamban, M.D.

107 Thoracic Trauma 348
Atima Chumpa, M.D.

108 Abdominal Trauma 353
Barbara M. Garcia Peña, M.D., M.P.H.

109 Genitourinary Trauma 358
Vincent J. Wang, M.D.

110 Facial Trauma 361
Ron L. Kaplan, M.D.

111 Eye Trauma 364
Cynthia Johnson Mollen, M.D.

112 Otolaryngologic Trauma 367
Jeffrey P. Louie, M.D.

113 Dental Trauma 369
Vincent J. Wang, M.D.

114 Burns 372
Andrea Stracciolini, M.D.

115 Orthopedic Trauma 375
Joyce Soprano, M.D.

116 Minor Trauma—Lacerations 380
Andrea Stracciolini, M.D.

SECTION V Surgical Emergencies

117 Minor Lesions 385
Vincent J. Wang, M.D.

118 Abdominal Emergencies 389
Barbara M. Garcia Peña, M.D., M.P.H.

119 Thoracic Emergencies 396
Vincent J. Wang, M.D.

120 Ophthalmic Emergencies 400
Cynthia Johnson Mollen, M.D.

121 Otolaryngologic Emergencies 403
Jeffrey P. Louie, M.D.

122 Urologic Emergencies 406
Vincent J. Wang, M.D.

123 Orthopedic Emergencies 408
Joyce Soprano, M.D.

124 Dental Emergencies 413
Vincent J. Wang, M.D.

125 Neurosurgical Emergencies, Nontraumatic 416
David Greenes, M.D.

126 Transplantation Emergencies 419
Dominic Chalut, M.D.

127 Approach to the Care of the Technology-Dependent Child 421
Jill C. Posner, M.D.

SECTION VI   Psychosocial Emergencies

128 Child Abuse 427
Kathy Boutis, M.D.

129 Psychiatric Emergencies 432
Thomas H. Chun, M.D.

130 Adolescent Emergencies 437
Christina Fong, M.B.B.S., M.P.H.

131 Behavioral Emergencies 442
Vincent J. Wang, M.D.

132 The ED Response to Incidents of Biologic and Chemical Terrorism 444
Vincent J. Wang, M.D.

Index 449

Contributing Authors

Bema K. Bonsu, MBChB, MD
Assistant Professor
Ohio State University School of Medicine
Children's Hospital
Attending Physician
Division of Emergency Medicine
Columbus, Ohio

Kathy Boutis, MD
Clinical Fellow in Pediatrics
Harvard Medical School
Fellow in Pediatric Emergency Medicine
Division of Emergency Medicine
Children's Hospital
Boston, Massachusetts

Jacqueline Bryngil, MD
Instructor in Pediatrics
Harvard Medical School
Assistant in Medicine
Children's Hospital
Boston, Massachusetts

Michele M. Burns, MD
Instructor in Pediatrics
Harvard Medical School
Assistant in Medicine
Children's Hospital
Boston, Massachusetts

Dominic Chalut, MD
Assistant Professor
McGill University
Associate Director
Division of Emergency Medicine
The Montreal Children's Hospital
Montreal, Quebec

Vincent W. Chiang, MD
Instructor in Pediatrics
Harvard Medical School
Attending Physician
Division of Emergency Medicine
Children's Hospital
Boston, Massachusetts

Atima Chumpa, MD
Instructor in Pediatrics
Harvard Medical School
Assistant in Medicine
Children's Hospital
Boston, Massachusetts

Thomas H. Chun, MD
Attending Physician
Pediatric Emergency Medicine
Department of Emergency Medicine
Hasbro Children's Hospital
Rhode Island Hospital
Providence, Rhode Island

Robert L. Cloutier, MD
Instructor in Pediatrics
University of Pennsylvania School of Medicine
Fellow in Pediatric Emergency Medicine
Children's Hospital of Philadelphia
Philadelphia, Pennsylvania

Karen Dull, MD
Clinical Fellow in Pediatrics
Harvard Medical School
Fellow in Pediatric Emergency Medicine
Division of Emergency Medicine
Children's Hospital
Boston, Massachusetts

Robert G. Flood, MD
Clinical Fellow in Pediatrics
Harvard Medical School
Fellow in Pediatric Emergency Medicine
Division of Emergency Medicine
Children's Hospital
Boston, Massachusetts

Christina Fong, MBBS, MPH
Consultant in A&E
Guy's and St. Thomas' Hospital
London, UK

David Greenes, MD
Instructor in Pediatrics
Harvard Medical School
Attending Physician
Division of Emergency Medicine
Children's Hospital
Boston, Massachusetts

Karen Dale Gruskin, MD
Instructor in Pediatrics
Harvard Medical School
Assistant in Medicine
Children's Hospital
Boston, Massachusetts
Director
Department of Pediatrics
Winchester Hospital
Winchester, Massachusetts

Cynthia R. Jacobstein, MD
Instructor in Pediatrics
University of Pennsylvania School of Medicine
Fellow in Pediatric Emergency Medicine
Children's Hospital of Philadelphia
Philadelphia, Pennsylvania

Ron L. Kaplan, MD
Instructor in Pediatrics
Harvard Medical School
Assistant in Medicine
Children's Hospital
Boston, Massachusetts

Jeffrey P. Louie, MD
Instructor in Pediatrics
University of Pennsylvania School of Medicine
Fellow in Pediatric Emergency Medicine
Children's Hospital of Philadelphia
Philadelphia, Pennsylvania

Cynthia Johnson Mollen, MD
Instructor in Pediatrics
University of Pennsylvania School of Medicine
Fellow in Pediatric Emergency Medicine
Children's Hospital of Philadelphia
Philadelphia, Pennsylvania

Barbara M. Garcia Peña, MD, MPH
Clinical Fellow in Pediatrics
Harvard Medical School
Fellow in Pediatric Emergency Medicine
Division of Emergency Medicine
Children's Hospital
Boston, Massachusetts

Stephen Porter, MD
Instructor in Pediatrics
Harvard Medical School
Assistant in Medicine
Children's Hospital
Boston, Massachusetts

Jill C. Posner, MD
Assistant Professor of Pediatrics
University of Pennsylvania School of Medicine
Attending Physician
Division of Emergency Medicine
Children's Hospital of Philadelphia
Philadelphia, Pennsylvania

Mark E. Ralston, MD, MPH
Director
Pediatric Emergency Medicine
Naval Medical Center
Portsmouth, Virginia

John J. Reeves, MD
Instructor in Pediatrics
Harvard Medical School
Assistant in Medicine
Children's Hospital
Boston, Massachusetts

Neil Schamban, MD
Clinical Fellow in Pediatrics
Harvard Medical School
Fellow in Pediatric Emergency Medicine
Division of Emergency Medicine
Children's Hospital
Boston, Massachusetts

Sujit Sharma, MD
Clinical Fellow in Pediatrics
Harvard Medical School
Fellow in Pediatric Emergency Medicine
Division of Emergency Medicine
Children's Hospital
Boston, Massachusetts

Joyce Soprano, MD
Instructor in Pediatrics
Harvard Medical School
Assistant in Medicine
Children's Hospital
Boston, Massachusetts

Andrea Stracciolini, MD
Instructor in Pediatrics
Harvard Medical School
Assistant in Medicine
Children's Hospital
Boston, Massachusetts

Barbara Walsh, MD
Clinical Fellow in Pediatrics
Harvard Medical School
Fellow in Pediatric Emergency Medicine
Division of Emergency Medicine
Children's Hospital
Boston, Massachusetts

Mark Waltzman, MD
Instructor in Pediatrics
Harvard Medical School
Assistant in Medicine
Children's Hospital
Boston, Massachusetts

Vincent J. Wang, MD
Assistant Professor of Clinical Pediatrics
Keck School fo Medicine of the University of
   Southern California
Attending Physician
Division of Emergency Medicine
Childrens Hospital Los Angeles
Los Angeles, California

Ben Willwerth, MD
Clinical Fellow in Pediatrics
Harvard Medical School
Fellow in Pediatric Emergency Medicine
Division of Emergency Medicine
Children's Hospital
Boston, Massachusetts

Foreword

The format of the *Review for Textbook of Pediatric Emergency Medicine* makes it easy for both medical students and busy practitioners to consult, and will serve physicians as a useful guide in the years to come beyond their academic course work. A series of questions, similarly constructed and addressing the same material as those about to appear on an upcoming examination, particularly if accompanied by explanations of the correct answers, should certainly contribute to an improved performance on the exam for several reasons. Many physicians find it difficult to dedicate long, uninterrupted blocks of time to studying and are thus unable to consistently review chapters in a textbook. On the other hand, one can try a few questions from this guide and read through the answers in 10 or 15 minutes. When starting an examination, understanding the mechanics of the questions may consume precious minutes. However, examinees who have recently challenged their knowledge in an identical drill will find themselves "in the groove" and able to focus on content much more rapidly. Lastly, frequent practice with questions enables readers to keep current on multiple topics simultaneously, and the reinforcement provided by seeing that they have chosen the correct answers builds confidence and points out areas that need to be pursued in more depth.

Despite the possible gains listed above, my enthusiasm for this book derives, however, not from its potential to boost test scores but rather from its ability to serve as a tool for continuing medical education. I have observed in myself an inverse relationship between age and the length of time that I am able to concentrate on didactic material, while remaining sufficiently alert so as to retain a small modicum of the information. Even when no external forces intrude into my milieu, I quickly find my attention drifting. Because I continue to learn at the same pace from my clinical experiences and conferences, I do not believe that my problem stems from neuronal atrophy. Instead, I would postulate that learning styles evolve as we mature. Although young medical students seem able to digest large volumes of theoretical information, older physicians need the motivation that comes from having to solve an urgent clinical problem. Such immediacy is provided by the question-and-answer format found in this textbook. Detailed case study scenarios replace the sterile quest for disconnected facts with the excitement of making a diagnosis and the struggle to find the optimal treatment.

Drs. Wang and Sharma, along with their colleagues from Boston and Philadelphia, have superbly addressed with this book of questions and answers the dual aims that I have discussed: testing and teaching. As fellows in training and recent graduates poised on the verge of certification, this group of authors has been able to take the perspective not just of anxious examinees waiting for the "big day," but also of practitioners striving to improve their fund of knowledge and clinical acumen. They have succeeded in both of their goals, creating a book that will be valued and enjoyed by physicians at every stage in their careers, caring for acutely ill and injured children.

I hold quite dear the textbook to which these questions directly relate, but I assure you that the issues addressed exist in any reliable reference and, more importantly, in the clinical arena. The spectrum of the material covered is extensive, and all those who exercise their diagnostic and therapeutic skills on these questions will most certainly enhance their expertise in pediatrics and emergency medicine.

Gary R. Fleisher, M.D.

Preface

As reflected in the *Textbook of Pediatric Emergency Medicine,* fourth edition, by Fleisher and Ludwig, the problems encountered when dealing with the acutely ill or injured child are extensive. Reviewing this diverse material is a daunting task. *Review for Textbook of Pediatric Emergency Medicine* is a question-and-answer study guide meant to facilitate this endeavor. As each chapter correlates directly with each of the 132 chapters in the textbook, the reader is able to focus on topics of his or her choice while being able to reference the material easily. The end result is over 1200 clinically oriented questions that review the full range of topics covered in the *Textbook of Pediatric Emergency Medicine*—from urgent care problems of a medical or surgical nature, to specific life-threatening emergencies.

The problems reviewed in this study guide are by no means limited to the Emergency Department setting. Rather, they represent the full spectrum of pediatric acute care issues encountered by various specialists and subspecialists, in particular, by emergency physicians, pediatric emergency physicians, pediatricians, and family practitioners.

The questions have been carefully crafted to maintain the highest standards. They resemble the questions used for board examinations in style and format. All questions are followed by answers with detailed explanations, thereby serving as an excellent review for physicians in training as well as those who are preparing for certification exams. For the established practitioner, the questions provide a stimulating self-assessment review of the most current approaches to management of the acutely ill or injured child. We have included a 50-question Pretest to serve as a stimulus for those who are interested in testing their knowledge on a smaller subset of random topics, as well as to provide insight into possible subjects in need of review.

This review book represents the combined efforts of current and recently graduated pediatric emergency medicine fellows from Children's Hospital, Boston, and Children's Hospital of Philadelphia. Many outstanding teachers and mentors who have dedicated their lives to the care of children helped to inspire each individual involved. It is our hope that this review book can convey some of the knowledge imparted to us while promoting better care for ill or injured children everywhere.

Sujit Sharma, M.D.
Second-year Fellow, Children's Hospital, Boston

Vincent J. Wang, M.D.
Former Chief Fellow, Children's Hospital, Boston*

*Presently, Attending Emergency Physician, Children's Hospital, Los Angeles

Acknowledgments

Our most sincere thanks go to Gary Fleisher, M.D., and Steve Ludwig, M.D. This book would not have been possible without their guidance and support.

Pre-test

VINCENT J. WANG, M.D., and SUJIT SHARMA, M.D.

QUESTIONS

1. A 2-month-old boy is brought to the ED because of difficulty breathing. He has had cough and rhinorrhea for several days. On examination, his vital signs are: T 37.9°C, HR 170, RR 12, and BP 80/50. He is tired appearing in the mother's arms. He has severe intercostal and subcostal retractions. He has bilateral wheezing on auscultation of his chest. Treatment includes:

   a. Reassurance and discharge to home on a humidifier
   b. Reassurance and discharge to home on albuterol syrup
   c. Obtaining a CBC, blood culture, urinalysis (UA), and urine culture
   d. Administration of dexamethasone IM
   e. Assisted bag-valve-mask ventilation

2. A 3-month-old girl is brought in to the ED for "wheezing." Over the past week her mother has noted increased work of breathing, which is more pronounced while the girl is feeding. The mother states that her child now takes approximately 30 minutes to consume 2 ounces of formula. She has had no fevers or cold symptoms. Her vital signs are: T 36.6°C, HR 174, RR 68, and BP 104/62. Her O_2 saturation is 94% on room air. She appears alert and nontoxic. You note intercostal retractions, with mild inspiratory and expiratory wheezes bilaterally. She has good distal pulses and appears well perfused. Her abdomen is soft and nontender, with a liver edge palpable 3 cm below the right costal margin. No spleen tip is palpated. This patient is most likely to benefit from:

   a. Nebulized albuterol
   b. IV normal saline 20 ml/kg
   c. IV furosemide
   d. Prostaglandin E_1
   e. Oral steroids

3. A 4-year-old girl is brought to the ED for epistaxis. She has had epistaxis for the past day now. The mother denies trauma or URI symptoms. The girl has otherwise been healthy, with no previous history of bleeding or bruising problems. On physical examination, she is alert and well appearing. Her mucous membranes are moist, but she has a dark red ecchymotic lesion on her upper gum. Her lungs are clear and her abdomen is soft. She also has scattered petechiae over her trunk and extremities. The most life-threatening complication of her disease is:

   a. High-output cardiac failure
   b. Intracranial hemorrhage
   c. Anemia
   d. Splenic sequestration
   e. Sepsis

4. An 18-month-old boy with Wernig-Hoffmann disease is brought to the ED for respiratory distress. He has had a worsening cough for the past 7 days, associated with fever. His vital signs are: T 38.2°C, HR 140, RR 8, and BP 100/60. He has severe retractions and appears tired. As you prepare to intubate him, you order the following group of medications:

   a. Atropine, lidocaine, thiopental, succinylcholine
   b. Atropine, midazolam, succinylcholine
   c. Atropine, thiopental, rocuronium
   d. Atropine, ketamine, succinylcholine
   e. Lidocaine, thiopental, rocuronium

5. A 4-year-old girl complains of finger pain. She has been complaining of pain of her left index finger for the past 2 days. There has been no fever and no recent trauma to the finger. On examination, her finger is erythematous over the distal tip. You palpate an area of fluctuance over her fingertip. Her fingernail is intact and without lesions. Treatment includes:

   a. Incision and drainage
   b. Radiography of her hand
   c. CBC and blood culture
   d. Trephination
   e. Removal of the fingernail

6. A 3-week-old girl is brought to the ED because of crying. She has been more fussy for the past 2 days. Her mother thought she felt warm but did not take her temperature. The girl has had occasional episodes of emesis. Her vital signs are: T 37.7°C, HR 150, RR 28, and BP 85/50. She is awake and crying. Her HEENT examination is normal. Her neck is supple, with no evidence of meningismus. Her chest is clear. Her abdomen is soft and nontender, without masses. Her extremities are well perfused, with no evidence of hair tourniquets. Fluorescein staining of her eyes is normal. Her UA and stool blood testing are normal. She has not stopped crying. Your next step in management is:

   a. Reassurance and discharge with follow-up
   b. Abdominal radiograph
   c. Lumbar puncture for cerebrospinal fluid (CSF)
   d. Changing her formula
   e. Skeletal series

7. An 18-month-old girl is brought to the ED for fever. She has had high fevers for 2 days. She is not drinking as well and seems more tired than usual. Her vital signs are: T 39.8°C, HR 150, RR 24, and BP 90/55. Her conjunctivae are clear and her tympanic membranes are normal. She has mild tonsillar swelling and four to five small vesicles with erythematous bases in the posterior aspect of the oropharynx. Her neck is supple and her chest is clear. Her abdomen is soft and nontender. She has no rashes. You diagnose her with:

   a. Roseola
   b. Streptococcal pharyngitis
   c. Gingivostomatitis
   d. Kawasaki disease
   e. Varicella (chickenpox)

8. A 2-year-old boy requires procedural sedation for fracture reduction. He has a history of asthma and is on the last day of a steroid taper. He also has a history of congenital dislocation of the hips. His examination is normal except for the displaced radius and ulna fracture on the right. Which medication do you choose for procedural sedation?

   a. Oral chloral hydrate
   b. IV ketamine
   c. IV fentanyl/midazolam
   d. IV pentobarbital
   e. Inhaled nitrous oxide

9. A 16-year-old boy complains of scrotal pain. He began having intermittent left-sided scrotal pain yesterday afternoon. He has not had fever, vomiting, or abdominal pain. On physical examination, his left hemiscrotum is swollen and diffusely tender. Both cremasteric reflexes are difficult to elicit. The most important test to perform at this point is:

   a. Urinalysis
   b. Testicular ultrasound
   c. Diagnostic needle aspiration
   d. Open surgical exploration
   e. Urethral swab

10. A 6-year-old boy complains of bilateral ear pain. He has had cough and rhinorrhea for the past 2 days. On examination, his temperature is 38°C and he has erythematous and bulging tympanic membranes bilaterally. You suggest the following treatment:

    a. No treatment is necessary
    b. Diphenydramine orally (PO)
    c. Cefaclor PO
    d. Amoxicillin PO
    e. Tetracycline PO

11. A 3-week-old boy is brought to the ED with vomiting, diarrhea, poor feeding, and jaundice. Opacification of the lenses is noted bilaterally on ocular exam. Which of the following findings is likely?

    a. Increased anion gap metabolic acidosis
    b. Pronounced indirect hyperbilirubinemia
    c. Glucosuria noted on urine analysis
    d. Hemolysis on peripheral blood smear
    e. Negative test for reducing substances in the urine

12. A 12-year-old boy comes to the ED after being hit in the mouth by a baseball bat. He says that his upper teeth suffered most of the damage. He denies loss of consciousness (LOC) or other symptoms. On examination, he has swelling of his upper lip, but no lacerations. His teeth are intact, but the upper incisors are displaced toward the pharynx at a 30-degree angle to the other teeth. Upon consultation with the dentist, you describe that the patient's teeth are:

    a. Subluxated
    b. Intruded
    c. Luxated
    d. Avulsed
    e. Fractured

13. A 3-year-old girl is brought to the ED because she had ingested an unknown quantity of acetaminophen. The ingestion occurred approximately 90 minutes ago. She is alert and crying. Her physical examination is normal. Immediate treatment at this time should be:

    a. Administration of syrup of ipecac
    b. Orogastric lavage
    c. Administration of activated charcoal
    d. Administration of N-acetylcysteine
    e. Administration of sodium bicarbonate

14. A 5-year-old girl with leukemia is brought to the ED with a diffuse vesiculobullous rash with areas of excoriation. Some of the lesions appear to be tear-shaped vesicles on an erythematous base. The child is somewhat ill appearing and has the following vital signs: T 38.2°C, HR 130, RR 20, and BP 100/76. It is expected that she is neutropenic, based on the timing of her last course of chemotherapy. Which of the following would be the most appropriate next step in management?

    a. Administer IV acyclovir
    b. Administer varicella immunoglobulin and IV antibiotics
    c. Administer IV acyclovir and IV antibiotics
    d. Administer IV acyclovir, varicella immunoglobulin, and IV antibiotics
    e. Administer varicella immunoglobulin and varicella vaccine

15. A 4-year-old child is brought to the ED for evaluation. She has been febrile for 2 weeks and has erythematous lips. The parents state that she had conjunctivitis, which was treated with eye ointment for 5 days, and an associated fine papular rash that is now gone. On physical examination, she is ill appearing, irritable, has an injected oropharynx, and a large left cervical node. Appropriate management includes:

    a. IV immune globulin and low-dose aspirin
    b. Low-dose aspirin alone
    c. High-dose steroids and high-dose aspirin
    d. IV immune globulin and high-dose aspirin
    e. High-dose steroids and low-dose aspirin

16. A mother describes a single oval lesion on the flank of her 5-year-old son. The lesion has been present for 2 weeks. He now has a diffuse papulosquamous rash consisting of small (1 cm) oval lesions that cover his entire back. Your management would be:

    a. Oral griseofulvin
    b. Topical ketoconazole
    c. No therapy
    d. Oral steroids
    e. Ear shampoo

17. A 5-month-old girl is brought into the ED after 24 hours of repeated vomiting and diarrhea. You are unable to obtain a blood pressure. She does not respond as the first two attempts are made at putting in a peripheral IV line. The next step in obtaining vascular access should be:

    a. Placement of an intraosseous needle
    b. Placement of a large-bore needle in the antecubital vein
    c. Placement of a catheter in the internal jugular vein
    d. Perform a femoral cutdown
    e. Perform a cutdown in a peripheral vein

18. A 5-day-old girl is brought to the ED appearing lethargic and pale. Her vital signs are: T 37.2°C, HR 186, RR 72 (labored), and BP 48/palpable. Capillary refill time is greater than 4 seconds and no rash is noted. A stat portable chest x-ray (CXR) shows cardiomegaly. You should administer:

    a. Dopamine
    b. Dobutamine
    c. Prostaglandin E_1
    d. Furosemide
    e. Epinephrine

19. A 7-month-old girl is brought to the ED because her parents note that she has not been using her right leg normally. On physical exam, she is afebrile and uncomfortable appearing. She has tenderness to palpation of the right lower leg. Plain radiographs of her tibia/fibula reveal a spiral fracture of the right tibia. On further questioning, her parents recall that earlier in the day they found the patient crying, with her right leg sticking out of the crib rails, but recall no other trauma. The most appropriate next step is:

    a. Obtain a skeletal survey
    b. Obtain a bone scan
    c. File a report with the Department of Social Services
    d. Place a posterior splint and arrange follow-up with orthopedics
    e. Place a long leg cast and discharge home

20. An 8-year-old boy comes to the ED comatose after being thrown from an automobile. His left pupil is 6 mm and nonreactive; his right pupil is 4 mm and reactive. Which of the following therapies would be contraindicated?

    a. Rapid-sequence intubation with ketamine and rocuronium
    b. Positive-pressure ventilation with mild hyperventilation
    c. IV mannitol administered at a dose of 1 g/kg
    d. Elevation of the head of the bed at an angle of 30 degrees
    e. Immobilization of the neck in a semi-rigid cervical collar

21. A 6-year-old girl is brought to the ED because of a mouse bite. She was feeding her pet mouse when it bit her on the forearm. She denies other trauma. On examination, she is well appearing, in no acute distress (NAD). She has two small puncture wounds on her forearm. Treatment includes:

    a. Irrigation and dressing only
    b. Amoxicillin-clavulanic acid PO
    c. Radiography of her radius and ulna
    d. Rabies immune globulin
    e. Send out test for tularemia antibodies

22. A 13-year-old boy is brought to the ED after being struck in the genital area by a baseball. He complains of scrotal pain and denies other injuries. On examination, he is alert but in pain. He has a contusion and abrasions over the glans penis and the penile shaft, with blood at the meatus. He has no testicular tenderness. The rest of his examination is normal. Further management at this point includes:

    a. Foley catheter insertion
    b. Pelvis radiography
    c. Retrograde urethrography
    d. Testicular ultrasound
    e. Abdominal CT scan

23. A 2-year-old boy is brought to the ED for breathing difficulty that has worsened over the past 6 hours. His mother reports that he has had cold symptoms and intermittent fevers over the past 2 days, as well as a "barky" cough. His vital signs are: T 38.9°C, HR 126, RR 32, and BP 108/65. You note subcostal retractions as well as inspiratory stridor at rest. Treatment should start with:

    a. Endotracheal intubation
    b. Nebulized albuterol
    c. IM dexamethasone
    d. Nebulized epinephrine
    e. Laryngotracheal bronchoscopy

24. A previously healthy 4-month-old boy is brought to the ED by the EMTs for generalized tonic-clonic seizures. He was given diazepam (Valium) rectally en route to the ED, but he is still actively seizing on arrival. His mother reports that he had been well previously, without any fever or vomiting. The patient has had some loose stools over the past 3 days, but he has been taking a good amount of water that his mother has been giving to prevent dehydration. He is afebrile now, with generalized tonic-clonic movements of upper and lower extremities. You should administer:

    a. Phenobarbital
    b. Furosemide
    c. Phenytoin
    d. Midazolam
    e. Hypertonic saline IV

25. A previously healthy 2-month-old girl is brought to the ED for irritability over the past 24 hours. Vital signs are as follows: T 36.2°C, HR 240, RR 64, and BP 101/58. Her O_2 saturation is 95% on room air. She appears lethargic and is not interested in feeding. Breath sounds are clear and no heart murmur is auscultated. The abdomen is soft and the liver edge is palpable 3 cm below the right costal margin. Which of the following should be done?

    a. Synchronized cardioversion
    b. IV normal saline 20 ml/kg
    c. Adenosine given orally
    d. Ice pack applied to face
    e. IV digoxin

26. A 3-year-old boy is referred to your ED because of a red neck mass. His mother noticed the mass 1 week ago; it has not changed since the time she initially noted it. The boy has had no fever, URI symptoms, or vomiting. The family owns a dog and a kitten. The mass is firm, mobile, and tender, with overlying erythema. The most appropriate therapy for this patient is:

    a. Observation alone
    b. Amoxicillin/clavulanate
    c. Erythromycin PO
    d. Incision and drainage
    e. Surgical excision

27. A 10-month-old boy is brought to the ED by his parents because he has had a subjective fever for the past 2 days and has now been refusing to crawl for the past 12 hours. He has had no recent URI symptoms, and his immunizations are up to date. On physical examination, he is noted to have a temperature of 38.9°C, but is in no acute distress. He is holding his right hip in a flexed, abducted, and externally rotated position. Severe discomfort is noted upon minimal movement of the right lower extremity. Which of the following would be the most appropriate next step in the management of this patient?

    a. Ibuprofen for 4–7 days
    b. CT scan of the right hip
    c. Arthrocentesis of the right hip
    d. Triple-phase bone scan
    e. MRI of the right hip

28. A 10-month-old girl is rushed to the ED after a seizure. Her parents found her with her eyes rolled back and with shaking of all four extremities while she had been taking a nap. The episode lasted 2–3 minutes. Other than a slight cold for the past 2 days, the patient had been well. On arrival to the ED, the patient is sleepy, but arouses to painful stimuli. She has a temperature of 40°C. Other than generalized hypotonia, her neurologic examination is nonfocal. The workup should include:

 a. No further tests
 b. Lumbar puncture
 c. EEG, lumbar puncture
 d. WBC count, blood culture, lumbar puncture
 e. Head CT scan, blood culture, lumbar puncture

29. A 13-year-old boy comes with his mother to the ED for evaluation of chest pain. He states that he has noted occasional sharp, stabbing pain that occurs intermittently while exercising. The pain only lasts a few seconds and is located in the area below his left nipple. He denies syncope or near syncope, but does think that his heart was going a little fast during these periods. Family history includes two grandparents that have recently died from "heart problems." The child has an unremarkable examination and a normal CXR and 12-lead ECG. What is most appropriate next step at this time?

 a. A cardiac stress test
 b. Echocardiogram
 c. No further evaluation is necessary
 d. Outpatient psychiatric evaluation
 e. 24-hour Holter monitor

30. A 9-year-old boy is involved in a high-speed motor vehicle collision. The patient is brought to the ED in a C-spine collar and on a backboard. The patient complains of neck pain. His examination reveals lower extremity weakness and paresthesias. His Glasgow Coma Scale score is 15 and his vital signs are stable. C-spine films do not reveal any bony abnormalities. Which of the following is most appropriate?

 a. Obtain flexion/extension views of the neck
 b. Begin immediate endotracheal intubation
 c. Administer 0.5 g/kg of mannitol IV
 d. Administer 30 mg/kg of methylprednisolone IV
 e. Order a psychiatric consult

31. A previously healthy 3-year-old boy is brought to the ED by his mother with complaints of headache and dizziness for the past day. The patient has been otherwise healthy, but history does reveal exposure to well water from a local farm. The boy is cyanotic and slightly lethargic on examination. He is in no respiratory distress, has no murmurs on cardiac auscultation, and has good peripheral perfusion. His O_2 saturation is 96% on room air. Which of the following is most likely to aid in diagnosing this patient's condition?

 a. Carboxyhemoglobin level
 b. CXR
 c. Echocardiogram
 d. Methemoglobin level
 e. Arterial blood gas (ABG)

32. A 5-year-old girl is brought to the ED for evaluation of a limp. Her mother reports that 2 weeks ago the child fell from her bunk bed, landing on her back. She appeared to be fine until 5 days ago, when she was noted to have difficulty walking. Other than a slight limp on the right, and mild tenderness over the lumbar spine, her examination is unremarkable. What test would be most helpful?

 a. CBC
 b. Spinal MRI
 c. Erythrocyte sedimentation rate (ESR)
 d. Bone scan
 e. Plain spine radiographs

33. A 16-year-old boy is involved in a high-speed, head-on automobile collision. On arrival to the ED he is noted to be anxious and is complaining of chest pain. Vital signs are: HR 108; RR 28, and BP 116/48. Which study would be MOST important to obtain next?

 a. Portable CXR
 b. 12-lead ECG, with rhythm strip
 c. Hemoglobin and hematocrit levels
 d. CT scan of the chest
 e. Cardiac ultrasound

34. A 7-year-old girl with a long-standing seizure disorder is brought to the ED by ambulance in status epilepticus. She developed sustained generalized tonic-clonic seizure activity 30 minutes prior to arrival. Ambulance personnel were unable to obtain IV access and gave no anticonvulsant medications prior to arrival. The patient is maintained on phenytoin and carbamazepine. On arrival to the ED, the girl has stable vital signs but she is having continued generalized tonic-clonic activity. You are unable to obtain IV access. The most appropriate management is:

    a. Lorazepam 0.1 mg/kg IM, repeated PRN (as needed)
    b. Diazepam 1.0 mg/kg PR (per rectum), followed by lorazepam 0.1 mg/kg IM
    c. Diazepam 0.5 mg/kg PR, followed by fosphenytoin 10 mg/kg IM
    d. Diazepam 0.5 mg/kg PR, followed by phenobarbital 10 mg/kg IM
    e. Paraldehyde 0.3 mg/kg PR, followed by fosphenytoin 10 mg/kg IM

35. A 3-year-old girl refuses to use her left arm. Her mother reports that the girl was in the midst of a temper tantrum and was pulling away from her grasp of the girl's hand. The girl has not used her left arm since then. She has been healthy, with no history of fever. On examination, she is well appearing and easily distractible. She is holding her left arm in a pronated and flexed position against her body. She has no swelling but does appear to have some tenderness in the region of her left elbow. You suspect:

    a. Radial head subluxation
    b. Monteggia fracture
    c. Supracondylar humeral fracture
    d. Elbow sprain
    e. Avulsion of her lateral epicondyle

36. A 6-month-old boy with a history of biliary atresia, which was recently repaired, comes to your ED for fever and abdominal pain. He has had fever and shaking chills for the past 6 hours. On examination, his vital signs are T 39°C, HR 160, RR 24, and BP 95/60. His conjunctivae are clear and his mucous membranes are dry. His chest is clear, and he appears to have right upper quadrant (RUQ) abdominal tenderness. His serum WBC count is 16,000. Which of the following laboratory tests would exclude the likely diagnosis?

    a. Serum bilirubin 2.5 mg/dl
    b. ALT 50 u/L
    c. AST 60 u/L
    d. Amylase 100 u/L
    e. None of these tests

37. Your ED is notified of a terrorist biological weapon of mass destruction (WMD) exposure at a local daycare center. The exposure occurred several hours ago and the terrorist organization is claiming responsibility for the exposure. As you prepare to triage and care for these patients, which of the following biological agents represents the greatest post-exposure risk for the health-care team?

    a. *Bacillis anthracis* (anthrax)
    b. *Yersinia pestis* (the plague)
    c. Staphylococcal enterotoxin B
    d. Human immunodeficiency virus (HIV)
    e. *Stachybotrys atra*

38. A 15-month-old girl is brought to the ED for fever and limp. She has had fever for 2 days and right hip pain for 2 days. Her vital signs are: T 38.7°C, HR 130, RR 28, and BP 90/60. She is ill appearing, with pain on range of motion of her right hip. Her WBC is 12,000 and her ESR is 60 mm/hour. Her hip ultrasound shows minimal fluid in her right hip space. Arthrocentesis removes 0.5 ml of fluid, which reveals a glucose level of 80 mg/dl and a WBC of 10,000, with mostly lymphocytes. The Gram stain is negative. Your next step in management is:

    a. Sending titers for *Borrelia burgdorferi*
    b. Hip arthrotomy and irrigation
    c. Discharge to home on oral cephalexin
    d. Technetium bone scan
    e. Discharge to home on ibuprofen

39. An 8-month-old boy is brought to the ED because of fever. He has had fever for 1 day, as high as 39°C. He has no other symptoms. His vital signs are: T 40°C, HR 150, RR 24, and BP 90/50. His physical examination is remarkable for a well-appearing, smiling boy in NAD. His chest is clear and his abdomen is benign. The rest of his physical examination is normal. Regarding management of this patient, which of the following statements is correct?

    a. He should be admitted for IV cefotaxime and observation
    b. CSF should be obtained for cell count, Gram stain, and culture
    c. The organism responsible for most occult bacteremia is *Haemophilus influenzae*
    d. He should be given ceftriaxone IM
    e. Bacteremia from group B *Streptococcus* would be unlikely

40. An obese 17-year-old female patient complains of abdominal pain. She complains of crampy abdominal pain for the past day, occurring intermittently. Upon examination, you note that she is crowning. After delivery, the infant is limp and cyanotic. Your next step in management after cutting the umbilical cord is:

    a. Drying and stimulation
    b. Administration of positive-pressure ventilation
    c. Endotracheal intubation
    d. Cardiac compressions
    e. Administration of naloxone

41. A 3-year-old girl is brought to the ED for fever and nasal discharge. She has had cough and fever for the past 3 days and has had copious greenish nasal discharge. She also complains of a sore throat. Her vital signs are: T 38.2°C, HR 110, RR 24, and BP 90/50. Upon percussion over her right supraorbital area, she seems to complain of pain. Her chest and throat are clear. Her physical examination is otherwise normal. Your diagnosis is:

    a. Viral upper respiratory infection (URI)
    b. Frontal sinusitis
    c. Streptococcal pharyngitis
    d. Sphenoid sinusitis
    e. Periorbital cellulitis

42. A 2-year-old girl is brought to the ED because of difficulty walking. She has been followed for mild lead poisoning for the past year. The house was appropriately treated. She has been otherwise healthy and has been developmentally normal. She did have chickenpox (varicella) 3 weeks ago, but has not had significant scarring from the lesions. She has been less active for the past few days, and the mother reports that the girl began "walking funny" 2 days ago. On examination, she is alert and playful. Her physical examination is remarkable for a mild truncal ataxia and imbalance when she walks. Your next step in management is to:

    a. Obtain a serum glucose level
    b. Obtain a urine toxicological screen
    c. Obtain a head CT scan
    d. Obtain a measurement of intracranial pressure (ICP)
    e. Discharge to home with reassurance

43. A 1-year-old boy is brought to the ED because of a cough and rhinorrhea. The anxious mother says that he has had frequent URI symptoms and is fearful that he is "just too sick." He has been feeding well and appears thin, but is well nourished. His vital signs are: T 38.1°C, HR 120, RR 28, and BP 90/50. His O_2 saturation is 98% on room air. His lungs are coarse, but without wheezing or rales. His abdomen is soft, and his heart rate is regular. You note that he has redundant tissue protruding from his rectum, but the mother says that his bowel movements have been normal, if not occasionally loose. Your management should include:

    a. Abdominal radiographs
    b. CBC
    c. Nasopharyngeal swab for culture
    d. Referral for sweat testing
    e. Aerosolized ribavirin

44. An 11-year-old boy complains of ankle pain. He says he was skateboarding when he fell, inverting his ankle. He has mild diffuse swelling and tenderness throughout the lateral aspect of his ankle. He complains of maximal tenderness over the distal fibula, 1 cm from the end. X-rays of his ankle show mild soft tissue swelling, but no evidence of fracture. Your management is:

    a. Compression wrap and ibuprofen
    b. Placement of a short leg cast
    c. Obtaining a comparison radiograph of the other ankle
    d. Scheduling a bone scan in the A.M.
    e. Obtaining a CBC and ESR

45. A 2-year-old girl is brought to the ED because of a fainting spell. She was with her older brother when she began crying. After crying for a few minutes, she stopped breathing, turned blue, and passed out. She awoke several seconds later, and resumed playing shortly thereafter. On examination, she is alert and playful. She has no evidence of trauma and her physical examination is normal. You should:

    a. Obtain an ECG
    b. Refer her for an EEG
    c. Obtain a serum glucose level
    d. Obtain an arterial blood gas
    e. Reassure the parents and discharge to home

46. A 5-year-old girl with a history of hydrocephalus and a ventriculoperitoneal shunt (VPS) is brought to the ED because of vomiting and diarrhea. Her last shunt revision was 3 years ago, when she presented with headache, vomiting, and lethargy. She has had three episodes of vomiting for each of the past 3 days and four to five episodes of diarrhea for 2 days. She has not tolerated anything by mouth today. Her vital signs are: T 38.1°C, HR 120, RR 20, and BP 95/60. On examination, she is well appearing but her eyes appear slightly sunken. The rest of her physical examination is normal. Your next step in management is:

    a. Obtain a head CT scan
    b. Obtain cell count, culture, and Gram stain of the CSF
    c. Administer an NS bolus
    d. Obtain a CBC and blood culture
    e. Discharge to home

47. In which of the following patients should you be concerned about nonaccidental trauma?

    a. A 14-month-old who has second-degree burns on his buttocks and the back of his legs
    b. A 5-year-old who has a femur fracture
    c. A 3-year-old Southeast Asian boy who has several discrete circular lesions on his back
    d. A 5-year-old with circular patches of alopecia
    e. A 2-year-old with a chin laceration

48. A 3-year-old girl with Angelman's syndrome is brought to the ED because she swallowed a nickel an hour ago. Upon examination, she is alert and in NAD. She is not drooling and has no respiratory compromise. Her breath sounds are clear. A radiograph reveals that the coin is in the stomach. Management includes:

    a. Admission for observation
    b. Endoscopic removal
    c. Exploratory laparotomy
    d. Whole bowel irrigation
    e. Discharge to home

49. A 4-year-old boy is brought to the ED after being rescued from a house fire. He was found hiding in the closet, curled up in a ball. He is lethargic, but responsive to pain. He has first-degree burns over his fingers, but there is no other evidence of cutaneous injury. The rest of his examination is normal. You confirm your diagnosis by obtaining:

    a. A lateral C-spine film
    b. Arterial blood gas
    c. Carboxyhemoglobin level
    d. Pulse oximetry
    e. Urine toxicological screening

50. A 5-year-old boy is brought to the ED after being stung by a bee while playing in the backyard. He complained of itching at first, then began having difficulty breathing. His vital signs are: T 37°C, HR 130, RR 24, and BP 80/40. On examination, he is alert and anxious appearing. He has lip and tongue swelling. His lungs are clear without wheezing, but he has stridor. He is tachycardic, and his abdomen is soft and nontender. Your immediate management is:

    a. Epinephrine 0.01 mg/kg SC
    b. Diphenhydramine 1 mg/kg IV
    c. Immediate intubation
    d. Tracheostomy
    e. NS bolus of 20 ml/kg IV

ANSWERS

1. e   Normal respiratory rates for 2-month-old infants should be between 24 and 40. A patient with respiratory distress will initially become tachypneic, but as the disease progresses and the infant's reserves diminish, the infant will tire and become bradypneic. An RR of 12 in a 2-month-old is very concerning and would prompt immediate airway management, including bag-valve-mask ventilation. Further airway support may be necessary if he does not improve. (Resuscitation—Pediatric Basic and Advanced Life Support, Chapter 1)

2. c   The history alone in this case is very suggestive of congestive heart failure. For a young infant, nursing or bottle feeding is the most vigorous activity in which he or she will engage. Respiratory complaints are almost always the presenting problem for children with congestive heart failure, so eliciting a detailed feeding history is crucial. Many congenital cardiac conditions present around this age, as the pulmonary vascular resistance has dropped significantly since the immediate newborn period. Wheezing can be one of the initial pulmonary findings in congestive heart failure. Cardiac murmurs may or may

not be heard, depending on the underlying defect. Hepatomegaly, however, strongly supports suspicions raised by history. A chest radiograph will show cardiomegaly. Furosemide would be the most appropriate treatment option because it will address the underlying problem of volume overload. Large fluid boluses would worsen the condition. Albuterol and steroids would be helpful if reactive airway disease were the cause of the wheezing. Prostaglandin E_1 is reserved for congenital cardiac conditions in which a proper blood flow through the heart depends on a patent ductus arteriosus. (Cardiac Emergencies, Chapter 82)

3. b   Idiopathic thrombocytopenic purpura (ITP) is the most common platelet disorder of childhood, typically presenting between the ages of 1 and 4 years. Clinical manifestations include petechiae, ecchymoses, epistaxis, gum bleeding (hemorrhagic bullae), hematuria, and, rarely, intracranial hemorrhage, which is the major life-threatening complication of ITP. High-output cardiac failure may occur with Kasabach-Merritt syndrome, anemia may occur with various hematological disorders, splenic sequestration is a complication of sickle cell disease, and sepsis is a complication of many oncologic diseases, as well as sickle cell disease. (Hematologic Emergencies, Chapter 87)

4. c   Wernig-Hoffmann disease is a degenerative disease of the motor neurons, and is also known as spinal muscular atrophy. Succinylcholine is contraindicated in patients with neuromuscular diseases because those patients may have acute increases in potassium. A nondepolarizing agent, such as rocuronium, should be used instead. Atropine should be used in children, especially under the age of 2 years, to help prevent bradycardia associated with intubation. Midazolam provides good sedation, as does ketamine. Ketamine, however, can cause acute increases in ICP, so it should not be used in situations where one is concerned that the ICP may be elevated. Ketamine is most often used in the intubation of asthmatic patients because it has bronchodilatory effects. Thiopental is also a good sedative agent to use for intubation. It has cerebroprotective effects, but it can cause decreases in blood pressure and should therefore be avoided in patients who are hemodynamically unstable. (Emergency Airway Management—Rapid-Sequence Intubation, Chapter 5)

5. a   Felons are infections of the distal pulp of the finger. Infections may involve abscess formation, as it does in this patient. Management includes incision and drainage, as well as oral antibiotics. There is no indication for radiography or blood tests. Trephination is indicated for subungual hematomas with less than 50% involvement of the fingernail bed. Removal of the fingernail is indicated for subungual hematomas with greater than 50% involvement of the fingernail bed, or with subungual lacerations or abscesses. (Minor Lesions and Injuries, Chapter 117)

6. c   Neonates may not mount a fever in response to meningeal inflammation. In this vignette, it is difficult to determine if the patient did have a fever prior to your assessment. Meningismus is difficult to ascertain in a neonate, and cannot be relied upon in your examination. Given her possible fever and her irritability, a lumbar puncture and fever evaluation are indicated. An abdominal radiograph may help determine if the patient has an intussusception, but this is less likely given her age and symptoms. Changing formulas has not been proven to be helpful in the treatment of colic—a diagnosis by exclusion. There is nothing in the history and examination to suggest nonaccidental trauma, which would warrant a skeletal series. (Crying, Chapter 17)

7. c   Gingivostomatitis may be caused by Coxsackie or herpes viruses. Patients develop high fevers and painful gum lesions, which may lead to poor oral intake. Lesions typically appear as vesicles or ulcers, associated with an erythematous base. Treatment is largely supportive, but many clinicians would prescribe various oral mixtures to alleviate pain. Roseola causes high fevers, followed by an erythematous rash after the fever dissipates. Streptococcal pharyngitis causes fever and throat pain, associated with erythema, exudate, and tonsillar hypertrophy; however, streptococcal pharyngitis is rare in this age group. Kawasaki disease typically presents with fevers of longer duration, conjunctivitis, a desquamating rash, adenopathy, and a strawberry-colored tongue. Even though varicella may cause fevers and vesicles, the lesions typically begin on the trunk rather than in the oropharynx; however, lesions may involve the oropharynx as the disease progresses. (Oral Lesions, Chapter 49)

8. c   Even though IV ketamine would work well for a fracture reduction (it produces great analgesia, amnesia, and sedation), the history of asthma is a relative contraindication. Although ketamine has brochodilatory effects and is recommended when intubating asthmatic patients, there is an increased risk of laryngospasm occurring during its use in the otherwise well patient with asthma who is undergoing

procedural sedation. Fentanyl/midazolam as a combination would be a better choice. There are no contraindications for this combination in a patient with a history of hip dislocation. Chloral hydrate and pentobarbital are sedatives, but they do not provide analgesia. Nitrous oxide works best in children who can cooperate with breathing from a mask, but it should be avoided in fractures that require significant reduction. (Sedation and Analgesia, Chapter 4)

9. b   The diagnosis of testicular torsion is often difficult. Torsion may be partial and intermittent, causing intermittent symptoms. The history is often complicated by an incidental history of trauma to the genitalia. The absence of cremasteric reflexes on the affected side is helpful for the diagnosis, but in this vignette, they are not helpful. A testicular ultrasound would help to differentiate between testicular torsion, torsion of an appendage, scrotal trauma, and epididymitis. A urinalysis would not be adequate or definitive. There is no indication for a diagnostic needle aspiration or urethral swab in this vignette. Surgical exploration would be indicated if the diagnosis were certain, but this is not the case. (Pain—Scrotal, Chapter 58)

10. d   Acute otitis media (AOM) may be unilateral or bilateral, and is often preceded by an upper respiratory infection. Amoxicillin remains the first medication recommended because of its efficacy and pleasant taste. Antihistamines have not been proven to be efficacious in the treatment of AOM. Cefaclor does not penetrate the middle ear cavity well enough to be efficacious for the treatment of AOM and is often associated with serum sickness. Tetracycline is not recommended in children with developing teeth (less than 9 years of age). (Pain—Earache, Chapter 55)

11. d   Gastrointestinal symptoms, failure to thrive, jaundice, and cataracts are findings associated with galactosemia. Galactosemia results in failure of conversion of dietary galactose to glucose and hypoglycemia. This results in the presence of reducing substances in the urine in the absence of glucosuria. A hyperchloremic, non-ion gap metabolic acidosis may be seen secondary to renal tubular dysfunction. The hyperbilirubinemia may initially be indirect, but a significant direct hyperbilirubinemia is characteristic after a week or two. Hemolysis may be a prominent finding, particularly in newborns. (Metabolic Emergencies (Inborn Errors of Metabolism), Chapter 98)

12. c   Luxation is defined as displacement of the tooth from the alveolar socket in any direction. Luxation is accompanied by extrusion from the socket. Subluxation injuries occur when the periodontal ligaments are damaged, causing excessive mobility, but no displacement within the dental arch. Intrusion injuries occur when the tooth is displaced into the socket. Avulsion injuries are teeth that are completely displaced from the socket. Fractures occur when the tooth is broken and may be associated with other injuries. (Dental Trauma, Chapter 113)

13. c   Acetaminophen remains a common toxicologic ingestion, with significant morbidity. There is almost no role for the administration of syrup of ipecac in the ED. Orogastric lavage may be performed if the ingestion occurred within 60 minutes of ingestion, but it carries its own risks. Administration of activated charcoal remains the mainstay treatment of most ED ingestions, including acetaminophen. Treatment of acetaminophen ingestions involves the administration of N-acetylcysteine, but this should not be instituted until a 4-hour acetaminophen level has been obtained. Administration of sodium bicarbonate is indicated for aspirin and tricyclic antidepressant overdoses, but not for acetaminophen overdoses. (Toxicologic Emergencies, Chapter 88)

14. c   Immunosuppression due to chemotherapy for leukemia puts this patient at high risk and warrants IV acyclovir for probable disseminated varicella. Given the patient's ill appearance and probable neutropenia, IV antibiotics should also be initiated after appropriate cultures are obtained. Scraping of the base of the lesions should also be obtained to confirm the diagnosis of varicella-zoster virus (VZV) and not herpes simplex virus (HSV), because the two can be easily confused clinically, although HSV is less likely to present with a diffuse rash. Bacterial superinfection of varicella lesions is common. Treatment with varicella-zoster immunoglobulin is reserved for patients with suspected exposures, but not for patients who have active disease. Concurrent chemotherapy should also be discontinued. (Rash–Vesicobullous, Chapter 67, and Oncologic Emergencies, Chapter 100)

15. d   The patient in this scenario is exhibiting four of the five features of Kawasaki disease. Kawasaki disease is a clinical diagnosis based on an unremitting fever of at least 5 days duration and four of the five following features: (1) rash; (2) nonexudative bulbar conjunctivitis with limbal sparing; (3) red cracked

lips, strawberry tongue, and erythematous oropharynx; (4) erythema, swelling, and/or induration of peripheral extremities; and (5) a solitary unilateral cervical lymph node greater than 1.5 cm in diameter. Children with this disease are commonly irritable and/or ill appearing. Initial therapy of choice is IV immune globulin and high-dose aspirin (80–100 mg/kg/day). The aspirin dose is usually decreased after the fever has subsided. Therapy is most beneficial when started within 10 days of onset of illness, but should not be withheld for patients presenting after this time. (Rash—Maculopapular, Chapter 62, and Rheumatologic Emergencies, Chapter 101)

16. c   A herald patch is seen in approximately 80% of children with pityriasis rosea. Another clue to the diagnosis is a distribution of the lesions along the dermatomes in the shape of a "Christmas tree, " although this finding is not always present. The disorder is a benign, self-limiting condition, thought to be of viral etiology. The initial herald patch may be confused with tinea corporis and the diffuse stage may be confused with secondary syphilis, drug-induced eruption, Mucha-Habermann disease, seborrheic dermatitis, nummular eczema, and psoriasis. No therapy is necessary. If itching is present it may be treated with oral antihistamines or topical 0.5% steroid cream. (Rash—Papulosquamous Lesions, Chapter 64)

17. a   If possible, a large-bore IV should be placed in a larger peripheral vein. If this is not possible after two attempts, an intraosseous line should be placed on the medial tibia, 2 cm below the tibial tuberosity and angled away from the growth plate. (Shock, Chapter 3)

18. c   This constellation of findings in a 5-day-old infant is consistent with cardiogenic shock related to closing of the ductus arteriosus. Disease states in which cardiac output from the left side of the heart is impeded (i.e., critical aortic stenosis) depend on a patent ductus arteriosus to allow blood to flow to the aorta from the pulmonary artery. These patients will therefore present rather acutely with cardiogenic shock when the ductus arteriosus closes, usually within the first 2 weeks of life. Other conditions one would expect to present similarly are hypoplastic left heart syndrome, interrupted aortic arch, and severe coarctation of the aorta. Because this patient has a ductal-dependent lesion, keeping the ductus arteriosus patent with prostaglandin E_1 is critical to her immediate survival. Other supportive medications, such as pressor agents and diuretics may be needed in the event that the heart has sustained significant damage; however, starting PGE_1 would be the priority. (Cardiac Emergencies, Chapter 82)

19. a   Spiral fractures of the tibia or femur in preambulatory children are suspicious for child abuse. In addition, the history of possible leg trauma in the crib is inconsistent with this injury. A skeletal survey is indicated for any child less than 2 years of age whom you suspect to have suffered nonaccidental trauma. A bone scan may be indicated to detect subtle rib fractures after a skeletal survey is completed. If further workup supports a suspicion of child abuse, a report of abuse or neglect should be filed with the Department of Social Services at that time. Although the definitive treatment for the fracture is either casting or splinting, the evaluation and diagnosis of other fractures takes precedence before definitive orthopedic care. (Orthopedic Trauma, Chapter 115, and Child Abuse, Chapter 128)

20. a   Rapid-sequence intubation is appropriate for a comatose, head-injured patient; however, ketamine would be contraindicated because it may elevate increased ICP. Other sedative agents, such as thiopental, midazolam, and fentanyl—which do not lead to elevations of ICP—would be preferred. The other therapies listed are all appropriate. Mild hyperventilation, administration of mannitol, and elevation of the head of the bed are all appropriate therapies for patients with clinical signs of increased ICP. Immobilization of the cervical spine is always appropriate in a trauma victim who is unconscious and therefore cannot cooperate with a complete physical examination to evaluate for cervical spine injury. (Neurotrauma, Chapter 105)

21. a   Domestic mouse bites are low-risk wounds, as would be wild mouse bites. Appropriate treatment would be irrigation and dressing only. There is no role for prophylactic antibiotics or radiography. Rabies immune globulin is not indicated for mouse bites. When tularemia is contracted from a bite, it is most commonly contracted from that of a rabbit. (Bites and Stings, Chapter 91)

22. c   Trauma to the external genitalia with blood at the meatus warrants a retrograde urethrogram to determine if there is any injury to the external urethra. Insertion of a Foley catheter is contraindicated because the insertion may convert a partial urethral tear into a complete one. Pelvic radiography is indi-

cated in high-impact traumatic injuries, which are more likely to be associated with pelvic fractures. Testicular ultrasounds are not indicated because there is no evidence of testicular injury. In the absence of abdominal symptoms, an abdominal CT scan is not necessary. (Genitourinary Trauma, Chapter 109)

23. d   This patient has laryngotracheobronchitis ("croup"). Although in most cases the disease is self-limited, responding well to supportive therapy alone, severe airway obstruction can occur. The presence of stridor at rest is a sign of more pronounced airway obstruction. Nebulized epinephrine (racemic) is the treatment of choice in this situation because it helps to diminish swelling directly at the site of inflammation. Although this patient would also benefit from the more prolonged effects of IM dexamethasone, giving this therapy alone would be inappropriate in this case scenario. Nebulized albuterol would be of no benefit. Endotracheal intubation would not be indicated in this case because there are no signs of impending respiratory failure. Bronchoscopy should be considered in cases of suspected or confirmed foreign body aspiration. (Stridor, Chapter 72)

24. e   Hyponatremia is one of the most common causes of seizures in patients less than 6 months of age. Young infants poorly tolerate dilute oral feedings because of their immature kidneys. A detailed history will lead one to the correct diagnosis in these cases. Treating the patient with hypertonic saline (3% sodium chloride) in a dose of 3–5 ml/kg will raise the serum sodium in small increments (2–4 mEq/l). The seizure is unlikely to respond to the antiepileptic drugs mentioned. Although a serum sodium level will confirm your diagnosis, waiting for a formal result may delay treatment. (Renal and Electrolyte Emergencies, Chapter 86)

25. a   This patient has supraventricular tachycardia (SVT). Patients often have irritability as a presenting symptom; however, SVT may progress to congestive heart failure over time if not treated. In asymptomatic patients, vagal maneuvers (such as ice applied over the face and mouth) can be attempted. Adenosine, given as a rapid IV push, should be given subsequently if vagal maneuvers do not work. In cases where patients start to show signs of cardiac decompensation, as in this case, synchronized cardioversion is the treatment of choice. Digoxin is used for chronic treatment of certain types of SVT, but it is not the treatment of choice in the acute care setting. A large fluid bolus in this case may worsen the patient's condition. (Tachycardia/Palpitations, Chapter 74, and Cardiac Emergencies, Chapter 82)

26. b   The patient in this scenario has lymphadenitis, which is most commonly caused by group A beta-hemolytic *Streptococcus* or *Staphylococcus aureus*. Amoxicillin/clavulanate is appropriate treatment for this infection. If there were no change in this child's condition after a few days of antibiotic therapy, one should consider cat-scratch disease. Cat-scratch disease is caused by *Bartonella henselae*, which can often be found in the saliva of kittens. There is not always a clear history of a scratch from the kitten. Lymphadenopathy from cat-scratch disease is usually a single node that is warm, tender, and indurated with overlying erythema. Titers can be sent to confirm this diagnosis. Treatment for well-appearing children is observation alone; rifampin, azithromycin, trimethoprim-sulfamethoxazole, and ciprofloxacin have been used with some effectiveness in children with systemic toxicity. Needle aspiration will provide relief in children with tender, suppurative nodes, but this is unnecessary otherwise. Surgical excision is unnecessary and can lead to formation of a draining sinus. (Neck Mass, Chapter 45, and Infectious Disease Emergencies, Chapter 84)

27. c   With a history of fever and pain with decreased range of motion of the hip, a septic joint is the most likely diagnosis. Other supporting evidence for this diagnosis would be an elevated ESR and leukocytosis. The definitive diagnosis, however, is made by arthrocentesis of the hip, at which time the synovial fluid may appear purulent, with WBC counts of 25,000–100,000/μl, a positive Gram stain (seen in 50% of the specimens collected), and positive culture (seen in 70–80% of the cultures). Although *Haemophilus influenzae*, *S. aureus*, and *Streptococcus pneumoniae* have been associated with septic joints, the most likely organism in this immunized patient is *S. aureus*. A triple-phase bone scan may be considered in the evaluation of acute osteomyelitis. A CT scan or MRI may be helpful in the evaluation of bony tumors and soft tissue collections, respectively; however, these imaging studies should be considered in this patient only after the diagnosis of a septic hip has been definitively excluded by arthrocentesis. Although nonsteroidal anti-inflammatory agents may be helpful for analgesia, this therapy alone would be more appropriate for transient synovitis of the hip. (Limp, Chapter 43) (Behrman RE, et al., eds. *Nelson Textbook of Pediatrics*, fifteenth edition. Philadelphia: W.B. Saunders, 1996.)

28. d   This patient had a simple febrile seizure (a single generalized seizure lasting less than 15 minutes). The patient frequently develops the seizure at the onset of a high fever. Lumbar puncture is recommended in patients less than 12 months old, in any case of suspected meningitis, and when the febrile seizure is complex. Head CT scan and EEG are not recommended in the workup of simple febrile seizures. The source of the fever should be evaluated based on the age of the patient and the height of the fever. In this patient, a WBC count and blood culture should be obtained to exclude occult bacteremia. Obtaining serum calcium, magnesium, and phosphorus levels is not indicated in this setting. (Neurologic Emergencies, Chapter 83)

29. c   Although the child has a number of concerning "red flags," such as symptoms during exercise and a fast heart rate, the overall impression is that of benign chest pain. The short duration of symptoms and the brief, sharp, inconsistent nature of the symptoms all suggest a benign precordial catch syndrome. This is very common in young healthy teens and adults. Although a CXR and an ECG are probably indicated, both would presumably be normal. The family history adds no information. (Pain—Chest, Chapter 52)

30. d   Neurological findings after a motor vehicle collision are worrisome for spinal cord injury. Treatment is directed at reducing swelling of the cord and improving neurological outcome. The therapy currently recommended is a loading dose of methylprednisolone, 30 mg/kg IV. Subsequent doses of 5.4 mg/kg/hour should be administered for the next 24 hours. Intubation is not necessary because the patient has no airway compromise and a GCS score of 15. Mannitol administration is used to decrease ICP. Flexion/extension views of the neck on plain film would be contraindicated because positioning the patient could worsen an underlying injury. The patient should remain in appropriate C-spine immobilization with appropriate C-spine precautions. (Neck Trauma, Chapter 106)

31. d   This child presents with signs and symptoms consistent with methemoglobinemia. Normal cardiac and respiratory findings help to rule out other organ systems as possible etiologies; however, a normal O_2 saturation in spite of obvious cyanosis is expected in methemoglobinemia because pulse oximetry does not recognize oxidized hemoglobin; rather, it distinguishes only between oxy- and deoxyhemoglobin. Pa_{O_2} measurement by arterial blood gas should also be normal because Pa_{O_2} is a measure of dissolved oxygen in the blood and does not reflect the amount of oxygen attached to hemoglobin. Even though patients with carbon monoxide poisoning may present with lethargy, they do not present with cyanosis; they classically have a cherry-red color to their skin. A carboxyhemoglobin level, therefore, would not be helpful. (Cyanosis, Chapter 16, and Hematologic Emergencies, Chapter 87)

32. b   The most concerning aspect of this child's history and examination is the delay in the onset of the limp. Although a limp immediately following a fall would more likely suggest a musculoskeletal etiology, this child's limp is more likely secondary to neurologic causes. Other neurological deficits may be seen but are not always present. Although all of the diagnoses could cause back pain and a limp, the history of trauma makes an epidural hematoma more likely. A herniated intervertebral disk is a rare diagnosis in a young child, but it would not be impossible. Of the selected tests given, a spinal MRI would be the most sensitive test to diagnose a compression injury from a spinal epidural hematoma. (Pain—Back, Chapter 51)

33. a   Given the limited information in this vignette, the patient could have a number of causes for his symptoms. Pneumothorax, hemothorax, aortic rupture, cardiac arrhythmia from cardiac contusion, pulmonary contusion, cardiac tamponade, ruptured esophagus, tracheobronchial disruption, rib fracture, vertebral injury, and simple chest wall contusion can all be caused by a rapid deceleration injury and blunt force trauma. A more thorough physical examination would clearly help to narrow the diagnostic possibilities. Of the choices, a CXR will give the most information in the shortest amount of time and will help to further direct care. A chest CT is rarely, if ever, the first test to obtain in trauma evaluation. The remaining choices would help to evaluate for specific causes of traumatic chest pain, but all will give only limited information. (Thoracic Trauma, Chapter 107)

34. c   Benzodiazepines are the first drug of choice for the treatment of status epilepticus. In the absence of IV access, diazepam can be given rectally at a dose of 0.5–1.0 mg/kg. Because the duration of action is less than 30 minutes, additional anticonvulsant medication is needed to prevent seizure recurrence. Because the patient is chronically on phenytoin, the second drug of choice in this case is fosphenytoin, which—unlike phenytoin—can be given IM. The initial dose of fosphenytoin should be 5–10 mg/kg

until the patient's serum phenytoin level is obtained. Lorazepam cannot be used IM, and rectal paraldehyde is recommended only when other agents are ineffective. (Seizures, Chapter 70, and Neurologic Emergencies, Chapter 83)

35. a   This patient has a classic history for a radial head subluxation, or nursemaid's elbow. Given the history and examination, fractures or avulsion injuries are unlikely. Sprains are rare in children and a diagnosis of exclusion, but given her history and examination, a nursemaid's elbow is more likely. (Immobile Arm, Chapter 36)

36. e   Acute cholangitis is a postsurgical emergency. Patients will typically develop RUQ abdominal pain, fever, and shaking chills, associated with jaundice. Jaundice may be absent, however, if the cholangitis evolves rapidly. Overwhelming sepsis may develop, usually with gram-negative organisms. The diagnosis is a clinical one, and normal laboratory values do not exclude the diagnosis. (Gastrointestinal Emergencies, Chapter 93)

37. e   *S. atra* is a fungus that produces trichothecene mycotoxins, which are dermally active fungal toxins. Health-care workers in contact with patients exposed to these toxins are potentially at risk for absorption of these toxins through the skin. *B. anthracis* and *Y. pestis,* in the context of WMD, are aerosolized agents. For optimal infectivity, these agents need to be aerosolized in 1–5 μm-sized particles, which is unlikely to occur by respiratory means. In addition, these agents are not volatile. Staphylococcal enterotoxin B is a foodborne, and potentially airborne, WMD. HIV cannot be transmitted via aerosolization or routine contact. (The Emergency Department Response to Incidents of Biologic and Chemical Terrorism, Chapter 132)

38. d   Given the patient's history, there is concern for septic arthritis, but with an arthrocentesis that appears to be inconsistent with the diagnosis, osteomyelitis is the next concerning diagnosis on the differential. Appropriate therapy at this time would be to obtain a bone scan or MRI of the hip to confirm this diagnosis. There is no indication for sending titers for *B. burgdorferi,* the etiologic agent for Lyme disease. With a normal arthrocentesis, a hip arthrotomy and irrigation are not necessary. (Joint Pain, Chapter 57)

39. e   Management of occult bacteremia remains controversial. The organism most frequently isolated is *Streptococcus pneumoniae,* with *Neisseria meningitidis* a distant second. Group B *Streptococcus* is frequently isolated from neonates, and would be extraordinarily rare in an 8-month-old child. If a child is over the age of 2–3 months, and is well appearing with no signs of meningeal irritation, CSF testing is not routinely indicated. Without further ancillary testing, antibiotics should not be routinely administered, nor should this patient be admitted for observation. (Infectious Disease Emergencies, Chapter 84)

40. a   The initial step in the resuscitation of a newborn baby is drying and stimulation of the baby. This should be done under a radiant warmer. With these measures, the newborn will often begin to make respiratory efforts and improve his circulation. If this is not successful, administration of oxygen, with or without positive-pressure ventilation, is indicated. Intubation and cardiac compressions would be next in the order of resuscitation. Administration of naloxone should be considered in any child whose mother may have received opioids or whose history is unknown or uncertain. Drying and stimulation should still be the first step in resuscitation, however. (Neonatal Resuscitation, Chapter 2)

41. a   Viral URIs can cause multiple symptoms in the upper respiratory system. Sinusitis should be suspected whenever the fever and symptoms are persistent (for more than 10 days) or severe. The frontal and sphenoid sinuses do not aerate until 4–7 years of age, however, and therefore cannot be infected in a 3-year-old patient. Pharyngitis is usually viral in this age group. Streptococcal pharyngitis does not usually occur until 6 years of age. In addition, this patient does not have signs suggestive of this diagnosis. Periorbital cellulitis will cause erythema periorbitally, but does not cause isolated supraorbital tenderness. It is difficult to determine true tenderness of the sinuses in a 3-year-old child. (Infectious Disease Emergencies, Chapter 84)

42. e   Acute ataxia may be caused by numerous etiologies. Given this patient's recent history of a varicella infection and her symptomatology lasting for several days, however, a post-varicella cerebellitis with ataxia is the most likely cause of her symptoms. If she had an acute onset of symptoms, with symptoms lasting hours instead of days, obtaining a serum glucose level (to help rule out alcohol ingestion) or a

urine toxicological screening would be indicated. With more chronic symptoms, or an atypical presentation of postinfectious cerebellitis, a head CT or MRI scan would be indicated to evaluate intracerebral or cerebellar causes of ataxia. Measurement of ICP should be preceded by an imaging study of the head. (Ataxia, Chapter 11, and Neurologic Emergencies, Chapter 83)

43. d Rectal prolapse has multiple causes, but its association with cystic fibrosis is frequent, and a sweat test is indicated for any child who has had rectal prolapse. The other interventions are not indicated. (Cystic Fibrosis, Chapter 96)

44. b Salter-Harris I fractures are fractures through the physis in a child whose physes have not closed. Radiographically, no fracture may be visible, and therefore the diagnosis is made by clinical suspicion. Because of his mechanism and the site of his maximal tenderness, this patient likely has a Salter-Harris I fracture of the distal fibula. The patient should be immobilized, either in a splint or a short leg cast, and referred to orthopedics. A compression wrap would be inadequate treatment. Obtaining a comparison view is helpful with the diagnosis of bowing fractures of a long bone. There is no indication for the last two choices. (Orthopedic Trauma, Chapter 115)

45. e Breath-holding spells can be frightening events for parents and caretakers, but given a classic history and description of the event, the diagnosis can be made with no further testing. Each of the other tests would be helpful to diagnose other causes of syncope. (Behavioral Emergencies, Chapter 131)

46. c Common things are common, even in light of uncommon diseases. Complications of a VPS include infection and obstruction. Infection usually occurs within 1 month of the most recent surgery, and becomes more rare as time elapses. Obstruction may cause a variety of symptoms—headache, vomiting, lethargy, irritability, and other symptoms. Given this patient's symptoms, however, and her normal neurological examination, an obstruction is less likely. She should receive hydration, whether orally or intravenously, to correct her dehydration. Her response to rehydration will determine if she can be discharged to home. (Neurosurgical Emergencies, Chapter 125)

47. a The pattern of these burns suggest immersion injuries from forcing a child into a hot tub of water and are suspicious of nonaccidental trauma. Normal burns should occur on one extremity, rather than the buttocks or the back of the legs. Femur fractures in children under the age of 2 are unusual as well because of the amount of force necessary to fracture the femur and the limited ability to ambulate in this age group. Choice "c" describes a practice called "cupping," which is a common cultural practice among Southeast Asians. Circular patches of alopecia are consistent with alopecia from tinea infections. Irregular patches would potentially be consistent with traction alopecia, a sign of nonaccidental trauma. Chin lacerations are common in 2-year-old children. (Child Abuse, Chapter 128, and Burns, Chapter 114)

48. e Patients with Angelman's syndrome ("Happy Puppet" syndrome) are not characterized by any gastrointestinal or respiratory abnormalities. Coins pass through the gastrointestinal tract remarkably well and therefore no further immediate treatment is necessary because the coin is beyond the esophagus. The parents can observe for the passage of the coin by checking the stools for the following weeks, but they should not feel pressured to do so. (Foreign Body—Ingestion/Aspiration, Chapter 29)

49. c Carbon monoxide poisoning may occur with any fire. Given the position in which the patient was found, it is unlikely that he suffered a traumatic injury; therefore, x-rays of his cervical spine are not warranted. An arterial blood gas may reveal that he has poor oxygenation or ventilation, but it will not lead to the diagnosis. Pulse oximetry may be falsely normal. Lethargy may be caused by toxic ingestions; therefore, obtaining urine screening for ingestions may be reasonable, but carbon monoxide poisoning is more likely. (Environmental Emergencies, Chapter 89).

50. a The initial management of a patient with anaphylaxis is the same as any patient with a life-threatening emergency (assessment and treatment of ABC—airway, breathing, and circulation, etc). This patient has stridor due to laryngoedema. The airway should be treated first, followed by treatment for other complications of anaphylaxis. Epinephrine should therefore be given to treat the laryngoedema. If the symptoms do not resolve with initial treatment, securing the airway would be the next priority. Treatment with diphenhydramine is important, but epinephrine will cause immediate relief of symptoms, whereas diphenhydramine will not. This patient is hypotensive, but the compromised airway needs to be addressed prior to circulation problems. (Allergic Emergencies, Chapter 92)

Abbreviations

Abbreviation	Explanation	Units of Measurement
ALT	alanine aminotransferase	
AST	aspartate aminotransferase	
BP	blood pressure	millimeters of mercury (mm Hg)
CBC	complete blood count	
cc	cubic centimeter	
CSF	cerebrospinal fluid	
C-spine	cervical spine	
CT	computed tomography	
CXR	chest radiograph	
dl	deciliter	
ECG	electrocardiogram	
ED	Emergency Department	
EEG	electroencephalogram	
ESR	erythrocyte sedimentation rate	millimeters per hour (mm/hr)
g	gram	
GCS	Glasgow Coma Scale	
hct	hematocrit	%
HEENT	head, eyes, ears, nose, throat	
Hgb	hemoglobin	grams/deciliter (g/dl)
hpf	per high-power field	
HR	heart rate	beats per minute
IM	intramuscular	
IV	intravenous	
kg	kilogram	
KUB	kidneys/ureter/bladder or abdominal plain film	
l	liter	
LOC	loss of consciousness	
MCV	mean corpuscular volume	fl
mg	milligram	
ml	milliliter	
MRI	magnetic resonance imaging	
μg	microgram; micron	
NAD	no acute distress	
NS	normal saline	
PO	per os (by mouth)	
RBC	red blood cells	per millimeters^3
RR	respiratory rate	breaths per minute
SC	subcutaneous	
SG	specific gravity	
T	temperature	degrees Celsius (°C)
T_4	thyroxine	micrograms per deciliter
TSH	thyroid-stimulating hormone	
UA	urinalysis	
URI	upper respiratory infection	
U/S	ultrasound	
WBC	white blood cells	per millimeters^3
x-ray	radiograph	

Life-Threatening Emergencies

Resuscitation—Pediatric Basic and Advanced Life Support

VINCENT J. WANG, M.D.

QUESTIONS

1. The paramedics bring a 4-month-old boy to the ED. He was found at home near the hospital, apneic and cyanotic. No other history is available. On examination, he is apneic and has circumoral cyanosis. His HR is 30. You immediately:

   a. Perform chest compressions
   b. Sweep the mouth for foreign bodies
   c. Perform back blows and chest compressions
   d. Hyperextend the neck to open the airway
   e. Perform the jaw-thrust maneuver

2. A 6-month-old girl is brought to the ED for respiratory distress. She has had cough and rhinorrhea for 3 days, and has been breathing faster for 1 day. On examination, she is alert, but anxious appearing. She has no cyanosis, but has an RR of 60 with moderate retractions. Her vital signs are: HR 140 and BP 100/60. Her pulse oximetry shows an O_2 saturation of 89%. Initial treatment is:

   a. O_2 via facemask
   b. O_2 via endotracheal (ET) tube
   c. Normal saline (NS) fluid bolus
   d. D5 ¼NS at a maintenance rate
   e. Obtain an arterial blood gas (ABG)

3. A 12-year-old girl has just been involved in a high-speed motor vehicular accident right outside of your hospital. She is brought to your ED almost immediately after the accident. No intervention has been performed. She is unconscious and apneic. With bagged ventilation, she has symmetric breath sounds that are equal. Initial management of the airway and cervical spine (C-spine) includes:

   a. Application of gentle anterior traction to maintain the C-spine in line
   b. Gentle flexion of the neck to open the airway
   c. Performing the jaw thrust maneuver to open the airway
   d. Using a soft C-spine collar for neck immobilization
   e. No C-spine precautions are necessary in this scenario

4. A 2-year-old girl has respiratory distress. Her family has recently emigrated from Central America. She has had high fevers for 1 day. She developed difficulty breathing just hours ago. On examination, she appears ill and is leaning forward and drooling. Initial treatment includes:

   a. Endotracheal (ET) intubation
   b. Ceftriaxone IV
   c. Dexamethasone IM
   d. Racemic epinephrine nebulizer treatment
   e. Warm soaks to the neck

5. Paramedics bring in a 6-year-old boy in status epilepticus. He has been seizing for 60 minutes. In the ED, he has received lorazepam multiple times, as well as phenobarbital to stop his seizures. He is now apneic. You prepare to intubate him with a(n):

   a. Uncuffed 4.5 mm ET tube
   b. Cuffed 4.5 mm ET tube
   c. Uncuffed 5.0 mm ET tube
   d. Cuffed 5.0 mm ET tube
   e. Uncuffed 5.5 mm ET tube

6. The 6-year-old boy in Question 5 is successfully intubated. The best method for immediate confirmation of ET tube placement is:

   a. Auscultating over the stomach
   b. Auscultating over both axillas
   c. Chest radiograph (CXR)
   d. End-tidal CO_2 monitoring
   e. Watching for humidified air in the ET tube

7. Appropriate ET tube selection for a 20-year-old male in respiratory failure is a(n):

   a. Uncuffed 8.0 mm ET tube
   b. Cuffed 8.0 mm ET tube
   c. Uncuffed 8.5 mm ET tube
   d. Cuffed 8.5 mm ET tube
   e. Uncuffed 9.0 mm ET tube

8. A 14-year-old girl with asthma and hypoxia requires minimal supplemental oxygen. Which of the following would be the best method to deliver oxygen to her?

   a. Oxygen hood
   b. Oxygen tent
   c. Nasal cannula
   d. Nonrebreathing mask
   e. ET intubation

9. A 15-year-old boy was pulled out of the bottom of a lake after being under water for several minutes. He is apneic and pulseless upon arrival to the ED. The best route for administration of fluids is via:

   a. Percutaneous intravenous central catheter (PICC)
   b. Radial arterial catheter
   c. Intraosseous cannula
   d. Saphenous vein catheter
   e. ET tube

10. A 2-year-old girl is brought to the ED with respiratory arrest. She becomes asystolic shortly after arrival. The patient is intubated and, despite administration of oxygen via ET tube, as well as adequate chest wall movement, the patient remains asystolic. The next treatment is:

    a. Re-intubation
    b. Atropine
    c. Epinephrine
    d. Dextrose 25%
    e. Bicarbonate

11. A 5-year-old girl is brought to the ED unconscious and asystolic. She had been trapped in a car trunk and was found an hour later. She is apneic and has no pulse. Which dose of epinephrine should be given initially?

    a. IV epinephrine as a continuous infusion at 1 µg/kg/min
    b. IV epinephrine 0.01 mg/kg as a single dose
    c. IV epinephrine 0.1 mg/kg as a single dose
    d. IV epinephrine 0.2 mg/kg as a single dose
    e. IV epinephrine 1 mg/kg as a single dose

12. A 4-year-old boy is brought to the ED for an allergic reaction. He has a known allergy to peanuts and accidentally ingested some peanuts approximately 15 minutes ago. Despite IV fluids and two appropriate doses of epinephrine, his BP remains at 65/30. The next best step in management is:

    a. IV diphenhydramine
    b. IV hydrocortisone
    c. IV cimetidine
    d. Dopamine as a continuous infusion IV
    e. Epinephrine as a continuous infusion IV

13. A 2-year-old girl is brought to the ED because she was found with an opened aspirin bottle. The mother is not sure how many tablets she had ingested. She has irregular respirations with a RR of 12 and a HR of 50. She is minimally responsive. Her ABG reveals a pH of 7.24, P_{CO_2} of 50, and HCO_3 of 10. The toxicologist recommends a continuous infusion of $NaHCO_3$ as treatment for the salicylate intoxication. You begin with:

    a. $NaHCO_3$ 1 meq/kg IV bolus
    b. $NaHCO_3$ continuous infusion titrated to effect
    c. IV epinephrine 0.01 mg/kg
    d. IV atropine 0.02 mg/kg
    e. Intubation

14. A 3-year-old girl drank a large quantity of over-the-counter cough syrup approximately 1 hour ago. The parents are certain that she has not ingested anything else. On examination, she is ataxic and lethargic. Her examination is otherwise normal. Initial treatment includes:

    a. Nasogastric (NG) lavage
    b. Activated charcoal
    c. Head computed tomography (CT) scan
    d. Dextrose 25%
    e. Lorazepam

15. A 12-year-old girl is brought to your ED in ventricular fibrillation. The transport physician had defibrillated her, and had given epinephrine and lidocaine without improvement. You make another attempt at defibrillation without success. The next step in the medical treatment of ventricular fibrillation is administration of:

    a. IV epinephrine 0.2 mg/kg
    b. IV atropine 0.02 mg/kg
    c. IV bretylium 5 mg/kg
    d. IV adenosine 0.1 mg/kg
    e. IV $NaHCO_3$ 1 mEq/kg

16. A 14-month-old boy is brought to the ED for fussiness. On auscultation of his chest, the triage nurse notes tachycardia. An ECG reveals a narrow, complex tachycardia at 260 beats per minute (bpm), without P waves. His vital signs are: T 38°C, HR 260, RR 28, and BP 100/55. Initial treatment is:

    a. Ice applied to the face
    b. Administration of IV adenosine 0.1 mg/kg
    c. Synchronized cardioversion
    d. Defibrillation
    e. Acetaminophen

17. An 8-month-old girl is brought to the ED for fussiness. Her findings on ECG are similar to the previous patient's findings. Her BP, however, is 60/30, and she is mottled. No further treatment has been instituted. Initial treatment is:

    a. Application of ice over her face
    b. Adenosine 0.1 mg/kg IV
    c. Adenosine 0.2 mg/kg IV
    d. Synchronized cardioversion
    e. Defibrillation

18. A 10-year-old boy has ventricular fibrillation. The patient's airway is adequate and he is currently well perfused. Cardiopulmonary resuscitation (CPR) is begun. Initial treatment includes:

    a. A precordial thump
    b. $NaHCO_3$
    c. Atropine
    d. Synchronized cardioversion
    e. Defibrillation

ANSWERS

1. e   The initial management in this vignette involves airway assessment. In infants, the mandibular block of tissue may obstruct the upper airway. The chin lift or jaw-thrust maneuver would be appropriate to alleviate this potential obstruction. Hyperextension is not indicated in a patient found unresponsive because of the risk of C-spine injuries. Sweeping the mouth with fingers or back blows and chest compressions are indicated in the case of an airway obstruction, but these maneuvers would be performed after the initial jaw-thrust maneuver. Chest compressions for cardiac resuscitation are not indicated initially but may be necessary after the airway has been secured.

2. a   Patients in respiratory distress should be assessed and given appropriate treatment for their degree of distress. This patient is maintaining her airway and does not appear to need assistance via endotracheal tube or bag-valve-mask ventilation. Oxygen via facemask or blowby is indicated. Patients who have respiratory distress may also be dehydrated because of their tachypnea, but this should be addressed after attending to her respiratory distress. An ABG is helpful in the assessment of respiratory distress, but should not be the first intervention performed.

3. c   In any case of trauma, a C-spine injury may complicate the management. Using a rigid C-spine collar is appropriate, but the rigid collar may need to be removed when intubating the patient. Use of a soft collar is not appropriate. Assigning a code team member to apply gentle cephalad traction to maintain the C-spine in line is an alternative to a rigid collar. Gentle flexion of the neck is not recommended due to the motion of the C-spine.

4. a   Epiglottitis is an infectious disease emergency. The patient should be calmed and no procedures should be done that might agitate the patient. The patient should be intubated as soon as possible in a controlled setting (e.g., the operating room). Ceftriaxone could be given for a bacterial infection, but it should not be administered to this patient before the airway is secured. Dexamethasone and racemic epinephrine nebulizer treatments are indicated for croup. Warm soaks will not help the patient, and may in fact exacerbate her condition. Lateral neck films may be obtained if the diagnosis is uncertain and the patient is reasonably stable.

5. e   The appropriate size endotracheal tube equals 4 + (age in years/4), up to a maximum of 8.0 mm, which is the size of an ET tube for a large adult. Children under the age of 10 years should be intubated with an uncuffed ET tube. Children 10 and over should be intubated with a cuffed ET tube.

6. d   The best immediate methods for confirming ET tube placement are end-tidal CO_2 monitoring and observing for symmetrical chest movement. Improvement of clinical status is also helpful. Because a child's small chest may transmit sounds throughout the chest, auscultation over the stomach and axillas is helpful but cannot be relied upon for confirmation. A chest radiograph will confirm the position, but it will often take several minutes to verify tube placement.

7. b   The appropriate size ET tube equals 4 + (age in years/4), up to a maximum of 8.0 mm, the size of an ET tube for a large adult. The age of this patient puts him above the calculated size, so a tube size of 8.0 mm is appropriate, unless he is small for his age. Children age 10 and older should be intubated with a cuffed ET tube.

8. c   For minimal supplemental oxygen in an older child, oxygen delivery via a nasal cannula is indicated. An oxygen hood is helpful for providing high concentrations of FiO_2 (fractional inspired oxygen concentration) to a newborn or infant. An oxygen tent is helpful for younger children requiring a stable environment for oxygen delivery, humidity, and temperature, and would not be indicated in this patient. A nonrebreathing mask could be used, but it would provide much more oxygen than is needed. Endotracheal intubation is indicated for complete airway control.

9. d   Ideal resuscitation lines are short IV catheters with a wide lumen diameter. The antecubital fossa is an adequate site for placement of these lines, but IV lines may be placed anywhere. A PICC line is a poor choice for resuscitation because it is a long catheter with a narrow lumen. Radial arterial catheterization is obtained for continuous blood pressure monitoring and access for blood draws. It cannot be used for administration of fluids. Similarly, an ET tube cannot be used for fluid administration, although it can be used for administration of certain medications. An intraosseous line would be difficult to place in a 15-year-old patient, and it would offer a limited flow rate.

10. c   Indications for the administration of epinephrine are asystole, symptomatic bradycardia, and hypotension not related to volume depletion. Epinephrine may also be given to change fine fibrillation to a coarse one prior to a defibrillation attempt. Given that the chest wall is moving in response to ventilation, there is no need to suspect that the patient is asystolic because of a blocked or dislodged ET tube. Atropine should be given for bradycardia, but not for asystole. Dextrose should be given for hypoglycemia. Sodium bicarbonate should be administered for specific causes once the airway has been secured. Asystole is not an indication for sodium bicarbonate administration without suspicion of an underlying treatable cause.

11. b   The initial dose of epinephrine should be 0.01 mg/kg. Even though there is no data supporting the use of high-dose epinephrine, it is our practice to administer a subsequent dose of 0.1 mg/kg if a second dose is necessary. A subsequent dose of 0.2 mg/kg may be given afterward if the patient is still unresponsive. The initial dose of epinephrine should not be given as a continuous infusion.

12. e   Despite appropriate fluid and epinephrine therapy, the patient continues to be symptomatic from anaphylaxis. Epinephrine is the ideal pressor agent for this scenario because it will treat the allergic reaction as well as provide blood pressure support. Diphenhydramine, cimetidine, and hydrocortisone are useful adjuncts for anaphylaxis, but the hypotension must be addressed immediately. Dopamine as a continuous infusion would be adequate for blood pressure support, but epinephrine would be a better choice.

13. e   There are multiple reasons to intubate this patient. She has irregular respirations and is obtunded. Even though rare, severe central nervous system (CNS) toxicity with aspirin is more common in younger children. The patient should be intubated as soon as possible because of this CNS depression. Treatment with $NaHCO_3$ for urinary alkalinization is indicated for mild to moderate ingestions. In this severe case, however, hemodialysis is warranted. In addition, treatment with $NaHCO_3$ should not be started until adequate ventilation is possible. Other treatment modalities, such as activated charcoal, are also indicated, but not if the patient is at risk for aspiration, as this patient is. The airway should be secured first. Epinephrine and atropine may be indicated, but the airway is the first priority.

14. d Over-the-counter cough syrups may contain 10% ethanol. Prescription cough syrups may contain other medications (e.g., codeine). Most of the treatment for an acute ethanol ingestion is supportive; however, patients may become significantly hypoglycemic from the ingestion, and this patient should therefore be given dextrose 0.5–1.0 g/kg. Activated charcoal is essentially ineffective in absorbing ethanol, and NG lavage 1 hour after the ingestion is unlikely to yield results. A head CT scan would be warranted if the patient had a witnessed fall, or was found unconscious. Lorazepam would potentially make her symptoms worse.

15. c At this point, bretylium at a dose of 5 mg/kg IV should be given. Defibrillation should be attempted after this intervention. If the defibrillation is not successful, the dose should be increased to 10 mg/kg IV and defibrillation should be reattempted.

16. a Patients in stable supraventricular tachycardia (SVT) may have vagal maneuvers attempted before attempting other treatments. A patient is considered to have stable SVT if the patient is well perfused and has a normal blood pressure. In adults, a carotid massage, Valsalva maneuver, or other vagal maneuvers may be attempted. In young children, placing ice over the face to induce the diving-seal reflex is usually the easiest vagal maneuver. Adenosine may be administered after vagal maneuvers have failed. Synchronized cardioversion is indicated in unstable SVT in patients who are poorly perfused and are hypotensive. Defibrillation is not indicated. Acetaminophen may be given for the fever, but it will not correct the SVT.

17. d This patient has unstable SVT and should receive synchronized cardioversion immediately.

18. e The initial dose of current for defibrillation is 2 joules/kg, repeated once if necessary. If this is unsuccessful, CPR should be continued and a second defibrillation attempt should be made at double the dose. This may be doubled again if necessary. A precordial thump is not indicated in children. Synchronized cardioversion should be used for SVT.

CHAPTER 2

Neonatal Resuscitation

JACQUELINE BRYNGIL, M.D.

QUESTIONS

1. You receive an ambulance call that they are bringing in a young woman who is pregnant and is complaining of contractions. Her vital signs in the field are HR 120, RR 20, BP 110/60. No other information is available. You prepare to receive the patient and a potential imminent delivery. Other associated conditions that would make this a "high-risk" delivery include each of the following, EXCEPT:

    a. Maternal history of diabetes
    b. Maternal use of cocaine
    c. Twin delivery
    d. Maternal history of smoking
    e. A repeat BP of 180/100

2. You are called to the resuscitation room to evaluate a newborn who was just delivered. The infant is a 36-week gestation neonate with respiratory distress. His vital signs are T 36.8°C, HR 180, RR 44, and BP 74/palpable. He has good respiratory effort and no stridor. The infant was delivered vaginally. You note that he appears slightly dusky. Your most appropriate next step in management of this infant is:

    a. Obtain a CXR
    b. Obtain an ABG
    c. Administer 100% oxygen
    d. Intubation
    e. Initiate chest compressions

3. A woman presents at 26 weeks in preterm labor. She has had no rupture of membranes and ultrasound (U/S) shows an appropriate-for-gestational-age infant with no evidence of fetal distress at this time. Your most appropriate course of action at this time is:

    a. Initiate vaginal delivery after administering betamethasone
    b. Perform emergent cesarean section after administering betamethasone
    c. Arrest of labor with beta-sympathomimetics and administer betamethasone
    d. IV administration of ampicillin
    e. Admit and observe

4. You are examining a 5-week-old boy in the ED who was recently discharged from the neonatal intensive care unit (NICU). The infant was born vaginally at 32 weeks' gestation and had Apgar scores of 4 and 7. He required brief intubation for persistent hypoxia and correction of early acidosis. His most recent CXR showed a ground-glass appearance and increased lung markings. You note a systolic to-and-fro murmur and mild hepatomegaly. This infant would respond most favorably to:

    a. Administration of 30 ml of packed red blood cells (PRBC)
    b. A fluid bolus of 20 ml/kg of normal saline
    c. Administration of theophylline
    d. Increasing his caloric intake
    e. Administration of a short course of indomethacin

5. You are present at an emergency delivery in your trauma room and are handed a limp, dusky newborn. Your most appropriate intervention at this time is:

    a. Initiate cardiac compressions
    b. Bag-valve-mask (BVM) ventilation with 100% O_2
    c. Dry and warm the infant
    d. Administer epinephrine
    e. Establish vascular access

6. During routine resuscitation of a full-term newborn in the ED, you note persistence of hypoxia and bradycardia of 90 bpm despite an adequate seal with the mask. Your colleague is using a self-inflating bag. Likely reasons for inadequate resuscitation in this situation include all of the following, EXCEPT:

    a. Presence of congenital heart disease
    b. Failure to depress the pop-off valve on the bag
    c. Inappropriate-sized equipment
    d. Presence of pneumothorax
    e. Gastric distension

ANSWERS

1. d   Many factors contribute to high-risk births (births in which the neonate may require resuscitation). Some more common factors are prematurity, multiple births, premature rupture of membranes (PROM), maternal drug abuse, maternal hypertension, and maternal diabetes. Maternal age less than 16 or greater than 35 years is also a risk factor for a high-risk birth. Even though maternal smoking is discouraged, this does not make the delivery a high-risk one.

2. c   When evaluating a child for respiratory distress, the appropriate order of assessment and management is ABC: Airway, Breathing, and Circulation. If you detect noisy respirations or a poor respiratory effort, you must first reposition the head. In this scenario, the patient's airway is not obstructed and the next appropriate step would be to administer 100% oxygen. Although a CXR and possibly an ABG are also indicated, they should be obtained after the initiation of treatment with oxygen. In a child with an HR above 80 bpm, chest compressions are not indicated.

3. c   Fetal lung maturation is not complete until approximately 34 weeks. In early labor, or in cases where preterm delivery of the infant is medically necessary, administration of steroids to the mother in the form of betamethasone is indicated to accelerate fetal lung maturation and to decrease the incidence of respiratory distress syndrome. In uncomplicated cases of spontaneous preterm labor, inhibition of labor with beta-sympathomimetic tocolytic agents is the treatment of choice. Had this infant exhibited signs of fetal distress, emergent cesarean section after administering betamethasone would be the appropriate choice of management. Vaginal delivery of a distressed newborn is never indicated. In this scenario, there is no rupture of membranes, and IV antibiotics would not be indicated. It would be inappropriate to admit and observe without initiating treatment to prevent the delivery of an infant with immature lungs.

4. e   In the infant with hyaline membrane disease (HMD), there is often a delay in the closure of the ductus arteriosus. Treatment of an infant with a symptomatic patent ductus arteriosus (PDA) includes administration of indomethacin followed by surgical closure if the indomethacin is unsuccessful. Symptoms of a PDA may include signs of failure, including hepatomegaly, increased pulmonary vascular markings on CXR, and a systolic to-and-fro murmur. Other factors that affect duct closure are perinatal hypoxia and acidosis. Administration of large fluid boluses or colloid solutions in this patient would likely increase the amount of failure. Theophylline, which is often used to treat apnea/bradycardia symptoms and bronchopulmonary dysplasia, is not helpful in HMD with a PDA. Although the patient has a higher caloric requirement, this will not alleviate the problem.

5. c   Most newborns respond with an increase in HR and RR after routine warming and drying. If the infant fails to respond to this initial measure, administration of 100% O_2 via bag-valve-mask (BVM) ventilation is indicated to stimulate respiratory efforts. Assessment of circulation should follow, and compressions should be initiated if the HR remains between 60 and 80 bpm or drops below 60 bpm. Vascular access and epinephrine administration may be required in the unresponsive newborn if the preceding interventions fail.

6. a   Adequate neonatal resuscitation depends on the availability of appropriately sized equipment and the delivery of enough pressure to the newborn to stimulate effective spontaneous breathing. Self-inflating bags often have a pop-off valve to prevent barotrauma; however, in the newborn, this may need to be occluded to deliver the pressure required for effective respirations. Factors that prevent adequate oxygenation and/or expansion of the lungs, such as a pneumothorax and gastric distension, must be recognized and corrected. Although congenital heart disease must always be a consideration, it is an unlikely reason for failed resuscitation in most full-term newborns.

CHAPTER **3**

Shock

KAREN DULL, M.D.

QUESTIONS

1. A previously healthy 15-month-old child is brought to the ED after 5 days of fever, diarrhea, and poor PO intake. His physical exam reveals a lethargic infant with HR 200, RR 54, BP 70/40, and a capillary refill time of 3 seconds. The most appropriate initial fluid management of this patient is:

   a. 20 ml/kg of lactated Ringer's solution given over 1 hour
   b. 10 ml/kg of PRBC given over 1 hour
   c. 20 ml/kg of 5% albumin given over 20 minutes
   d. 20 ml/kg of NS as rapidly as possible
   e. 20 ml/kg of NS over 1 hour

2. A 4-day-old boy born at term to a 25-year-old mother is brought to the ED limp and pale with a temperature of 38.9°C. Which of the following initial vital signs most likely indicates impending cardiac arrest?

   a. HR 60
   b. O_2 saturation of 92%
   c. BP 60/40
   d. HR 200
   e. RR 70

3. A 3-day-old previously healthy boy is brought to the ED with "heavy breathing," listlessness, and pallor, which had developed over the last hour. He was the product of an uncomplicated term pregnancy and delivery. Your exam reveals a listless, ashen baby with poor tone and decreased femoral pulses. He is afebrile, with vital signs of HR 180, RR 44, and BP 85/40. Lung examination reveals scattered rales. A III/VI systolic murmur can be heard at the fourth left costal margin. Chest x-ray (CXR) shows increased pulmonary vascular markings with fluid in the fissures. Immediate management must include:

   a. Dobutamine
   b. Prostaglandin
   c. Albuterol
   d. Epinephrine
   e. Dopamine

4. A 13-month-old girl is brought to the ED with a 1-month history of weight loss and tachypnea with feeding. On exam HR is 210, RR 100, and BP 50/25. She is listless and mottled, and her capillary refill time is 3 seconds. She has a III/VI systolic murmur, best heard over the left lower sternal border (LLSB). Her liver is palpable at her umbilicus and she has diffuse rales throughout. The most appropriate initial IV therapy includes:

   a. 0.01 mg/kg epinephrine IV
   b. 10 µg/kg/min dopamine IV
   c. 2 µg/kg/min dobutamine IV
   d. 5 mg/kg dopamine IV
   e. 0.1 mg/kg/min norepinephrine IV

5. A 5-year-old girl with acute lymphoblastic leukemia (ALL) who had just finished a course of chemotherapy is brought to the ED with fever to 40°C associated with chills. Her exam is significant for mild listlessness and pallor. Which of the following predicts a poor response to therapy?

   a. HR 180
   b. RR 60
   c. Hypotension
   d. Capillary refill time of 3 seconds
   e. Irritability

6. A 5-month-old girl is brought into the ED after 24 hours of repeated vomiting and diarrhea. You are unable to obtain a blood pressure. She does not respond as the first two attempts are made at putting in a peripheral IV line. The next step in obtaining vascular access should be:

   a. Placement of an intraosseous needle on the medial tibia 2 cm below the tibial tuberosity
   b. Placement of a large-bore needle in the antecubital vein
   c. Placement of a catheter in the internal jugular vein
   d. Perform a femoral cutdown
   e. Perform a cutdown in a peripheral vein

7. A 13-year-old girl with recent menses and tampon use comes into the ED with fever and rash for the last 3 days. She has received 50 ml/kg of NS in the first hour of her initial treatment. Her BP is 80/40, HR 150. She is alert with cool extremities and a capillary refill time of 3 seconds. The next step in her management should be:

   a. Start dopamine at 5 μg/kg/min
   b. Start epinephrine at 0.1 μg/kg/min
   c. Give another 20 ml/kg bolus over the next hour
   d. Repeat 20 ml/kg NS bolus as long as there is no pulmonary edema on CXR
   e. Start dobutamine at 2–5 μg/kg/min

8. A 6-year-old child is brought to the ED unresponsive with cold, blue extremities, a rectal temperature of 41°C, and blood oozing from her mouth. Which of the following is a true statement regarding this patient?

   a. You would expect her to have increased fibrinogen
   b. You would expect her to have decreased fibrin split products
   c. She should be treated with platelets only if her platelet count is less than 20,000/mm³
   d. 10 ml/kg of fresh frozen plasma should be given IV
   e. She most likely will have a normal prothrombin time/partial thromboplastin time (PT/PTT)

9. A 2-week-old girl is brought to the ED with fever of 38.9°C and poor feeding for 48 hours. Physical exam is significant for RR 80, HR 200, O_2 saturation 92% on 100% FIO_2, poor tone, and gray skin. Which of the following would be an appropriate therapy after the IV access has been obtained?

   a. Obtain a blood culture, catheterized urine culture, and lumbar puncture (LP), followed by ampicillin and gentamicin
   b. Obtain a blood culture and catheterized urine culture, give ampicillin and gentamicin, then perform the lumbar puncture later
   c. Obtain a blood culture and a catheterized urine culture, give ampicillin and gentamicin, and order latex agglutination tests on the urine
   d. Obtain a blood culture and catheterized urine culture, give IV cefuroxime, and perform a lumbar puncture later
   e. Obtain a blood culture and catheterized urinalysis (UA), give ceftriaxone and obtain a head CT to rule out high intracranial pressure (ICP)

ANSWERS

1. d   The child described in the scenario has hypovolemic shock. The initial therapy should include 20 cc/kg of normal saline (NS) or lactated Ringer's solution, infused as rapidly as possible. The child should then be reassessed for signs of improved intravascular volume. It has been shown that children who receive at least 40 cc/kg of resuscitative fluid within the first hour have better survival and do not have an increased risk of either cardiogenic pulmonary edema or adult respiratory distress syndrome (ARDS).

2. a   The infant in the vignette has neonatal sepsis, probably due to group B streptococci. Cardiac output is determined by stroke volume and heart rate. To increase cardiac output, infants increase heart rate rather than stroke volume because they have limited ability to increase stroke volume. Infants can tolerate higher heart rates than adults because ventricular filling time is less critical to total cardiac output. The usual HR for a 4-day-old infant is 120–160 beats per minute (bpm). A heart rate of 60 bpm in the setting of sepsis indicates severe myocardial toxicity and impending cardiac arrest.

3. b   Acute onset of cardiogenic shock associated with depressed femoral pulses suggests left-sided outflow tract obstructive cardiac disease. Such infants depend on a patent ductus arteriosus for distal perfusion. If the ductus closes, sudden shock may ensue. In those cases, prostaglandin E_2 (PGE$_2$) infusion is life saving by its ability to reopen the ductus and restore peripheral perfusion.

4. c   Dobutamine should be considered initially in patients with cardiogenic shock because it is a selective stimulant of B$_1$ receptors. It serves as an excellent afterload reducer without increasing the heart rate. Starting doses are 2–5 μg/kg/min.

5. c   Compensated shock in children is characterized by tachycardia, tachypnea, delayed capillary refill time, orthostatic changes in blood pressure, and irritability. Tachycardia occurs to increase cardiac output. Delayed capillary refill occurs as increased sympathetic tone causes peripheral vasoconstriction. Late or uncompensated shock occurs when the normal compensatory mechanisms fail to perfuse end organs

(brain, heart, and kidneys). Hypotension is a sign of uncompensated shock and generally requires more aggressive resuscitation. Tachypnea and tachycardia become more enhanced. Capillary refill time becomes increasingly delayed (more than 4 seconds). The skin may be mottled or pale, with cool extremities.

6. a   If possible, a large-bore needle should be placed in a larger peripheral vein. If this is not possible after two attempts, an intraosseous line should be placed on the medial tibia 2 cm below the tibial tuberosity, angled away from the growth plate.

7. a   Dopamine would be the first choice to improve cardiac function and improve circulation for patients who have a moderate degree of hypotension after initial fluid resuscitation. Significant inotropic and vasopressor effects are seen with doses of 5–10 μg/kg/min. Patients with severe cardiovascular dysfunction require epinephrine infusion. Dobutamine should never be the initial treatment for septic shock because it can cause hypotension.

8. d   Shock can lead to the consumption of coagulation factors and platelets. Disseminated intravascular coagulation is characterized by thrombocytopenia, increased fibrin degradation, decreased fibrinogen, and prolonged prothrombin and partial thromboplastin times. Treatment includes platelet transfusion for a platelet count of less than 50,000 or active bleeding. Fresh frozen plasma (FFP) should be given to correct prolonged PT/PTT.

9. b   The infant in the vignette is too unstable for a lumbar puncture; however, antibiotic therapy should not be delayed. Lumbar puncture performed at a later time will reveal pleocytosis if meningitis is present. Ampicillin and gentamicin will provide coverage for group B streptococci, *E. coli*, and *Listeria*, which are the most common bacterial causes of neonatal sepsis and meningitis.

CHAPTER 4

Sedation and Analgesia

ATIMA CHUMPA, M.D.

QUESTIONS

1. A 3-year-old girl injured her distal forearm when she fell off of a swing. Radiographs reveal a displaced distal radius fracture that requires closed reduction in the ED. There was no head injury and she has a noncontributory past medical history. Among the following agents, which is the most appropriate for procedural sedation in this patient?

   a. Nitrous oxide
   b. Pentobarbital
   c. Ketamine
   d. Midazolam
   e. Chloral hydrate

2. In which of the following cases would pentobarbital be an ideal choice for procedural sedation?

   a. A 4-year-old boy who is undergoing closed reduction for a radius fracture
   b. A 10-year-old girl who is undergoing chest tube placement for a pneumothorax
   c. A 3-year-old boy who needs a head CT scan for evaluation of an afebrile seizure
   d. A 2-year-old girl who is undergoing a laceration repair of the lower lip
   e. A 12-month-old boy who is undergoing an abscess drainage in the buttock

3. A 12-year-old girl has a displaced distal radius and ulna fracture requiring closed reduction. The injury occurred when she fell while in-line skating. She has no significant past medical history. You are considering nitrous oxide for sedation. Using nitrous oxide, you would:

   a. Administer it in combination with oxygen (20% nitrous oxide, 80% oxygen)
   b. Expect that the effect will wear off immediately after it is discontinued
   c. Expect that the patient will not remember pain during the procedure
   d. Administer it in combination with an opioid agent
   e. Recognize that the risk of regurgitation and aspiration is high

4. A 3-year-old boy sustained an injury to his finger when it was caught in a door. He has an actively bleeding nailbed laceration. Which of the following local anesthetics is the most appropriate to use?

   a. Lidocaine with epinephrine
   b. LET (solution of 4% lidocaine, 0.1% epinephrine, 0.5% tetracaine)
   c. TAC (solution of 2% tetracaine 25 ml, 1:1000 epinephrine 50 ml, and cocaine 11.8 g)
   d. EMLA (eutectic mixture of local anesthetics)
   e. Bupivacaine

5. A 6-year-old boy sustained a displaced distal radius and ulna fracture when he fell while in-line skating. He requires closed reduction in the ED. His past medical history is noncontributory, but he currently has an upper respiratory tract infection (URI). Which of the following sedatives and analgesics would you select for this patient?

   a. Ketamine, midazolam, and atropine
   b. Fentanyl and midazolam
   c. Meperidine, promethazine, and chlorpromazine
   d. Pentobarbital
   e. Chloral hydrate

6. After administering a total of 6 mg/kg of IV pentobarbital IV to a 28-month-old girl who is undergoing head CT imaging, her O_2 saturation has dropped to 85% on room air, and she is noted to have a RR of 4. She has poor air entry on chest auscultation. You deliver assisted ventilation via bag-valve-mask. Her O_2 saturation improves to 90% on room air without improvement in RR. At this point, you would immediately:

   a. Administer naloxone
   b. Administer flumazenil
   c. Prepare for intubation
   d. Obtain a CXR
   e. Obtain an ABG

7. A 13-month-old boy with a large abscess on his buttock was referred by his primary care doctor for incision and drainage. You decide to use IV fentanyl and midazolam for procedural sedation. You place EMLA cream prior to IV insertion as per the mother's request. Fentanyl and midazolam are administered IV at 2 μg/kg and 0.05 mg/kg respectively. You administer 1% lidocaine without epinephrine around the abscess. While you are making the incision to drain the abscess, the patient develops generalized tonic-clonic seizure activity. You suspect that this is caused by:

   a. EMLA
   b. Lidocaine
   c. Fentanyl
   d. Midazolam
   e. Head injury

8. A 2-year-old girl sustained a laceration above her eyelid when she tripped and fell while walking. You administer IV ketamine and midazolam for procedural sedation. While repairing the laceration, she develops stridor with suprasternal retractions and poor air entry. Her O_2 saturation is 89% on room air with no improvement with blowby O_2. You would immediately:

   a. Administer succinylcholine
   b. Perform endotracheal intubation
   c. Administer flumazenil
   d. Deliver positive-pressure ventilation
   e. Administer racemic epinephrine

9. In which of the following cases can TAC be used safely and effectively?

   a. A 4-year-old boy with a through and through laceration of the nares
   b. A 3-year-old girl with an eyelid laceration
   c. A 2-year-old girl with a vermilion border laceration
   d. A 3-year-old girl with a dog-bite wound on her cheek
   e. A 2-year-old with a nailbed laceration

10. A 2-year-old boy comes to your ED with a first-time seizure. You order a head CT scan. His vital signs are: T 37.2°C, HR 120, RR 36, and BP 98/60. His neurological examination is normal. You administer 75 mg/kg of chloral hydrate orally. Thirty minutes after choral hydrate administration, he remains noncooperative. At this point you would:

   a. Repeat another dose of chloral hydrate
   b. Wait until it takes effect
   c. Place an IV and administer pentobarbital
   d. Immediately take him to head CT
   e. Administer midazolam orally

ANSWERS

1. c   Ketamine is commonly used for painful procedures (e.g., laceration repair and fracture reduction). It is generally given with atropine and midazolam to reduce excessive salivation and to blunt unpleasant dreams caused by ketamine. Nitrous oxide is also commonly used for painful procedures in the ED. It provides analgesia, amnesia, and sedation with a dissociative effect. Because nitrous oxide is administered via a mask, it is best for children 8 years and older who can cooperate and understand the procedure. Pentobarbital, midazolam, and chloral hydrate do not provide analgesia and are not recommended for this painful procedure.

2. c   Pentobarbital is a sedative with no analgesic properties. Sedation occurs rapidly after IV administration. It is ideal for nonpainful procedures (e.g., sedation for imaging studies), but because it does not have analgesic properties, it is not recommended for painful procedures.

3. c   Nitrous oxide has sedative, analgesic, and amnestic properties. It also has a dissociative effect on patients. Patients may complain of pain, but they do not seem to remember it. The onset of action is approximately 5 minutes after administration is initiated and takes approximately 5 minutes from the time the administration is stopped for the effects to wear off. When used with a mixture of more than 20% oxygen, it does not produce serious side effects. When used in a 50/50 mixture with oxygen, it provides analgesia, not anesthesia. The patient usually remains awake, is able to follow commands, and maintains protective airway reflexes. Opioids should not be given when administering nitrous oxide because the combination may produce a deeper level of sedation.

4. e   Bupivacaine is similar to lidocaine, but it has a longer duration of action, lasting for up to 6 hours. Lidocaine without epinephrine would also be reasonable for the preceding scenario. Lidocaine with ep-

inephrine should not be used in areas supplied by end arteries because epinephrine causes vasoconstriction and will potentially cut off the blood supply to those areas. LET and TAC are used effectively on facial or scalp lacerations in areas where there is increased vascularity. EMLA is not meant for use on open wounds and must be applied to the skin for 60 minutes before it is effective; therefore EMLA is not practical in this case.

5. b The combination of fentanyl and midazolam would provide the most effective and safest sedation for this painful procedure. Fentanyl provides analgesic and sedative effects, whereas midazolam provides sedative, anxiolytic, and amnestic effects. Ketamine should not be used in children who have upper respiratory tract infections because the intercurrent illness increases the risk of laryngospasm. The combination of meperidine, promethazine, and chlorpromazine is not recommended for sedation in the ED, because it can produce deep and prolonged sedation with respiratory depression as well as dystonic reactions in some patients. Pentobarbital and chloral hydrate do not provide analgesia and therefore should not be given to children undergoing painful procedures.

6. c Pentobarbital has its greatest use for nonpainful procedures. Like other barbiturates, pentobarbital may cause respiratory depression. Physicians must be prepared to give assisted ventilation and to intubate the patient if necessary. There are no reversal agents for pentobarbital.

7. b Lidocaine may cause seizures, cardiac arrest, and coma if the patient inadvertently receives a toxic amount of lidocaine, or if lidocaine is injected directly into blood vessels. The maximal dose of lidocaine is 7 mg/kg. Physicians should aspirate back while infiltrating lidocaine to ensure that it is not being administered directly into a vessel.

8. d The event described in this case is consistent with laryngospasm, which is a rare adverse effect of ketamine. Neonates and children with upper respiratory tract infections are at greater risk for developing laryngospasm; therefore, ketamine should be avoided in these children. Positive-pressure ventilation should be delivered if the patient develops laryngospasm or symptoms of inadequate ventilation. Intubation may be necessary if this first intervention is not adequate.

9. d TAC has been shown to be as effective as lidocaine for most wounds on the face and scalp, but it is less effective for wounds on the trunk and extremities. The major problem associated with TAC is the risk of cocaine toxicity, which can lead to seizures and death. TAC, therefore, should not be applied near mucous membranes, where rapid absorption can occur. TAC can also cause corneal abrasions and should not be used near the eye.

10. b Chloral hydrate is a pure sedative hypnotic without analgesic properties. It is useful for painless procedures (e.g., imaging studies). It can be given orally at 20–75 mg/kg. In this case, the patient received the optimal dosage; however, it may take longer for chloral hydrate to take effect. The sedation effect is variable; in some patients the peak effect may take 40–60 minutes or longer to accomplish. Chloral hydrate is a relatively safe drug; however, respiratory depression may occur in patients with sleep apnea or those who receive other concomitant sedatives.

CHAPTER **5**

Emergency Airway Management— Rapid-Sequence Intubation

ATIMA CHUMPA, M.D.

QUESTIONS

1. A 3-month-old boy is brought to the ED by his mother after she noted that he became lethargic and difficult to arouse. On arrival, his vital signs are: T 37°C, BP 62/34, HR 144, RR 4, and O_2 saturation 89% on room air. On your exam, he has a parietal hematoma, bulging anterior fontanel, and bruises over the lower extremities. After assisted ventilation with bag-valve-mask (BVM), you decide to intubate him. Which of the following agents are the most appropriate for rapid-sequence intubation (RSI) in this patient?

   a. Atropine, thiopental, succinylcholine
   b. Midazolam, succinylcholine
   c. Atropine, ketamine, vecuronium
   d. Atropine, thiopental, vecuronium
   e. Ketamine, succinylcholine

2. A 6-year-old girl with a history of severe asthma has difficulty breathing. She has been treated by her primary care physician with inhaled albuterol and prednisone. On exam, she has suprasternal and intercostal retractions, poor air entry, and inspiratory and expiratory wheezing. Her O_2 saturation on 100% oxygen is 80%; ABG shows pH 7.08 and P_{CO_2} 85. You are going to intubate her. Which of the following is the sedative/anesthetic of choice?

   a. Thiopental
   b. Ketamine
   c. Midazolam
   d. Fentanyl
   e. Diazepam

3. Which of the following endotracheal (ET) tubes would you select for the patient in Question 2?

   a. 4.0 mm, uncuffed
   b. 4.5 mm, cuffed
   c. 5.0 mm, cuffed
   d. 5.5 mm, uncuffed
   e. 6.0 mm, uncuffed

4. In which of the following cases can ketamine be used safely for rapid-sequence intubation (RSI)?

   a. A 7-year-old boy who presents to the ED after falling from a tree and is unconscious upon arrival
   b. A 15-year-old boy who has been stabbed in the chest and has BP 80/40 and a depressed mental status upon arrival
   c. A 16-year-old girl with a history of hallucinations and a tricyclic antidepressant overdose
   d. An 8-year-old boy with a history of chronic renal failure and hypertension who presents with depressed mental status
   e. A 10-year-old boy who has sustained multiple trauma, including facial lacerations and an open right globe injury

5. After administration of fentanyl during RSI in a 16-year-old girl with a history of asthma, her O$_2$ saturation drops and she becomes difficult to ventilate manually with a BVM. On auscultation, you are unable to hear breath sounds. All of the following statements are true, EXCEPT:

    a. This condition can be treated by administering a paralytic agent
    b. This condition can be treated by administering naloxone
    c. This condition is associated with a high dose of fentanyl
    d. This condition is associated with the rate of fentanyl administration
    e. This condition often develops in patients with pulmonary diseases

6. A 5-year-old boy who sustained multiple injuries in a motor vehicle accident is brought to the ED unresponsive, with vital signs of HR 110 and BP 86/48. Which of the following combination agents is the most appropriate for RSI?

    a. Atropine, thiopental, rocuronium
    b. Atropine, ketamine, succinylcholine
    c. Lidocaine, etomidate, succinylcholine
    d. Atropine, lidocaine, thiopental, succinylcholine
    e. Atropine, lidocaine, etomidate, rocuronium

7. You will be administering lidocaine, etomidate, and succinylcholine to a 17-year-old boy with a brain tumor, depressed mental status, and absent gag reflex. Which of the following steps should be considered prior to giving these drugs?

    a. Administering atropine 0.02 mg/kg
    b. Administering vecuronium 0.01 mg/kg
    c. Administering succinylcholine 0.5 mg/kg
    d. Administering succinylcholine 0.1 mg/kg
    e. Administering thiopental 2 mg/kg

8. Ten minutes after RSI with atropine, ketamine, and succinylcholine in a 10-year-old girl with status asthmaticus, the patient is noted to become flushed, with a temperature of 43°C. As quickly as possible, you should:

    a. Administer IV diphenhydramine
    b. Administer IV dantrolene
    c. Administer IV antibiotics
    d. Administer PR acetaminophen
    e. Administer a 20 ml/kg NS bolus

9. You are intubating an 18-month-old boy with status epilepticus with atropine, thiopental, and succinylcholine. Which of the following are the correct steps for RSI?

    a. Atropine, preoxygenation, succinylcholine, thiopental, intubation
    b. Atropine, preoxygenation, thiopental, succinylcholine, intubation
    c. Preoxygenation, atropine, Sellick maneuver, succinylcholine, thiopental, intubation
    d. Preoxygenation, thiopental, atropine, succinylcholine, intubation
    e. Sellick maneuver, preoxygenation, atropine, thiopental, succinylcholine, intubation

ANSWERS

1. **d**   The most likely cause of respiratory depression in this patient is an intracranial injury. Thiopental has a cerebral protective effect—it reduces intracranial pressure (ICP), cerebral metabolism, and oxygen demand; therefore, it is the sedative of choice for RSI in patients with head injury. It can, however, cause hypotension and is not recommended for hypotensive, hypovolemic patients. Succinylcholine provides the fastest intubating condition among all paralytic agents; however, it is contraindicated in patients with extensive crush injuries or burns sustained more than 7 days previously. Vecuronium, even though it has a slower onset, is safe to use in variety of conditions. Ketamine causes increased ICP and is contraindicated in patients with head injuries. Atropine should be used for RSI in all infants to prevent bradycardia.

2. **b**   Ketamine has a bronchodilating effect and is the sedative of choice for RSI in patients with status asthmaticus. Thiopental can cause bronchospasm and should not be used in this patient. Other sedatives do not have a bronchodilating effect.

3. d   The ET tube size can be calculated by using the formula, (age/4) + 4. An uncuffed ET tube should be used in patients under the age of 8 years. The anatomy of the larynx in this age group is funnel shaped, with narrowest portion at the cricoid ring; therefore, the cuff is not required for these children.

4. b   In addition to the bronchodilating effect, ketamine also results in sympathetic stimulation and increased systemic blood pressure. Ketamine use is recommended for RSI in patients with status asthmaticus and hypotension. Ketamine can cause increased ICP, increased intraocular pressure, hallucinations, and hypertension; therefore, it is contraindicated in other cases listed in Question 4.

5. e   The condition described in this case is chest wall rigidity caused by fentanyl. It is associated with a higher dose of fentanyl and rapid rate of administration. It can be treated with a muscle relaxant or naloxone. There is no evidence that the risk of developing chest wall rigidity is increased with underlying pulmonary conditions.

6. e   This patient presents with hypotension and suspected head injury. Ketamine causes sympathetic stimulation and can increase blood pressure; however, it can also increase ICP and is therefore contraindicated. Etomidate has less cardiovascular depression compared with the barbiturates and does not raise ICP. Thiopental should not be used in this case because it causes vasodilatation and myocardial depression and can further reduce the blood pressure. Succinylcholine, even though it can cause increased ICP, is not contraindicated in patients with head injury. Succinylcholine or rocuronium may be used in this patient. Lidocaine reduces ICP and should be given in patients with head injury. Atropine should be given in children undergoing RSI.

7. b   Succinylcholine may cause fasciculations, muscle pain, rhabdomyolysis, and myoglobinuria. This effect is most pronounced in muscular individuals. To prevent fasciculation, defasciculation is recommended. It can be accomplished by administering one tenth the paralyzing dose of a nondepolarizing muscle relaxant 1–3 minutes prior to succinylcholine administration. Defasciculation is not necessary in children less than 5 years old.

8. b   The condition described in this scenario is consistent with malignant hyperthermia. Malignant hyperthermia is a metabolic reaction reported with succinylcholine that is characterized by profoundly increased temperature. It may also be associated with disseminated intravascular coagulation, metabolic acidosis, and rhabdomyolysis. In addition to instituting aggressive cooling measures for malignant hyperthermia, dantrolene, 1 mg/kg, can be administered every 1–5 minutes until the symptoms are resolved.

9. c   RSI starts with preoxygenation with spontaneous inspiration or mask ventilating with 100% oxygen for 2–5 minutes to increase the oxygen reserve. Atropine should then be administered in all children during RSI to prevent bradycardia resulting from intubation. Atropine also reduces oral secretion. A good mask seal and ability to intubate the patient should be ascertained before proceeding to the next step. Sellick maneuver should then be performed to prevent passive gastric regurgitation and aspiration. This can be accomplished by applying the pressure on the cricoid ring sufficient to occlude the esophageal lumen without compressing the airway. This should be maintained until tracheal intubation is confirmed. BVM ventilation should be avoided during RSI to prevent regurgitation and aspiration. Should the patient require BVM ventilation, Sellick maneuver should be used during BVM ventilation. Next, a sedative and a paralytic agent can be administered in a rapid sequence. Some experts recommend giving sedatives before paralytics; others prefer the reverse. After the sedative and paralytic have taken full effect, intubation can then be accomplished.

CHAPTER 6

Prehospital Care

SUJIT SHARMA, M.D.

QUESTIONS

1. Regarding the provision of prehospital care to ill or injured patients, which of the following statements about "first responders" is true?

    a. They do not require any formal training
    b. They are trained to perform initial patient assessment
    c. They are not trained in basic life support (BLS)
    d. They generally do not provide patient transport
    e. They are trained to provide spinal immobilization

2. Which of the following statements regarding the role of basic life support/emergency medical technicians (EMTs) is true?

    a. They are not trained to assess severity of a patient's condition
    b. They may not apply antishock trousers (MAST)
    c. They are trained in recognition and treatment of cardiac arrhythmias
    d. They are trained in ventilatory assistance, including intubation
    e. They are trained to recognize altered mental status as well as shock

3. Which of the following statements is true with regard to the duty of a prehospital care provider to provide care to ill or injured patients in the field?

    a. Prehospital care providers are not legally responsible for their actions
    b. Prehospital care providers are required to provide care for patients even if they may be at risk for personal injury
    c. Children must be treated for any emergency condition, unless parents are refusing treatment
    d. Parents may not be asked to sign a form that would release the care provider from responsibility if they are refusing treatment
    e. Prehospital care providers are protected by Good Samaritan laws

4. Which of the following statements regarding documentation for prehospital care providers is true?

    a. These documents do not become part of the child's record
    b. They are not required to report suspected child abuse
    c. They are required to report illegal drug use
    d. These documents cannot be used as evidence
    e. These documents are not considered confidential

5. Which of the following statements is true with regard to the capabilities of advanced life support (ALS) providers?

    a. They are trained in the recognition of arrhythmias, but not in treatment
    b. They are not trained to perform chest decompression
    c. They are trained in peripheral vein cannulation, but not intraosseous placement
    d. They are trained in respiratory support, including endotracheal and nasotracheal intubation
    e. They are not trained to administer drugs for toxicological emergencies

ANSWERS

1. d   Although the term *first responder* can generically refer to any person who first arrives at the scene, a formal first responder course has been developed nationally to train individuals in basic life support (BLS). Training is also provided to clear an obstructed airway, control life-threatening hemorrhage, and perform emergent splinting of extremities. Spinal immobilization and patient assessment are beyond the capabilities of first responders. They are not trained to provide patient transport in ambulances, although this may vary in rural areas.

2. e   Basic life support providers, in most regions known as EMTs, are trained to provide all the services of a first responder as well as to evaluate the severity of a patient's condition, provide simple interventions (e.g., spinal immobilization and application of MAST), and transport patients. Beyond basic assessments taught in BLS, they are trained to recognize respiratory distress, altered mental status, and shock. Providing ventilatory assistance is within their capabilities; however, endotracheal intubation and the recognition/treatment of specific arrhythmias is not.

3. c   Prehospital care providers act in an official capacity and are paid for what they do, so they are legally responsible for their actions and are not protected by Good Samaritan laws. They are required to provide treatment for any child if an emergency exists. If the parents refuse treatment, they may be asked to sign a waiver of responsibility. If there is a risk of personal injury, a prehospital care provider is not required to provide care.

4. c   Detailed documentation is a very important part of providing prehospital care, because the information does become part of the child's record and can be used as evidence. The information is considered confidential. Prehospital care providers are also required to report any suspicion of child abuse, gunshot wounds, and illegal drug use.

5. d   ALS providers are capable of more advanced skills than EMTs. These skills include advanced diagnostic skills, recognition and treatment of arrhythmias, and the treatment of many other emergent medical conditions (e.g., toxicologic emergencies). Their capabilities in respiratory support include assisted ventilation, including both endotracheal and nasotracheal intubation, as well as chest decompression. Peripheral/central venous cannulation and intraosseous access are also part of their training.

CHAPTER 7

Transport

JEFFREY P. LOUIE, M.D.

QUESTIONS

1. The Federal Emergency Treatment and Active Labor Act (EMTALA) was written to provide guidelines and management of interfacility transportation of patients. Which statement best defines the purpose of the EMTALA?

   a. To ensure that the receiving hospital has helicopter services available 24 hours/day
   b. EMTALA states that transport teams consist of at least one physician
   c. It is the referring facility's responsibility to decide on the mode of transportation (ground or air)
   d. The referring facility may discuss with the patient the risk and benefits of transfer, which may include the financial ramifications
   e. The transport of an unstable patient is prohibited and the referring facility must stabilize the patient prior to transport

2. A 10-year-old boy is at a referring facility and is having an asthma exacerbation. The physician on duty wishes to transfer him to an appropriate hospital with a pediatric pulmonologist. The medical command physician suggests some medical management advice. Which statement is true regarding the process and management of that patient?

   a. The referring facility is legally mandated to carry out all of the receiving facility's management decisions prior to transportation
   b. Once the receiving facility has been contacted by the referring facility, it now assumes most of the medical-legal responsibility for the patient
   c. The referring hospital still carries some medical-legal responsibility even after the transport team has left that hospital
   d. Management of conflicts between the transport team and referring hospital should be resolved by the medical command physician
   e. Once the transport team arrives at the referring hospital, the decision to depart is determined by the referring facility

3. A 15-year-old is 3 hours away from the receiving hospital. The patient has a closed head injury and has been intubated. It is decided by the referring facility to transport this patient by helicopter. Which of the following statements is true regarding air transports?

   a. Helicopter transports usually fly more than 5000 feet above sea level
   b. There are no contraindications to air transports with the advent of pressurized helicopter cabins
   c. At lower altitudes, gas (air) expands, thus it is during landing that most complications occur
   d. Patients who are intubated because of underlying lung disease and hypoxia may become more hypoxic at high altitudes
   e. Intubated patients with cuffed tubes are not at risk for tracheal necrosis

4. A physician requests transfer of a patient in her ED. She has a new-onset diabetic in diabetic ketoacidosis (DKA) and feels that a pediatric endocrinologist should manage this patient. All of the following would be valid reasons to transfer this patient, EXCEPT:

   a. Need for advanced level of care
   b. A second opinion
   c. Frustrated parents
   d. Insurance issues
   e. The family has no insurance

5. The transport team is notified of an intubated asthmatic with a right chest tube in place at a referring facility. An issue arises as to whether to transfer this patient by ground ambulance or by helicopter. Which of the following concerns is most valid?

   a. The patient should be transported by ground, because flying in a helicopter will put the patient at risk for a pneumothorax

   b. The patient should be flown, because traffic will increase the ground transport time by 45 minutes

   c. The patient should be sent by ground, because a member of the transport team is prone to air sickness

   d. The patient should not be flown, because if the patient develops a pneumothorax, nothing can be done

   e. The patient should be ground transported, because the pneumothorax may expand at high altitude

ANSWERS

1. c   The referring physician decides the mode of transportation. EMTALA is a federal regulation written to provide guidelines for the referring and receiving hospitals. It states that the referring hospital must do everything possible to stabilize the patient's medical condition prior to transport. The referring hospital may not transfer a patient against his/her will unless the referring facility cannot provide the appropriate level of care, and must obtain consent to transfer from the patient or parents. In addition, it is the referring hospital's responsibility to inform the patient of the risk and benefits of a transfer. This discussion should not include the financial ramifications of the decision. The referring hospital is responsible for selecting an appropriate means of transport. The receiving hospital can accept a patient if it has the appropriate level of care. The ability of the patient to pay for medical care may not be considered by either the referring or receiving facility. EMTALA does not state that the receiving hospital should have helicopter services; however, tertiary hospitals normally have helicopter services available. EMTALA does not require that a physician be present on each transport team. Finally, it is the receiving facility's decision to accept or decline an unstable patient.

2. d   Any conflicts should be managed by the receiving hospital's medical command, who should then talk to the referring physician. In most cases, the level of medical and legal responsibility increases as the receiving facility becomes more involved with the patient, and any medical recommendations from the receiving hospital are considered advice that the referring facility will decide to implement. Once the transport team departs the referring hospital, however, the receiving facility now assumes all medical and legal responsibility. The decision to leave a referring facility is made by the transport team in conjunction with the medical command physician.

3. d   An increase in altitude will bring with it a decrease in ambient oxygen as well as a potential increase in the size of air spaces. Thus, patients who are hypoxic at sea level will become more hypoxic at higher altitudes, secondary to Dalton's law. Gas expands as the altitude increases (Boyle's law); thus, patients with a pneumothorax or a pneumocephalus are at increased risk for morbidity and mortality. Cuff tubes should be slightly deflated to prevent tracheal necrosis. Bladder Foley catheters must also be adjusted. Most helicopters do not have pressurized cabins, because they do not fly at more than 1000 feet above sea level. Other patients at risk for air transport complications are divers who have the "bends" or patients with bowel obstruction.

4. e   Patients are not to be transferred to another facility for financial reimbursement issues or as an attempt to avoid an initial assessment. Procedures for stabilization and interventions are outlined in COBRA and EMTALA regulations.

5. b Deciding whether or not to transport a patient by ground or air can be difficult. This patient is severely ill, and a rapid transport is necessary to facilitate tertiary care; thus, flying is the best option. Air transport by helicopter is low altitude transport and will not put a patient at risk for a pneumothorax, nor will it exacerbate it. If a patient does develop a pneumothorax, needle decompression can be done. A chest tube can be placed, although it may be physically difficult to perform, given the confined environment.

CHAPTER **8**

Myocardial Infarction

NEIL SCHAMBAN, M.D.

QUESTIONS

1. A 65-year-old man in the waiting room with his 5-year-old granddaughter tells the triage nurse he has chest pain. The triage nurse relays this information to you and asks you what you would like to do. Your management goals are to:

   a. Immediately administer nitroglycerin for pain control

   b. Stabilize the patient and establish cardiac versus noncardiac chest pain while arranging transport

   c. Administer ibuprofen for analgesia while the patient and his granddaughter wait in triage

   d. Arrange for immediate transport to an adult tertiary care facility

   e. Immediately administer PO aspirin (acetylsalicylic acid—ASA)

2. An 80-year-old man with diabetes collapses on the floor in the ED while watching the suture repair of his grandson's forehead. He is pale, diaphoretic, and mildly short of breath. He is given oxygen and feels slightly better. An ECG is obtained. Of the following findings, which are most consistent with a myocardial infarction (MI)?

   a. A 2-mm ST-segment elevation diffusely throughout the ECG

   b. Tall R waves in the anterior leads with concomitant deep S waves

   c. Deep S wave in I with an inverted T wave and Q wave in lead III

   d. A 3-mm ST elevation in leads V1–V3 with ST depression in AVL and I

   e. Sinus tachycardia with a left anterior hemiblock

3. You are called to a Code Blue in the parking lot of your ED. When you arrive, you find a 50-year-old obese male in supine position and having difficulty breathing. Which of the following symptoms are most consistent with cardiac chest pain?

   a. Shortness of breath with pain radiating in between the scapulae

   b. Right scapular pain with right upper quadrant pain

   c. Sharp, pleuritic midsternal chest pain associated with anxiety, tachypnea, and shortness of breath

   d. Left hand tingling, chest pressure, and left jaw pain associated with diaphoresis

   e. Sharp, reproducible left chest wall pain

4. A 50-year-old male complains of sudden onset of shortness of breath with exertion while walking up stairs. He experienced mild diaphoresis, but all of his symptoms are now resolved. He has not had chest pain. He smokes one pack per day and has a history of non–insulin-dependent diabetes mellitus. Which of the following would be an appropriate management plan?

   a. Reassure the patient that this is typical for an anxiety reaction and discharge home

   b. Give the patient 30 cc of Maalox with viscous lidocaine and suggest outpatient follow-up

   c. Perform initial stabilization, obtain an ECG, and arrange transport

   d. Administer IM ketorolac for suspected costochondritis and discharge home with close follow-up

   e. Administer 2.5 mg of nebulized albuterol for exacerbation of chronic obstructive pulmonary disease (COPD)

5. The same patient in the previous question now complains of substernal pain radiating to the neck and jaw. The ECG demonstrates three ST-segment elevations in V1–V3. Vital signs are HR 110, BP 160/90, and RR 30. Appropriate management steps would include:

    a. Give ASA, sublingual (SL) nitroglycerin, calcium channel blocker, and arrange for overnight observation

    b. Administer morphine sulfate and SL nitroglycerin until pain free. Give aspirin PO and arrange for outpatient stress testing the next day

    c. Administer aspirin PO. Place the patient on oxygen. Give morphine sulfate and SL nitroglycerin until pain free. Make immediate arrangements for thrombolysis

    d. Place patient on O_2, give an ACE inhibitor with calcium channel blocker. Administer IV nitroprusside and esmolol with arrangements for immediate intracoronary thrombolysis

    e. Administer morphine for pain. Follow up with primary care physician in 1–2 days

ANSWERS

1. b   Chest pain has many etiologies in the older adult patient. Myocardial ischemia is a diagnosis that must be considered in every case. The initial step is always stabilization (IV, oxygen, and monitor). The history and ECG should be obtained while the patient is being stabilized in order to differentiate between cardiac and noncardiac chest pain. Once cardiac chest pain is suspected, therapy can be initiated and transport arranged. Specific therapy should not be initiated prior to appropriate clinical suspicion and stabilization. Certain noncardiac conditions that present with chest pain can be worsened with therapy (e.g., aspirin and heparin) directed at myocardial ischemia, whereas basic therapies for myocardial ischemia are contraindicated in an acute aortic dissection secondary to the bleeding risk. Nitroglycerin is relatively contraindicated in a right ventricular MI secondary to volume-sensitive hypotension. Other common causes of chest pain include pneumonia, pulmonary embolus, and pneumothorax.

2. d   ECG is diagnostic only 40–65% of the time for acute MI in cases that present with chest pain. When ECG changes are present, the most specific indicator for acute MI is ST elevation in a specific arterial distribution with reciprocal ST depression. In this case, the pattern is most consistent with an acute anterior MI. Diffuse ST elevation is commonly seen with pericarditis and not with an MI. Tall R waves with deep S waves reflect hypertensive, not ischemic, changes. The pattern described in Answer "c" is the classic pattern for pulmonary embolus. Sinus tachycardia with a left anterior hemiblock can be a normal finding.

3. d   Classic cardiac chest pain typically is midsternal pressure with radiation to the left hand and jaw. Associated symptoms of diaphoresis and pallor are common. Shortness of breath and pain radiating to the scapula in Answer "a" are classic for an aortic dissection. Answer "c" reflects symptoms most consistent with a pulmonary embolus. Sharp, reproducible chest wall pain (Answer "e") is typical for costochondritis.

4. c   Beware of diabetics! Cardiac ischemia may present as shortness of breath with no other symptoms. The only appropriate management in this setting is hospital admission with presumed diagnosis of myocardial ischemia. Administration of beta agonists would be absolutely contraindicated.

5. c   The patient described is having an acute MI. Ultimately, the patient should receive intravenous thrombolytics or undergo cardiac catheterization ASAP. The mainstay of therapy until such arrangements are made includes IV, O_2, and monitoring. Nitroglycerin and morphine sulfate can be given for

pain control. ASA should always be given. (The only contraindication is severe anaphylaxis). Heparin and beta blockade should be considered as well. Calcium channel blockers and ACE (angiotensin-converting enzyme) inhibitors have no role in the acute MI, and may be dangerous. Intracoronary thrombolysis is no longer used. The currently accepted definitive measures include IV thrombolysis, cardiac catheterization with stent or balloon angioplasty, and surgical coronary bypass.

SECTION II **Signs and Symptoms**

CHAPTER 9

Abdominal Distension

BARBARA M. GARCIA PEÑA, M.D., M.P.H.

QUESTIONS

1. A 4-day-old infant develops abdominal distension. According to his parents, he is more sleepy and cranky than usual. He has not been vomiting. His stools are yellow and seedy. On exam, his vital signs are: T 37°C, HR 130, RR 24, BP 80/40. He has moderate abdominal distension. The most likely cause for the abdominal distension is:

   a. Intussusception
   b. Volvulus
   c. Constipation
   d. Sepsis
   e. Gastroenteritis

2. The mother of a 5-year-old boy complains that he has developed diffuse abdominal distension and vomiting. He has a past history of appendectomy 2 years ago. The most appropriate diagnostic study would be:

   a. Upper gastrointestinal (GI) series
   b. Barium enema examination
   c. Prone cross-table lateral radiograph
   d. Abdominal CT
   e. Abdominal ultrasound (U/S)

3. A 15-year-old girl with bulimia nervosa comes to the ED with increasing abdominal distension. On examination she is quiet, afebrile, and has tympanitic distension with absent bowel sounds. Her abdomen is nontender and there is no palpable mass. The most likely etiology for her abdominal distension is:

   a. Peritoneal irritation with pancreatic enzymes
   b. Bowel perforation
   c. Hypokalemia
   d. Sepsis
   e. Bowel obstruction

4. A 3-year-old African-American boy comes to the ED with massive abdominal distension. On examination, he is afebrile, tachycardic, tachypneic, and ill-appearing. He has a II/VI systolic murmur, heard best at the right upper sternal border. Abdominal examination shows a markedly distended abdomen with tenderness in the left upper quadrant. The spleen is palpable 4 cm below the left costal margin. The liver is of normal size. The best diagnostic test would be:

   a. Abdominal CT
   b. Abdominal U/S
   c. KUB (kidneys/ureter/bladder or abdominal plain film)
   d. Peripheral blood smear
   e. Hematocrit (hct)

5. A 5-year-old girl comes to the ED with gradual abdominal distension. She has not had fever or vomiting. She sometimes stools in her underwear and has irregular stooling patterns, but does have a bowel movement almost every day. On examination, she is afebrile with stable vital signs. Her abdomen is moderately distended, but soft. The most likely cause for the distension is:

   a. Bacterial overgrowth
   b. Cystic fibrosis
   c. Celiac disease
   d. Parasites
   e. Obstipation

6. A 4-month-old girl is brought to the ED with abdominal distension and increased irritability over the past week. She has had no fever, vomiting, or diarrhea. On examination, she is afebrile, with HR 170 and RR 70. Her examination is unremarkable except for a II/VI holosystolic murmur, heard at the left lower sternal border, and abdominal distension. Her liver is palpable 5 cm below the right costal margin. Which of the following diagnostic tests is most indicated at this time?

   a. Liver function tests (LFTs)
   b. CXR
   c. Urine amino acids
   d. Abdominal CT
   e. Abdominal U/S

7. A 2-day-old boy presents to the ED because his mother is concerned regarding his "big belly." He is otherwise well. On physical examination, he is afebrile with stable vital signs. His abdomen is markedly distended with a questionable palpable mass in the left upper quadrant. What is the most likely cause of the abdominal distension?

   a. Obstructive uropathy
   b. Neoplasm
   c. Constipation
   d. Bowel duplication
   e. Mesenteric cysts

8. A 16-year-old girl complains of gradually worsening abdominal distension. She is previously healthy, but has had irregular menstrual periods. Her last period was 2 months ago, which is not uncommon for her. She has had vomiting, but no diarrhea or fever. On examination, she is afebrile with stable vital signs. Her examination is otherwise unremarkable except for midline abdominal distension. Which is the most appropriate next step in diagnosis?

   a. KUB
   b. Pelvic U/S
   c. Pelvic CT
   d. LFTs
   e. Urine human chorionic gonadotropin (HCG)

9. A 15-year-old girl complains of abdominal distension. She has been healthy with regular menstrual periods in the past. She states that she has had severe, diffuse abdominal pain and vomiting, but no diarrhea or fever. On examination, she is afebrile with stable vital signs. Her examination is otherwise unremarkable except for abdominal distension and left lower quadrant abdominal tenderness. Her pregnancy test is negative. Which of the following is the most appropriate next step in diagnosis?

   a. Barium enema
   b. Pelvic U/S
   c. Pelvic CT
   d. Pelvic MRI
   e. LFTs

10. A 14-year-old girl complains of gradual abdominal distension over the past year. She is otherwise healthy, but has not started menstruating. She has no other symptoms. Physical examination reveals a young girl with stable vital signs and no fever. Her abdomen is mildly distended in the lower midline area. Before further examination or diagnostic evaluation, your leading diagnosis is:

   a. Pregnancy
   b. Ovarian cyst
   c. Hematocolpos
   d. Neoplasm
   e. Omental cyst

11. A 4-year-old boy is brought to the ED with respiratory distress and abdominal distension. On examination, he is afebrile with HR 100, RR 40, BP 90/60, and O_2 saturation 96% on room air. Lung examination shows decreased aeration at the bases. His abdomen is markedly distended and tympanitic. After assessing and stabilizing his airway, breathing, and circulation, which of the following should be done next?

   a. Paracentesis
   b. Emergent thoracotomy
   c. Emergent CT scan
   d. Turning the child to a lateral decubitus position
   e. Passage of a nasogastric or orogastric tube

ANSWERS

1. d   There are many causes of abdominal distension in childhood. In infancy, however, sepsis is the most common cause of painless abdominal distension, even in the absence of fever. Although intussusception and volvulus are relatively common in infants and must be carefully considered, the patient in this vignette appears relatively well, without vomiting and abdominal cramping, which are symptoms more characteristic of these causes. Constipation is unlikely, as the patient is having yellow, seedy stools characteristic of breast-fed infants. In addition, constipation rarely, if ever, occurs at age 4 days. Gastroenteritis usually does not cause abdominal distension in the neonate.

2. c The patient in this scenario has signs of mechanical obstruction. This may occur in children of all ages due to adhesions from previous abdominal surgery. The most appropriate study to evaluate for mechanical obstruction is the prone cross-table lateral radiograph of the abdomen. The lack of air in the rectum and sigmoid colon supports the diagnosis of mechanical obstruction.

3. c Abdominal distension without tenderness in an afebrile girl suggests an ileus due to poisoning (methyldopa), botulism, or an electrolyte disturbance (e.g., hypokalemia). The only abdominal finding is usually distension. Peritoneal irritation with bile, blood, or pancreatic enzymes would produce signs such as guarding and rebound. The presence of fever without peritoneal signs suggests systemic infection, anticholinergic poisoning, or intestinal inflammation. Aerophagia is unlikely, as the patient has not been screaming and has absent bowel sounds.

4. d In the toxic child, splenomegaly without hepatomegaly suggests sickle cell sequestration crises, malaria, or intraparenchymal bleeding with an intact capsule. Because there is no history of trauma, fever, or travel to a foreign country, the latter two are unlikely and U/S, CT, or KUB would be unhelpful. A low hct would only suggest anemia without a specific cause. Hence, the diagnostic study of choice would be a peripheral blood smear to evaluate for sickling.

5. e Obstipation is a very common cause for abdominal distension. For this diagnosis, there is usually a history of irregular stooling, chronic constipation, or encopresis. The underlying cause for the obstipation may be a pathologic process such as Hirschsprung's disease or hypothyroidism, or it may reflect a severe functional disturbance. Stools that are diarrheal, bulky, or foul-smelling suggest malabsorption due to bacterial overgrowth, cystic fibrosis, parasites, or celiac disease.

6. b The infant in this vignette is showing signs of congestive heart failure (CHF), most likely due to a VSD (ventricular septal defect). The presence of a murmur and her enlarged liver leads one to the diagnosis. LFTs, abdominal U/S, and CT would be unhelpful, as the underlying diagnosis lies in the cardiac examination. Urine amino acids are not indicated because a metabolic disorder is unlikely.

7. a The most common cause of abdominal distension in the newborn period is obstructive uropathy. The other choices are seen much less frequently as causes of abdominal distension in infancy.

8. e The most likely cause of the midline abdominal distension in this girl is pregnancy, until proven otherwise. Before any radiographic imaging is performed, the patient's pregnancy status should be determined. LFTs would also be unhelpful, as she is nontender in the right upper quadrant, without evidence of liver dysfunction.

9. b The young lady has a torsed ovarian cyst. Ovarian, as well as mesenteric, omental, or peritoneal cysts generally present with a subacute history of abdominal distension. The exception to this is a large torsed ovarian cyst that usually produces marked abdominal pain and vomiting. Abdominal U/S identifies intraabdominal cysts readily, and this would be the diagnostic study of choice in this scenario. An MRI or CT might not identify the torsed cyst. Barium enema is not indicated in this patient. LFTs and urinalysis would be unhelpful and the patient does not show signs of liver pathology or urinary tract infection/pyelonephritis.

10. c A 14-year-old female who has not started menstruating has primary amenorrhea. This, in combination with a midline slow-growing pelvic mass, leads one to the diagnosis of hematometrocolpos, which can be made with pelvic examination. She does not have pain, so an ovarian cyst or omental cyst is unlikely. A neoplasm is also unlikely in the absence of other symptoms. In addition, pregnancy is unlikely with a 1-year history of gradual distension.

11. e Abdominal distension may cause a marked decrease in diaphragmatic excursion. The first step in management of all children with abdominal distension is the assessment and stabilization of the child's respiratory status. Passage of a nasogastric or orogastric tube oftentimes results in a marked improvement in the child's overall respiratory status. Endotracheal intubation is not presently indicated, as the patient is maintaining his own airway and breathing spontaneously with good oxygenation saturation. Paracentesis would not be indicated, as the distension may be caused by ileus or aerophagia. A CT scan would not be helpful in alleviating the child's respiratory distress.

CHAPTER **10**

Apnea

JILL C. POSNER, M.D.

QUESTIONS

1. A 5-week-old male infant is brought to the ED 24 hours after a single brief, 15-second episode of eyes rolling back into his head and extremity limpness that resolved spontaneously with mild stimulation. The patient had eaten 3 hours prior to the event. He presents at the urging of the primary care provider who evaluated him earlier today. If the infant had experienced an acute life-threatening event (ALTE), which of the following statements are true?

   a. He is likely to have an identifiable etiology
   b. He has an increased risk of developing sudden infant death syndrome (SIDS)
   c. He should be started empirically on antireflux measures
   d. He must have demonstrated cyanosis, by definition
   e. He will most likely have an unremarkable physical examination and normal lab findings

2. The parents of a 2-month-old full-term girl report that during sleep, the infant "stopped breathing, turned blue, and was unresponsive," despite 15–20 seconds of vigorous stimulation. She has had no fevers and has otherwise been feeding well. Physical examination in the ED shows: T 37.4°C, HR 140, RR 36, BP 90/45. She is alert, vigorous, and there are no abnormal findings. The management is to:

   a. Provide reassurance and discharge the infant
   b. Prescribe a home cardiorespiratory monitor and discharge the patient
   c. Admit the infant to the hospital
   d. Obtain a full complement of blood, cerebrospinal fluid (CSF), and radiographic studies
   e. Obtain an emergent head CT scan

3. A 15-month-old boy is brought to the ED after having an episode in which he became apneic, cyanotic, and had some shaking of the extremities. The mother had just denied the child a cookie before dinner when the event occurred. In the ED, his physical examination is normal. The most likely diagnosis is:

   a. Seizure disorder
   b. Breath-holding spell
   c. Toxic ingestion
   d. ALTE
   e. Gastroesophageal reflux

4. A 6-month-old full-term girl is brought to the ED after she "stopped breathing." Further history reveals that during feeding she began to cough, arch her back, and turn red. She has otherwise been healthy. Vital signs show: T 37.8°C, HR 120, RR 28, and BP 94/48. The physical examination is normal. The management is:

   a. Admit the patient for a pneumogram
   b. Obtain an ABG
   c. Perform a full evaluation for sepsis
   d. Reassure the parents and discharge the patient
   e. Obtain a barium swallow

5. A 3-month-old former 28-week premature infant is brought to the ED with a 2-day history of tachypnea and poor feeding. The mother reports that the infant had briefly "stopped breathing" on two occasions during that day. In the ED, physical examination reveals T 38.8°C, HR 176, RR 60, and BP 88/44, with an O_2 saturation of 92% on room air. The infant has several witnessed, brief episodes of apnea without cyanosis. The fontanel is sunken, mucous membranes are dry, and his capillary refill time is 3 seconds. His cardiac rhythm is tachycardic with no murmur auscultated. There are suprasternal and subcostal retractions with rhonchi and wheezes heard in all lung fields. There is no hepatosplenomegaly. The most likely diagnosis is:

a. Congenital heart disease
b. Supraventricular tachycardia
c. *Streptococcus pneumoniae* meningitis
d. Respiratory syncytial virus (RSV) bronchiolitis
e. Gastroesophageal reflux

ANSWERS

1. e   An ALTE is defined as severe apnea associated with a change in color, muscle tone, or mental status. A history of perioral or facial cyanosis certainly heightens the degree of concern that a significant event occurred; however, the absence of cyanosis or the presence of facial "redness" should not provide reassurance. Even though the differential diagnosis for an infant who has an ALTE is extensive, no cause is identified in about half of patients. There has been no clear relationship established between "idiopathic ALTE" and SIDS. Many infants will be brought to the ED with a history concerning for a significant event yet have a normal physical examination. These cases can be particularly challenging for the ED physician. Laboratory and other diagnostic tests should be obtained as clinically indicated. In most cases, it is prudent to admit the patient to the hospital for further diagnostic evaluation and observation. Infants at greatest risk are predominantly those under the age of 4 months.

2. c   The role of the ED physician in caring for these types of infants is to identify any persistent life-threatening problems, to assess the severity of the event, and to determine the need for further diagnostic evaluation. It is not uncommon for the infant to appear completely normal upon arrival to the ED following a significant event as described by the caretaker. A careful history and physical examination are of paramount importance and will provide the majority of the information that is sought by the ED physician. If historical information suggests that a significant apneic event has occurred, the infant may be at risk for recurrence. A normal physical exam does not provide assurance that the event will not recur. Although a more aggressive search for an underlying cause may be necessary, the use of laboratory and radiographic studies should be selective and guided by the clinical scenario. Hospital admission should be arranged for observation and further diagnostic evaluation. The decision to prescribe a home cardiorespiratory monitor should not be made in the ED.

3. b   Breath-holding spells (or attacks) are common in young children and can be a source of great anxiety to parents. Both forms, pallid and cyanotic, are manifest by a short period of apnea. The key to making the diagnosis is in obtaining the history of a precipitating factor. The child with cyanotic spells usually begins crying when angered or frustrated, holds his breath until he becomes cyanotic, and then loses consciousness. The spell can often mimic seizures with opisthotonic posturing and brief extremity shaking. Pallid spells are usually precipitated by a sudden pain or fright; the child cries one or two gasps, then falls limp without significant cyanosis. The prognosis for children with breath-holding spells is excellent and there is no increased incidence of epilepsy. Reassurance is the treatment and most children cease to have attacks by school age.

4. d   Choking episodes are common among infants and can be a frightening experience for a parent. The key to making the diagnosis lies in the history. A minute-by-minute recount of the event with open-ended questions such as "and then what happened" will help gather the history without making suggestions. Laboratory and other studies should be obtained only when clinically indicated. An arterial blood gas (ABG) should not be used as a screening test for a serious event. Parental reassurance and counseling will be sufficient in most cases of infant choking episodes. Parents should be given specific instructions regarding indications for returning to the ED and for primary care provider follow-up.

5. d   The differential diagnosis for apnea in an infant is broad. It includes serious systemic diseases such as sepsis, seizures, and cardiogenic shock, as well as less acute but equally serious diagnoses such as gastroesophageal reflux or idiopathic apnea. It is clear that the patient in the scenario has an ongoing life-threatening cause for his apnea and warrants immediate intervention and diagnostic evaluation. Although all of the answers provided are etiologies of apnea, this patient seems to be in extremis due to an infectious process. The fever, hypoxemia, work of breathing, and wheezes are suggestive of bronchiolitis. Respiratory syncytial virus (RSV) may cause apnea in premature infants or those who have preexisting lung disease or congenital heart disease. In addition, it has been postulated that RSV may have a central respiratory inhibitory effect causing apnea in some young-term infants. Meningitis remains on the differential diagnosis; however, patients with meningitis and an open fontanel usually demonstrate at least some degree of fullness. Given this patient's degree of extremis, many would advocate that a lumbar puncture be performed to eliminate meningitis as an etiology, even though the possibility of meningitis is small in a patient with an oxygen saturation of 92%. Congenital heart disease would be more likely to present with a cardiac murmur and hepatomegaly in addition to the respiratory findings in this patient. Similarly, most infants with supraventricular tachycardia will have a heart rate of at least 200–220 bpm. Gastroesophageal reflux is unlikely given the description of the clinical scenario.

CHAPTER 11

Ataxia

JOYCE SOPRANO, M.D.

QUESTIONS

1. A 2-year-old girl is brought to the ED with a 1-day history of stumbling while walking. Her parents report that she awoke that morning with mild unsteadiness that worsened throughout the day such that she is now refusing to walk. Other than chickenpox (varicella) 3 weeks ago, she has been well until today. On physical examination, she is afebrile and well appearing. She has mild head titubation and an ataxic gait. The strength in her lower extremities is normal. The most likely additional finding is:

   a. A large mass in the posterior fossa on head CT scan
   b. An elevated blood ethanol level
   c. Acute otitis media
   d. Mild elevations of CSF lymphocytes and protein
   e. Absent ankle reflexes

2. A 7-year-old boy is brought to the ED for evaluation of intermittent stumbling. His parents report that several times in the past 3 months he has had episodes of unsteady gait that last 5–10 minutes, followed by a severe posterior headache. He has had vomiting associated with some of the episodes. The episodes seem to be increasing in frequency and severity. He has otherwise been developing normally. His physical examination is unremarkable. The most appropriate next step is:

   a. Discharge on ibuprofen
   b. Obtain a head CT scan
   c. Perform a lumbar puncture (LP)
   d. Obtain an EEG
   e. Send a serum copper level

3. A 3-year-old boy is brought to the ED with a 2-day history of fever to 40°C. His parents noticed that he had developed an unsteady gait over the past day, and seemed to be increasingly lethargic over the past few hours. On physical examination, he is arousable to painful stimuli only and his vital signs are HR 60, systolic BP 140, and T 40°C. After obtaining IV access, the most appropriate next step is:

   a. Push ceftriaxone
   b. Administer IV phenytoin
   c. Give NS 20 ml/kg IV bolus
   d. Obtain an emergent head CT scan
   e. Perform a lumbar puncture

4. A 15-year-old previously healthy female patient is brought to the ED by ambulance from her school, where she was found stumbling in the hallways. On physical examination, she is sleepy but arousable, her vital signs are normal, and she has an ataxic gait. She is unable to recall events prior to her arrival in the ED. Which of the following is the most important next step in the management of this patient?

   a. Psychiatric consultation
   b. LP
   c. Head CT scan
   d. EEG
   e. Serum ethanol level

ANSWERS

1. d   This clinical scenario is most consistent with acute cerebellar ataxia, or postinfectious cerebellitis, which commonly follows 2–3 weeks after primary varicella infection. The CSF in this disorder generally shows mild elevations in lymphocytes and protein. Patients with posterior fossa tumors would be expected to have other signs of increased ICP on physical exam. Ethanol intoxication would be expected to cause sedation as well as ataxia. Although otitis media could cause slight unsteadiness, labyrinthitis with this degree of ataxia is unusual in young children. Guillain–Barré syndrome severe enough to cause ataxia and areflexia would be unlikely with normal strength in the legs.

2. b   This clinical scenario could be consistent with many of the causes of intermittent ataxia, including migraine and epilepsy, or with causes of progressive chronic ataxia, including posterior fossa tumors, metabolic disorders, and degenerative disorders of the cerebellum. The initial step in the work-up should be to obtain a head CT scan to evaluate for structural abnormalities. The other tests would then be performed if the CT scan were normal. Although this patient may be suffering from migraine headaches, other, more serious conditions should be excluded first.

3. a   This patient has signs of increased ICP, including bradycardia, hypertension, and obtundation. The high fever makes infections etiologies such as meningitis or encephalitis likely. These would be diagnosed by lumbar puncture; however, because there are signs of raised ICP, LP should be avoided until results of a head CT scan have been obtained. Prior to obtaining the CT scan, blood cultures should be obtained and broad-spectrum IV antibiotics should be given to begin presumptive treatment of meningitis. Intravenous fluid boluses should be avoided in cases of elevated ICP. The presence or absence of papilledema would not change the initial management in this scenario.

4. c   The most common causes of acute ataxia in an adolescent include traumatic intracranial injury or concussion, intracranial hemorrhage, central nervous system infection, drug intoxication, and conversion reaction. The most critical diagnoses to exclude are traumatic injury and hemorrhage; thus, an emergent head CT scan should be obtained immediately. If the CT scan is normal, blood and urine should then be obtained for toxic screens. The absence of fever makes infectious etiologies unlikely; thus, LP is not necessary in the initial management. Epilepsy is an unlikely cause of acute ataxia; thus, EEG should not be obtained emergently. Psychiatric consultation to evaluate for possible conversion reaction should be obtained if the remainder of the evaluation is normal.

CHAPTER 12

Breast Lesions

MARK WALTZMAN, M.D.

QUESTIONS

1. A 1-week-old boy is brought to the ED because the parents are concerned about enlargement and redness of the right perinipple area. He is afebrile, with a physical examination significant for an erythematous, tender, swollen right breast without nipple discharge. Appropriate management includes:

   a. Warm compress and outpatient follow-up
   b. Warm compress, oral antibiotics, and outpatient follow-up
   c. Complete sepsis evaluation and admission for IV antibiotics
   d. Complete sepsis evaluation, drainage of the site, and admission for IV antibiotics
   e. Aspiration of the site and oral antibiotics

2. A 17-year-old obese girl with asthma comes to the ED for complaints of warmth, tenderness, and dimpling of the skin in the periphery of the left breast. Therapy should include:

   a. 1% hydrocortisone cream
   b. Talcum powder to the area
   c. Amoxicillin orally
   d. Dicloxacillin orally
   e. Incision and drainage of the area

3. A 19-year-old female patient comes to the ED with a complaint of a painful mass in the upper outer quadrant of the breast. Her menstrual period is due. Exam reveals a nodular lesion in the upper outer quadrant of the breast as well as a greenish-brown discharge from the nipple. Treatment should include:

   a. Ibuprofen
   b. Oral contraceptive pills
   c. Mammography
   d. Oral antibiotics
   e. Warm compresses

4. An 18-year-old female patient comes to the ED with pain, warmth, and erythema around the right nipple. She is postpartum 3 weeks and has been breast feeding. Physical exam reveals a fluctuant area around the right nipple. Treatment should include all of the following EXCEPT:

   a. Discontinuation of all breast feeding
   b. Discontinuation of breast feeding from the affected breast only
   c. Oral antibiotics
   d. Warm compresses
   e. Incision and drainage

ANSWERS

1. **c**   Infection of the breast may take the form of cellulitis (mastitis) or an abscess. There is a bimodal age occurrence: neonates and again in postpubertal females. Neonatal breast infection is most often seen in the first few weeks of life when the breast bud is enlarged due to maternal estrogen stimulation. *Staphylococcus aureus* is the most common organism, but *E. coli* has also been found. Neonatal mastitis generally mandates a complete sepsis evaluation and IV antibiotics for at least 48 hours due to the likelihood of bacteremia in this age group.

2. **d**   Mastitis in postpubertal female patients is often seen in women who are overweight, have large breasts, or have conditions such as diabetes, rheumatoid arthritis, history of steroid treatment, granulomatous disease, or who have had local trauma. Local signs and symptoms include warmth, pain, tenderness, erythema, dimpling of the skin, and purulent nipple discharge. Fever may or may not be present. The organism most often isolated is *S. aureus.* Enterococci, anaerobic streptococci, and *Bacteroides* species occur less commonly. Treatment should be initiated with antistaphylococcal drugs such as cephalexin or dicloxacillin. Patients should be instructed to keep the area as clean and dry possible, wear a clean cotton bra to avoid excessive sweating, and avoid skin creams or talcum powders. They should be re-evaluated in 24–48 hours to assure that the infection is clearing. Incision and drainage are only occasionally necessary.

3. **a**   Fibrocystic disease is generally seen in women in their teens and twenties. It usually causes cyclically painful masses that are sometimes bilateral and are frequently most prominent in the upper outer quadrant of the breast. The masses often change in size or degree of nodularity during the course of the menstrual cycle, with the worst degree of pain premenstrual. Nipple discharge may be present and is nonbloody, green, or brown. These lesions are not considered to be premalignant. There is no specific treatment, but avoidance of caffeine and treatment with nonsteroidal anti-inflammatory drugs (NSAIDs) have been recommended for symptomatic relief.

4. **a**   Mastitis that occurs within several days of delivery is likely to be due to *S. aureus,* which may be transmitted from infant to infant and then to the nursing mother through cracked skin in the nipple. Therapy consists of warm compresses, continued breastfeeding, and antistaphylococcal antibiotics. Mastitis that occurs 2 or more weeks following delivery is either the result of poor hygiene or inadequate emptying of the breast with subsequent mild stasis, engorgement, and colonization of bacteria within the milk. If an abscess develops it usually requires both antibiotics and drainage, often by aspiration, for cure. Breastfeeding can proceed in the opposite breast, but not from the breast with an abscess due to the risk of the neonate acquiring infection.

CHAPTER **13**

Coma and Altered Level of Consciousness

JOYCE SOPRANO, M.D.

QUESTIONS

1. A 3-year-old boy is brought to the ED by ambulance. His parents report that several hours previously he had tripped while walking up cement stairs and struck the left side of his head on the ground. He had no loss of consciousness (LOC), but later began getting sleepy, vomited several times, and seemed unsteady when he walked. On physical examination, he opens his eyes and withdraws his extremities only to painful stimuli. He moans but does not say words. His Glasgow Coma Scale (GCS) score is:

   a. 5
   b. 6
   c. 7
   d. 8
   e. 9

2. Shortly after the initial evaluation of this patient, you are unable to obtain any response to painful stimuli. He has vital signs of HR 60, RR 14 and irregular, and BP 140/90. His left pupil is 6 mm and poorly responsive to light, and the right pupil is 3 mm and responsive. He has extensor posturing of the arms and legs. The most appropriate initial management is:

   a. Obtain an emergent head CT scan
   b. Give IV fosphenytoin
   c. Perform rapid-sequence intubation
   d. Obtain a neurosurgical consultation
   e. Give IV hydralazine

3. A 7-year-old girl with a history of congenital hydrocephalus and a ventriculoperitoneal shunt is brought to the ED for unresponsiveness. Her mother reports that the patient had been sick with a fever and vomiting for several days, then was found poorly responsive in bed that morning. She has a seizure disorder for which she takes phenytoin and valproic acid. On physical examination, her vital signs are: T 38.3°C, HR 110, BP 90/65, and RR 20. She is arousable to painful stimuli. Her pupils are 4 mm and reactive, she has increased tone and reflexes throughout, and has coarse breath sounds. The first step in management should be:

   a. Give IV fosphenytoin
   b. Obtain a head CT scan
   c. Obtain CSF sample from the shunt reservoir
   d. Obtain a CXR
   e. Obtain an EEG

4. A 4-year-old boy is brought to the ED for lethargy. He has had a fever for 24 hours, with increasing lethargy and onset of vomiting in the past several hours. Other than a history of chronic otitis media he has been healthy. While in triage he has a focal seizure of the right arm and leg that lasts 1–2 minutes. On physical examination, he is obtunded with a T of 39.4°C, HR 120, RR 30, and BP 97/63. His eyes are deviated to the left side and his pupils are equal and sluggishly reactive. He has increased tone and reflexes on the right arm and leg. After obtaining IV access and administering anticonvulsant medications, the most appropriate next step is:

   a. Perform a lumbar puncture
   b. Administer IV ceftriaxone and acyclovir
   c. Obtain a head CT scan
   d. Obtain an EEG
   e. Administer NS 20 ml/kg IV bolus

5. A 2-year-old near-drowning victim is brought to the ED by ambulance. She was found pulseless and apneic by ambulance personnel 3–4 minutes after being removed from a swimming pool by her parents. She was intubated and CPR was performed until a spontaneous pulse was obtained. In the ED, she has T 32°C and a GCS of 3. The most likely additional finding is:

a. Pinpoint unreactive pupils
b. Roving conjugate eye movements
c. Blinking with corneal touch
d. Nystagmus with the oculovestibular response
e. Absent oculocephalic reflexes

6. A 17-year-old male is found poorly responsive outside a nightclub. On arrival to the ED, he is afebrile with HR 80, RR 12, and BP 120/80. He responds to painful stimuli. His pupils are 2 mm and reactive. Which of the following is appropriate in the initial management of this patient?

a. Administer IV naloxone
b. Administer IV flumazenil
c. Administer PO ipecac
d. Perform gastric lavage via a nasogastric tube
e. Obtain an ECG

ANSWERS

1. d   This head injury patient has a Glasgow Coma Scale of 8: 2 points for opening his eyes to painful stimuli, 2 points for nonspecific verbal output, and 4 points for withdrawing his extremities to painful stimuli.

2. c   This patient has vital signs and a neurologic exam that are consistent with increased intracranial pressure (ICP) and probable herniation. The initial steps in management should be to secure the airway and assist breathing. Rapid-sequence intubation with medications to prevent rises in ICP is indicated. Emergent head CT scan and neurosurgical consultation should then be obtained. Antihypertensives are contraindicated in patients with increased ICP, because the elevated blood pressure may be a physiological response to maintain cerebral perfusion pressure.

3. b   This patient has several possible reasons for having altered level of consciousness, including ventriculoperitoneal (VP) shunt malfunction, seizure with a postictal period, supratherapeutic anticonvulsant levels, and CNS infection. The most critical problem to exclude in this clinical scenario is a VP shunt malfunction with hydrocephalus and raised ICP. Head CT scan should therefore be obtained first. If head CT scan does not indicate a malfunction of the VP shunt, CSF should be obtained to exclude a CNS or shunt infection. Anticonvulsant levels and a CXR should be obtained at that point as well. Emergent EEG is not necessary in this patient with a known seizure disorder.

4. b   This patient most likely has a CNS infection as the cause of his fever, seizure, and altered level of consciousness. Etiologies include meningitis, encephalitis, and brain abscess. The focal seizure and neurologic deficits suggest the possibility of a focal process (e.g., an abscess or herpes encephalitis). His altered level of consciousness may be due to increased ICP; thus, a head CT scan should be obtained prior to lumbar puncture. Intravenous antibiotics and acyclovir should be administered empirically prior to the head CT scan. Until increased ICP is excluded, IV boluses should be avoided as long as the patient is not hypotensive. Although EEG may be helpful later, it is not indicated in the initial management of this patient.

5. e   This patient is most likely comatose due to a severe anoxic brain injury. This usually causes loss of brainstem reflexes, including the oculocephalic reflex. Conjugate eye movements are usually absent. Corneal reflexes are absent; thus, there would be no blinking with corneal touch. You would expect loss of nystagmus with the oculovestibular reflex. Pupils are usually enlarged and unreactive after massive CNS injury.

6. a   In a comatose patient in whom you suspect a toxic ingestion, naloxone may be given empirically. Flumazenil is indicated only in pure benzodiazepine ingestion in a patient who has no history of seizures; it is contraindicated in a unknown ingestion. In order to prevent aspiration of stomach contents, ipecac should never be given to a patient with depressed consciousness, and gastric lavage should be performed only after the airway is secured with an endotracheal tube. ECG may be obtained after the initial attempts to secure the airway and reverse the cause of the altered level of consciousness.

CHAPTER **14**

Constipation

VINCENT J. WANG, M.D.

QUESTIONS

1. A 6-month-old boy is brought to the ED because of infrequent stools. The mother says that he has always had infrequent stools, stooling once per week. He has also been a slow feeder. On physical examination, his vital signs are: T 35.9°C, HR 60, RR 20, and BP 90/60. He is awake and looking around. His chest is clear, no murmurs are auscultated, and his abdomen is soft and nondistended. You do not palpate any masses. His rectal vault contains soft stool. He appears to be hypotonic throughout his body without any fasciculations. The most helpful diagnostic test is:

   a. Rectal biopsy
   b. Serum T_4/TSH (thyroid-stimulating hormone)
   c. Electrocardiogram
   d. Abdominal CT scan
   e. Electromyography

2. An 8-year-old boy is brought to the ED because of abdominal pain. He has had intermittent abdominal pain for the past several months. He has not had fever or vomiting, but he does complain of occasional nausea. He says that he has had normal bowel movements. On physical examination, he is well appearing, in NAD (no acute distress). He is obese, and his abdomen is nontender. His rectal examination reveals hard stool in the vault. Treatment for the likely cause of his symptoms might include any of the following, EXCEPT:

   a. Digital disimpaction
   b. Phosphate enemas
   c. Increasing fluid intake
   d. Tap water enemas
   e. Dietary changes

3. A 10-month-old girl is brought to the ED for constipation. She was diagnosed with constipation several months ago and has required frequent glycerin suppositories. She has not had fever and has always fed poorly. On physical examination, she is awake and alert, and appears small for age. Her abdomen is slightly distended and you palpate a mass in the left lower quadrant. Her rectal examination reveals no stool in the ampulla. Definitive diagnostic testing includes:

   a. Rectal biopsy
   b. Abdominal CT scan
   c. Electromyography
   d. Serum ferritin level
   e. Serum calcium level

4. A 3-year-old boy is brought to the ED for constipation. He has had no stools for the past 5 days. He has had cough and rhinorrhea for the past week and has been taking albuterol syrup for his symptoms. His vital signs are: T 38°C, HR 110, RR 24, and BP 100/60. On physical examination, he is alert, in NAD. His mucous membranes are moist. His chest is clear and his abdomen is soft and nontender. His rectal examination reveals no stool in the vault. Treatment includes:

   a. IV hydration
   b. Discontinuation of albuterol
   c. Fleet's enema
   d. Dietary changes
   e. No treatment is necessary

5. A 6-year-old girl is brought to the ED for constipation. The mother reports that she normally passes stool once per day, but for the past week has done it only once. She has no other symptoms, but the last time she had a bowel movement she appeared to be in pain, and the mother noticed streaks of blood in the stool. What physical examination finding are you likely to find in this patient?

   a. Increased rectal tone
   b. Ptosis
   c. Anal fissure
   d. Bradycardia
   e. Low weight for age

6. A 4-month-old boy is brought to the ED because of constipation. He has had less frequent stooling over the past week. He has not had fever or other symptoms. His review of systems reveals that he is an otherwise well child, but because of his parents' "naturalism beliefs," he has not received any immunizations, and eats only naturally sweetened foods. The parents do not have any medical problems. On physical examination, his vital signs are: T 37°C, HR 120, RR 24, and BP 85/50. He looks around and appears to be alert and awake, but he has generalized weakness and hypotonia. His respirations are shallow. On circumspection, his parents report that he has always been weak, but has appeared alert and attentive. Which of the following questions in your history is likely to be positive?

   a. Has he been fed unpasteurized honey?
   b. Did he have decreased fetal movements?
   c. Does he seem to become more tired with activity?
   d. Does he sweat while feeding?
   e. Did he pass normal stools after birth?

7. A 14-year-old girl is brought to the ED because of constipation and abdominal distension. She has had increasing difficulty passing stool, and feels like she is straining when she does. She denies sexual activity and says that she has not had her menstrual period yet. She has not had fevers or weight loss. On physical examination, she is alert but uncomfortable appearing. Her abdomen is slightly distended and you palpate a midline, lower abdominal mass. You note a dark red sac protruding from within the vaginal orifice. There is no discharge. Treatment includes:

   a. Midline incision of the sac
   b. Application of estrogen cream
   c. Hysterectomy
   d. Laser fulguration
   e. Prenatal counseling

ANSWERS

1. b Hypothyroidism is a systemic cause of constipation that should not be overlooked. A rectal biopsy would be warranted if the Hirschsprung's disease were suspected, but this would be unlikely given the other systemic signs and symptoms. Complete heart block could be the cause of the bradycardia; however, this too is unlikely given the systemic signs. An abdominal CT scan to evaluate abdominal masses is unlikely to be helpful given this presentation. A neuromuscular disease, such as Werdnig-Hoffmann disease or botulism, is unlikely to be the case given the constellation of symptoms and the lack of fasciculations; therefore, electromyography is not indicated.

2. d Functional constipation is the most common cause of chronic constipation. Even though he reports having normal bowel movements, the practitioner should investigate the frequency and consistency of his stools. Given that this is a chronic problem, "normal" for him may be infrequent, hard stools. Each of the answer choices is appropriate therapy, except for choice D. Tap water enemas are potentially hazardous.

3. a Hirschsprung's disease is a cause of chronic constipation that is often diagnosed as a neonate, but is most frequently diagnosed later in the first year of life. Associated symptoms for late diagnoses are as described in the vignette. There may also be a history of increasing difficulty passing stools. A barium enema may demonstrate an abrupt change in the bowel size between the aganglionic and ganglionic segments. Manometric studies are also helpful, but the definitive test is a rectal biopsy that demon-

strates aganglionic cells. Abdominal CT scan would be warranted to evaluate a pelvic mass. Electromyography would be indicated for neuromuscular disease. Iron can cause constipation, but it would be unlikely in this scenario, and a serum ferritin level would be unlikely to be elevated. Hyperparathyroidism may cause constipation, but is also unlikely in this scenario.

4. e   Viral illnesses are the most common cause of acute constipation. This type of illness will frequently cause a nonspecific ileus and a decrease in stool frequency. Even though dehydration is a common cause of constipation (lack of PO intake), this patient does not have signs and symptoms of dehydration. The use of albuterol is not associated with constipation. The absence of stool in the vault and the acuity of the symptoms would suggest that this is not chronic constipation.

5. c   Rectal pain from an anal fissure may cause constipation because of painful voiding. The associated findings of pain while voiding and blood-streaked stools support this diagnosis. Increased rectal tone would not be likely in any patient with constipation. Ptosis may accompany neuromuscular causes of constipation. Bradycardia may be associated with hypothyroidism. Patients with chronic causes of constipation may have poor weight gain. The latter three causes are unlikely, given her presentation.

6. b   Werdnig-Hoffman disease (spinal muscular atrophy Type 1) is a disorder of the motor cells of the cranial nerve nuclei and the anterior horn cells. This is the most severe form of spinal muscular atrophy. Patients will typically present early in life, often with reports of decreased fetal movements during the last trimester. Hypotonia and weakness are long-standing and generalized. Even though botulism may manifest with weakness, symptoms are typically acute with a progressive descending paralysis. Tiredness with activity would be characteristic with myasthenia gravis (MG); however, neonatal MG is unlikely given that the mother does not have MG, and he is unlikely to have other forms of MG. Sweating with feeds would suggest cardiorespiratory disease, and abnormal stooling after birth would suggest Hirschsprung's disease, but these would be unlikely given the other signs and symptoms.

7. a   Hydrometrocolpos results from the collection of fluid and menstrual flow behind an imperforate hymen. Patients may present in childhood, or after they have begun menses. The accumulation of fluid can result in a lower abdominal mass that may obstruct bowel and bladder voiding. Application of estrogen cream is the appropriate treatment for a urethral prolapse, but this usually occurs in a younger child, with a prolapsed mass from the urethra, rather than the vaginal orifice. A hysterectomy might be indicated for a uterine mass, such as a tumor, but this would be a last option treatment. In addition, even though a uterine tumor is a possible diagnosis, this would be much less likely than hydrometrocolpos. Laser fulguration would be indicated for perianal warts, and is not indicated here. Pregnancy should be considered in the differential diagnosis, but the vaginal examination argues against this.

Ddx: Constipation
- Hypothyroidism
- Functional
- Acute Viral illness
- Hirschsprung's
- SMA, I (W-H)
- Mech. Obstx
- Botulism ——> Acute, progressive, descending paralysis
- Dehydration
- Anal fissures
- Diet Δ

CHAPTER **15**

Cough

BEMA K. BONSU, MBChB, M.D.

QUESTIONS

1. A 37-day-old infant is brought to the ED for a persistent cough for 5 days. He was born by spontaneous vaginal delivery following a normal pregnancy. He had mild conjunctivitis at about 2 weeks of age, but has otherwise been well. He has been afebrile during this illness, but has been breathing slightly faster than usual. His mother denies any other symptoms. On physical examination, his vital signs are T 37.4°C, HR 120, RR 90, and BP 85/62. He is nontoxic in appearance and appears well hydrated. He has a staccato cough and has mild intercostal recessions. He has good air exchange, but you auscultate a few scattered rales. You obtain a CXR that shows increased pulmonary markings bilaterally and a patchy infiltrate in the right upper lobe. Your next step is:

   a. Discharge to home on oral amoxicillin
   b. Admit for IV ampicillin
   c. Admit for nebulized albuterol
   d. Admit for IV erythromycin
   e. Admit for a swallow study

2. A 2-year-old previously healthy boy is brought to the ED because of a 6-month history of recurrent cough. His mother has noticed that his cough is worse and lasts longer "when he has a cold." His cough has been persistent for 2 weeks and is described as a dry staccato cough that is worse at night, but is also exacerbated by activity over the daytime. He does not have a runny nose and has not been sneezing. He has not had fever and otherwise appears well. There has been no exposure to tuberculosis, and no one in his immediate family has allergies or a chronic cough. On examination the patient is afebrile and has an RR of 16. He is not in respiratory distress, and auscultation of his chest reveals no abnormalities. He has no gallops or murmurs. The rest of his exam is normal. A CXR is normal. Your next step is to:

   a. Prescribe codeine elixir
   b. Perform a PPD (purified protein derivative) skin test
   c. Initiate a trial of albuterol
   d. Obtain sinus radiographs
   e. Prescribe 5 days of azithromycin

3. A migrant family brings their 9-month-old girl to your ED with a 7-day history of worsening cough following a 3-day history of rhinorrhea. She has several severe bouts of cough per day associated with circumoral cyanosis. She appears exhausted after each bout and is drinking less. Her father has had a persistent cough for about 10 days. She had been afebrile, but now has a temperature to 38.9°C. She had been growing well previously but has only received one set of immunizations. On examination she appears ill, but is nontoxic. She is mildly dehydrated and is in mild respiratory distress. Her RR is 52 and her HR is 120. As you place your tongue depressor in her mouth she gags and has a prolonged bout of coughing, after which she makes an inspiratory sound and appears exhausted. A CXR reveals a left upper lobe infiltrate. Your next step is to:

   a. Arrange for bronchoscopy
   b. Administer inhaled racemic epinephrine
   c. Discharge on high dose oral amoxicillin
   d. Prescribe oral erythromycin
   e. Admit for parenteral antibiotics

4. A 7-year-old girl with attention deficit hyperactivity disorder is brought to your ED with a 3-month history of facial tics and a cough. She has been on methylphenidate (Ritalin) for 5 months. Her facial tics and cough are present only when she is awake. Although the cough is annoying, it does not appear to bother her. She is occasionally able to suppress her cough. There is no family history of asthma or allergies. She denies chest pain, coryza, or sneezing. Her chest exam is normal and the examination of her throat reveals no abnormalities. A CXR is unremarkable. Your next step is to:

   a. Discontinue her methylphenidate
   b. Start oral codeine
   c. Place a PPD skin test
   d. Give inhaled albuterol
   e. Discharge with a diagnosis of psychogenic cough

5. A 2-year-old boy has had a persistent cough for 2 days. It started with a brief choking incident while he was playing at home. The child appeared well afterward. He has had mild rhinorrhea and hoarseness since the incident but is otherwise asymptomatic. He is not drooling and continues to feed well. On examination in the ED his temperature is 37.6°C, and he is in no respiratory distress. He appears to have mild stridor and a barky cough. He receives racemic epinephrine but his stridor does not improve. X-rays of his neck and chest reveal no infiltrates and are otherwise normal. Your next step is to:

a. Administer IM dexamethasone
b. Arrange for laryngoscopy
c. Discharge with croup instructions
d. Discharge on an antitussive medication
e. Obtain a barium swallow

6. A 4-year-old fully immunized girl is brought to the ED for fever, a croupy cough, drooling, and stridor. She is ill appearing but does not appear toxic and is not in acute distress. She has had coryza and a sore throat for a day but has otherwise been asymptomatic. She has no rashes and her parents deny any recent choking episodes. You administer racemic epinephrine with minimal improvement. You order a lateral neck x-ray that is negative for a foreign body. The supraglottic shadows are normal, but the upper airway has irregular margins. There is no steeple sign. Your next step is to:

a. Admit the patient for parenteral antibiotics
b. Administer IM dexamethasone
c. Admit to the operating suite for immediate intubation
d. Diagnose spasmodic croup and discharge on standard treatment
e. Administer IV diphenhydramine

7. A 9-year-old boy is brought to your ED with fever to 40°C, a persistent cough, chest pain, sore throat, and a headache. His cough is his most prominent symptom and is dry and persistent. On examination his temperature is 39.2°C, and he appears somewhat ill. His throat is red but he has no exudate or lesions. He has no rhinorrhea and his conjunctivae are not injected. He is not tachypneic, but examination of his chest reveals rales in his left lower lobe. No pleural rubs are noted on his examination. A CXR reveals diffuse, patchy infiltrates with a small left pleural effusion. You discharge him home on:

a. Oral amoxicillin
b. IV ceftriaxone and then home on oral cephalexin
c. Oral azithromycin
d. Oral clindamycin
e. Oral trimethoprim-sulfamethoxazole

ANSWERS

1. d   Chlamydia pneumonitis is suggested by this infant's presentation. This is an atypical pneumonia usually affecting infants 1–3 months of age, who present with a persistent cough and tachypnea without fever. In about 50% of children there may be a preceding bout of conjunctivitis. Although mortality is low, some infants will have a rocky course marked by severe hypoxemia; therefore, all such children need to be admitted to the hospital for observation and IV erythromycin. If obtained, a CBC may show eosinophilia in about 75% of patients. Patients presenting with isolated chlamydia conjunctivitis also need to be treated with systemic antibiotics. Sepsis and meningitis would be unlikely in this patient because of the duration of symptoms and because of the absence of fever or suggestive symptoms. In addition, ampicillin alone would be inadequate antibiotic coverage.

2. c   Although a history of chronic cough should raise the possibility of tuberculosis, the lack of risk factors and a negative CXR would argue against this diagnosis. An atypical pneumonia in the absence of CXR findings would be unlikely. Pertussis (treatment with azithromycin) would similarly be unlikely because of the duration of symptoms. Sinus radiographs are nonspecific and would not be indicated in the absence of other URI symptoms. Codeine elixir is not recommended to suppress cough symptoms. This child's symptoms would fit a diagnosis of cough variant asthma and the normal chest examina-

tion, and negative CXR would not rule out this diagnosis. Nocturnal exacerbation is common, as is a relationship to activity. Particularly suggestive would be a family history of asthma or a move to a new environment that has the usual triggers of asthma [e.g., smoke (even if smoking occurs outside the home) or a pet]. A trial of beta agonists is indicated in this patient and is more likely to be successful than a cough suppressant.

3. **e**   This child probably has pertussis complicated by bacterial pneumonia. This is suggested by her immunization status as well as her history and presentation. All children with pertussis complicated by pneumonia need to be admitted for parenteral antibiotics. Although radiographic changes are uncommon with uncomplicated pertussis, any child with suggestive symptoms and a new fever should have a radiograph of the chest. If the CXR is consistent with pneumonia, such patients need to be admitted to the hospital for parenteral antibiotics. Oral erythromycin should be reserved for the well-appearing child with uncomplicated pertussis. Foreign body aspirations are less likely in this age group. The inspiratory sound heard by the physician is probably the classic "whoop" described for pertussis and should not be mistaken for stridor associated with viral croup. Because this child's symptoms are not consistent with viral croup, racemic epinephrine is not indicated.

4. **a**   This child has Tourette's syndrome precipitated by the use of methylphenidate. The cough in this vignette is probably a verbal tic and will not respond to oral codeine. Although disappearance of the cough with sleep and the ability to suppress it may suggest a psychogenic origin, these tics are not voluntary. There is no suggestion of reactive airway disease (the resolution of her cough with sleep would argue against this diagnosis), and pulmonary tuberculosis without radiographic findings would be unlikely. Methylphenidate should be discontinued and substituted, even though her verbal tics may persist despite these measures.

5. **b**   Cough, hoarseness, or stridor after a choking episode signifies a foreign body aspiration until ruled out. Patients may be acutely symptomatic or may have a more benign presentation. Negative radiographs do not exclude the diagnosis, and this child needs laryngoscopic evaluation to rule out the diagnosis. Although this presentation mimics viral croup, the negative x-rays make this diagnosis less likely. Furthermore, the physician should not diagnose viral croup without an attempt to rule out a foreign body aspiration. A barium swallow would be useful if this patient presented with symptoms suggestive of an esophageal foreign body such as drooling, odynophagia, or dysphagia, but had a negative CXR. It should be noted, however, that a foreign body in the esophagus can lead to partial airway obstruction and should be excluded if upper airway evaluation is negative in the presence of suggestive symptoms.

6. **a**   Not all croup is viral croup. The "bumpy airway" noted on the lateral radiograph likely represents a pseudomembrane in bacterial tracheitis. This condition is uncommon, but it should be in the differential diagnosis of any highly febrile child (temperature greater than 39°C) with a slower onset of illness who appears sicker than the average child with viral croup. Respiratory distress is invariably present and the clinical presentation may mimic viral croup closely. In more toxic-appearing patients the absence of supraglottic radiologic findings rules out a diagnosis of epiglotittis. It is unclear if this condition is a bacterial complication of croup or a primary bacterial infection, but the causative organism is usually *S. aureus*. Because of the potential for rapid airway compromise, all such patients need to be admitted to the intensive care unit (ICU) for close observation and parenteral antistaphylococcal antibiotics.

7. **c**   Between 5 and 15 years of age *Mycoplasma pneumoniae* is the most common cause of community-acquired pneumonia. It is an atypical pneumonia, and children usually present with cough as their most significant complaint. Sore throat, headache, and pleuritic chest pain are commonly associated symptoms. Chest auscultatory findings may be minimal, but the CXR usually reveals a pneumonia. Macrolides are the antibiotics of choice, and both erythromycin and azithromycin would be efficacious. The alternative would be doxycycline. All of the other antibiotics would be poor choices for *Mycoplasma* infections.

CHAPTER 16

Cyanosis

SUJIT SHARMA, M.D.

QUESTIONS

1. A previously healthy 3-year-old male is brought to the ED by his mother with complaints of headache and dizziness for the past day. The patient has been otherwise healthy, but history does reveal exposure to well water from a local farm. The boy is cyanotic and slightly lethargic on exam. He is in no respiratory distress, has no murmurs on cardiac auscultation, and has good peripheral perfusion. Saturated O_2 is 96% on room air. Which of the following is most likely to aid in diagnosing this patient's condition?

   a. Carboxyhemoglobin level
   b. Chest x-ray (CXR)
   c. Echocardiogram
   d. Methemoglobin level
   e. Arterial blood gas (ABG)

2. A 4-month-old female infant is brought in by her parents for concerns of "dark" lips that they have noted over the past week. On exam she appears slightly lethargic, with a bluish appearance to the lips and tongue. Vital signs show: RR 44, HR 148, and BP 102/61. Saturated O_2 is 80% on room air. Cardiac auscultation reveals a harsh systolic murmur. Which of the following conditions is the patient most likely to be suffering from?

   a. Transposition of the great arteries
   b. Total anomalous pulmonary venous return (TAPVR)
   c. Ventricular septal defect (VSD)
   d. Tetralogy of Fallot
   e. Truncus arteriosus

3. A 15-month-old previously healthy male is brought to the ED with coughing that began acutely 2 hours earlier. On exam his vital signs are: T 37°C, HR 148, RR 44, and BP 108/64. He appears slightly cyanotic with a saturated O_2 of 82% on room air. Auscultation of the chest reveals expiratory wheezes on the right side with diminished air entry when compared with the left. Which of the following treatments would be most helpful for this patient?

   a. Oral amoxicillin
   b. Rigid bronchoscopy
   c. Inhaled albuterol
   d. Oral prednisone
   e. Inhaled budesonide

4. A previously healthy 18-month-old girl is brought into the ED for an episode of "turning blue" at home. The episode lasted less than 1 minute. The patient is alert and playful and has a normal physical exam. She does not appear cyanotic and has a saturated O_2 of 100% on room air. The parents do relay to you that she was crying vigorously just prior to the episode. Which of the following would be most appropriate?

   a. Echocardiogram
   b. AP/lateral chest radiographs
   c. Reassurance to the parents
   d. Neurology consultation
   e. Methemoglobin level

ANSWERS

1. **d**   This child presents with signs and symptoms consistent with methemoglobinemia. Normal cardiac and respiratory findings help to rule out those organ systems as possible etiologies; however, a normal saturated O_2 in spite of obvious cyanosis is expected in methemoglobinemia because pulse oximetry does not recognize oxidized hemoglobin, but rather distinguishes only between oxy- and deoxyhemoglobin. PaO_2 measurement by arterial blood gas (ABG) should also be normal because this is a measure of dissolved oxygen in the blood and does not reflect the amount of oxygen attached to hemoglobin. Even though patients with carbon monoxide poisoning may present with lethargy, they do not present with cyanosis, and classically have a cherry-red color to their skin. A carboxyhemoglobin level would therefore not be helpful.

2. **d**   This cyanotic patient presents with signs consistent with a cyanotic congenital heart defect as the cause of her cyanosis. Tetralogy of Fallot is the most common cyanotic congenital heart defect. It is associated with a systolic murmur caused by pulmonary outflow obstruction and usually presents after the newborn period. Transposition of the great arteries is the most common cyanotic congenital heart defect that presents in the newborn period. Although less common, truncus arteriosus and TAPVR (total anomalous pulmonary venous return) are cyanotic heart defects. Ventricular septal defect (VSD) is not associated with cyanosis.

3. **b**   The history and physical findings in this 15-month-old patient suggest foreign body aspiration. Radiographic imaging would help to confirm your suspicions; however, essential intervention would be rigid bronchoscopy. Measures aimed at treating reactive airway disease or infection are unlikely to be of benefit.

4. **c**   This patient's presentation is most consistent with a breath-holding spell as the cause of the brief episode of cyanosis, as elicited mainly by the history. Testing for pathology involving the heart and/or lungs is unnecessary in this situation. Patients with methemoglobinemia would appear cyanotic at presentation. Further neurological evaluation is not needed in the case of breath-holding spells if one is confident with the diagnosis because reassurance and parental counseling are usually adequate.

CHAPTER 17

Crying and Colic in Early Infancy

VINCENT J. WANG, M.D.

QUESTIONS

1. A 2-week-old boy has been crying more than usual, according to the parents. He has been feeding well and has not been vomiting. He is afebrile and his physical examination is normal. His urinalysis and stool heme testing are normal. Initial appropriate diagnostic testing includes:

   a. Sepsis evaluation
   b. Fluoroscein staining of the eyes
   c. Air contrast enema
   d. Testicular ultrasound (U/S)
   e. Upper gastrointestinal (GI) series

2. A 2-month-old girl has had inconsolable crying for several hours. She has been well otherwise and went to her pediatrician today for her 2-month visit and immunizations. On examination, her temperature is 37°C. Her physical examination is normal. Her urinalysis is normal and heme testing of her stool is negative. Appropriate therapy/intervention at this time includes:

   a. Reassurance of the parents
   b. Obtain CSF culture and cell count
   c. Perform an air contrast enema
   d. Obtain a surgical consultation
   e. Changing the girl's formula

3. A 5-month-old boy has had episodic crying for 1 day. He has had intermittent episodes of harsh crying interspersed with periods of normal behavior. He is afebrile. His abdomen is soft and without masses. His stool heme test is positive for blood. The test most likely to reveal the diagnosis is:

   a. Air contrast enema
   b. Upper GI series
   c. Urinalysis
   d. Testicular U/S
   e. Skeletal series

4. A 6-month-old girl has been crying more often for the past 2 days. The mother says she has been afebrile and has been well otherwise. She is alert, but is somewhat malnourished. Her examination is significant for healing bruises over her shins. She has mild tenderness over her right upper arm. Appropriate treatment at this time includes:

   a. Reassurance
   b. Abdominal CT scan
   c. Upper GI series
   d. Skeletal series
   e. Ibuprofen

5. A 5-week-old girl presents with persistent crying. She has been crying intermittently for 2 weeks. She has been afebrile and her examination is normal. Screening tests are all normal. Treatment includes:

   a. Simethicone
   b. Dicyclomine hydrochloride
   c. Changing her formula
   d. Inpatient observation
   e. Reassurance

ANSWERS

1. b   Corneal abrasions are common causes of crying in the newborn. Initial diagnostic testing should include fluoroscein staining in newborns with crying. If negative, the other tests may be considered if the history suggests another problem.

2. a   Screaming spells after pertussis vaccinations are a common cause of crying if temporally associated with the vaccination. Crying spells typically occur within a day of the immunization. Reassurance should be offered if no other source of crying has been found. Obtaining a CSF specimen is diagnostic for meningitis, another cause of irritability in infants, but the patient has not had fever and has a normal physical exam. Crying may be caused by intussusception, but the patient is young for this diagnosis and the history is not consistent with this diagnosis. Changing the formula has not been proven to be helpful treatment for colic.

3. a   Intussusception is the most common cause of abdominal obstruction in infants and children. The child will classically present with intermittent episodes of crying, interspersed with periods of normal behavior. Currant jelly stool is a late finding, but the stool may be heme-positive earlier in the course. An air contrast enema would diagnose this condition, as well as treat it. An upper GI series could be used to diagnose a malrotation of the bowel. In the absence of scrotal or testicular pain, the diagnosis of testicular torsion by testicular ultrasound is unlikely. A skeletal series would be helpful for occult nonaccidental trauma, and is not indicated here.

4. d   Nonaccidental trauma may cause intermittent crying, especially when associated with recent trauma. A skeletal series is indicated to determine occult fractures. Whereas a toddler may have bruising over his or her shins, a 6-month-old is not able to ambulate and should not have bruising over her shins. In addition, pain over other sites suggests this diagnosis.

5. e   Colic is diagnosed on history in the presence of a normal examination. Parental counseling and reassurance is the best treatment for colic. Dicyclomine hydrochloride is the only medication proven to be effective, but it has been associated with apnea; therefore, its use is discouraged. Simethicone has never proven to be effective. Changing formulas has been effective for patients who have cow's milk protein intolerance, but this represents only a small subset of patients with colic.

CHAPTER 18

Dehydration

RON L. KAPLAN, M.D.

QUESTIONS

The following case relates to Questions 1–3: A 1-week-old girl is brought to the ED with excessive sleepiness, irritability, poor feeding, and with decreased urine output. She is afebrile with HR 180, RR 52, and BP 70/48. She is pale with doughy skin, sunken anterior fontanel, and dry mucosa. Distal pulses are slightly diminished and capillary refill time is 3–4 seconds. Bedside glucose level is 80 mg/dl.

1. Initial IV fluid resuscitation should be:

   a. D5 LR 20 ml/kg bolus
   b. D5 ½NS at twice maintenance
   c. ½NS 20 ml/kg bolus
   d. NS 20 ml/kg bolus
   e. D5 ½NS 20 ml/kg bolus

2. After the preceding treatment the exam is essentially unchanged with HR 174, BP 74/50, slightly diminished distal pulses, and 3–4-second capillary refill time. The following electrolytes are obtained: Na 188 mEq/l, K 3.8 mEq/l, Cl 130 mEq/l, CO_2 12 mEq/l, glucose 62 mg/dl. IV fluid resuscitation should continue with:

   a. ¼NS at twice maintenance
   b. ½NS at twice maintenance
   c. ½NS 20 ml/kg bolus
   d. NS 20 ml/kg bolus
   e. D5 ½NS at twice maintenance

3. Additional treatment along with fluid resuscitation should include:

   a. IV bicarbonate
   b. IV D25W
   c. IV antibiotics
   d. IV dopamine
   e. IV hydrocortisone

4. A 1-year-old boy with stomatitis is brought to the ED with fever, decreased intake, fussiness, decreased tearing, and decreased urine output. He is refusing to take all oral fluids. The following vital signs are obtained: T 39.2°C, HR 158, RR 36, and BP 94/67. Weight is 9 kg. His eyes are slightly sunken and mucous membranes are dry. Distal pulses are strong and capillary refill time is 2–3 seconds. Serum electrolytes are: Na 139 mEq/l; K 4.2 mEq/l; Cl 105 mEq/l; HCO_3 15 mEq/l. What should be used to provide maintenance and replacement fluids:

   a. D5 ¼NS at 40 ml/hour
   b. D5 ½NS at 40 ml/hour
   c. D5 ¼NS at 80 ml/hour
   d. D5 NS at 80 ml/hour
   e. D5 LR at 80 ml/hour

5. A 2-year-old girl is brought to the ED with low-grade fever and vomiting and diarrhea for 2 days. She last vomited several hours ago and has had a few sips of juice since then. She appears well with slightly decreased tearing and a slightly dry mouth. Vital signs are normal. She has strong distal pulses and brisk capillary refill. What is the most appropriate treatment:

   a. Trial of oral rehydration
   b. IV NS 20 ml/kg bolus
   c. IV D5 ¼NS at twice maintenance
   d. IV D5 ½NS at twice maintenance
   e. IV D5 NS at twice maintenance

ANSWERS

1. **d**   This infant has signs of significant dehydration, including tachycardia, sunken fontanel, sunken eyes, dry mucosa, and poor peripheral perfusion as evidenced by diminished pulses and delayed capillary refill. Blood pressure is maintained, but hypotension is a late finding suggestive of impending circulatory failure. The excessive irritability and doughy skin are seen particularly with hypernatremic dehydration. Regardless of the cause or type of dehydration, volume expansion with isotonic crystalloid such as normal saline is the treatment of choice. Dextrose-containing solutions should not be used for volume expansion, and are indicated only for the treatment of hypoglycemia.

2. **d**   Restoration of circulating volume must be achieved with isotonic fluids regardless of the type of dehydration. This infant with hypernatremic dehydration still has signs of intravascular depletion after the initial fluid bolus, so this should be repeated until the intravascular volume has been restored. Because the sodium concentration of normal saline is less than the patient's sodium, this should still result in some lowering of the patient's sodium as well. Definitive treatment of the hypernatremia is undertaken once the circulating volume has been restored.

3. **c**   Sepsis and meningitis must be considered in the differential diagnosis of the ill-appearing neonate, and empiric treatment with IV antibiotics should be instituted after appropriate cultures have been obtained. Bicarbonate is indicated only in the treatment of severe metabolic acidosis that does not improve despite appropriate volume expansion. Dextrose is indicated for the treatment of hypoglycemia. Dopamine is used to treat persistent hypotension despite fluid resuscitation, and hydrocortisone would be indicated if one were considering congenital adrenal hyperplasia as the cause of this patient's illness.

4. **c**   This child's dehydration is likely the result of decreased intake due to stomatitis and increased insensible losses associated with fever. The mild tachycardia, slightly sunken eyes and dry mucosa, and capillary refill time of 2–3 seconds are consistent with moderate, or approximately 10%, dehydration. Again, isotonic crystalloid as a 20 ml/kg bolus would be the appropriate choice for initial volume expansion. D5 ¼NS or D5 ½NS is usually used as maintenance and replacement solution, depending on the patient's weight and serum electrolytes. Assuming this child is 10% dehydrated gives a dry weight of 10 kg, the fluid deficit would be estimated at 1000 ml. If one counts the initial fluid bolus that this child is most likely to receive (approximately 20 ml/kg of NS), then the remaining deficit is 800 ml. In the case of isotonic dehydration half of this deficit can be given over the first 8 hours; the remaining half over the next 16 hours. In the first eight hours, therefore, 400 ml of replacement fluid is given in addition to the maintenance requirements. Maintenance would be 40 ml/hour in a 10-kg child. To give an additional 400 ml over 8 hours would add 50 ml/hour to this rate, for a total of approximately 90 ml/hour. Choosing a rate of twice maintenance often approximates the calculated rate.

5. **a**   This patient has signs of mild dehydration and she now appears to be able to take oral fluids. A trial of oral rehydration is indicated in this case. If vomiting persists or diarrhea is excessive, IV fluids may be required.

CHAPTER 19

Diarrhea

MARK WALTZMAN, M.D.

QUESTIONS

1. A 4-year-old girl has been on several courses of amoxicillin over the past month for otitis media. The child now comes to the ED with abdominal distension and bloody diarrhea. All of the following would be appropriate for diagnosis and management, EXCEPT:

   a. IV fluids
   b. Metronidazole
   c. Clindamycin
   d. Sigmoidoscopy
   e. Stool culture

2. A 3-year-old boy comes to the ED with a 5-day history of passage of frequent, watery, nonbloody stools, and crampy abdominal pain. He has been voiding well, has been taking POs well, and has had no emesis. His vital signs are: T 36°C, HR 100, RR 20, and BP 100/60. His abdomen is soft and nontender. Therapy should include:

   a. Metronidazole
   b. Trimethoprim-sufamethoxazole
   c. Sigmoidoscopy
   d. Oral glucose electrolyte solution
   e. Loperamide *anti motility*

3. A 1-year-old boy with trisomy 21 comes to the ED for evaluation of diarrhea. He has had a history of alternating constipation and diarrhea since birth. His abdomen appears distended. On rectal exam there is a dilated rectal vault without stool present. Management should include:

   a. Metronidazole
   b. Abdominal CT
   c. Barium enema
   d. Cathartics
   e. Sigmoidoscopy

4. A 3-year-old girl comes to the ED for evaluation of diarrhea. She has had a history of alternating constipation and diarrhea since 18 months of age. On rectal exam there is a dilated rectal vault with firm stool present. Management should include:

   a. Metronidazole
   b. Abdominal CT
   c. Barium enema
   d. Cathartics
   e. Sigmoidoscopy

ANSWERS

1. c   A serious disorder that may cause bloody diarrhea is pseudomembranous colitis. This disease results from an overgrowth of toxin-producing clostridial organisms in the bowel and must be considered after a course of antibiotic therapy, which can destroy the normal flora of the gut. It may occur at any age, but it is not common in early childhood. Although the incidence of pseudomembranous colitis is highest after treatment with an infrequently prescribed antibiotic, clindamycin, any of the antibacterial drugs may be the culprit. Amoxicillin, because of its frequent use, is responsible for most childhood cases. The patient clinically appears ill, with prostration, abdominal distension, and bloody stools. Microscopic examination of the feces, sigmoidoscopy, stool culture, and analysis for toxin are useful diagnostic tests. Treatment includes symptomatic therapy as well as metronidazole or vancomycin orally.

2. d   Afebrile children with nonbloody diarrhea are usually judged to have viral enteritis. Those who receive antibiotic agents, such as amoxicillin, may be suffering from a drug-related gastrointestinal disturbance, but not usually from pseudomembranous colitis. Therapy is supportive. Oral therapy is indicated in a well-hydrated, well-appearing child. Optimal oral therapy emphasizes the use of appropriate glucose and electrolyte solutions as well as the early reintroduction of feeding. Antibiotics and sigmoidoscopy play no role in the treatment of typically viral gastroenteritis in the well-appearing child. Loperamide or other antimotility agents are not indicated in the treatment of childhood diarrhea.

3. c   The role of the emergency physician in the evaluation of the child with chronic diarrhea is to select out those few children who have urgent conditions and refer the remainder to their regular source of care. In the infant in particular, consideration must be given to Hirschsprung's disease and to cystic fibrosis. A rectal exam should be performed on the child with chronic diarrhea. With overflow stools secondary to prolonged constipation, the rectal ampulla contains a large amount of hard stool, but it is often empty in the patient with Hirschsprung's disease. Diagnosis of Hirschsprung's disease is made with rectal biopsy; however, barium enema is sometimes useful in defining a transition zone between the ganglionic and aganglionic segment of intestine.

4. d   As noted earlier, the role of the emergency physician in the evaluation of the child with chronic diarrhea is to select out those few children who have urgent conditions and refer the remainder to their regular source of care. This child's presentation is consistent with functional constipation. Constipation with overflow stools is treated by removing the obstruction (the impacted stool) and maintaining passage of stool until the dilated ampulla returns to normal caliber.

CHAPTER 20

Disturbed Child

THOMAS H. CHUN, M.D.

QUESTIONS

1. A 14-year-old boy is brought to your ED for evaluation of behavior changes. On examination, he exhibits impaired reality testing, inappropriate affect, poor behavior control, and abnormal relating abilities. Other findings that would be suggestive to you of an organic (as compared with a primarily psychiatric) etiology for his psychotic symptoms include:

    a. A history of a prodromal phase and gradual onset of symptoms
    b. Visual hallucinations or impaired recent memory
    c. Normal vital signs and absence of autonomic instability
    d. Intact orientation to person, place, and time
    e. Intact cognition and intellectual ability

2. A 16-year-old girl is brought to the ED after attempting to cut her wrists. She and her parents endorse a 3-month history of irritable mood, escalating arguments with her parents, insomnia, social isolation and withdrawal from her friends, and a 10-kg weight loss. The most important step in the initial ED management of this patient would include:

    a. Obtaining appropriate mental health consultation and/or follow-up
    b. Starting psychotropic medication (i.e., because many of these medications have delayed efficacy)
    c. Medical evaluation of the patient
    d. Admission to a hospital as a "cooling-off" period
    e. Laboratory evaluations to rule out organic causes

3. A 7-year-old boy is brought to the ED for severe temper tantrums. His mother states that he has a past history of head banging, severe enough to "give himself a concussion." She describes him as uncontrollable and extremely destructive during these tantrums. On examination in the ED, he is alert, oriented, and cooperative with the examination. He engages appropriately with and seems eager to please the examiner. The manner of interaction appears to be normal for his age and expected development. To complete this patient's mental status examination (MSE) adequately, the ED physician should:

    a. Rely on what has already been performed
    b. Informally test for intelligence quotient (IQ)
    c. Assess school performance
    d. Test constructional abilities using cards and blocks
    e. Screen for depression

4. A 15-year-old boy confides to his best friend that he is so bored with life that he has thought about killing himself. The friend tells the boy's parents, who bring him to the ED for evaluation. They are concerned about his listening to aggressive music, and his stepfather wants him committed to a psychiatric facility. His primary care physician states that he seems like a "well child." In deciding on a disposition for this patient, the factor(s) that is/are most important in guiding this decision is:

    a. Whether the patient is suicidal or homicidal
    b. Whether the patient and family can safely manage the problem as an outpatient
    c. The disposition the patient most prefers
    d. The disposition the family most prefers
    e. The disposition the patient's primary care physician recommends

ANSWERS

1. b   Ruling out possible organic causes of a patient's psychiatric symptoms is one of the most important roles of an ED physician. Table 20.2 in the *Textbook of Pediatric Emergency Medicine,* fourth edition, summarizes the differences commonly seen in organically versus psychiatrically induced psychosis. Acute onset, no history of prodromal symptoms, presence of autonomic symptoms, abnormal vital signs, disturbed orientation, impaired recent memory or intellectual abilities, and visual or tactile hallucinations are suggestive of organically induced psychosis. The list of medical causes for psychiatric symptoms is vast. Tables 20.3 and 20.4 are abbreviated lists of such causes. Any suspicion of an organic etiology requires a full medical evaluation and likely hospitalization in a medical facility.

2. c   The goals of evaluating a patient with behavioral disturbance are threefold. The first is detecting any life-threatening conditions and determining if a medical or organic condition is the cause of the symptoms. Many medical conditions can present with primarily psychiatric symptomatology. Failure to detect an underlying organic condition can result in significant patient harm by exposing the patient to inappropriate therapies or by delaying appropriate treatment. The majority of pediatric psychiatric patients can be "medically cleared" by a careful and thorough history and physical examination. This patient appears to be clinically depressed; however, ruling out hypothyroidism, eating disorders and their sequelae, and substance abuse are important medical considerations for this girl.

    The other two goals are to evaluate the patient for the presence of suicidal or homicidal ideation and to assess the family functioning and social support. A complete evaluation of all three areas is necessary to make appropriate diagnostic, therapeutic, and disposition decisions. Mental health consultation, psychotropic medications, and hospitalization are not always warranted and may or may not be helpful. Laboratory evaluation should be ordered on the basis of clinical suspicion and is not mandatory for every behaviorally disturbed patient.

3. a   ED physicians should be familiar with the elements of a mental status examination (MSE). A formal MSE entails evaluation of orientation, memory, cognitive function (e.g., intelligence, fund of knowledge, ability to reason, etc.), activity level, ability to relate to others, mood, affect, thought content and process, and insight. It also includes identifying a patient's strengths and weaknesses, which are often critical in determining disposition. In the pediatric population, a formal MSE is rarely required. Essentially all MSE data can be garnered in the course of interviewing the child or adolescent about why they are in the ED, and by asking about their home, school, and social life, their interests and hobbies, and so on. Interviewing strategies should include using open-ended, nonjudgmental questions and developmentally appropriate language. IQ and formal psychological testing (e.g., cards and blocks) are not part of the MSE. Assessment of school performance and depression screening are important parts of any psychiatric evaluation, but are not aspects of a formal MSE.

4. b   Even though all of these factors should be weighed in disposition decisions, the most important factors are the severity of symptoms and the patient's and his family's ability to manage the problem on an outpatient basis. The entire focus of an ED psychiatric evaluation should be to make this determination. Not all patients with suicidal or homicidal ideation need to be admitted. Patients who were not and are not actively suicidal or homicidal can be considered for discharge, if adequate safety and supervision at home and timely outpatient follow-up can be arranged. Even if a mental health professional has evaluated a patient, ED physicians maintain joint responsibility for these patients. It is thus important that ED physicians personally assess these two areas in all psychiatric patients and concur with the consultant's recommendations.

CHAPTER 21

Dizziness

JOYCE SOPRANO, M.D.

QUESTIONS

1. A 7-year-old boy is brought to the ED after awakening with dizziness. His parents report that other than a slight cold the preceding week, he had been feeling well until this morning, when he awoke with severe dizziness and vomiting. On physical examination, he is afebrile and his vital signs are normal. He is lying still on the stretcher with his eyes closed. When he sits up, he develops vomiting and nystagmus. The remainder of his examination is normal. The most appropriate next step is:

   a. Obtain an emergent head CT scan
   b. Start broad-spectrum IV antibiotics
   c. Start broad-spectrum PO antibiotics
   d. Start PO prednisone and dimenhydrinate
   e. Obtain electronystagmography

2. A 13-year-old girl is referred to you for dizziness. She reports that over the past several months she has had recurrent episodes of severe dizziness followed shortly afterward by throbbing pain in the back of her head. Her mother recalls that the patient's speech seemed slurred several times during the dizziness. Between episodes she has no symptoms. Her physical examination is normal. The most important next step is:

   a. Obtain a head CT scan
   b. Obtain a brain MRI
   c. Obtain an EEG
   d. Perform a lumbar puncture
   e. Obtain an otorhinolaryngology consultation

3. A 9-year-old boy is brought to the ED with dizziness. Several hours before admission he fell while skateboarding, striking the left side of his head on the ground. He had no loss of consciousness (LOC), but has had worsening dizziness and nausea since. On physical examination, he has slight nystagmus with the slow component toward the left. He has a contusion over the left temporoparietal skull. The most appropriate next step is:

   a. Discharge home and have his parents awaken him every 2 hours
   b. Obtain a head CT scan
   c. Obtain a temporal bone CT scan
   d. Obtain both head and temporal bone CT scans
   e. Obtain an EEG

4. A 3-year-old girl is seen in the ED for recurrent "attacks." Her parents report that she becomes pale, vomits, and her eyes "twitch" several times each month. The episodes last only a few minutes and she has no LOC. She seems to be normal between episodes. Her physical examination is normal. The most likely diagnosis is:

   a. Benign paroxysmal vertigo
   b. Paroxysmal torticollis of infancy
   c. Ménière's disease
   d. Vestibular seizures
   e. Vestibular neuronitis

5. A 16-year-old girl is brought to the ED by ambulance from school, where she complained of dizziness. She reports that while playing basketball she felt dizzy and thought she was going to "pass out." She denies current illness, recent trauma, or drug use. On physical examination, she is afebrile, and has HR 120, RR 30, and BP 110/60. Her neurologic examination is normal, including no evidence of nystagmus. The most appropriate combination of tests to evaluate this patient is:

   a. Head CT scan, urine toxic screen, qualitative human chorionic gonadotropin (HCG), hematocrit (hct), blood glucose
   b. Head CT scan, qualitative HCG, blood glucose
   c. Head CT scan, ECG, qualitative HCG, hct
   d. ECG, qualitative HCG, hct, blood glucose
   e. ECG, urine toxic screen, qualitative HCG, hct, blood glucose

ANSWERS

1. **d** This clinical scenario is most consistent with vestibular neuronitis, which is a viral infection of the labyrinth or vestibular nerve that presents with acute vertigo. Prednisone may shorten the course of the condition, and the antihistamine dimenhydrinate may decrease the vertigo. Because there was no mention of middle ear infection on the physical examination, antibiotics are not indicated. If there had been a history of trauma or recurrent symptoms, head CT scan would be indicated. Electronystagmography may separate central from peripheral vestibular disorders when the diagnosis is uncertain, but that would not be indicated in this case.

2. **b** This patient's symptoms are suggestive of recurrent basilar migraine, with vertigo and dysarthria followed by a throbbing occipital headache. Other brain stem and cerebellar processes (e.g., tumor and infarction) should be excluded with brain MRI. Head CT is insufficient to detect small brainstem lesions. If MRI is normal, an EEG may be obtained at that time to exclude vestibular seizures, although this diagnosis is unlikely because the patient reports no alteration of consciousness during the episodes. The patient is unlikely to have multiple sclerosis with a normal neurologic examination; however, if the MRI is suggestive of this disease, lumbar puncture may be performed at that time. Because she has a normal ear examination and her symptoms are suggestive of a central cause of vertigo, otorhinolaryngology consultation is unlikely to aid in the diagnosis.

3. **d** This patient may have posttraumatic vestibular dysfunction from a fracture through the temporal bone. His examination suggests a peripheral cause of the nystagmus because the slow component is toward the area of suspected trauma. Patients with trauma-related vestibular dysfunction should be evaluated with a temporal bone CT scan that may reveal a temporal bone fracture. Head CT scan should also be obtained to evaluate for other intracranial injuries. EEG is not indicated in the initial management of head injury. Any patient with neurologic dysfunction after a head injury should not be discharged prior to brain imaging.

4. **a** This clinical scenario is consistent with benign paroxysmal vertigo, with recurrent brief attacks of vestibular dysfunction without alteration of consciousness. Paroxysmal torticollis of infancy is seen in younger infants, but it may be a prelude to benign paroxysmal vertigo. Ménière's disease, a disorder of recurrent attacks of vertigo, tinnitus, and hearing loss, is uncommon prior to age 10 years. Vestibular seizures have associated alteration of consciousness. Vestibular neuronitis is an acute infection with symptoms that last 1–3 weeks.

5. **e** This patient has pseudovertigo, with lightheadedness and presyncope, but no signs of vestibular dysfunction. In this adolescent patient, likely causes of pseudovertigo include anxiety, anemia, pregnancy, hypoglycemia, and toxic ingestion. Thus, the initial workup should include a urine toxic screen, qualitative HCG, hematocrit, and blood glucose. Although cardiac arrhythmia is less likely, an ECG should be performed to exclude this potentially dangerous condition. Head CT scan is not indicated in the initial management of pseudovertigo if the patient has a normal neurologic examination.

CHAPTER 22

Edema

VINCENT J. WANG, M.D.

QUESTIONS

1. A 3-year-old boy comes to the ED with left lower leg swelling. He was running in the fields near his home. On examination, he is well appearing and ambulates without difficulty. He has a punctate lesion on the sole of his left foot. There is edema around his foot and ankle, but no warmth. He has no other complaints. Appropriate treatment includes:

   a. IV cefazolin
   b. IV ceftriaxone
   c. PO cephalexin
   d. PO diphenhydramine
   e. Splinting

2. A 9-year-old girl has developed right-sided periorbital edema. She has had cough, greenish rhinorrhea, and fever for several days. On examination she is well appearing with right periorbital edema and erythema. She has no proptosis and her extraocular movements are normal. She has no surrounding erythema or other lesions. The most helpful diagnostic imaging would include:

   a. Sinus imaging
   b. CT of the head with IV contrast
   c. CT of the head with facial bone cuts
   d. Panorex films (dentition)
   e. Skull series

3. A 6-year-old boy is referred to the ED for evaluation of generalized edema. You would be unlikely to find edema at which of the following sites:

   a. Periorbital areas
   b. Scrotum
   c. Hips
   d. Lower back
   e. Feet

4. A 4-year-old African-American girl is referred to you for evaluation of generalized edema. She had an upper respiratory infection (URI) several weeks ago. She is otherwise well now, but the mother noticed that she appears to have gained weight over the past few days. On examination, she is alert and well appearing. She has moderate periorbital swelling, labial swelling, and lower extremity swelling, without erythema. The most useful diagnostic test to confirm the diagnosis is:

   a. Urinalysis
   b. CBC
   c. Serum magnesium level
   d. Hemoglobin electrophoresis
   e. Test dose of epinephrine

5. A 1-year-old boy with a history of failure to thrive has worsening poor feeding and lethargy. He has been ill over the past few days. On examination, he is ill appearing, with tachycardia and tachypnea. His heart sounds are normal. His liver edge is palpable 4 cm below the right costal margin. He has edema of his lower extremities. Appropriate treatment includes:

   a. Pericardiocentesis
   b. Administration of normal saline
   c. Administration of albumin 5%
   d. Administration of epinephrine
   e. Administration of furosemide

ANSWERS

1. **d** The boy presents after a probable insect bite, noted as the punctate lesion on the sole of his foot. Symptoms of surrounding edema, without warmth, fever, erythema, or linear streaking, suggest that this is an allergic reaction from the insect bite rather than a cellulitis. Normal ambulation suggests an etiology other than trauma or joint infection. Without systemic symptoms, oral diphenhydramine and supportive care would be appropriate treatment.

2. **a** The girl presents with symptoms of a periorbital cellulitis complicated with an acute sinusitis. Sinus radiography or sinus CT would help with the diagnosis. In cases of orbital cellulitis, CT of the orbits would be imperative; however, her clinical symptoms do not suggest this. Panorex films are helpful if you suspect the etiology of facial swelling is dental in origin. Skull-series radiographs would aid in the diagnosis of a skull fracture.

3. **c** Generalized edema will be most evident in the dependent portions of the body, including the lower back and the extremities. Edema may also be present in areas of increased distensibility (e.g., the periorbital areas, scrotum, labia, or ears).

4. **a** The patient's symptoms suggest that she has nephrotic syndrome. The urinalysis will confirm this diagnosis with the presence of large quantities of protein in the urine. In addition, the serum albumin level is decreased, the serum cholesterol and triglyceride levels are increased, and the total serum calcium level is decreased. A CBC would substantiate an infectious process, but this would still be a clinical diagnosis, which is not suggested in this scenario. Hemoglobin electrophoresis would be helpful if you suspected sickle cell disease, which may present with digit swelling. Sickle cell disease, however, does not present with generalized edema. A test dose of epinephrine could be used to differentiate an allergic reaction from other causes of edema, but it is not indicated here.

5. **e** The patient's presentation suggests that he has undiagnosed cardiac disease and is presenting with congestive heart failure (CHF). Pericardiocentesis would be indicated with a pericardial tamponade. Administration of normal saline or albumin would likely exacerbate the patient's symptoms. Epinephrine is not indicated in this case. Judicious administration of a diuretic would help alleviate the patient's symptoms.

CHAPTER 23

Epistaxis

DOMINIC CHALUT, M.D.

QUESTIONS

1. A 4-year-old boy is brought to the ED because of a 2-hour history of profuse bilateral epistaxis (nosebleed) not responding to local pressure. The parents observed hematemesis twice. The vital signs are: RR 18, HR 120, and BP 130/85. The child is pale-looking. The exam of Little's area shows no obvious bleeding site. The bleeding is most likely caused by:

   a. Kiesselbach's plexus trauma
   b. Allergic rhinitis
   c. Foreign body
   d. Posterior nasal bleed
   e. Rhinitis sicca

2. A 16-year-old girl is brought to the ED with a recurrent episode of epistaxis easily controllable by local pressure. The epistaxis occurs approximately once per month. She is otherwise healthy, has no history of bleeding diathesis, and takes no medication. Her recurrent epistaxis is compatible with:

   a. Wegener's granulomatosis
   b. Vicarious menstruation
   c. von Willebrand's disease
   d. Allergic rhinitis
   e. Rhinitis sicca

3. A 2-year-old boy is brought to the ED for a nosebleed that occurred this morning. It has now stopped. This is the first episode noted by the parents. The child had upper respiratory tract (URI) symptoms for the last 24 hours. He is otherwise healthy. On examination, a bleeding site is identified on the anterior septum. What investigation should be done?

   a. CBC
   b. CBC/PT-PTT
   c. CBC/PT-PTT/ristocetin aggregation study
   d. CBC/PT-PTT/ristocetin aggregation study/level of Factor VIIIc and VIIIag
   e. None

4. A 10-year-old girl had nasal packing 24 hours ago for epistaxis. She presents with abrupt onset of high fever, vomiting, diarrhea, headache, myalgias, and diffuse erythema. Her vital signs are: RR 24, HR 160, and BP 85/40. What is the most likely diagnosis?

   a. Influenza
   b. Toxic shock syndrome
   c. Meningococcemia
   d. Scarlet fever
   e. Erythema multiforme

5. A 17-year-old boy complains of epistaxis. He has had allergic rhinitis, with a recent exacerbation. On examination, he has a slow but active source of bleeding on the right. Which therapy is most likely to achieve hemostasis?

   a. Cotton pledgets moistened with xylocaine
   b. Cotton pledgets moistened with normal saline
   c. Cotton roll under the lower lip
   d. Cotton pledgets moistened with drops of epinephrine
   e. Cotton pledgets moistened with petroleum jelly

6. A 5-year-old boy known to have classic hemophilia has severe epistaxis. The child is hemodynamically stable. What would be the best therapy?

   a. Nasal packing
   b. Silver nitrate cauterization
   c. Factor VIII infusion
   d. Factor IX infusion
   e. Surgical ligation of vessels

ANSWERS

1. d   Blood seen in the oropharynx, blood in both nares, difficulty controlling bleeding despite adequate anterior pressure, and a normal anterior exam are more characteristic of a posterior nasal bleed. Although rare in a young child, a hypertensive patient may be more prone to this bleeding. We would expect to see blood in Little's area with Kiesselbach's plexus trauma. Allergic rhinitis and rhinitis sicca are usually milder bleeds of the anterior nasal chambers. Bleeding is usually well controlled with local pressure, and the most common site of bleeding is in the Little's area. A foreign body in the nares is usually associated with some purulent discharge.

2. b   Vicarious menstruation refers to a condition occasionally found in adolescent girls in which monthly epistaxis, related to vascular congestion of the nasal mucosa, occurs concurrently with menses and is presumably related to cyclic changes in hormone levels. Allergic rhinitis and rhinitis sicca should not be so regular on a monthly basis, but more seasonal, with the first being associated with exposure to allergens and the latter being more frequent during the winter season, when the humidity in the air is lower. Von Willebrand's disease is usually associated with mucosal bleeding, excessive bruising, and menorrhagia. Wegener's granulomatosis is a progressive, destructive process characterized by persistent nasal discharge, crusted and pustular lesions, swelling, induration, and finally, ulceration of midline structures of the face.

3. e   In children without clinical evidence of severe blood loss who have no suspicion of systemic factors, and for whom an anterior site of bleeding is identified, reassurance and education regarding appropriate at-home management need to be provided. In von Willebrand's disease, both Factors VIIIc and VIIIag are depressed and the platelets do not aggregate when ristocetin is added to platelet-rich plasma. A patient with von Willebrand's disease usually presents with recurrent epistaxis, mucosal bleeding, excessive bruising, and (in girls) with menorrhagia. (Corrigan JJ. "Von Willebrand Disease." *Nelson Textbook of Pediatrics,* fifteenth edition, Philadelphia: W. B. Saunders; 1996, p. 1428.)

4. b   The advent of expandable nasal tampons had simplified nasal packing for the emergency physician. They pose the risk of toxic shock syndrome, however, necessitating careful patient instructions and follow-up. This patient is in shock (hypotensive and tachycardic); influenza, scarlet fever, and erythema multiforme are unlikely to cause shock. Meningococcemia could present with shock, although petechiae and/or purpura are usually present on physical exam. The clinical picture presented (i.e., fever, vomiting, diarrhea, headache, myalgia, diffuse erythema, and shock) is typical of toxic shock syndrome, especially in a patient who has had nasal packing.

5. d   The use of cotton pledgets moistened with epinephrine (1:1000) or application of topical thrombin will help achieve hemostasis. Epinephrine (1:10,000) would be too dilute. If a roll of cotton is used, it needs to be inserted underneath the upper lip to compress the labial artery.

6. c   For children with nosebleeds from a hemorrhagic diathesis, the underlying disorder must be corrected. In classic hemophilia, or hemophilia A, the level of Factor VIIIc is reduced to 0–5% of normal. Therapy with Factor VIII concentrates permit achieving hemostasis. In hemophilia B, the Factor IX is deficient. Nasal packing, silver nitrate cauterization, and surgical ligation of vessels would not correct the underlying disorder. (Corrigan JJ. "Factor VIII Deficiency." *Nelson Textbook of Pediatrics,* fifteenth edition, Philadelphia: W. B. Saunders; 1996, pp. 1424–1427.)

CHAPTER **24**

Eye—Red

ANDREA STRACCIOLINI, M.D.

QUESTIONS

1. A 16-year-old girl comes to the ED with an acutely red, painful eye. She states that she awoke this morning with yellow drainage from her eye. She denies fever, trauma, or a foreign body sensation in the eye. She states that she did not put her contacts in this morning because she was in too much pain. Evaluation of this patient should include:

   a. Slit lamp examination
   b. Fluorescein staining
   c. Visual acuity check
   d. Ophthalmology evaluation
   e. All of the above

2. A 14-year-old boy was hit in the right eye while playing basketball earlier in the day. He is brought to the ED with an acutely red and painful eye. On physical examination, his extraocular muscles are normal, and the pupils are reactive bilaterally. There is no blood in the anterior chamber, fluorescein staining of his eye is negative, and there is no foreign body seen. The right pupil is slightly smaller than the left. Evaluation and treatment of this patient should include:

   a. Ophthalmology referral
   b. Systemic antibiotics
   c. Topical steroids
   d. Eye patching
   e. Erythromycin ointment

3. A 7-year-old boy comes to the ED with a painful and red left eye. On examination, you note a focal nodular elevation with overlying inflammation on the sclera. The eye is tender and there is a bluish hue to the inflamed area. On slit lamp examination, there are no cells seen in the anterior chamber. The likely diagnosis is:

   a. Iritis
   b. Scleritis
   c. Conjunctivitis
   d. Glaucoma
   e. Foreign body

4. A 16-year-old girl comes to the ED with a painful red eye. She tells you that she has had similar symptoms in the past, which have always resolved spontaneously. She denies pain or discharge. She wears contact lenses. On fluorescein staining of the cornea you see a linear branching pattern. The next step in caring for this patient is:

   a. Topical acyclovir
   b. Topical gentamicin
   c. Topical prednisone
   d. Hospital admission
   e. Eye patch

5. A 6-year-old girl complains of a sandy foreign body sensation of her eyes. The child has had a low-grade fever and eye pain for the past 24 hours. On physical examination there is marked eyelid swelling bilaterally with significant scleral injection, pseudomembranes, and preauricular adenopathy. The only discharge is significant tearing of both eyes. Your most likely diagnosis is:

   a. Foreign body
   b. Corneal abrasion
   c. Allergic conjunctivitis
   d. Periorbital cellulitis
   e. Keratoconjunctivitis

6. A 12-year-old girl is brought to the ED with the chief complaint of itching, tearing eyes. On physical examination, you note a blisterlike elevation of the conjunctiva. There is mild periocular swelling bilaterally. There is no history of fever, significant drainage, or pain. The correct treatment at this time is:

   a. Topical antihistamine
   b. Topical antibiotic
   c. Topical steroids
   d. Eye patch
   e. None of the above

7. An 18-year-old boy tells you that his eyes feel dry occasionally, and that they often feel like they have sand in them. He also complains of photophobia and says that the symptoms are worse after prolonged reading or watching TV. On examination, you note erythema of all four eyelid margins and flaking/crusting at the base of the eyelashes. Fluorescein staining of his eyes is negative for a corneal abrasion. The most likely diagnosis is:

a. Blepharitis
b. Allergic conjunctivitis
c. Keratoconjunctivitis
d. Foreign body
e. Uveitis

8. A 3-year-old girl comes to the ED with the following symptoms: redness, increased tearing, and photophobia. You note that the child also has heterochromia. There is no history of fever, discharge, or change in vision. Evaluation of this patient is likely to reveal:

a. CSF pleocytosis
b. Elevated intraocular pressure
c. Fluorescein uptake
d. Cobblestoning
e. Anterior chamber WBCs

ANSWERS

1. e   Any child who is a regular contact lens wearer, even if the lens is not in the eye at the time of the examination, should be referred to an ophthalmologist within 24 hours if they complain of a persistent red eye. Red and often painful eyes of a contact lens wearer may represent a potentially blinding corneal infection. A slit lamp examination should be performed to look for cells in the chambers of the eye. Fluorescein staining is necessary to rule out corneal abrasions or ulcers that are especially prone in contact lens wearers. A visual acuity evaluation is appropriate in the ED evaluation of any patient who has eye complaints.

2. a   Traumatic injury may result in a red eye because of a corneal or conjunctival abrasion, hyphema, iritis, or, rarely, traumatic glaucoma. In the absence of a corneal or conjunctival abrasion, foreign body, or trichiasis (eyelashes that turn against the ocular surface), the painful red eye following trauma represents iritis. This may not develop for up to 72 hours following the trauma. Photophobia and blurred vision also may occur, and the affected pupil may be smaller. A cloudy inferior cornea caused by deposition of inflammatory cells and debris on the inner surface can be seen. All patients with iritis, regardless of the etiology, require ophthalmologic referral, although immediate consultation is not necessary. Topical steroids should not ordinarily be prescribed by the non-ophthalmologist. Antibiotics (systemic or topical) are not indicated in this patient because infection is not suspected. Eye patching might be helpful if the diagnosis was corneal abrasion.

3. b   Episcleritis and scleritis may cause a painful red eye. Scleritis is often associated with an underlying systemic disease, particularly the collagen vascular disorders. Episcleritis is usually an isolated ocular abnormality. Both may present with focal or diffuse inflammation. A nodular elevation may be seen involving the sclera. The eye may be tender and there may be a bluish hue to the inflamed area. There may also be pain on attempted movement of the eye. Diagnosis requires slit lamp examination. Iritis is diagnosed by slit lamp examination by noting the presence of inflammatory cells in the anterior chamber. Infectious conjunctivitis does not present with these symptoms. There is often diffuse injection of the sclera and discharge. Glaucoma is uncommon in children. Congenital glaucoma is usually not associated with a red eye or pain. Young children with acute glaucoma often have enlarged eyes (buphthalmos) with tearing, photophobia, and sometimes heterochromia. There was no foreign body mentioned on examination; thus, this is not the diagnosis.

4. a   Another cause of painful ocular inflammation is herpetic corneal infection. Herpes simplex or varicella-zoster viruses may cause this. There is usually no concomitant dermatologic manifestation except during chickenpox (varicella), when a unilateral or bilateral lesion may be seen on the conjunctiva, usually near, but not on, the cornea. There may be focal injection. This infection usually requires no treatment. Patients with herpetic corneal ulcers may have a history of recurrent symptoms, but herpes can occasionally be painless because of induced corneal hypoesthesia. These disorders are virtually always unilateral. Fluorescein staining of the cornea reveals a linear branching pattern. Corneal abrasions are not recurrent and do not have a branching pattern on fluorescein examination. Corneal ulcers are seen

with contact lens wearers, but they have different manifestations. Herpetic corneal ulcers require urgent treatment to prevent corneal scarring and visual loss. All patients who may have herpetic corneal lesions need an ophthalmologic evaluation in the ED and immediate treatment. Topical antibiotics are appropriate for bacterial conjunctivitis. Eye patching and topical treatment with an anesthetic are appropriate treatments for corneal abrasions. Topical steroids are not indicated in this case because you suspect a herpes infection of the cornea, and because steroids should not be prescribed by ED physicians without ophthalmologic consultation.

5. e Eye pain and marked lid swelling may be associated with epidemic keratoconjunctivitis (EKC) caused by adenovirus. Patients may describe that they have a sandy foreign body sensation as opposed to true ocular pain. Pseudomembranes are fairly diagnostic. Low-grade fever and tender preauricular adenopathy may also occur, making it difficult to distinguish EKC from periorbital cellulitis. EKC usually affects the eyes bilaterally. There may be prominent photophobia and tearing, which is not usually seen in cellulitis. Corneal abrasions or the presence of a foreign body are diagnoses with unilateral symptoms, and should be easily diagnosed with fluorescein staining and physical examination. Allergic conjunctivitis is not associated with fever or adenopathy.

6. a Itching is an important symptom when a patient presents with red eyes. When associated with swelling of the conjunctiva and a blisterlike elevation, allergic conjunctivitis is the likely diagnosis. The causative agent is often unknown. There may be associated periocular swelling, along with photophobia, tearing, and lid swelling. Treatment may include antihistamines and/or vasoconstrictors. Blepharitis does not present with a blisterlike elevation. Bacterial and viral infections are often associated with a yellow discharge and also do not present with swollen conjunctivae. Itching is not usually an associated symptom; thus, there is no role for antibiotic treatment at this time.

7. a Blepharitis is an idiopathic disorder in which there is suboptimal flow of secretions. The deficiency of flow results in an abnormal tear film and corneal dessication. As with this patient, symptoms are aggravated by prolonged staring. The most characteristic sign is erythema of all four eyelid margins and flaking and crusting at the base of the eyelashes. Allergic conjunctivitis is associated with itchiness of the eyes and swelling of the conjunctiva. A foreign body can be detected on physical examination, and uveitis is diagnosed via slit lamp examination detecting cells in the anterior chamber. Keratoconjunctivitis does not present with this symptomatology.

8. b Glaucoma in children is rare. Congenital glaucoma is usually not associated with a red eye or pain. Young children with glaucoma often have enlarged eyes (buphthalmos) with tearing, photophobia, and possibly heterochromia. Purulent discharge is seen with bacterial infections of the eyes. Acute acquired glaucoma causes a painful red eye, possibly associated with corneal clouding and decreased visual acuity. Intraocular pressure must be measured in all cases in which glaucoma is suspected.

CHAPTER 25

Eye—Strabismus

MARK E. RALSTON, M.D., M.P.H.

QUESTIONS

1. A 7-year-old boy falls 6 feet off playground equipment, hitting his head. In the ED, he is alert but states that he sees "two of everything." You detect a vertical misalignment of his eyes, specifically a tendency of the right eye to remain in relative upgaze. You diagnose a traumatic palsy of the:

   a. Sixth cranial nerve (VI) innervating the lateral rectus muscle
   b. Fourth cranial nerve (IV) innervating the superior oblique muscle
   c. Third cranial nerve (III) innervating the medial rectus muscle
   d. Third cranial nerve (III) innervating the inferior oblique muscle
   e. Third cranial nerve (III) innervating the inferior rectus muscle

2. A 6-month-old boy is found to have a limitation of lateral gaze in his left eye on a visit to the ED for evaluation of fever. Your differential diagnosis includes all of the following EXCEPT:

   a. Pontine glioma
   b. Gradenigo's syndrome
   c. Parinaud's syndrome
   d. Duane's syndrome
   e. Benign sixth nerve palsy

3. A 16-year-old boy is hit in his right eye in a fight at school. On the phone, the school nurse gives a general description of the injury, which you speculate may be a blow-out fracture. Once the boy is in the ED, you are most likely to detect diplopia when you ask him to look in which of the following directions:

   a. Upward
   b. Downward and laterally
   c. Laterally
   d. Downward and medially
   e. Medially

4. A 2-year-old boy falls out of a shopping cart, hitting his head on the tile floor of the grocery store. He is brought by his mother to the ED 2 hours later with a left parietal scalp hematoma, Glasgow Coma Scale (GCS) score of 6, and bilateral 3 mm reactive pupils. While transporting the boy to the radiology department for a head CT after a rapid sequence induction and intubation, the neurosurgery resident detects the development of a complete left third nerve palsy. Examination of the eye shows:

   a. Eye positioned up and adducted with pupillary dilatation
   b. Eye positioned down and abducted with pupillary constriction
   c. Eye positioned up and abducted with pupillary dilatation
   d. Eye positioned down and abducted with pupillary dilatation
   e. Eye positioned down and adducted with pupillary constriction

5. A healthy 3-month-old girl is brought to the ED for evaluation of "crossed eyes" by her concerned parents, who ask for a referral to ophthalmology. The infant has a flat, broad nasal bridge with prominent epicanthal folds. You perform the Hirschberg corneal light reflex test, which centers the light reflex in both eyes. You explain to the parents:

   a. The child will be seen immediately by the ophthalmology service
   b. The child will need to begin a daily routine of eye patching
   c. Corrective eye muscle surgery successfully treats this condition
   d. A routine consult to ophthalmology has been requested
   e. The examination is normal; ophthalmology referral is not necessary

6. A 2-year-old boy is brought into the resuscitation room for evaluation of obtundation and vomiting. There is no history of trauma. The patient scores 6 on the pediatric GCS. Funduscopic examination reveals bilateral papilledema. You perform the doll's-eyes maneuver (oculocephalic reflex), which you are asked to explain en route to the CT suite after a rapid sequence induction and intubation. All of the following statements about the doll's-eyes maneuver are correct, EXCEPT:

a. The maneuver tests the integrity of cranial nerves III, VI, and VIII

b. The maneuver is abnormal if the eyes move opposite to the direction of the head

c. An abnormal response is suggestive of a destructive pontine-midbrain lesion

d. Ice water calorics (oculovestibular reflex) ascertain the same information

e. A normal response may be abolished by barbiturate poisoning

7. A 3-year-old boy is brought to the ED for evaluation of an outward drift of his left eye, especially when he is tired. After a careful eye examination, you recommend referral to a pediatric ophthalmologist. In your differential diagnosis of exodeviations, you include all of the following, EXCEPT:

a. Intermittent exotropia
b. Orbital tumor
c. Hyperthyroidism
d. Möbius's syndrome
e. Orbital cellulitis

ANSWERS

1. b   The fourth cranial nerve is the only ocular cranial nerve that completely decussates and has a dorsal projection over the midbrain. It also has the longest intracranial course of the ocular cranial nerves. These anatomical features renders the fourth cranial nerve especially vulnerable to head trauma.

2. c   The sixth cranial nerve innervates the ipsilateral lateral rectus muscle that turns the eye laterally. Its intracranial course renders it vulnerable to vascular or neoplastic changes in the midbrain (pontine glioma), increased intracranial pressure (e.g., head trauma), anterior midline craniofacial tumors, otitis media and petrositis (Gradenigo's syndrome), and cavernous sinus abnormalities. Duane's syndrome is a congenital condition that affects ipsilateral eye abduction. A benign sixth nerve palsy, painless and acquired in children, is frequently preceded by a febrile illness or URI. It may be recurrent, but it usually resolves completely. Parinaud's syndrome is a palsy of vertical gaze, either isolated (producing impaired conjugate upward eye movement) or associated with pupillary or nuclear oculomotor (third cranial nerve) paresis. It indicates a lesion that exerts pressure on the mesencephalic tegmentum, typically tumors of the pineal gland or third ventricle.

3. a   Blow-out fractures usually involve the weakest portion of the orbit, the floor. If the inferior rectus muscle is entrapped within the fracture, upward gaze is impaired. The eye may also occasionally have limitation of movement in the direction of the fracture. All patients with orbital fractures must receive a complete ophthalmic examination in order to detect possible accompanying ocular injury. Orbital fractures rarely involve the lateral wall. Fractures of the superior wall may allow communication inside the cranial cavity.

4. d   A complete third nerve palsy is characterized by an eye that is positioned down (due to the unopposed action of the superior oblique muscle) and abducted (due to the unopposed action of the lateral rectus muscle). There is associated ipsilateral ptosis and pupillary dilatation. The findings are explained by compression of the third nerve due to temporal lobe (uncal) herniation through the hiatus of the tentorium.

5. e   Pseudostrabismus (pseudoesotropia) is one of the most common reasons for infant referral to a pediatric ophthalmologist. The observer is given a false impression of convergent deviation of the eyes due to the broad, flat nasal bridge and prominent epicanthal folds of infants that obscure more white sclera nasally than temporally. Pseudostrabismus is differentiated from true misalignment (strabismus) of the eyes when the Hirschberg corneal light reflex test is centered in both eyes and no refixation movement

occurs in the cover–uncover test. If strabismus is present, the reflected corneal light reflex is asymmetric, appearing offcenter in one eye.

6. b   The doll's-eyes maneuver is normal if the eyes move in the orbits in the direction opposite to the rotating head, maintaining their position relative to the environment. Absence or asymmetry of eye movements constitute an abnormal doll's-eyes maneuver. If there is any question of cervical spine injury, the doll's-eyes maneuver should not be performed.

7. d   Möbius's syndrome is characterized by congenital facial paresis and defective abduction (producing esotropia), which may be unilateral or bilateral. All other conditions are associated with exotropia. This patient likely has intermittent exotropia, the most common exodeviation in childhood, which has a typical onset between age 6 months and 4 years. The outward drift of one eye occurs when the child is fixating at distance and is more frequent during periods of fatigue or illness. Eye muscle surgery may be performed based on the amount and frequency of the deviation.

CHAPTER 26

Eye—Unequal Pupils

MARK E. RALSTON, M.D., M.P.H.

QUESTIONS

1. A 17-year-old girl is brought to the ED with a concern that her pupils are unequal in size. She is completely asymptomatic and has no current or past medical problems. Right and left pupils measure 4.0 mm and 5.5 mm, respectively, and constrict equally to light both directly and consensually. Relative difference in pupillary size does not change in dim versus bright light. You reassure the patient that approximately _____ % of the population has a normal variation in pupillary size exceeding _____ mm.

   a. 50, 1
   b. 20, 0.4
   c. 20, 0.2
   d. 10, 1
   e. 10, 0.4

2. The pupillary dilatation, or "blown pupil," which the boy in Question 4 (Chapter 25) developed, is specifically due to impairment of:

   a. Ipsilateral optic nerve
   b. Ipsilateral parasympathetic fibers
   c. Contralateral optic tract
   d. Contralateral fourth cranial nerve
   e. Ipsilateral sympathetic fibers

3. A 12-month-old boy is brought to the ED after his mother discovers a hard, nontender mass on the left side of his neck. Skin examination reveals several firm, blue-tinged subcutaneous nodules resembling blueberry muffins. You detect miosis, ptosis, and mild enophthalmos of the left eye. You are concerned about a lesion in:

   a. Orbit
   b. Parasympathetic preganglionic fibers
   c. Lung apex
   d. Cervical sympathetic ganglion
   e. Thoracic duct

4. You could confirm the ophthalmic diagnosis of the boy in Question 3 by instillation of 1–2 drops of 4% cocaine into each eye with the following result:

   a. Miotic pupil dilates within 20–45 minutes; normal pupil constricts within 20–45 minutes
   b. Miotic pupil fails to dilate; normal pupil dilates within 20–45 minutes
   c. Miotic pupil fails to dilate; normal pupil constricts within 20–45 minutes
   d. Miotic pupil dilates within 20–45 minutes; normal pupil fails to dilate
   e. Miotic pupil constricts further within 20–45 minutes; normal pupil fails to dilate

5. The most common cause of a dilated nonreactive pupil in children is:

   a. Transtentorial herniation
   b. Internal ophthalmoplegia secondary to central or peripheral lesion
   c. Tonic pupil
   d. Iridoplegia secondary to ocular trauma
   e. Pharmacologic blockade

6. You detect a Marcus Gunn pupil in a 2-year-old girl with paralytic strabismus and amblyopia who is brought to the ED for evaluation of fever. On rounds you are asked about the cause of the patient's pupillary sign. All of the following statements about the Marcus Gunn pupil sign are correct, EXCEPT:

   a. The sign indicates an asymmetric, prechiasmatic, afferent conduction defect
   b. The sign is associated with a "jaw-winking" phenomenon
   c. Bright light presented to the normal eye causes both pupils to constrict
   d. The sign is a sensitive indicator of optic nerve and retinal disease
   e. Bright light presented to the affected eye causes both pupils to dilate

7. An 8-year-old boy is poked by a stick in his right eye at school. In the ED, you observe a ruptured globe and an eccentrically placed, teardrop-shaped pupil. You immediately consult ophthalmology for further management. Causes of pupillary distortion and displacement in children include all of the following, EXCEPT:

a. Wilson's disease
b. Iris prolapse
c. Iris tear
d. Persistent pupillary membrane
e. Synechiae

ANSWERS

1. b Physiologic anisocoria is the condition featured in this patient. If pupils are abnormally asymmetric in size, the larger pupil is abnormal if the relative difference in size increases in bright light (larger pupil constricts defectively), but the smaller pupil is abnormal if the relative difference increases in dim light (smaller pupil dilates defectively).

2. b The pupillary dilatation observed in the uncal (transtentorial) herniation syndrome is caused by compression of postganglionic parasympathetic fibers that are carried on the surface of the third nerve and innervate the sphincter pupillae muscle. As the parasympathetic fibers become compressed and impaired, ptosis develops (due to dysfunction of the levator palpebrae muscle of the upper eyelid) and the pupil dilates and becomes nonreactive (due to unopposed action of postganglionic sympathetic fibers innervating the dilator pupillae muscle).

3. d Horner's syndrome (miosis, ptosis, anhidrosis) results from interruption of sympathetic fibers and may be a presenting sign of tumor in the cervical region, particularly neuroblastoma (e.g., arising from a cervical sympathetic ganglion). The subcutaneous "blueberry muffin" nodules are characteristic of metastatic neuroblastoma.

4. b Cocaine prevents norepinephrine reuptake at the terminal myoneural junction of the dilator pupillae muscle that is innervated by sympathetic postganglionic fibers. Pupillary dilatation caused by the direct effect of norepinephrine is a normal response to cocaine. Failure of the miotic pupil to dilate in response to cocaine implies interruption of normal sympathetic innervation and is diagnostic of Horner's syndrome.

5. e All are causes of a dilated nonreactive pupil. Pharmacologic blockade, particularly by purposeful or accidental instillation of a cycloplegic agent (e.g., atropine and related agents), represents the most common cause in children. Instillation of 1–2 drops of 0.5–1% pilocarpine (cholinergic agent) will differentiate neurologic iridoplegia from pharmacologic blockade. Pilocarpine will cause constriction of the pupil within minutes in the case of neurologic iridoplegia, but it has no effect on the pupil dilated with atropine. Tonic pupil (Adie's pupil) is a dilated pupil that constricts slowly to light and accommodation, then redilates in a slow, tonic fashion. Tonic pupil is usually unilateral and is the result of cholinergic supersensitivity following postganglionic denervation and imperfect renervation of the sphincter pupillae muscle. One drop of dilute (0.125%) pilocarpine will cause brisk pupillary constriction. Primary causes of tonic pupil in children are infectious processes (predominantly viral syndromes) and trauma.

6. b The Marcus Gunn pupil sign is not to be confused with the Marcus Gunn "jaw-winking" phenomenon, which is characterized by paradoxical retraction of a ptotic lid evoked by jaw movement.

7. a Dyscoria (abnormal pupillary shape) and correctopia (abnormal pupillary position) occur frequently as a result of ocular trauma and may be signs of iris prolapse in perforating injuries or tears of the iris. Synechiae are adhesions of the iris to either the lens or cornea. In some cases of persistent pupillary membrane, dense remnant strands of tissue traverse and distort the pupil. The classic ophthalmic sign in Wilson's disease is the Kayser-Fleischer ring, which is a golden brown ring in the peripheral cornea resulting from copper accumulation in Descemet's membrane.

CHAPTER 27

Eye—Visual Disturbances

MARK E. RALSTON, M.D., M.P.H.

QUESTIONS

1. A 16-year-old girl with previously normal vision is evaluated in the ED for sudden blurring of her vision. Examination reveals no evidence of trauma. Ocular movements are intact, but you detect diplopia on direct confrontation of her right eye (left eye completely covered). You suspect:

   a. Orbital cellulitis
   b. Hysterical reaction
   c. Ophthalmoplegic migraine
   d. Brain tumor
   e. Herpes zoster

2. A 9-year-old baseball player is hit in his left eye with a baseball. Ocular examination in the ED reveals a hyphema and lens dislocation. Late complications of this injury include all of the following, EXCEPT:

   a. Glaucoma
   b. Commotio retinae
   c. Optic atrophy
   d. Retinal detachment
   e. Cataract

3. In the United States, the most common corneal infection causing permanent visual impairment is due to:

   a. *Neisseria gonorrhea*
   b. Herpes zoster
   c. *Chlamydia trachomatis*
   d. Herpes simplex
   e. Fungal infection

4. A 10-year-old boy is brought to the ED for evaluation of sudden-onset pain, redness, increased tearing, blurring of vision, and photophobia in his right eye. He suffers from recurrent episodes of arthritis, mostly involving the hip girdle and sacroiliac joints. You perform a thorough slit lamp examination, expecting to find all of the following, EXCEPT:

   a. Retinal neovascularization
   b. Iris congestion
   c. Ciliary flush
   d. Aqueous humor "flare"
   e. Keratic precipitates

5. A 2-year-old boy has rubbed his eyes with a solution that you determine to be a caustic alkali. Your management should include all of the following, EXCEPT:

   a. Irrigate eyes with copious quantities of tepid water or saline after topical anesthesia
   b. Irrigate until symptom relief and normalization of tear pH (near pH 7)
   c. Instill a neutralizing solution to achieve a tear pH of 7
   d. Perform a fluorescein examination of each eye after irrigation is complete
   e. Refer the boy to an ophthalmologist if you find serious conjunctival or corneal injury

6. A 17-year-old African-American girl develops sudden, painless loss of vision in her left eye. Direct ophthalmoscopic examination reveals a cherry-red fovea, pale white optic disc, and marked arterial narrowing. Pupillary evaluation demonstrates an afferent pupillary defect (Marcus-Gunn pupil). The differential diagnosis of this condition includes all of the following, EXCEPT:

   a. Migraine
   b. Sickle cell hemoglobinopathy
   c. Subacute bacterial endocarditis
   d. Retinitis pigmentosa
   e. Systemic lupus erythematosus

7. A 16-year-old soccer player suffers a head injury with transient LOC at the scene. In the ED, the patient demonstrates total vision loss. Neurological examination (including funduscopic evaluation) is otherwise normal. A head CT shows no abnormalities. Regarding the blindness, you advise the parents:

   a. It may improve to light perception only over a period of days to weeks
   b. It is permanent
   c. It is usually due to a hysterical reaction
   d. It will require immediate intervention by an ophthalmologist
   e. It will resolve completely within minutes to hours

8. A 13-year-old girl sustains sudden deterioration of vision in her right eye. There is no history of trauma. In the ED, the fundus is partially obscured by blood clots that are visible within the vitreous humor. Your differential diagnosis for vitreous hemorrhage includes all of the following, EXCEPT:

   a. Diabetes mellitus
   b. Hypertension
   c. Leukemia
   d. Central retinal vein occlusion
   e. Carbon monoxide poisoning

9. An 18-year-old male with history of depression complains of visual haziness "like standing in a snowfield" approximately 30 hours after ingesting a solvent-containing wood alcohol. Funduscopic examination reveals optic disc hyperemia, venous engorgement, and papilledema. Anion and osmolar gaps are elevated. Therapy for this ingestion attempts to prevent blindness by blocking the production of which of the following:

   a. Formic acid
   b. Formaldehyde
   c. Alcohol dehydrogenase
   d. Aldehyde dehydrogenase
   e. Lactic acid

ANSWERS

1. b Sudden-onset monocular diplopia may result from lens dislocation or a defect in the media or macula. In most cases, no disease can be found to explain monocular diplopia and it usually signifies hysteria. Orbital cellulitis, ophthalmoplegic migraine, tumor, and herpes zoster may cause external ophthalmoplegia (paralysis of individual ocular muscles) that results in binocular diplopia.

2. b Commotio retinae, or retinal edema, is a relatively early complication (usually occurring within 24 hours) following blunt ocular trauma. Traumatic cataracts form usually within days of injury, but onset may be delayed for years.

3. d Worldwide, trachoma (*Chlamydia trachomatis*) is the most frequent corneal infection causing permanent visual impairment. A thorough slit lamp examination will reveal the characteristic dendritic ulcers of herpes simplex on a fluorescein-stained cornea. Steroid-containing eye medications should not be used unless herpes simplex has been excluded in a patient presenting with a red eye. Consider recurrent herpes infection in the red eye of a patient with previous herpes simplex keratitis.

4. a Acute anterior uveitis, caused by juvenile rheumatoid arthritis (pauciarticular type II) in this patient, is often obscure. Other etiologies include trauma, Kawasaki disease, sarcoidosis, corneal abrasion, foreign body, herpetic keratitis, and bacterial or fungal corneal ulcer. Signs of anterior uveitis include conjunctival hyperemia particularly in the perilimbal region (ciliary flush), inflammatory deposits on the posterior surface of the cornea (keratic precipitates, or KP), cells and protein ("flare") in the aqueous humor, iris congestion, and, sometimes, neovascularization of the iris (not retinal neovascularization). In posterior uveitis, eye pain and photophobia may be less severe, but visual impairment may be more pronounced compared with anterior uveitis. The two most common causes of posterior uveitis in children are toxoplasmosis and toxocariasis.

5. c Use of neutralizing solutions is not recommended.

6. d Causes of retinal artery occlusion include systemic lupus erythematosis (non-infective emboli), subacute bacterial endocarditis (infective emboli), sickle cell hemoglobinopathy (emboli of sickled RBC, hemolyzed RBC debris, blood coagulants, or bone marrow), and migraine (arterial spasm). The extent of visual loss varies depending on involvement of the central retinal artery (total loss) or branch occlusion (visual field defect). Retinal artery occlusion is an absolute ophthalmologic emergency necessitating immediate ophthalmologic consultation. Visual symptoms characteristic of optic neuritis (e.g., due to multiple sclerosis) include pain on eye movement, diplopia, disturbance of color vision, gradual blurring of vision, and sudden visual loss. Retinitis pigmentosa is a progressive retinal degenerative condition typically involving impairment of night vision and gradual loss of peripheral vision.

7. e Cortical blindness due to injury to the visual cortex of the brain has been observed even in the setting of trivial head trauma. It may involve total loss of vision and is often associated with an otherwise normal physical examination. The entire course is usually brief, with full restoration of vision within minutes to hours.

8. e The multiple causes of vitreous hemorrhage include penetrating or blunt trauma, diabetes mellitus, hypertension, sickle cell disease, leukemia, retinal tear, retinoblastoma, central retinal occlusion, persistent hyperplastic primary vitreous, and familial exudative vitreoretinopathy. Carbon monoxide poisoning may cause visual loss but is not associated with vitreous hemorrhage.

9. a Methanol (wood alcohol) is commonly found in many solvents, paint removers, windshield washing solutions, and duplicating fluids. Its metabolic products may cause metabolic acidosis, blindness, and death after a characteristic latent period of 6–30 hours. Methanol is metabolized first to formaldehyde by alcohol dehydrogenase, then to formic acid by aldehyde dehydrogenase. Blindness is caused primarily by formic acid.

CHAPTER 28

Fever

BEMA K. BONSU, MBChB, M.D.

QUESTIONS

1. A 3-week-old male infant is brought to your ED with a 2-day history of fever. He was born by uncomplicated spontaneous vaginal delivery at 37 weeks gestation following a normal pregnancy. At his 2-week check-up he was noted to be gaining weight appropriately. His vital signs are: T 38.9°C, HR 140, RR 40, and BP 90/60. The patient is sleepy but arousable. His left tympanic membrane appears slightly dull and his neck is supple, without signs of meningeal irritation. His peripheral WBC is 16,000. His urinalysis shows 3 leukocytes per high-power field (hpf). Blood and urine cultures were obtained. Your management at this point should consist of:

   a. Discharge on antipyretics with close follow-up
   b. Discharge on oral amoxicillin with close follow-up
   c. Lumbar puncture and admission for parenteral antibiotics
   d. CXR to rule out pneumonia
   e. Stool for analysis and culture, and outpatient follow-up

2. A 19-month-old boy is brought to your ED with a 3-day history of fever associated with a runny nose. He appears well. His temperature by infrared tympanic thermometry is 39.8°C. His chest is clear to auscultation, his abdomen is soft, and he is circumcised. No bacterial source can be found for his fever. A CBC reveals a WBC of 8200, with a manual differential of 60% neutrophils and 27% bands. A blood culture is sent to the laboratory. Appropriate management at this point will be to:

   a. Obtain a urine sample
   b. Administer IM ceftriaxone
   c. Perform a lumbar puncture
   d. Obtain a CXR
   e. Discharge on antipyretics

3. A 3-year-old boy is brought to your ED following a brief generalized seizure. He has been developing normally and this is his first seizure. He developed a runny nose on the day of his admission. He appeared playful just prior to his seizure. His temperature on arrival is 39.5°C. After being observed in the ED for about 45 minutes the patient starts to arouse. He appears fussy, but is consolable. No focal neurologic deficits can be found. He resists all attempts to examine him so that meningeal signs cannot be adequately assessed. The appropriate next step is to:

   a. Repeat the examination in 1 hour
   b. Perform a lumbar puncture
   c. Load the patient with phenytoin 20 mg/kg
   d. Order a CT scan of the patient's head
   e. Obtain a CBC and blood culture

4. A 7-week-old girl is referred in to your ED for evaluation of a rectal temperature of 39.2°C. She has no bacterial source of infection on physical examination. Her urinalysis is negative, her peripheral WBC is 9000, with 70% neutrophils, 28% lymphocytes, and 2% bands, and her lumbar puncture reveals a leukocyte count of 8 cells/mm³. Blood, urine, and CSF cultures are sent to the laboratory. Acceptable options for the management of this child would include any one of the following, EXCEPT:

   a. IM ceftriaxone in the ED
   b. Admission to the hospital for IV antibiotics
   c. Discharge with follow-up in 24 hours
   d. Admission to the hospital for observation
   e. Discharge on amoxicillin

5. A 9-month-old boy has a 3-day history of fever and rhinorrhea, followed by increasing work of breathing and tachypnea. On exam his eyes are closed and he is drinking a bottle of formula. His axillary temperature is 39.2°C, and his RR is 60, but is taking a bottle comfortably. His O$_2$ saturation on room air is 96%. He has mild intercostal recessions, but is not flaring or grunting. He has copious rhinorrhea and a staccato cough. On examination of his chest, you note prolonged expiration with end expiratory wheezes. Dipstick of the urine is negative. Your initial management should be to:

   a. Obtain a CBC and blood culture
   b. Administer nebulized albuterol and oral steroids
   c. Discharge on antipyretics
   d. Catheterize the patient for urine and send for culture
   e. Obtain a lateral neck radiograph

6. A 9-month-old boy returns to the ED 24 hours after evaluation for fever. He has been ill for 3 days with high spiking fevers. At his first visit he received 15 mg/kg of amoxicillin orally for an "early left otitis media" and was discharged on the same medication (45 mg/kg/day given three times per day). He was also started on oral acetaminophen at 10 mg/kg per dose every 6 hours. He now presents with increasing fussiness. On examination his temperature is 38.7°C. He appears irritable and tired, grunts occasionally, and fusses more when his mother picks him up. His left ear is slightly erythematous, but it insufflates well. He has no nuchal rigidity and Kernig's and Brudzinski's signs are negative. His chest is clear to auscultation and his abdomen is soft. Your next step in management should be to:

   a. Discharge on an increased dose of amoxicillin at 80 mg/kg/day
   b. Administer antipyrine/benzocaine (Auralgan) to his left auditory canal
   c. Increase acetaminophen to 15 mg/kg per dose
   d. Perform lumbar puncture
   e. Obtain a blood culture and discharge on amoxicillin-clavulanate

7. A mother comes to your ED over the winter months stating that her 2-month-old daughter "feels warm to touch." She did not take her temperature but remembers that she was advised to seek medical evaluation whenever her baby developed a fever. The baby is wrapped up in four blankets and feels warm to touch. Axillary temperature at triage prior to unbundling the baby is 38.1°C. You unbundle the baby and after 3 minutes obtain a rectal temperature of 37.9°C. The baby appears well and is nursing comfortably. She has a diaper rash, but her exam is otherwise unrevealing. Your next step is:

   a. To obtain a screening CBC and urinalysis
   b. To observe the infant in the ED and verify normothermia after 1 hour
   c. To do a full sepsis work-up (CBC, blood culture, urinalysis, urine culture, and spinal tap)
   d. To give an antipyretic and verify normothermia two more times before discharge
   e. To evaluate for Münchausen's syndrome by proxy

8. Five days into treatment for chickenpox (varicella), a 3-year-old girl develops a high spiking fever to 40°C. On physical examination she does not appear to be in distress and is breathing comfortably. A few of her lesions are beginning to scab, but none appears infected. A thorough examination of her extremities and vertebrae reveals no tenderness to palpation or motion. Her abdomen is soft and you find no source for her fever on completing your examination. Her peripheral WBC is 11,500/mm^3, and her sedimentation rate (ESR) is 21. As the treating ED physician you determine that the test most likely to identify the source of her fever is:

   a. A bone scan
   b. Blood culture
   c. Urine culture
   d. Spinal tap
   e. CXR

9. A 12-year-old boy is brought to the ED with a fever. On exam he is febrile to 41.5°C. He has been taking "a lot" of Excedrin-PM (methapyrilene) tablets frequently for a severe headache that developed earlier that day. He is slightly delirious and his skin is hot and dry. His throat is red and parched. He has not voided in about 12 hours. He does not appear to have an intercurrent illness. Your management at this time includes all the following, EXCEPT:

   a. Cooling blankets
   b. Throat cultures
   c. Gastric lavage
   d. Activated charcoal
   e. Physostigmine

10. A 19-day-old previously healthy neonate develops bloody stools associated with fever to 39°C. She continues to feed well and has had no emesis. Her mother denies any rashes or URI symptoms. She has not been "gassy," and has not been treated recently with an antibiotic. Her rectal temperature is 39.2°C. She appears well. Her abdomen is soft, nondistended, and nontender. Careful examination of her anus reveals no fissures or abrasions. An acute abdominal series shows a few fluid-filled loops of bowel, but no evidence of obstruction. Stool is guaiac positive and reveals leukocytes. Your next step should be:

    a. Obtain stool and blood cultures
    b. Change the child's formula to one that is soy based
    c. Obtain a surgical consult
    d. Discharge on acetaminophen and iron
    e. Send stool for *Clostridium difficile* culture

11. On a busy night in December, a 19-month-old Asian-American child is brought to your ED with fever and a transient papular rash. It is well past her bedtime and she has been crying. Two hours later, as she is led to an examining room, her nurse notices a diffuse petechial rash on her face and neck that was not present when she was initially brought to the ED. Her temperature is 39°C, HR 100, and BP 98/65. You are called to evaluate this child. She appears tired but is not toxic in appearance. She is minimally fussy but smiles when you make funny faces at her. Both tympanic membranes are slightly red, but insufflate well. There are no skin lesions elsewhere and she has no other source for her fever. Your most appropriate next step would be to:

    a. Discharge with close follow-up
    b. Obtain a CBC and blood culture while observing in the ED for 1–2 hours
    c. Perform a lumbar puncture and start IV ceftriaxone pending laboratory results
    d. Discharge on oral amoxicillin
    e. Check for hyponatremia

12. On day 7 of life a neonate is brought to your ED with fevers to 38.8°C and lethargy. Over the last 24 hours he has been feeding poorly. On examination you notice a few vesicles on his scalp at the site where scalp electrodes were placed during labor. His 19-year-old mother did not have any antenatal visits. Your next step is to:

    a. Prescribe topical mupirocin
    b. Prescribe oral cephalexin
    c. Discharge with close follow-up
    d. Initiate IV acyclovir
    e. Initiate IV ampicillin and gentamicin

13. A 22-month-old boy is brought to the ED with a 2-day history of fever to 38.9°C and drooling. You notice on examination that he tilts his head to the left and resists attempts to move his head to the midline. His mother states that he fell off the couch a week before presentation, cried for about 10 minutes, but seemed well thereafter. Examination reveals a slightly ill-appearing child who is drooling and has torticollis. His pharynx is mildly erythematous but is otherwise without abnormality. His examination reveals no other findings. The most likely diagnosis is:

    a. Rotatory subluxation
    b. Peritonsillar abscess
    c. Meningitis
    d. Retropharyngeal abscess
    e. Benign muscular torticollis

14. A fair-skinned 9-year-old boy is brought by ambulance to your ED delirious and with a fever to 42°C. He has been out playing baseball on a hot summer afternoon. He developed a mild upper respiratory illness 1 day prior to his presentation. On examination he is obtunded and twitching occasionally. His blood pressure is 80/60 and his skin is hot and dry. He appears to have weakness on the right side of his body. The most important step in initial management is giving:

    a. Oral acetaminophen
    b. Oral ibuprofen
    c. IV ceftriaxone
    d. Ice water baths
    e. IV ketoralac

15. A 2-year-old Caucasian girl is brought to the ED for high-grade fevers for 6 days. She has been exposed to an adult with streptococcal pharyngitis within the last 3 days. She has a faint maculopapular rash. She refuses to walk and appears to have swollen hands and feet. She has conjunctival injection and a markedly inflamed oral cavity. Her CBC reveals a hematocrit of 39, WBC of 14,000, and a platelet count of 510,000. Her urinalysis reveals numerous leukocytes. Your next step is:

    a. IM penicillin
    b. IV immunoglobulin
    c. Bone scan
    d. IV oxacillin
    e. IV ampicillin and gentamicin

16. A 3-year-old girl is brought to the ED with a maculopapular rash. She has had low-grade fevers to 38.4°C for 4 days and an increasingly severe cough. Her rash started on her face but has progressed to her torso. Following the appearance of her rash, her temperatures have increased to 40°C. Her conjunctivae are injected and her pharynx is erythematous. Her parents have been without medical insurance since she was about 10 months of age. You diagnose:

    a. Roseola infantum
    b. Erythema infectiosum
    c. Rubeola
    d. Rocky Mountain spotted fever (RMSF)
    e. Meningococemia

17. A 4-year-old boy who lives in the south-central United States is brought to the ED with fever and rash for about 24 hours duration. His rash started as a macular eruption on his wrists and ankles but has progressed proximally and has become petechial in nature. He is toxic in appearance and is very irritable to your exam. Temperature is 39.8°C, HR 124, RR 20, and BP 100/60. Laboratory tests reveal the following results: Peripheral WBC of 13,000, platelet count of 130,000, hematocrit 41, Na 129, K 4.1, Cl 101, HCO_3 19, PT 11.1, and PTT 21. Your next step in management is to:

    a. Consult hematology
    b. Administer IV tetracycline
    c. Administer IV steroids
    d. Administer IV chloramphenicol
    e. Administer IV immunoglobulin

18. You call a 13-month-old child back to the ED 24 hours after fever evaluation because of a positive blood culture (*S. pneumoniae*). His peripheral white count was 16,000 at the first ED encounter. Following that visit he was discharged on amoxicillin (80 mg/kg/day) for otitis media. On arrival, the patient has a temperature of 38.8°C and appears ill. Your management includes:

    a. No further tests; discharge on amoxicillin and antipyretics
    b. Repeat blood culture and discharge on amoxicillin and antipyretics
    c. Spinal tap and repeat blood culture; discharge on amoxicillin for 10 days if spinal fluid is normal
    d. Spinal tap, CXR, and repeat blood culture; admit for parenteral antibiotics
    e. Repeat CBC and administer ceftriaxone if the WBC is greater than 15,000

19. An 18-month-old girl is brought to the ED with high-grade fevers and refusal to eat. Her temperature has been as high as 40°C, and she is drooling. On examination her gums are inflamed and she has shallow ulcers on her gums, the tip of her tongue, and buccal mucosa. She has no lesions on her tonsillar pillars or posterior pharynx. She has markedly tender anterior cervical lymph nodes. You diagnose:

    a. Herpangina
    b. Aphthous ulcers
    c. Acute necrotizing ulcerative gingivitis (ANUG)
    d. Acute herpetic gingivostomatitis
    e. Stevens-Johnson syndrome

20. A 17-year-old boy complains of high fevers, diarrhea, and dizziness. He was involved in a motor vehicle accident 3 days previously and sustained a nasal fracture and septal hematoma. The hematoma was drained and his nose was packed to prevent recurrence of the hematoma. On examination the patient still has the nasal pack in place. He has some periorbital ecchymosis around his left eye. He appears severely ill. His temperature is 39.2°C, BP 80/50, HR 130, RR 18, and capillary refill time is 4 seconds. His exam is otherwise unremarkable. Your next step is to:

    a. Give a 20 ml/kg bolus of NS and discharge
    b. Remove the packing, start IV fluids, and admit for IV oxacillin
    c. Send stool for culture, rehydrate, and admit for observation
    d. Head CT to rule out an intracranial abscess
    e. Blood culture and admission for IV ampicillin

21. A 5-year-old boy with asthma is brought to the ED in severe distress and with a fever to 38.2°C. You obtain a CXR that shows right middle lobe atelectasis. He appears to be tiring out, so you decide to intubate him. After preoxygenating him, you perform a rapid-sequence intubation with succinylcholine and thiopental. Fifteen minutes after intubating this patient he develops a temperature of 42°C. Your next step is to administer:

    a. IV ketorolac and sponge down with cold water
    b. Rectal acetaminophen and sponge down with cold water
    c. A defasciculating dose of pancuronium and sponge down with cold water
    d. IV dantrolene and sponge down with cold water
    e. IV phenytoin and sponge down with cold water

22. The 6-year-old daughter of Nigerian immigrants visited her extended family for a month in Lagos (West Africa) for the first time. Within 2 weeks of her return to the United States she develops a high spiking fever with severe prostration. She has no past medical history and does not have sickle cell disease. She denies URI or GI symptoms. She complains of headaches and myalgias but denies URI symptoms. Her stools are soft but neither bloody nor watery. Her vital signs are: T 40°C, HR 120, RR 20, and BP 110/90. She has no neck stiffness and is able to flex and extend her neck fully. Kernig's sign is negative. Her tympanic membranes and throat are unremarkable. Chest is clear and her abdomen is soft and nontender. The rest of her physical examination is unrevealing. Your next step is to:

a. Discharge on antipyretics
b. Perform a lumbar puncture
c. Obtain blood for smear and Giemsa staining
d. Check her stools for parasites
e. Obtain blood culture

ANSWERS

1. c   The current standard of care for febrile infants less than 1 month of age is based more on consensus than on "hard" evidence. The initial evaluation consists of a blood culture, urine culture, and spinal fluid culture. Stool culture and CXR are obtained only if the patient has watery stools or respiratory symptoms, respectively. A normal physical exam, a minor source of infection (e.g., an ear infection), and/or normal screening tests (CBC and urinalysis) do not rule out serious bacterial infection. Young infants are admitted for parenteral antibiotics effective against gram-negative enteric rods and group B *Streptococcus*. Coverage for *Listeria monocytogenes* (ampicillin) is recommended where the risk for infection by this organism is relatively high (e.g., in high prevalence areas, in premature babies, and in neonates less than 1 week of age). After 1 week of life, *Listeria* almost invariably presents as meningitis. The lowest CSF cell count recorded in three of the largest series of infants (48 total cases) with *Listeria* meningitis was 80 white cells per mm^3. Thus the risk of *Listeria* infection may be low if preliminary CSF analysis in a neonate older than 1–2 weeks does not show pleocytosis. There has been a decline in human listeriosis in the United States, and Sadow et al. have more recently proposed eliminating ampicillin from the antibiotic regimen for neonatal sepsis in areas of low *Listeria* prevalence, for patients who are 15 days or older, and in patients without a CSF pleocytosis. (Tappero JW, Schuchat A, Deaver KA, et al. Reduction in the incidence of human listerosis in the United States. JAMA 1995;273:1118–1122. Kessler KL, Dajani AS. *Listeria* meningitis in infants and children. Ped Inf Dis J 1990;9(1):61–63. Visintine AM, Oleske JM, Nahmias AJ. *Listeria monocytogenes* infection in infants and children. Am J Dis Child 1977;131:393–397. Lavetter A, Leedom JM, Mathies AW, et al. Meningitis due to *Listeria monocytogenes*. A review of 25 cases. N Engl J Med 1971;285:598–603. Sadow KB, Derr R, Teach SJ. Bacterial infections in infants 60 days and younger. Epidemiology, resistance and implications for treatment. Arch Pediatr Adolesc Med. 1999;153:611–614.)

2. e   A 19-month-old boy who is circumcised is at extremely low risk for a urinary tract infection. A peripheral WBC of 15,000 cells/mm^3 stratifies young children into risk categories for occult bacteremia. Febrile children 3–36 months of age with a temperature of 39°C or greater and a peripheral WBC above 15,000 cells/mm^3 have a 1 in 20 chance of having *S. pneumoniae* bacteremia. A high percentage of bands on peripheral blood smear as an isolated finding is not a good discriminator between patients with or without bacteremia. In addition there is a significant amount of interobserver variability when bands are counted manually, making such counts less useful. A high absolute neutrophil count (greater than 10,000) may be a more specific indicator of bacteremia than a high peripheral WBC (15,000 cells/mm^3). Lumbar puncture and CXRs are not indicated in the absence of suggestive toxicity, irritability, or respi-

ratory symptoms. (Lee GM, Harper MB. Risk of bacteremia for febrile young children in the post-*Haemophilus influenzae* type b era. Arch Pediatr Adolesc Med 1998;152:624–628. Kuppermann N, Fleisher GR, Jaffe DM. Predictors of occult pneumococcal bacteremia in young febrile children. Ann Emerg Med 1998;31(6):679–687. Jaffe DM, Fleisher GR. Temperature and total white blood cell count as indicators of bacteremia. Pediatrics 1991;87(5):670–674.)

3. a The description of this child's seizure meets criteria for a simple febrile seizure. It was single, brief, generalized, nonfocal, and followed a brief illness. It is not unusual for children to have a brief period of irritability when recovering from a febrile seizure; however, if this period of fussiness persists, a diagnosis of bacterial meningitis should be considered. Thus, the child in this vignette should not be discharged from the ED until a more adequate clinical assessment has been obtained. Such assessment may be aided by antipyretics. It should be noted that even though meningitis can present with febrile seizures, these seizures are usually atypical and would be unlikely in a child noted to be playful just prior to the seizure. Thus, immediate lumbar puncture, though acceptable in this patient, can probably be deferred for an hour or so, especially if doing so enables the physician to get a more thorough exam. A CT is not indicated in the absence of focal findings, and occult bacteremia evaluation (CBC and blood culture) is unlikely to be useful at 3 years of age. Phenytoin is not recommended for a first febrile seizure. (Al-Eissa YA. Lumbar puncture in the clinical evaluation of children with seizures associated with fever. Pediatr Emerg Care 1995;11(6):347–350.)

4. e Prior to 1992, the standard of care for children under 3 months of age with fever in most academic institutions was a full sepsis workup and hospital admission for parenteral antibiotics, pending culture results. Given the overall cost of inpatient admission, a number of researchers have developed criteria that identify children at low risk for serious or invasive bacterial infection who can be managed as outpatients. Baskin et al. have shown that children 1–3 months of age, who are well appearing and have normal urinalysis, CSF analysis, and a peripheral WBC less than 20,000 can be safely managed at home, provided they receive two doses of ceftriaxone 24 hours apart. Although this strategy excluded all patients with bacterial meningitis, it missed some infants with bacteremia or urinary tract infection (UTI). However, none of the infants with missed bacterial infections suffered an adverse outcome while on outpatient antibiotic treatment. Baker et al. used more stringent criteria and have identified infants at low risk who can be managed at home without antibiotics, as long as close follow-up is assured. The bottom line is, because no strategy is foolproof, no young infant should be discharged from the ED without firm plans for close follow-up. Oral amoxicillin is not acceptable and would not be adequate treatment in this age group. (Baskin M, O'Rourke EJ, Fleisher GR. Outpatient treatment of febrile infants 28–90 days of age with intramuscular administration of ceftriaxone. J Pediatr 1992;120(1):22–27. Baker MD, Bell LM, Avner JR. Outpatient management without antibiotics of fever in selected infants. N Eng J Med 1993;329:1437–1441.)

5. c The child in this vignette probably has bronchiolitis. Recent studies by Kupperman et al. and Greenes et al. have found that highly febrile children 3–36 months who have recognizable viral infections (e.g., bronchiolitis, croup, varicella, or stomatitis) are at low risk (as low as 0.2%) for occult bacteremia or urine infections (1.9% overall, but less in males). Thus, such children for the most part do not need to be routinely evaluated for occult bacteremia or UTI. Nebulized albuterol and steroids (by any route) have not been found to be useful in the management of bronchiolitis. Upper airway obstruction would present with stridor (not wheezing), thus making a lateral neck radiograph unnecessary. (Kuppermann N, Bank DE, Walton EA, Senac MO, Jr., McCaslin I. Risk for bacteremia and urinary tract infections in young febrile children with bronchiolitis. Arch Pediatr Adolesc Med. 1997;151(12):1207–1214. Greenes DS, Harper MB. Low risk of bacteremia in febrile children with recognizable viral syndromes. Pediatr Inf Dis J. 1999;18(3):258–61.)

6. d Paradoxical irritability, persistent irritability, and grunting in a young child recently treated with an antibiotic should always raise the possibility of a serious bacterial infection (e.g., bacterial meningitis). It is likely that this child has partially treated meningitis, even in the absence of meningismus, because such signs may be absent in younger infants. In comparing antibiotic-pretreated to untreated children Rothrock et al. showed that pretreated children had a lower frequency of altered mental status and fever (over 38.3°C noted in the treating facility), but had a higher frequency of vomiting. At diagnosis the frequency of fever (by history), seizures, and focal findings was similar between the two groups, as were clinically diagnostic findings such as Kernig's sign and nuchal rigidity. These researchers concluded that

the clinical presentation of bacterial meningitis for patients pretreated with antibiotics was less overt. It is unclear if this finding is secondary to the effect of antibiotics or is inherent to the type of bacterial meningitis (i.e., fulminant versus nonfulminant). Thus, all febrile children pretreated with antibiotics that present with persistent irritability, especially if such irritability is worsened (paradoxically) by efforts to console, should have a spinal tap unless the ED physician can justify not performing this procedure. The ear findings in this child are "soft" and should not dissuade the emergency physician from looking for more serious sources of infection. Furthermore, in a retrospective study Schutzman et al. have shown a similar rate of occult bacteremia in children with versus those without clinically diagnosed acute otitis media. There are no prospective studies validating these results, and it is unclear if a diagnostic bias (i.e., toward giving a diagnostic label such as otitis media in children with "fever without a source") may have explained these findings. (Rothrock SG, Green SM, et al. Pediatric bacterial meningitis: is prior antibiotic therapy associated with an altered clinical presentation? Ann Emerg Med 1992;21:146–152. Schutzman SA, Petrycki S, Fleisher GR. Bacteremia with otitis media. Pediatrics 1991;87:48–53.)

7. b   Fever measured at home by thermometer is more likely to be replicated in the ED when compared with that measured by touch. Infants who are overbundled at home may develop minimally elevated temperatures. If they appear completely well on arrival in the ED, they should have their temperature repeated a number of times while being observed. A well-appearing infant who is febrile by touch alone and is overbundled, but who is subsequently found to be afebrile (on repeated temperature measurements in the ED) can be discharged home safely, provided no antipyretic medications or interventions have been provided either at home or in the ED. Such children can be discharged to home with careful instructions to return if they become symptomatic (i.e., measured fever, lethargy, irritability, disturbed sleep, or poor feeding). Parents should be taught how to measure and interpret their child's temperature. If antipyretics have been provided by the caregiver or in the ED, a longer period of observation is warranted; conversely, the ED physician may be compelled to "bite the bullet" and perform a full sepsis evaluation. (Bonadio WA, Hegenbarth M, Zachariason M. Correlating reported fever in young infants with subsequent temperature patterns and rate of serious bacterial infections. Pediatr Infect Dis J 1990;9:158–160.)

8. b   Any child with chickenpox who has a recurrence of high fever (especially if fever occurs between days 4 and 6) without source may have bacteremia or focal infection from group A beta-hemolytic *Streptococcus* (GABHS). Several studies have reported a rise in the frequency and severity of GABHS, and Doctor et al. have more recently reported a sevenfold increase in the frequency of serious GABHS infection complicating primary varicella since 1993 at the Children's Hospital in Boston. Even though osteomyelitis, arthritis, and pneumonia are possibilities in this case, these complications should be clinically evident in a 3-year-old child. In addition, although the diagnosis of urinary tract infection should be considered in any young female child with a fever, the most parsimonious explanation for this child's fever would be an infectious complication of varicella such as GABHS bacteremia or focal infection. It should be noted that such bacteremia can occur without a clear focus in the skin, or without leukocytosis. (Doctor A, Harper MB, Fleisher GR. Group A beta-hemolytic streptococcal bacteremia: Historical overview, changing incidence, and recent association with varicella. Pediatrics 1995;96(3): 428–33. Cowan MR, Primm PA, Abramo TJ, Wiebe RA. Serious group A β-hemolytic streptococcal infections complicating varicella. Ann Emerg Med 1993;23:818–823.)

9. b   This child's presentation is consistent with central anticholinergic poisoning, probably secondary to methapyrilene in Excedrin. Although streptococcal pharyngitis is a possibility, it does not explain all the patient's symptoms. Unlike most toxic ingestions, in this case there is clear indication for delayed decontamination in anticholinergic toxicity because of the associated delayed gastric emptying. Gastric lavage and charcoal can be administered and may be effective up to 8 hours and 24 hours postingestion, respectively. Treatment for hyperpyrexia is indicated in this patient, and physostigmine (0.02 mg/kg) would reverse the effects of pure anticholinergic toxicity. It should not be given if cyclic antidepressant toxicity is suspected. (Toxicologic emergencies. In: Fleisher GR, Ludwig S, eds. *Textbook of Pediatric Emergency Medicine.* Kearney TE. "Physostigmine" in therapeutic drugs and antidotes. In: *Poisonings and Drug Overdose,* third edition. Olson KR, ed. Stamford, CT: Appleton & Lange, 1999:402–403.)

10. a   This neonate likely has *Salmonella* enterocolitis. *Salmonella* is responsible for more than 90% of bacterial enteritis in infants. In a study by Torrey et al., 6% of infants with *Salmonella* gastroenteritis devel-

oped bacteremia. Even though there is no clear evidence to suggest that antibiotic treatment of young infants with proven *Salmonella* enteritis or bacteremia prevents invasive disease, the current recommendation is to treat *Salmonella* bacteremia with appropriate antibiotics (i.e., ampicillin or amoxicillin for 5 days pending susceptibility testing). If *Salmonella* meningitis develops, treatment with a third-generation cephalosporin (ceftriaxone or cefotaxime) is recommended for a minimum of 4 weeks. Ampicillin, chloramphenicol, and treatment duration of less or equal to 3 weeks have all been associated with an increased frequency of relapse. Although an acute abdomen (e.g., malrotation with volvulus) is possible, the general condition of the child plus the negative radiographs (to a lesser extent) argue against this diagnosis. Formula intolerance is unlikely to present with an acute febrile illness and is usually associated with bloating and flatulence. *C. difficile* is a common commensal organism in young infants; therefore, its presence in the stool without corroborating evidence (e.g., antecedent antibiotic use) would be unlikely. (Infectious disease emergencies. In: Fleisher GR, Ludwig S, eds. *Textbook of Pediatric Emergency Medicine*, fourth edition. Torrey S, Fleisher GR, Jaffe D. Incidence of *Salmonella* bacteremia in infants with *Salmonella* gastroenteritis. J Peds 1986;108:718–721.)

11. b   The combination of fever and petechiae always raises the possibility of meningococcal bacteremia. Seven to 10% of hospitalized patients with fever and petechiae have been found to have meningococcemia. More recently, Mandl et al. have found that less than 1 in 50 children 3–36 months of age evaluated in an outpatient setting for fever and petechiae has bacteremia or sepsis, and about 1 in 200 has meningococcemia. Streptococcal pharyngitis was the most commonly associated bacterial infection in children over 18 months of age, presumably causing 26% of cases in this age group. The clinical appearance (toxic versus nontoxic) and peripheral WBC were found to be of discriminative value in terms of identifying patients at risk of serious bacterial infections. None of 357 well-appearing patients had serious invasive bacteremia (upper confidence limit 1%) versus 6 of 53 ill-appearing children, whereas all children with serious invasive bacteremia looked ill and had an abnormal CBC (greater than 15,000 or less than 5,000 white cells/mm^3). Furthermore, both children with meningococcemia had purpura. The child in this vignette probably has petechiae from crying (given her clinical appearance and the distribution of her rash). It would be prudent, however, to observe such a child in the ED for a few hours to rule out an evolving illness and to obtain a CBC and blood culture. A progressive rash, worsening toxicity, abnormal CBC, and/or abnormal coagulation profile (PT greater than 13.5) would increase the risk of impending or actual sepsis and argue for presumptive parenteral antibiotics and admission. In cases of unsuspected meningococcal disease (UMD), however, Kuppermann et al. demonstrated that the only hematological parameter that differed significantly was the band count. Given the low incidence, however, the predictive value of the band count is low. Although oral amoxicillin could theoretically treat early meningococcal bacteremia, the high risk (50%) of invasive complications would make such empiric treatment risky. Unpublished data suggests that empiric antibiotic treatment of patients with UMD improves outcome, but the data did not isolate the use oral antibiotics alone. Rickettsial infections such as Rocky Mountain spotted fever (RMSF) can present with petechial rashes; however, children are usually sicker and the progression of the rash is typically from the distal extremities toward the trunk. Though present in classic cases of RMSF, hyponatremia and thrombocytopenia are neither sensitive nor specific to this disease and thus are not very useful. (Infectious disease emergencies. In: Fleisher GR, Ludwig S, eds. *Textbook of Pediatric Emergency Medicine*, fourth edition. Mandl KD, Stack AM, Fleisher GR. Incidence of bacteremia in infants and children with fever and petechiae. J Peds 1997;131(3):398–404. Baker RC, Sequin JH, Leslie N, et al. Fever and petechiae in children. Pediatrics 1989;84:1051–55. Kuppermann N, Malley R, Inkelis SH, Fleisher GR. Clinical and hematologic features do not reliably identify children with unsuspected meningococcal disease. Pediatrics 1999;103(2):e20. Wang VJ, Malley R, Fleisher GR, Inkelis SH, Kuppermann N. Antibiotic treatment of patients with unsuspected meningococcal disease. Abstract presentation at the annual meeting of the Society for Pediatric Research, New Orleans, May 1998.)

12. d   Fever associated with a vesicular eruption noted less than 30 days after birth should always increase suspicion for neonatal herpes simplex. The herpetic lesions are more commonly found where there is a break in the skin, but they may be found anywhere. Such children need intravenous acyclovir therapy because of actual or potential invasive (especially CNS) disease. Erythema toxicum is not associated with fever. Impetigo and folliculitis can mimic neonatal herpes, but should be considered diagnoses of exclusion. Fever in a neonate should warrant admission with IV antibiotics, but with a likely source, acyclovir is a more appropriate treatment choice, although some would argue that the patient should be

started on antibiotics as well as acyclovir. Topical or oral antibiotics alone would be unacceptable. (Dermatology. In: Fleisher GR, Ludwig S, eds. *Textbook of Pediatric Emergency Medicine*, fourth edition.)

13. d   The most likely diagnosis in this child is a retropharyngeal abscess. In fact, fever and torticollis in a young child should always raise the possibility of this disease, especially if the patient is drooling or has difficulty swallowing. Retropharyngeal abscess is caused by enlargement and suppuration of the lymph nodes in the posterior pharynx. This condition is less common in older children because these nodes tend to regress with age. Peritonsillar abscess is more commonly found in older children and is usually a complication of streptococcal pharyngitis. These children present with severe sore throat, trismus, and drooling. The pharynx usually reveals enlarged tonsils as well as anterior displacement, and inflammation of the tonsillar pillars, usually unilaterally. Rotatory subluxation of C1/C2 (RSC) usually occurs after trauma or as an enthesitis associated with an infection of structures in the neck. The remote history of trauma in this patient makes the diagnosis of RSC unlikely. True torticollis would be an uncommon presentation of meningitis, which would more likely present with neck pain and stiffness associated with involuntary muscle spasm on neck flexion.

14. d   The history is consistent with a heat-related illness. Antipyretics are of unproven value and other (usually external) means of reducing temperature must be employed. There are three main types of heat-related illness: heat cramps, heat exhaustion, and heat stroke. This patient probably has had a heat stroke given the height of fever and the presence of circulatory collapse and neurologic dysfunction. Treatment includes removal of clothes, followed by active cooling (with ice-water baths) and fluid replacement. Phenothiazines may be used to prevent shivering but need to be used with caution in the presence of hypotension.

15. b   Kawasaki's disease is a multisystem illness of uncertain etiology characterized by several days of high fevers, mucositis (inflamed cracked lips, erythematous pharynx, and strawberry tongue), non-exudative, limbal-sparing conjunctivitis, periarticular swelling (involving the hands and feet), rash, and palmar erythema with subsequent desquamation. Although this disease has been called *mucocutaneous lymph-node syndrome,* cervical lymph-node enlargement is one of the less common manifestations. Even though not included in the list of features that define this syndrome, irritability has been noted in many reports and in clinical practice. The pyuria noted on this patient's urinalysis is sterile (part of vasculitis) and should not be confused with leukocytes secondary to a UTI. Close to 1–2 weeks after onset of symptoms, many patients develop thrombocytosis. About 20% of untreated patients will develop coronary aneurysms; treatment with IV immunoglobulin and salicylates reduces this rate to 4%. Mortality is less than 0.1% in the United States and results from myocarditis or myocardial infarction (MI). Streptococcal scarlet fever can present with pharyngitis, fever, and a rash; however, the rash is usually papular or sandpapery (scarlatiniform rashes also occur with Kawasaki's disease) and pyuria and swelling of the hands and feet would be highly atypical. (Rheumatologic emergencies. In Fleisher GR, Ludwig S, eds. *Textbook of Pediatric Emergency Medicine,* fourth edition. Newburger JW, Takahashi M, Burns JC, et al. The treatment of Kawasaki syndrome with intravenous gamma globulin. New Engl J Med 1986;315:341. Kawasaki Disease. 1997 Redbook: Report of committee on infectious diseases, twenty-fourth edition. American Academy of Pediatrics. 1997:316–319.)

16. c   Rubeola is a now-rare viral infection characterized by a maculopapular rash, pharyngitis, and conjunctivitis. In developing countries and in un-immunized children living in the United States, the disease is still a threat. It is heralded by low-grade fever and mild constitutional symptoms lasting 4–5 days. A maculopapular rash appears on day 3–5 and progresses caudally from the head. It is followed by a heightening of fever, which is a feature that helps differentiate this illness from roseola infantum. About 24 hours prior to appearance of the rash, patients develop an enanthem (Koplik's spots) that may persist for up to 72 hours. Erythema infectiosum is not usually associated with high-grade fevers, and the rash of RMSF usually shows a different progression. Meningococcemia is not usually associated with marked mucosal involvement, even though there are reports of conjunctivitis associated with this disease. Conjunctival petechiae and purpura may also accompany meningococcemia and may conceivably be mistaken for conjunctivitis. (Infectious disease emergencies. In: Fleisher GR, Ludwig S, eds. *Textbook of Pediatric Emergency Medicine.* Measles. 1997 Redbook: Report of committee on infectious diseases, twenty-fourth edition. American Academy of Pediatrics. 1997:344–357.)

17. d   IV chloramphenicol or IV doxycycline are the treatments of choice for RMSF. A low serum sodium concentration and thrombocytopenia make the diagnosis more likely, but neither finding is sensitive or

specific. Although tetracyclines are relatively contraindicated in children less than 8 years of age toxicity from this class of antibiotics appears to be related to dose, type, and frequency of administration. Doxycycline is relatively safe and is recommended by some experts even in younger children with suspected RMSF, because it may offer an advantage over chloramphenicol in the treatment of ehrlichiosis, which is a condition that may mimic RMSF. Chloramphenicol has been associated with the rare but fatal complication of aplastic anemia, but it is probably the antibiotic of choice among the alternatives given. Untreated, up to 30% of individuals infected with RMSF will die; the overall case fatality rate for patients diagnosed with RMSF is 3.9% (in part due to delay in diagnosis and treatment). RMSF should be highly suspected when characteristic features develop in children who live or visit the south Atlantic, southeastern, or south-central states during the tick season (usually summer). It should be noted however that the disease has been reported in almost all states of the United States. (Infectious disease emergencies. In: Fleisher GR, Ludwig S, eds. *Textbook of Pediatric Emergency Medicine*, fourth edition. Rocky Mountain Spotted Fever. 1997 Redbook: Report of committee on infectious diseases, twenty-fourth edition. American Academy of Pediatrics. 1997:452–454.)

18. d   The persistence of fever despite antibiotic treatment in a patient with documented pneumococcal bacteremia suggests either ongoing bacteremia or the presence of invasive bacterial disease such as pneumonia, osteomyelitis, septic arthritis, or meningitis. The risk of invasive disease is increased if the child looks unwell. Thus, persistent fever after empiric antibiotic treatment in a patient with documented pneumococcal bacteremia needs to be evaluated to reduce the risk of tissue invasion or to detect complications as early as possible. This evaluation consists of a careful examination to exclude pneumonia, osteomyelitis, septic arthritis, and meningitis as complications. The current recommendations are that any young child with pneumococcal bacteremia who appears ill or toxic on re-evaluation needs a full sepsis evaluation and a lumbar puncture. Although the management of febrile well-appearing children with documented pneumococcal bacteremia varies, all ill-appearing children should be admitted to the hospital for parenteral antibiotics (usually cefotaxime or ceftriaxone). If a diagnosis of meningitis is suggested by the CSF profile, IV vancomycin should be added. Discharge on oral antibiotics and antipyretics without excluding meningitis could lead to a further delay in diagnosis and potentially increase the severity of sequelae. There is no evidence that a low peripheral WBC after initiating treatment excludes a diagnosis of persistent bacteremia or invasive disease; thus, the CBC should not be used as a decision-making tool once bacteremia has been documented. (Infectious disease emergencies. In: Fleisher GR, Ludwig S, eds. *Textbook of Pediatric Emergency Medicine*, fourth edition. Baraff LJ, Bass JW, et al. Practice guideline for the management of infants and children 0 to 36 months of age with fever without source. Pediatrics 1993;92:1–12.)

19. d   This 18-month-old has acute primary herpetic gingivostomatitis. This can be a severe disease characterized by high-grade fever associated with vesicles and ulcers on the gums, lips, tongue, and anterior pharynx. Lesions rarely involve the posterior pharynx, a feature that helps differentiate this condition from herpangina. Tender anterior cervical adenopathy is common and there is usually a marked decrease in oral intake. All dehydrated children need to be admitted for IV hydration. Two placebo-controlled trials have supported the use of oral acyclovir but the role of topical acyclovir in primary herpetic gingivostomatitis is less clear. Aphthous ulcers are not usually associated with fever, and Stevens-Johnson syndrome (which can be a complication of herpetic stomatitis) is associated with a more severe mucositis involving oral and conjunctival surfaces. ANUG is found in adolescents and is uncommon in young children. It is characterized by gingivitis and point tenderness with flattening of the interdental gingivae; it is not usually associated with fever. (Dental emergencies. In: Fleisher GR, Ludwig S, eds. *Textbook of Pediatric Emergency Medicine*, fourth edition. Ducoulombier H, Cousin J, Dewilde A, et al. A controlled clinical trial versus placebo of acyclovir in the treatment of herpetic gingivostomatitis in children (in French). Ann Pediatr (Paris) 1988;35:212–216. Aoki FY, Law BJ, Hammond GW, et al. Acyclovir suspension for treatment of acute herpes simplex virus gingivostomatitis in children: A placebo controlled, double-blind trial. Abstracts for the thirty-third interscience conference on Antimicrobial Agents and Chemotherapy 1993: 399.)

20. b   This 17-year-old probably has toxic shock syndrome, which is a complication of nasal packing or nasal tampons. Some authorities suggest antistaphylococcal treatment for all patients who require nasal packing for more than a day. This condition presents with GI symptoms, high fever, and hypotension. The treatment is removal of the offending agent and treatment with fluids and antistaphylococcal antibiotics. (Epistaxis. In: Fleisher GR, Ludwig S, eds. *Textbook of Pediatric Emergency Medicine*, fourth

edition. Fairbanks DN. Complications of nasal packing. Otolaryngol Head Neck Surg 1986;94(3) 412–415. Nahass RG, Gocke DJ. Toxic shock syndrome associated with use of a nasal tampon. Am J Med 1988;84 (3 pt 2):629–31.)

21. d   Succinylcholine has been associated with malignant hyperthermia. This is a life-threatening condition that should be treated promptly with IV dantrolene (1–2 mg/kg rapidly every 5–10 minutes to a maximum of 10mg/kg) and aggressive measures to reduce temperature. There is no role for antipyretics and a defasciculating dose of pancuronium will not aid in temperature control. A seizure would be unlikely in the presence of muscle paralysis and would be unlikely to raise the temperature that high; thus phenytoin would not be indicated in this setting. (Kearney TE. "Dantrolene." In Therapeutic drugs and antidotes. In: *Poisonings and drug overdose,* third edition. Olson KR, ed. Stamford, CT: Appleton & Lange, 1999:354–355.)

22. c   Malaria should be part of the differential for any febrile child who has recently lived in a tropical or sub-Saharan region of the world such as West Africa. This infection is caused by the *Plasmodium* parasite and is carried by mosquitoes. It is characterized by high fevers, rigors, myalgias, and, occasionally, by severe prostration. The diagnosis is made by Giemsa stain of a smear of blood, which reveals ring forms in the erythrocytes if malaria is present. Treatment includes oral chloroquine, IV quinidine, or IV quinine with the addition of tetracycline, Fansidar®, or mefloquine in areas with chloroquine resistance. Parasitic colitis would be unlikely without bloody diarrhea and meningitis would be unlikely without meningeal signs in a 6-year-old child. Although sepsis is clearly a possibility in this patient, a blood smear (thick smear for qualitative and thin smear for quantitative diagnosis) would more rapidly reveal or exclude the diagnosis of malaria and should be given higher priority. (Malaria. 1997 Redbook: Report of committee on infectious diseases, twenty-fourth edition. American Academy of Pediatrics 1997:335–343.)

CHAPTER **29**

Foreign Body— Ingestion/Aspiration

ANDREA STRACCIOLINI, M.D.

QUESTIONS

1. A 2-year-old girl is brought to the ED with a history of drooling, vomiting, and refusal to eat or drink. The child is alert and interactive. There are no signs of respiratory distress or stridor. On physical examination the child is afebrile, and the lungs are clear to auscultation. Her O$_2$ saturation on room air is 99%. On further history the mother states that the child was playing in the house with a can of change earlier in the day. The appropriate next step in evaluation of this patient is:

   a. Radiograph
   b. GI consult
   c. Direct laryngoscopy
   d. Airway fluoroscopy
   e. Endoscopy

2. An 18-month-old boy is brought to the ED because he had had a choking episode while playing with his father's calculator. The child began drooling and developed increased work of breathing. On physical examination, the child is afebrile with RR 32. The child is in moderate distress, sitting up with expiratory stridor. The lungs are clear to auscultation and have good aeration. The next best step in caring for this patient is:

   a. Airway fluoroscopy
   b. Otorhinolaryngology consultation for removal
   c. Direct laryngoscopy, intubation
   d. Foley catheter removal
   e. Balloon-tipped catheter removal

3. A 3-year-old boy was seen putting a screw into his mouth. The parents bring him to the ED because they are concerned that he swallowed it. There is no history of choking and the child has no respiratory distress. The child is otherwise well. On x-ray you see a 5.5-cm screw in the stomach. The correct treatment for this child is:

   a. Parental stool examinations
   b. Endoscopic removal
   c. Daily x-rays
   d. Admission, abdominal exams
   e. Discharge with follow-up

4. A 2½-year-old girl was observed playing with her grandfather's jar full of change. Her parents found her with two pennies and a quarter in her mouth. They are suspicious that she swallowed a coin. X-ray reveals a likely quarter in the child's stomach. The best management plan is:

   a. Administration of ipecac orally
   b. Endoscopic removal
   c. Serial abdominal x-rays
   d. Parental stool examinations
   e. No intervention

5. An 18-month-old boy comes to the ED with a history of choking while eating popcorn. The child is alert and playful. His RR is 58, and his O$_2$ saturation on room air is 100%. There are no retractions, wheezes, or stridor on exam. The breath sounds are symmetric. The inspiratory and expiratory x-rays are normal. The appropriate next step in treating this patient is:

   a. Discharge to home with follow up
   b. Lateral decubitus x-ray
   c. Admission and observation
   d. Airway fluoroscopy
   e. Immediate bronchoscopy

ANSWERS

1. a   Coins account for 50–75% of childhood esophageal foreign bodies, and pennies predominate. Foreign bodies of the esophagus lodge at three levels: the cricopharyngeus muscle in the thoracic inlet (60–80%), gastroesophageal junction (10–20%), and aortic arch (5–20%). The history and exam suggest an esophageal foreign body. The initial evaluation with a CXR to include the upper abdomen and oropharynx is appropriate as the first screen for a radiopaque esophageal or gastric foreign body. The combination of a soft-tissue lateral neck and a wide CXR that includes the oropharynx and abdomen is alternatively used as an initial "foreign body search." Airway fluoroscopy is useful in the evaluation of a child that you suspect aspirated a foreign body. GI consultation and endoscopy are appropriate after the diagnosis is made. There is no role for direct laryngoscopy.

2. b   Disc batteries are frequently within reach of children. The history and examination described suggest a foreign body ingestion; in this case, likely a disc battery from the calculator. These batteries cause corrosive injury to the hollow viscera. Disc batteries that lodge in the esophagus should be removed promptly because of the potential to erode rapidly through the esophagus. Foley catheter and balloon-tipped catheter removal are techniques that have been used with some success, but they are generally reserved for rounded esophageal foreign bodies (coins) in a stable child. These techniques would not be indicated in this child, who needs immediate attention and removal of the disc battery. There is no role for airway fluoroscopy and direct laryngoscopy in the patient described in this case.

3. b   Most foreign bodies of the stomach and lower GI tract can be managed expectantly. Long objects (more than 5 cm long) should be removed from the stomach because they are unable to negotiate the turns of the duodenum and other tight bends in the lower GI tract. Sewing needles also have increased propensity for perforation. Serial abdominal x-rays every 3–5 days can be obtained when an object is likely to or has passed out of the stomach to a place where journey through the GI tract is questionable. Parental stool examinations for a foreign body are unpleasant tasks, often abandoned. Inability to retrieve the foreign body after 1 week or more of stool examination often heightens parental concern.

4. e   As mentioned in the preceding explanation, most foreign bodies of the stomach can be conservatively managed. Most rounded objects such as coins will traverse the GI tract in 3–8 days without any complication. Some objects occasionally remain in the stomach for a long duration of time. A prolonged time, up to weeks, should be allowed for passage of inert objects before surgical or endoscopic removal is needed. Parental stool examination is often frustrating and anxiety provoking, and is not recommended.

5. d   The initial step in evaluating a child for foreign body aspiration is expiratory and inspiratory chest x-rays. Further evaluation is warranted if these studies are normal and the clinical suspicion of aspiration is high, as they are in this child with tachypnea and a remarkable history. Discharge and admission for observation are therefore incorrect choices. Airway fluoroscopy is an appropriate next step, looking for air trapping and evidence of mediastinal shift away from the foreign body. In some cases in which the CXRs are positive, or there are physical findings (unilateral wheeze, decreased aeration) and a good aspiration history, the patient may go directly to bronchoscopy. Lateral decubitus films are unlikely to be helpful in conjunction with normal inspiratory and expiratory films. However, when inspiratory and expiratory films cannot be obtained, as in the case with young children, lateral decubitus films may be helpful.

CHAPTER 30

Gastrointestinal Bleeding

RON L. KAPLAN, M.D.

QUESTIONS

1. A 6-year-old boy has had low-grade fever and vomiting for several hours. He is brought to the ED because his parents noted a few flecks of coffee-ground material in his last episode of emesis. He has had several sips of liquids since then with no further emesis. He was previously well with no significant past medical history. He has a temperature of 38.2°C and vital signs are all normal. He is generally well appearing, and physical exam is unremarkable. The most appropriate test to obtain next is:

   a. Abdominal x-rays
   b. CBC and electrolytes
   c. Stool hemoccult
   d. Nasogastric lavage with saline
   e. Upper GI series

The following case relates to Questions 2 and 3: A 2-day-old male born at home presents to the ED with blood noted in his stool the previous night. This morning he vomited and had blood noted in the vomitus and in his nose. He is pale and mottled with grunting respirations, HR 194, and BP 42/26.

2. Which laboratory study is most likely to be abnormal?

   a. Platelet count
   b. Prothrombin time (PT)
   c. Partial thromboplastin time (PTT)
   d. Apt test
   e. Hematocrit (hct)

3. Which of the following immediate treatments is most important?

   a. Fresh frozen plasma (FFP)
   b. Vitamin K
   c. IV dopamine
   d. Crystalloid followed by O-negative blood
   e. Factor VIII concentrate

4. A 1-week-old presents to the ED with progressive bilious emesis, lethargy, abdominal distension, and maroon-colored stool. After stabilization and nasogastric tube placement, which of the following is indicated next:

   a. Emergent surgical intervention
   b. Abdominal x-rays
   c. Upper GI series
   d. Air contrast enema
   e. Endoscopy

5. A 6-month-old presents to the ED with episodic irritability and agitation followed by periods of lethargy. He is afebrile with normal vital signs, sleeping but arousable. Abdomen is soft, with no masses. Stool is heme positive. Which diagnostic procedure is indicated next?

   a. Gastric lavage with saline
   b. Abdominal CT scan
   c. Contrast enema
   d. Colonoscopy
   e. Upper endoscopy

The following case relates to Questions 6 and 7: A previously well 18-month-old presents to the ED with sudden massive rectal bleeding.

6. After stabilization and resuscitation, which of the following is indicated next?

   a. Abdominal x-rays
   b. Nasogastric lavage with saline
   c. Air contrast enema
   d. Technetium scan
   e. Colonoscopy

7. What is the most likely diagnosis?

   a. Intussusception
   b. Inflammatory bowel disease
   c. Juvenile polyp
   d. Hemolytic uremic syndrome (HUS)
   e. Meckel's diverticulum

The following case relates to Questions 8–10: A 4-year-old with asthma has been treated with albuterol and prednisolone for 2 days. He presents to the ED with persistent severe cough and posttussive emesis. Coffee-ground material has been noted in his emesis, and stools are dark and tarry. He is well appearing with normal vital signs, hemodynamically stable.

8. Which diagnostic procedure is indicated next?

   a. Abdominal x-rays
   b. Nasogastric lavage with saline
   c. Upper GI series
   d. Endoscopy
   e. Barium enema

9. He suddenly starts to cough and vomits coffee-ground material with streaks of bright red blood. A nasogastric tube is placed, with return of grossly bloody gastric contents. IV access is established, labs are sent, and fluids are started. Which procedure is indicated next?

   a. Abdominal x-rays
   b. Upper GI series
   c. Endoscopy
   d. Abdominal ultrasound
   e. Abdominal CT scan

10. What is the most likely diagnosis?

   a. Gastric ulcer
   b. Esophageal varices
   c. Esophagitis
   d. Gastric outlet obstruction
   e. Mallory-Weiss tear

ANSWERS

1. c The majority of children with gastrointestinal bleeding have acute, self-limited processes. This patient presents with gastroenteritis. The coffee-ground material suggests an upper GI source of bleeding. If the stool is negative for occult blood and the history and physical are otherwise unremarkable, further studies may not be necessary.

2. b This infant has hemorrhagic disease of the newborn caused by vitamin K deficiency. This results in deficiency of the vitamin K–dependent clotting factors and prolongation of the prothrombin time. The Apt test distinguishes maternal from fetal red blood cells in cases of swallowed maternal blood. The hematocrit may be low or may be unchanged initially in patients with acute hemorrhage who have not yet received fluid resuscitation.

3. d This infant is in hemorrhagic shock. The hypotension suggests severe hemorrhage and impending circulatory failure, and blood transfusion is needed as fast as possible. This is most rapidly achieved by transfusing O-negative blood because waiting for typed and cross-matched blood can result in fatal delays. Crystalloid should be pushed as fast as possible while awaiting the blood. Fresh frozen plasma may also be useful adjunctive therapy, and vitamin K administration is necessary in order to correct the underlying deficiency. Factor VIII therapy would be indicated in patients with hemophilia. Dopamine is not indicated in the face of hemorrhagic shock.

4. a This infant has midgut volvulus until proven otherwise. He is clearly obstructed, and the maroon-colored stool suggests vascular compromise. Immediate surgical intervention is indicated, and waiting to obtain other studies may result in fatal complications.

5. c This child has a history consistent with intussusception. The classic triad of signs and symptoms include colicky abdominal pain, sausage-shaped mass, and currant jelly stool. There may be associated vomiting. The lack of a mass, vomiting, and currant jelly stool should not detract from the diagnosis in this patient with a history suggestive of intussusception. Currant jelly stool is only seen late and implies vascular compromise. Air contrast enema is the diagnostic procedure of choice, and it often results in successful reduction of the intussusception.

6. b Brisk rectal bleeding typically occurs in patients with a lower GI lesion, but it may be seen in some patients with massive upper GI bleeding as well. The presence of blood in the intestine shortens intestinal transit time, so bright red blood may be seen. It is therefore necessary to perform gastric lavage on patients with significant rectal bleeding to rule out an upper GI source.

7. e Meckel's diverticulum is the most common cause of massive rectal bleeding in children in this age group. Polyps may cause painless rectal bleeding, but significant hemorrhage usually does not occur. Intussusception, inflammatory bowel disease, and HUS (hemolytic urea syndrome) can all cause lower GI bleeding, but they would be expected to have other associated findings.

8. b The presence of coffee-ground emesis and melena suggests an upper GI source of bleeding. Gastric lavage with saline, looking for the presence of coffee-ground material or gross blood, is the next step in the evaluation. An upper GI series is indicated for patients with a grossly positive lavage if there is no further active bleeding, and endoscopy is indicated for persistent or recurrent bleeding.

9. c This patient is having a persistent upper GI hemorrhage. Volume resuscitation is necessary and endoscopy is indicated to identify and control the source of bleeding.

10. e The history of upper GI bleeding associated with severe cough is most consistent with a Mallory-Weiss tear. Gastric irritation associated with steroid use may also cause upper GI bleeding, but this is unlikely in this case because the patient has only been on steroids for 2 days. Esophageal varices are a common cause of upper GI bleeding among patients with liver disease. Significant hemorrhage would be unlikely among patients with esophagitis.

CHAPTER 31

Groin Masses

VINCENT J. WANG, M.D.

QUESTIONS

1. A 16-year-old sexually active boy complains of "groin lumps." He has no other medical problems and says he has never had a sexually transmitted disease (STD) before. He has a cluster of painful vesicles and ulcers on the glans penis. Both testes are descended in the scrotal sac. He has several enlarged mobile masses bilaterally in the groin region. Management includes:

   a. Penicillin
   b. Ceftriaxone
   c. Acyclovir
   d. Doxycycline
   e. Lymph node biopsy

2. A 17-year-old sexually active girl complains of unilateral groin swelling. On examination of her labia minora, she has a deep and painful ulcer with ragged edges and a friable base. The base is covered with a yellow exudate. She has left-sided adenopathy, which is mildly tender. Management includes:

   a. Penicillin
   b. Ceftriaxone
   c. Acyclovir
   d. Trimethoprim-sulfamethoxazole
   e. Lymph node biopsy

3. A 2-month-old boy is referred to you for evaluation of a right-sided groin mass. He was born without complications at 32 weeks gestational age. He has been feeding well and has not had other symptoms. On examination, you palpate a normal testicle on the left side, but none palpable on the right. He has a nontender, mobile mass in the right inguinal region. Immediate treatment includes:

   a. Biopsy of the mass
   b. Operative reduction
   c. Trimethoprim-sulfamethoxazole
   d. Sitz baths
   e. Reassurance and outpatient follow-up

4. After you diagnose a 2-year-old boy with an undescended right testis, you stress the importance of outpatient follow-up with a urologist or general surgeon because the patient is at risk for all of the following, EXCEPT:

   a. Infertility
   b. Delayed sexual development
   c. Cancer
   d. Testicular torsion
   e. Hernia

5. A 16-year-old girl has been vomiting and has a painful left-sided groin mass. She is afebrile, but ill appearing. She has a prominence of her left groin area. The mass is 3 cm in diameter, firm, and tender. It is not mobile. She has no other lesions and denies sexual activity or recent travel. Treatment includes:

   a. Warm soaks
   b. Penicillin
   c. Ceftriaxone
   d. Biopsy
   e. Surgical exploration

ANSWERS

1. c   Venereal disease is a common cause of lymphadenopathy in a sexually active adolescent. Herpes may present with painful vesicles or ulcerations on the genitalia, accompanied with painful adenopathy. Acyclovir will shorten the duration of symptoms and decrease viral shedding. The chancre of primary syphilis is indurated, with firm borders and a shallow, smooth base. This is generally painless. Chancroid may present with painful ulcers, ragged edges, and a deep friable base. Adenitis is common, but it is usually unilateral. Lymphogranuloma venereum causes painless papules, vesicles, or ulcers. Adenitis is usually unilateral.

2. b   Chancroid is caused by *Haemophilus ducreyi*, and presents with the symptoms described. The patient may be treated with azithromycin orally or ceftriaxone intramuscularly.

3. e   This patient has a retractile or undescended testis. A retractile testis is pulled into an abnormally high position because of a hyperactive cremasteric reflex. The testis can usually be milked back into the scrotum by the examiner. Undescended testes are more common in premature babies. Nearly all infants under 900 g are cryptorchid, whereas 0.7% are at 1 year of age. Appropriate treatment for this patient is observation alone for a retractile testis. For an undescended testis, treatment is observation and possible repair between the ages of 1 and 2 years, if the testicle does not descend. Biopsy is not indicated in either case. Operative reduction would be indicated if the history and findings were suggestive of an incarcerated inguinal hernia. Trimethoprim-sulfamethoxazole and sitz baths are not indicated.

4. b   Cryptorchid patients may develop testicular atrophy, infertility, cancer, testicular torsion, or traumatic injury. They are also at increased risk for the development of a hernia. Germ cell depletion, Leydig cell atrophy, smaller seminiferous tubules, and peritubular fibrosis may also occur, but there is no evidence that sexual development will be delayed.

5. e   An incarcerated inguinal hernia is a surgical emergency. The inability to move the mass or reduce it confirms the diagnosis of incarceration, and the patient should be reduced intraoperatively, if it cannot be done in the ED.

CHAPTER 32

Hearing Loss

MARK E. RALSTON, M.D., M.P.H.

QUESTIONS

1. A 24-month-old boy with past medical history of recurrent otitis media is evaluated in the ED for rhinorrhea and cough. The mother reports the child has two words in his vocabulary and asks for an evaluation of his hearing. Examination of the right tympanic membrane reveals a white saclike structure that is draining a shiny, greasy, foul-smelling fluid. You diagnose:

   a. Acute otitis media with perforation
   b. Otitis externa
   c. Cholesteatoma
   d. Otitis media with effusion
   e. Recurrent acute otitis media

2. An 8-year-old boy presents to the ED with acute onset hearing loss in his right ear. With a 512 Hz tuning fork, you diagnose conductive hearing loss, distinguishing it from sensorineural hearing loss by:

   a. Weber's test: lateralizes to right ear; Rinne test positive: AC > BC in right ear (BC = bone conduction; AC = air conduction)
   b. Weber's test: lateralizes to left ear; Rinne test positive: AC > BC in right ear
   c. Weber's test: lateralizes to right ear; Rinne test negative: BC > AC in right ear
   d. Weber's test: lateralizes to left ear; Rinne test negative: BC > AC in right ear

3. A 1-year-old boy with congenital sensorineural hearing loss is being evaluated in triage for spontaneous gross hematuria. You are paged by the nurse, who reports the child is hypertensive on repeated evaluations with the appropriately sized cuff. As you walk to triage, you suspect the child's diagnosis to be:

   a. Systemic lupus erythematosus (SLE)
   b. Acute poststreptococcal glomerulonephritis
   c. Idiopathic hypercalciuria
   d. Alport's syndrome
   e. IgA nephropathy

4. A 12-year-old girl sustains a basilar skull fracture in a motor vehicle collision. In the ED you detect a unilateral conductive hearing loss. Possible causes of this condition in this child include all of the following, EXCEPT:

   a. Perilymphatic fistula
   b. Ossicular disruption
   c. Tympanic membrane perforation
   d. Cerebrospinal fluid (CSF) otorrhea
   e. Hemotympanum

5. A 2-year-old girl arrives in the ED in status epilepticus. After stabilization of the patient, you learn from the mother that the child has a congenital hearing loss. You order an ECG, expecting to find:

   a. Type II second-degree AV (atrioventricular) block
   b. Third-degree (complete) AV block
   c. Premature ventricular contractions
   d. Prolonged QT interval
   e. Premature atrial contractions

6. A 15-month-old boy is suspected of having a problem with his hearing because he fails to respond appropriately to noises. Causes of conductive hearing loss at this age include all of the following, EXCEPT:

   a. Cerumen impaction
   b. Foreign body
   c. Acute otitis media
   d. Otitis media with effusion
   e. TORCH infection

7. A previously healthy 17-year-old boy develops sudden-onset hearing loss and ringing in his right ear while scuba diving. In the ED he is severely vertiginous. You detect nystagmus. Otoscopic examination is normal. Tuning-fork examination is Rinne positive in the right ear, with lateralization of Weber's test to the left ear. You refer him to the otolaryngology service for further evaluation of suspected:

a. Air embolism
b. Perilymphatic fistula
c. Labyrinthitis
d. Nitrogen narcosis
e. Tympanic membrane perforation

8. A previously healthy 16-year-old girl is seen for fever and acute-onset vertigo with associated vomiting and tinnitus. Your tuning fork examination reveals a sensorineural hearing loss. Neurological evaluation is otherwise normal. Meningeal signs are absent. The most likely cause of her condition is:

a. Cerebrovascular accident
b. Viral labyrinthitis
c. Migraine
d. Acoustic neuroma
e. Hypothyroidism

9. A 14-year-old girl is brought to the ED for evaluation of headache and unsteadiness. Further questioning reveals a history of gradual deterioration of her hearing. Neurological examination is remarkable for right facial weakness and ataxia. Family history is positive for neurofibromatosis in the father. You search for café-au-lait spots but find none. You obtain a CT scan specifically looking for:

a. Meningioma
b. Cerebellar astrocytoma
c. Acoustic neuroma
d. Brainstem glioma
e. Medulloblastoma

10. An 18-year-old boy is found to have a high-frequency sensorineural hearing loss on a recruitment physical examination for the U.S. Navy. In the ED, you learn from his worried parents that he listens to loud music with headphones for hours every day. Otoscopic examination is normal. You explain on rounds that severe and permanent hearing loss can follow brief exposures to sound intensity exceeding _____ decibels, and chronic exposure to sound intensity exceeding _____ decibels.

a. 100, 50
b. 140, 50
c. 140, 80
d. 180, 100
e. 220, 150

ANSWERS

1. c A cholesteatoma may develop in children with recurrent acute otitis media with a marginal tympanic membrane perforation and cause a conductive hearing loss. Squamous epithelium of the external auditory canal grows through the perforation into the attic of the middle ear compartment, producing an epidermal inclusion cyst. It is lined by keratinized, stratified, squamous epithelium and contains desquamated epithelium or keratin. If tympanomastoid surgery is delayed, a cholesteatoma can erode other temporal bone structures and invade the intracranial cavity.

2. c *Weber's test.* A vibrating tuning fork placed on the midforehead is heard louder on the side of the conductive hearing loss (which shuts out the masking effect of room noises) and opposite the side of the sensorineural hearing loss. *Rinne test.* A vibrating tuning fork is placed against the mastoid until the sound ceases (bone conduction), at which point the still-vibrating tuning fork is held next to the ipsilateral ear until the sound ceases (air conduction). In conductive hearing loss, bone conduction persists longer than air conduction (Rinne negative). In sensorineural hearing loss, air conduction persists longer than bone conduction (Rinne positive).

3. d Alport's syndrome is an *X*-linked dominant disorder that commonly presents as asymptomatic microscopic hematuria, but recurrent episodes of gross hematuria are not uncommon. A minority of patients also have sensorineural hearing loss, which may begin in the high-frequency range, but progresses to involve speech frequencies and can result in deafness.

4. a If a basilar skull fracture involves the temporal bone, inner and/or middle ear compartments may be disrupted with concomitant sensorineural and/or conductive hearing loss, respectively. Causes of conductive hearing loss include ossicular disruption, tympanic membrane perforation, CSF otorrhea, and hemotympanum. Perilymphatic fistula is an anomalous connection between the middle and inner ear compartments associated with sensorineural hearing loss.

5.　d　Patients with Jervell-Lange-Nielsen syndrome, which is a prolonged QT syndrome associated with congenital sensorineural hearing loss, are at high risk for ventricular arrhythmias (precipitating cerebral hypoxia and seizures in this patient), including a particular form of ventricular arrhythmia known as *torsade de pointes.*

6.　e　Sensorineural hearing loss has been described with all of the congenital infections referred to by the acronym TORCH, representing toxoplasmosis, other agents, rubella, cytomegalovirus, and herpes simplex. The acronym has been modified to STORCH to include congenital syphilis, which is also a cause of sensorineural hearing loss.

7.　b　Perilymphatic fistula may occur following sudden barotrauma (i.e., any condition that abruptly increases the pressure within the middle ear or inner ear compartments). Potential causes of perilymphatic fistula include vigorous physical exertion, deep water diving, playing a wind instrument, and flying in an airplane. The leak is typically at either oval or round windows and should be repaired before the sensorineural hearing loss becomes irreversible. Air embolism, nitrogen narcosis, and tympanic membrane perforation are not associated with sensorineural hearing loss. Labyrinthitis produces a sensorineural hearing loss, but it does not occur in the setting of barotrauma.

8.　b　Viral labyrinthitis is the most frequent cause of acquired sensorineural hearing loss in children without a history of trauma. Typical symptoms are related to inflammation of the inner ear and include tinnitus, vertigo, and vomiting. Neurological examination is without focal abnormalities. Specific causes include adenovirus, parainfluenza viruses, herpes simplex, cytomegalovirus, mumps, and rubeola. Cerebrovascular accident, migraine, acoustic neuroma, and hypothyroidism do not fit the presentation of fever and acute-onset sensorineural hearing loss.

9.　c　Bilateral acoustic neuromas represent the most characteristic finding in neurofibromatosis, NF-2. Signs of a cerebellopontine angle mass (e.g., sensorineural hearing loss, facial weakness, ataxia, or headache) are more commonly present in the second and third decades of life although they may appear in childhood. Café-au-lait spots and skin neurofibromas (absent in this patient) are classic features in NF-1, but they are much less common in NF-2.

10.　c　Acoustic trauma, resulting from exposure to high-intensity sound (e.g., loud music, fireworks, machinery, gunfire) is a cause of acquired sensorineural hearing loss. Manifested by a depression at 4000 Hz on the audiometric examination, noise-induced hearing loss is often temporary, but it can become permanent if the exposure is chronic.

CHAPTER 33

Heart Murmurs

SUJIT SHARMA, M.D.

QUESTIONS

1. A healthy-appearing 2-month-old male is brought to the ED with a monilial diaper rash. On examination you note a systolic murmur at the left upper sternal border that transmits well to the back. The following vital signs are recorded: T 36.9°C, HR 164, RR 42, and BP 92/54. Saturated O_2 is 98% on room air. The remainder of the physical examination is normal. Which of the following would be most appropriate?

   a. Cardiology consultation
   b. Echocardiogram
   c. Primary care follow-up
   d. Oral furosemide
   e. Oral digoxin

2. A previously healthy 8-year-old boy comes to the ED with complaints of a sore throat for 1 day. His vital signs show T 39.2°C, HR 128, RR 24, and BP 112/68. He appears well on exam, with a pharynx that is erythematous and exudative. A soft systolic murmur is appreciated at the left upper sternal border. The remainder of his examination is unremarkable. Which of the following would be the most appropriate?

   a. Throat culture and outpatient treatment
   b. Cardiology consultation
   c. Echocardiogram
   d. Admission and IV antibiotics
   e. Serial blood cultures

3. A 3-year-old African-American girl is brought to the ED with a complaint of pain in the right knee for several hours. She is afebrile but mildly tachycardic. The knee appears normal on exam, but she is mildly tender from the thigh to the calf. You hear a II/VI systolic murmur on exam. No other gross abnormalities are noted. Which of the following is most likely to be helpful in finding a cause for the murmur?

   a. CBC
   b. ESR
   c. ANA
   d. Twelve-lead ECG
   e. Echocardiogram

4. A 5-month-old boy is being seen in the ED for oral thrush. On physical examination a systolic ejection murmur is heard along the right sternal border. The patient is well appearing with the following vital signs: HR 136, RR 36, and BP 94/56. Saturated O_2 is 89% on room air. He has an otherwise unremarkable physical exam. Which of the following is most likely to elucidate the cause for his murmur?

   a. Methemoglobin level
   b. Echocardiogram
   c. CBC
   d. CXR
   e. 12-lead ECG

ANSWERS

1. c   The murmur heard in this well-appearing child is most consistent with peripheral pulmonic stenosis. This is a normal murmur, caused by angulation of the distal pulmonary arteries. The absence of cyanosis or signs of congestive heart failure supports outpatient follow-up, and obviates the need for any treatment or further diagnostic studies/consultative help.

2. a   This patient has a hyperdynamic flow murmur, most likely due to fever and tachycardia related to an ongoing streptococcal pharyngitis. Further workup for acute rheumatic fever or infective endocarditis is not necessary, given this presentation and otherwise unremarkable examination.

3. a   One has to be concerned about sickle cell anemia as a cause for knee pain in a patient with this type of presentation. Without any other clinical evidence to point toward a rheumatic process, a CBC would be most beneficial, because this patient's murmur could be most likely related to anemia.

4. b   This patient has a heart murmur as well as mild cyanosis, which are most likely due to an underlying cyanotic congenital heart disease (e.g., tetralogy of Fallot). Although a CXR as well as an ECG may show mild abnormalities, an echocardiogram would be the study of choice to fully elucidate the pathology. A CBC would not be a helpful diagnostic tool in this patient, and patients with methemoglobinemia do not have lowering of their saturated O_2 despite obvious cyanosis.

CHAPTER 34

Hematuria

VINCENT J. WANG, M.D.

QUESTIONS

1. A 6-year-old girl has had pink-colored urine today. She has had left-sided flank pain and fever for 1–2 days. On examination, she is well appearing, but she has mild tenderness in the left costovertebral angle (CVA) area. Her examination is otherwise normal. Her urinalysis shows 5–10 WBC/hpf (per high-power field) and TNTC RBC/hpf ("too numerous to count"). Appropriate evaluation includes:

   a. Ordering a CT scan
   b. Performing ultrasonography
   c. Obtaining a urine calcium level
   d. Repeating the urinalysis tomorrow
   e. Obtaining a urine culture

2. A 3-month-old boy, formerly 24 weeks premature at birth, is referred to the ED for evaluation of hematuria. He has bronchopulmonary dysplasia and has been on aminophylline and furosemide since shortly after birth. His mother noted red-colored urine in the diaper. He is otherwise well appearing. Appropriate initial evaluation or management includes:

   a. Discontinuing aminophylline
   b. Discontinuing furosemide
   c. Performing a urine microscopy
   d. Obtaining an ultrasound (U/S) of the kidneys
   e. Obtaining a CT scan of the kidneys

3. A 3-year-old boy is sent by his daycare center for hematuria. He is malnourished and has multiple contusions over his arms and legs, at various stages of healing. He has a large contusion over his lower back. His urine microscopy reveals 50 RBCs per hpf, and is otherwise normal. Appropriate evaluation includes:

   a. CT scan
   b. Ultrasonography
   c. Intravenous pyelogram
   d. Prothrombin (PT) level
   e. Repeat urine via catheterization

4. A 9-year-old boy complains of difficulty voiding and abdominal pain. He has been well until the past few weeks, when he developed difficulty voiding. He complains of increasingly dull abdominal discomfort that is relieved by voiding. On examination, he is alert and well appearing. His abdomen is soft and nontender after voiding. His urinalysis reveals 10–20 RBCs per hpf. Appropriate evaluation includes:

   a. Outpatient repeat urinalysis
   b. Urine calcium/creatinine ratio
   c. Urine oxalate levels
   d. Angiography
   e. Renal ultrasound

5. A 2-year-old girl reportedly had blood in her diaper at daycare. She is referred to your ED for possible abuse. In the knee-chest position, you notice a hemorrhagic mass when you spread the labia. There are no other signs of trauma. Treatment includes:

   a. Application of hydrocortisone cream
   b. Application of estrogen cream
   c. Application of neosporin/polymyxin cream
   d. Application of nystatin cream
   e. Consultation with social services

6. A 6-year-old boy has swelling of his legs and feet. He was treated for pharyngitis approximately 10 days ago. He is alert, but ill appearing. His HR is 120 and his BP is 140/100. His lungs are clear and his abdomen is soft. He has mild periorbital and lower extremity edema. His BUN (blood urea nitrogen) is 30 mg/dl and his serum creatinine (Cr) is 1.9 mg/dl. Findings on his urinalysis consistent with his disease are:

   a. Specific gravity less than 1.010
   b. Absence of proteinuria
   c. Blood clots
   d. RBC casts
   e. Bright red color

7. A 16-year-old girl is referred from a pediatrician for hematuria. She has recently immigrated to the United States. She has had cough for several years and has had chronic malaise, both of which are seemingly worse over the past few weeks. She was evaluated in her pediatrician's office and was noted to have a blood on a dipstick evaluation of her urine. She also had a CXR that was significant for a focal consolidation in the left upper lobe, with a fluid level. Treatment for this patient includes:

a. Repeat urinalysis in a few days
b. Hemodialysis
c. Administration of methylprednisolone
d. Administration of isoniazid
e. Administration of ampicillin

ANSWERS

1. e   A urinary tract infection (UTI) is one of the most common causes of hematuria. Her symptoms suggest that a UTI is the cause of her hematuria. A urine culture will be the definitive evaluation for this diagnosis. CT scanning is the test of choice for nephrolithiasis, which is not indicated here. CT scanning would also be appropriate in cases of trauma and hematuria. Ultrasonography would be a reasonable test to evaluate anatomy for congenital anomalies and to evaluate possible tumors or masses. Hypercalciuria may cause hematuria, but the clinical picture is usually in a patient who is asymptomatic. In an asymptomatic patient with a suspicious urinalysis, a repeat urinalysis may be warranted.

2. c   Although furosemide may be the etiology of nephrolithiasis, which may cause hematuria, initial evaluation should include a urine microscopy on an appropriately obtained urine sample. Red-colored urine found in a diaper may be urine mixed with blood from an anal fissure; therefore, a catheterized or suprapubic specimen should be obtained. A urine dipstick is not adequate because both myoglobinuria and hemoglobinuria would be positive on a dipstick test. Discontinuation of furosemide (and use of another diuretic) may be warranted, but not initially. Likewise, ultrasound and CT scanning may be indicated in the evaluation, but not initially.

3. a   This patient is the victim of nonaccidental trauma and child neglect. He has sustained trauma to his back, potentially affecting his kidneys. A threshold of 20 RBC/hpf has been suggested as a lower limit to warrant further evaluation for renal trauma. A CT scan would be the test of choice because of its sensitivity, and because it will also evaluate other organs, including the liver, spleen, or duodenum. Although ultrasound is helpful, it is only 70% as sensitive as the CT scan. An IV pyelogram is the test of choice in an emergent situation, when there is insufficient time to obtain a CT scan. A PT level might be helpful if a coagulopathy was the diagnosis in question, but this is not likely to be helpful with the general malnourished condition. In a 3-year-old boy, urinary catheterization is not routinely necessary to confirm hematuria.

4. e   This patient has hematuria associated with signs of obstruction. Ultrasonography would be indicated to evaluate for anatomic anomalies or extrinsic causes of compression. Wilm's tumor will cause hematuria in 12–25% of cases. Even though nephrolithiasis might cause abdominal pain and difficulty voiding, the pain is characteristically described as severe, often causing the patient to writhe in pain. A repeat urinalysis is not indicated given his symptoms. Urine calcium/creatinine and oxalate levels would be helpful to diagnose nephrolithiasis. Angiography may define renal flow, but it may not reveal an extrinsic source of obstruction.

5. b   Urethral prolapse may cause hematuria or vulvar bleeding. Varying amounts of urethral tissue may extrude through the meatal opening. The tissue appears hemorrhagic, edematous, and boggy, but the condition is relatively benign. Treatment includes application of premarin cream until the prolapse resolves. Sitz baths are unlikely to cure the problem, but may relieve associated dysuria. There is no role

for neomyxin/polysporin, hydrocortisone, or nystatin cream. Surgical excision may be required for resolution. Consultation with social services is not indicated.

6. d   Formerly the most common cause of hematuria in childhood, acute poststreptococcal glomerulonephritis (APGN) typically presents with hypertension, edema, renal insufficiency, and hematuria approximately 1–2 weeks after a streptococcal infection. APGN is a glomerular source of bleeding. The antecedent streptococcal infection usually involves a nephritogenic strain of group A beta-hemolytic *Streptococcus,* causing a pharyngitis or a skin infection. The nephritis will typically present with a urine appearance that is smoky or tea colored, with RBC cell casts, proteinuria, cellular casts, and dysmorphic RBCs. There may be renal insufficiency, and the C3 level will be depressed. Nonglomerular bleeding will have a urine appearance of red or pink urine, associated with blood clots, and an absence of proteinuria. The morphology of the erythrocytes (RBCs) is normal. Treatment is largely supportive.

7. d   Tuberculosis is a common cause of hematuria in adults, but less so for children because of the incubation period required for renal involvement. Tuberculosis must be suspected given the history and findings on examination. It is unlikely that this patient will develop renal insufficiency; therefore, hemodialysis is not necessary. Methylprednisolone may be used for autoimmune disorders causing hematuria (e.g., systemic lupus erythematosus), but it would be harmful in this vignette. Although the radiographic finding might represent a bacterial pneumonia, the history is more consistent with tuberculosis, and ampicillin is not helpful.

CHAPTER **35**

Hypertension

VINCENT J. WANG, M.D.

QUESTIONS

1. A 2-year-old boy is brought to the ED because of fever and cough. His initial vital signs are: T 40°C, HR 120, RR 20, and BP 130/90. His examination is normal except for rales at the right base. Explanations for his elevated BP include:

   a. The BP is normal for his age
   b. The BP cuff is too large
   c. The patient was crying during the BP measurement
   d. The BP increases incrementally for each degree of temperature elevation
   e. A pneumonia may cause elevations in BP

2. A 10-year-old boy has a BP of 130/85. He is otherwise completely well. His evaluation and initial ancillary testing does not reveal an identifiable source. Appropriate treatment includes:

   a. Discharge to home and follow-up with his primary care provider
   b. Intra-arterial BP measurements
   c. Outpatient treatment with furosemide
   d. Outpatient treatment with labatolol
   e. Admission for further diagnostic evaluation

3. A 3-year-old girl complains of headaches and has a resting BP of 125/90. She is otherwise healthy, with no current medical problems. Her neonatal history is significant for polycythemia, requiring a partial exchange transfusion. Your examination of her, which is thorough and pertinent to specific causes, is completely normal. Definitive diagnostic evaluation includes:

   a. Toxicologic screening
   b. Echocardiogram
   c. Head CT scan
   d. Urine catecholamine testing
   e. Renal angiography

4. A 5-year-old boy is referred to you for evaluation of his BP. He has a resting BP of 120/75. He is otherwise healthy and without complaints. His physical examination is significant for diminished femoral pulses, and his lower extremity BP 100/60 on the right and 96/58 on the left. Appropriate evaluation includes:

   a. Outpatient serial BP measurements
   b. Echocardiogram
   c. Urine catecholamine testing
   d. Duplex ultrasound imaging of the calves
   e. Renal angiography

5. A 14-year-old girl complains of a headache. The triage nurse obtains BP 240/140, and this is promptly brought to your attention. She has had a history of frequent UTIs and asthma. She is ill appearing on examination. Her serum testing reveals: Na 140, K 3.9, Cl 110, HCO$_3$ 24, BUN 50, Cr 3.5, and glucose 110. She begins seizing. Your choice of antihypertensive treatment includes:

   a. Sodium nitroprusside
   b. Nifedipine
   c. Hydralazine
   d. Labetalol
   e. Clonidine

6. A 12-year-old boy is referred by his primary care physician for a BP of 200/120. He complains of intermittent episodes of headache, sweating, palpitations, and flushing. He has lost weight over the preceding months. He is anxious appearing and his HR is 140 on examination. He begins seizing. The best choice of antihypertensive medication includes:

   a. Labetalol
   b. Nicardipine
   c. Phentolamine
   d. Diazoxide
   e. Hydralazine

7. A 16-year-old boy with chronic renal failure and depression is brought to the ED after an overdose. He normally takes nifedipine orally, but took the entire bottle of nifedipine capsules 1–2 hours ago. He is slow to react and has a BP of 70/40. The best choice of treatment includes IV:

   a. Epinephrine
   b. Phentolamine
   c. Potassium
   d. Calcium
   e. Glucose

ANSWERS

1. c It will be difficult to obtain a BP in a crying child, and, if obtained, it may be falsely elevated. Reasons for falsely elevated BP measurements include patients in pain, patients who are crying, and BP measurements made with cuff sizes that are too small. There is no association between hypertension and temperature, or hypertension and pneumonia.

2. a In a patient with significant but moderate hypertension, appropriate management is a thorough history and evaluation identifying risk factors, underlying medical causes, and complications of hypertension. If these are normal, the patient should be discharged to outpatient follow-up with the primary care provider for serial BP measurements. There is no role for invasive BP measurements. Outpatient medical therapy should not be instituted from the ED visit. Admission is unnecessary in an asymptomatic patient.

3. e Common causes of hypertension in children under 6 years of age include renal parenchymal diseases, coarctation of the aorta, and renal artery stenosis. Given the significant neonatal history, requiring exchange transfusion (via umbilical artery catheterization), the evaluation of renal artery stenosis should proceed. Even though coarctation of the aorta is a possible cause, the history and physical examination indicate another etiology. Toxicologic screening would be indicated in an adolescent who you suspected ingested amphetamines or other substances that could cause hypertension. A head CT scan is not indicated. This patient does not exhibit systemic symptoms of a pheochromocytoma or neuroblastoma, which may also secrete catecholamines; thus, urine catecholamine screening is less likely to be helpful.

4. b This patient has a coarctation of the aorta. Appropriate evaluation would include an echocardiogram. Given his diminished femoral pulses, serially repeated BP measurements are not adequate. Urine catecholamine screening and renal angiography are not indicated. Duplex ultrasound imaging is appropriate for deep venous thromboses, but not for the evaluation of coarctation of the aorta.

5. a Sodium nitroprusside is a powerful vasodilator with nearly immediate onset of effect. This would be appropriate treatment in this hypertensive crisis. Nifedipine and hydralazine are effective medications for hypertensive urgencies, but should not be used in hypertensive emergencies because their onset of effect is longer. Labetalol can be used for hypertensive emergencies, but relative contraindications for its use include patients with asthma, pheochromocytoma, heart block, or congestive heart failure.

6. c This patient has hypertension because of an underlying pheochromocytoma. The best antihypertensive medication, therefore, is phentolamine for its alpha-blocking properties. Labetalol is contraindicated in this condition. Nicardipine and diazoxide are appropriate for other hypertensive emergencies, but they are not the best choice for this scenario. Hydralazine may be used in a hypertensive urgency.

7. d Complications of antihypertensive therapy may occur, especially in the outpatient setting. Nifedipine is a calcium channel blocker and will cause vasodilation. In a nifedipine overdose, calcium should be given if the patient is symptomatic. Epinephrine will improve blood pressure, but calcium is a better choice. There is no role for phentolamine, potassium, or glucose administration.

CHAPTER **36**

Immobile Arm

VINCENT J. WANG, M.D.

QUESTIONS

1. A 2-year-old boy was playing at home when he reportedly fell onto his arm. He has not used his right arm since then. He has been healthy with no history of fever. On examination, he is well appearing and easily distractible. He is holding his right arm in a pronated and flexed position against his body. He has no tenderness of his upper extremities. Appropriate management includes:

   a. Obtaining radiographs of his entire right upper extremity
   b. Obtaining a radiograph of his right elbow
   c. Placing a clavicle strap
   d. Obtaining an antinuclear antibody (ANA) test
   e. Supinating and flexing his forearm

2. A 9-month-old girl, recently immigrated from Sudan, presents with irritability. She cries whenever someone holds her hands. There is no history of trauma or fever. On examination, she is alert, but crying. She has pain on movement of her left upper extremity, especially when her hand is palpated. She has mild puffiness of her left hand and fingers. There is no warmth, erythema, or deformity. The definitive diagnostic test would be:

   a. Radiograph of the left arm
   b. CBC
   c. ANA
   d. Hemoglobin electrophoresis
   e. Thick smear

3. A 4-year-old girl complains of elbow and knee pain for the past year. She has had low-grade fevers and malaise, but no history of trauma. Her mother says the pain and stiffness seem worse in the mornings. On examination, she is well appearing and in no acute distress. She has stiffness and swelling of both of her elbows and her left knee. She has mild warmth over the joints, but no erythema. Definitive diagnostic testing includes:

   a. Radiographs of the elbows
   b. Rheumatoid factor
   c. ANA
   d. Hemoglobin electrophoresis
   e. None of the above

4. A 5-year-old boy complains of left elbow pain. He had been climbing on the monkey bars when he fell onto his left arm. He complains of pain over his left elbow. On examination, he has mild swelling of his left elbow. He has pain on range of motion, but has normal neurovascular function. Radiographs of his elbow reveal no bony abnormalities, but there is a lucency in the soft tissues, posterior to the distal humerus. Appropriate treatment includes:

   a. Immobilization and orthopedic evaluation
   b. Immobilization and outpatient follow-up as needed
   c. Placing an Ace wrap
   d. Recommending a biopsy of the site
   e. Immediate operative reduction

5. A 4-year-old girl complains of left arm pain. She has been complaining of pain for several weeks now, despite "normal" examinations by her physician. She is otherwise healthy with no other medical problems. On examination, she has mild tenderness over the distal humerus. There is no swelling, erythema, or warmth. A radiograph of her humerus reveals a 1-cm lesion in the distal humerus. The lesion is ovoid and eccentrically located, with a sclerotic medullary border. Appropriate management includes:

   a. Consulting social services
   b. Obtaining a skeletal series
   c. Casting the arm
   d. Performing a bone marrow biopsy
   e. Administering analgesics only

6. A 7-year-old girl has swelling over her right distal radius after falling while rollerblading. She has point tenderness at this site. Her radiograph is normal, with no evidence of fracture. Appropriate treatment includes:

   a. Casting her forearm
   b. Administering analgesics and reassuring the patient
   c. Performing fluoroscopy of the distal radius
   d. Obtaining radiographs of her elbow
   e. Obtaining a CBC and ESR (erythrocyte sedimentation rate)

ANSWERS

1. e   Even though this patient does not present with the classic history of a "nursemaid's elbow" (axial traction), some patients will have a radial head subluxation with an antecedent history of falling onto the arm. The patient will typically hold his arm in a pronated and flexed position against his body. There will be minimal to no tenderness of his arm, and no erythema, warmth, or fever. If this is the case, attempts at manual reduction are appropriate. A supination and flexion maneuver has classically been taught for reduction. One study of a hyperpronation maneuver has reported improved success. (Macias CG, Bothner J, Wiebe R. A comparison of supination/flexion to hyperpronation in the reduction of radial head subluxations. Pediatrics 1998;102(1):e10.) Radiographs would be appropriate if a fracture was suspected or if reduction had failed. Radiographs of the entire upper extremity may be necessary if the examination is difficult or equivocal. A clavicle strap is indicated for clavicular fractures, but this is not the case. An ANA would aid with the diagnosis of a rheumatologic process.

2. d   Any child of African ethnicity with unexplained limb pain should be screened for sickle-cell disease. Screening is routinely performed at birth in some regions of the United States. Dactylitis may be the first presentation of sickle-cell disease in a child, but patients with sickle-cell disease may also present with bony or joint pain consistent with vaso-occlusive crises. Given the history and physical examination, it is unlikely that this patient has a fracture, infection, or neurologic process. This patient may have an early manifestation of juvenile rheumatoid arthritis (JRA) or systemic lupus erythematosus (SLE), but larger joints are usually affected. A thick smear would be appropriate for the diagnosis of malaria, which may cause irritability accompanied by fever, but not limb pain.

3. e   Pauciarticular-onset JRA is the most common form of JRA, affecting 30–40% of patients. It is characterized by arthritis affecting four or fewer joints over the first 6-month period. Unlike other forms of JRA, as many as 90% of patients will be ANA positive, but this test is not definitive. Clinical findings are similar to polyarticular onset JRA. Other laboratory findings are anemia, elevation of ESR and C-reactive protein, and a leukemoid reaction of the WBCs. Rheumatoid factor is not helpful. Even though ancillary testing will support the diagnosis, the diagnosis of JRA is primarily based on clinical suspicion.

4. a   This patient most likely has a nondisplaced supracondylar humeral fracture. The lucency behind the posterior aspect of the distal humerus is the "posterior fat pad" sign, which is suggestive of an occult fracture. Immobilization and orthopedic evaluation is indicated. Operative reduction is not necessary for this degree of injury (Grade I), but may be necessary with displacement (Grades II and III).

5. e   Benign fibrous cortical defects are usually incidental findings that may occur in up to 40% of children. They are most commonly found in the metaphyses of long bones. Most are asymptomatic, but some patients may present with chronic bone pain or a pathologic fracture. Treatment is usually unnecessary because most will regress spontaneously. Curettage or steroid injections are occasionally performed for fractures or persistent symptoms. (Pappo AS. "Benign Tumors." In: Behrman et al., eds. *Nelson Textbook of Pediatrics,* fifteenth edition. Philadelphia: W.B. Saunders, 1996;461:1475–1477.) This finding is not consistent with nonaccidental trauma; therefore, a social services consult and skeletal series are not necessary. Casting is not necessary unless there was a pathologic fracture associated with the defect. Likewise, bone marrow biopsy is unnecessary because this is not a malignant lesion.

6. a   Salter-Harris I fractures are fractures through the epiphyseal growth plate. Radiographic findings may be absent, requiring clinical suspicion for diagnosis. Point tenderness over a growth plate suggests this type of fracture. Immobilization, either by splinting or casting the injured site, is indicated. Analgesics and reassurance are not adequate. Fluoroscopy is not necessary. Referred pain from the elbow is unlikely, given the mechanism of the injury and the physical findings. Infection is also unlikely, given the scenario, and therefore a CBC and ESR are not indicated.

CHAPTER 37

Injury—Ankle

VINCENT J. WANG, M.D.

QUESTIONS

1. An 8-year-old girl complains of ankle pain. She had jumped down from a tree and had twisted her ankle by inverting it. She has moderate swelling and tenderness over the distal fibula, with the point of maximal tenderness 1–2 cm proximal to the end of the fibula. Radiographs of her ankle are normal. Your next step in management includes:

   a. Ibuprofen, an Ace wrap, and discharge to home
   b. Obtaining stress views of the distal fibula
   c. Immobilization and orthopedic evaluation
   d. Operative immobilization with pinning
   e. Obtaining an CBC and ESR

2. A 13-year-old boy complains of ankle pain. He had jumped over a fence and landed on his ankle awkwardly. He complains of moderate swelling and pain over the ankle diffusely, but on your examination you are able to localize the tenderness to the lateral aspect of the tibial physis. Radiographs of the ankle reveal slight widening of the lateral aspect of the tibial physis, but no fractures. You suspect that he has a(n):

   a. Juvenile Tillaux fracture
   b. Triplanar fracture
   c. Salter-Harris V fracture of the distal physis
   d. Hill-Sachs fracture
   e. Ankle sprain

3. A 14-year-old boy has ankle pain and swelling. He had fallen from a ledge, but had landed on his feet. He complains of severe pain and swelling over his left ankle. He has moderate swelling over the entire ankle, with diffuse tenderness. His ankle radiographs reveal a fracture line through the anterolateral tibial epiphysis. A second fracture line lies through the medial part of the epiphysis. A third fracture line runs through the tibial shaft. Further appropriate diagnostic imaging includes:

   a. Stress films
   b. Ankle arthrography
   c. Computed tomography (CT scan)
   d. Ultrasonography
   e. Bone scan

4. An 18-year-old girl complains of right ankle pain after playing basketball. She had inverted her ankle during the game. On examination, she has mild swelling over the lateral ankle. She has tenderness anterior to the distal fibula, but no fibular tenderness. She bears weight, with a mild limp, and has no ankle instability. Her neurovascular examination is normal. Treatment includes:

   a. Obtaining a CBC and ESR
   b. Ibuprofen, an Ace wrap, and discharge to home
   c. Obtaining a radiograph of her ankle
   d. Immobilization and orthopedic evaluation
   e. Operative immobilization with pinning

5. A 17-year-old girl complains of left ankle pain after playing soccer. She had inverted her ankle and complains of severe pain and swelling over her lateral ankle. On examination, she has moderate swelling and diffuse tenderness over her lateral ankle. Her anterior drawer test reveals 1-cm laxity anteriorly and her talar tilt test reveals minimal laxity. Radiographs of her ankle are normal and her physes are fused. Your diagnosis is:

   a. Salter-Harris I fracture of the distal fibula
   b. Grade III sprain of the deltoid ligament
   c. Grade II sprain of the posterior talofibular ligament
   d. Grade III sprain of the anterior talofibular ligament
   e. Disruption of the tibiofibular syndesmosis

6. A 16-year-old boy complains of right ankle pain after crashing his motorcycle. On examination, he has a gross deformity of his ankle, with posterior displacement of the foot. He has no palpable dorsalis pedis pulse and his toes are cold and pale. Immediate treatment includes:

   a. Immobilization and orthopedic evaluation
   b. Doppler ultrasonography
   c. Longitudinal traction to the foot
   d. Immediate operative intervention
   e. Normal saline (NS) bolus IV

7. A 5-year-old girl complains of ankle pain. She was jumping on a bed two days ago, and has been complaining of lateral ankle pain since then. She refuses to walk. On examination, her temperature is 38.2°C, and she has mild tenderness, but no swelling over the distal fibula. You note warmth of the area, but no erythema, WBC 11,000, ESR 50 mm/hr, and her ankle radiographs are normal. Your next step in management is:

   a. Discharge to home on analgesic medications
   b. Immobilization and outpatient orthopedic referral if the pain persists
   c. Stress views of the ankle
   d. Bone scan
   e. Arthrocentesis

ANSWERS

1. c   Salter-Harris I fractures of the physes are characterized by fractures through the growth plate, and may have no radiographic abnormalities. The diagnosis is made on clinical suspicion in a child whose growth plates have not fused. Significant tenderness and swelling over a physis in this scenario is suggestive of a Salter-Harris I fracture. Appropriate treatment involves immobilization with splinting or casting, and orthopedic evaluation.

2. a   Juvenile Tillaux fractures result from external rotation injuries and are an example of transitional fractures. Closure of the distal tibial physis typically begins in the center of the bone, spreading medially, posteriorly, and finally laterally. The lateral aspect of the distal tibial physis is less stable for approximately 18 months after the medial tibial physis begins to close. A juvenile Tillaux fracture involves a fracture through the lateral border of the tibia because it is torn off by the anterior tibiofibular ligament. It is a Salter-Harris III fracture that may be difficult to diagnose because routine x-rays may not show the fracture line well. The only radiographic sign may be minimal widening of the lateral tibial physis, but a faint vertical fracture line may also be seen through the epiphysis.

3. c   Triplanar fractures are another example of a transitional fracture. It is a combination of a juvenile Tillaux fracture and a Salter-Harris II fracture of the distal tibia. CT scanning of the fracture is often necessary to fully evaluate these fractures. The other studies are not indicated.

4. b   Ankle sprains are more common in adults and in children whose physes have fused. She has tenderness over her anterior talofibular ligament, without ankle instability; therefore, she has a Grade I ankle sprain. According to the Ottawa ankle rules, she does not require radiographic imaging.

5. d   The presence of a laxity on the anterior drawer test and instability on the talar tilt test suggests an isolated injury of the anterior talofibular ligament, which is the weakest of the lateral ligaments. Salter-Harris I fractures are fractures through the physis, which is fused in this patient. The deltoid ligament is on the medial aspect of the ankle. The posterior talofibular ligament is the strongest of the three lateral ligaments, and injury would manifest as laxity on extreme dorsiflexion of the ankle.

6. c   Vascular compromise from a posterior dislocation of the ankle is an orthopedic emergency that must be reduced immediately. Reduction may be attempted by applying longitudinal traction to the foot. If this is not successful, application of longitudinal traction should be combined with pulling the foot in a posterior to anterior direction.

7. d   Osteomyelitis may manifest as described in this vignette. The ESR is a helpful, but nonspecific, marker of inflammation, but it does support this diagnosis. A normal CBC and radiograph do not exclude this diagnosis, and if clinical suspicion is high, a bone scan or an MRI is indicated, despite these normal values. Without ankle swelling or effusion, arthrocentesis is not indicated. Stress views are not indicated, given the clinical symptoms.

CHAPTER 38

Injury—Head

DAVID GREENES, M.D.

QUESTIONS

1. A 12-year-old boy was a passenger in a high-speed motor vehicle accident. On arrival to the ED, he appears to be sleeping, but he opens his eyes when you speak to him. Upon your command, he is able to squeeze your fingers or lift his legs. When asked if he knows where he is, he says he thinks he's in an ambulance. You record his Glasgow Coma Scale (GCS) score as:

   a. 11
   b. 12
   c. 13
   d. 14
   e. 15

2. An 18-month-old boy is brought to the ED after falling 10 feet from an open window. On physical examination, you immediately note periorbital ecchymoses ("raccoon's eyes"). Which of the following other physical examination findings would be least expected in this patient?

   a. Ecchymosis overlying the mastoid bone
   b. Bleeding from the right ear
   c. Retinal hemorrhages
   d. Clear rhinorrhea
   e. Right facial droop

3. A 5-year-old boy fell off his bicycle and struck his head 2 hours ago. He had loss of consciousness (LOC) for approximately 10 seconds and does not remember the event. He initially complained of headache and vomited once. By the time of your examination, he is feeling much better, with a normal examination of the head and a completely normal neurologic examination. Of the following, which is the most appropriate course of action?

   a. Observe in the ED for 2–4 hours
   b. Discharge to home with instructions
   c. Admit to hospital for 24 hour observation
   d. Obtain skull radiographs
   e. Consult a neurosurgeon

4. Which of the following head-injured patients, all of whom have normal neurologic examinations, would be the most appropriate candidate for skull radiographs?

   a. A 4-year-old boy with hemotympanum and Battle's sign
   b. A 7-year-old girl with an occipital scalp hematoma
   c. A 6-month-old boy with a parietal scalp hematoma
   d. A 9-month-old boy with palpable depression of skull vertex
   e. A 2-year-old boy who fell 5 feet but has normal head examination

5. A 7-year-old boy fell 6 feet from a tree house to the ground. He is brought to the ED 2 hours after the fall. Which of the following historical features is most concerning for cerebral contusion or intracranial hematoma?

   a. A brief convulsion immediately upon impact
   b. LOC for 10 seconds
   c. Two episodes of emesis
   d. A brief convulsion that occurred 10 minutes ago
   e. Amnesia for the fall

ANSWERS

1. c The Glasgow Coma Scale (GCS) is an assessment tool used to describe a patient's level of neurologic functioning, ascribing a score between 3 and 15. Three separate subscales are used to assess the patient's eye opening, motor activity, and verbal skills. The full scale is available for review in Table 38.1 in the *Textbook of Pediatric Emergency Medicine*, fourth edition. The patient described would receive an eye opening score of 3 ("opens eyes to voice"), motor score of 6 ("follows commands"), and a verbal score of 4 ("answers questions, but confused"), for a total score of 13.

2. c Periorbital ecchymoses, or "raccoon's eyes" are classic physical examination findings in cases of basilar skull fracture. Basilar skull fractures lead to unique clinical signs because of injury to the paranasal sinuses and mastoid air cells adjacent to the basal skull, because of injury to the cranial nerves coursing through the basal skull, or because of injury to the blood vessels that pass through the basal skull. If the dura is lacerated, cerebrospinal fluid (CSF) leaks can occur as well.

   Ecchymosis or swelling overlying the mastoid (Battle's sign) indicates injury to the mastoid air cells. Hemotympanum, or blood from the external ear, also indicates injury to the mastoid or to the adjacent basal portion of the temporal bone. Clear rhinorrhea in this setting may indicate leakage of cerebrospinal fluid (CSF) through a dural tear and into fractured paranasal sinuses. Right facial droop indicates a seventh nerve injury, which is seen in some cases of basilar skull fractures.

   Retinal hemorrhages result from severe shear forces, and they are virtually pathognomonic for the shaking-impact syndrome seen in abused children. Retinal hemorrhages would not be expected in a typical case of basilar skull fracture.

3. a This child has clearly suffered a nontrivial head injury, with a history of LOC, headache, and vomiting. Because this child is improving, the most likely diagnosis is concussion, with no focal intracranial injury; nonetheless, the clinician needs to recognize the potential for intracranial injury in this situation. Although most children with clinically significant intracranial injuries are symptomatic from the time of the trauma, a small subset of children do not become symptomatic until several hours later. It would be inappropriate, therefore, to discharge the patient at this time, with no further evaluation for possible intracranial injury. One option would be to perform a head CT, and to discharge the patient to home if the CT is normal. Another appropriate option, however, is to observe the child for 4–6 hours after the injury. If the patient has no clinical deterioration during this time period, it is highly unlikely that the patient will have significant deterioration later. In most routine cases of concussion, it is unnecessary to admit the child to the hospital for a prolonged period of observation. With a well-appearing patient who has no evidence of a surgical lesion, it is unnecessary to consult a neurosurgeon at this time. Skull radiographs would not provide information about the intracranial contents and would be unlikely to be helpful.

4. c For most head-injured patients, the decision should be whether to perform a head CT or to perform no imaging at all. In the case of suspected basilar skull fracture (a) or clinically evident depressed skull fracture (d), head CT should be pursued to afford a view of both the skull as well as the adjacent intracranial structures, which may also be injured. In well-appearing children beyond infancy (b and e), head CT is usually not necessary, even in cases in which scalp hematoma is present. In c, however, it is reasonable to pursue skull radiographs as the initial imaging study. Head-injured infants may have intracranial injury with few, if any, clinical signs, especially if they have an associated skull fracture. Although one could use head CT as the initial imaging study for all head-injured infants, head CT has the disadvantage of requiring sedation for many infants. Many clinicians, therefore, use skull radiographs as an initial imaging test for well-appearing head-injured infants, especially if they have a scalp hematoma. Those patients with skull fractures identified on plain radiographs should then have a head CT to evaluate for associated intracranial injury. Well-appearing infants without skull fracture are quite unlikely to have a clinically important intracranial injury and may be safely managed without head CT.

5. d Posttraumatic seizures may be classified as immediate, early, or late. Immediate posttraumatic seizures result from the direct application of energy to the brain cortex as a result of the traumatic impact. These seizures occur within seconds of the trauma. Although immediate seizures indicate a high-force blow to the brain, they are not necessarily associated with focal intracranial pathology. In contrast, early posttraumatic seizures, occurring minutes to hours after the trauma, are frequently a manifesta-

tion of an irritable focus in the brain, often associated with cerebral contusion or intracranial bleeding. Early seizures should be considered to be an indication for immediate head CT. Brief LOC, amnesia for the traumatic event, and self-limited vomiting all may be associated with more serious head injuries, but they are not uncommon in patients with minor head injury. If a patient appears well when examined, these historical features do not necessarily indicate a high risk for intracranial pathology.

CHAPTER **39**

Injury—Knee

ANDREA STRACCIOLINI, M.D.

QUESTIONS

1. A 10-year-old boy complains of severe pain and swelling over the distal left femur that occurred after he fell from the jungle gym at school. He is refusing to bear weight. On physical examination he has focal tenderness and swelling over the distal femur. His neurovascular examination is intact. Plain radiographs of the femur and knee (including a sunrise view) are normal. The most likely diagnosis in this child is:

   a. Salter-Harris fracture
   b. Torn anterior cruciate ligament (ACL)
   c. Patellar fracture
   d. Epicondylar fracture
   e. Supracondylar fracture

2. A 14-year-old boy comes to the ED after injuring his knee while playing football. The knee is significantly swollen and he is unable to bear weight. On physical examination, he is afebrile and there is diffuse swelling of his knee. The Lachman test is positive. His knee radiographs reveal no fractures. The ED management of this injury includes:

   a. Knee immobilization
   b. Immediate orthopedic consultation
   c. Arthrocentesis
   d. MRI
   e. Arthroscopy

3. A 16-year-old female dancer comes to the ED after an acute injury to her knee. She tells you that she heard a ripping sound and felt a popping sensation. She initially had significant pain, but the pain has now resolved. On physical exam the knee is not swollen, erythematous, or deformed. Range of motion is entirely normal. The most likely diagnosis is:

   a. Patellar subluxation
   b. Medial meniscal tear
   c. ACL sprain
   d. Posterior cruciate ligament (PCL) sprain
   e. Salter-Harris I fracture

4. A high school football player injures his left knee during practice. He says that he planted his foot on the ground and turned to catch a pass. He felt a "pop," subsequently followed by left knee pain. The knee swelled immediately and he was unable to finish practice. He has not been able to bear weight on the leg following the injury. The most likely injury is:

   a. A medial collateral ligament (MCL) sprain
   b. A lateral meniscal tear
   c. A sprain of the lateral collateral ligament (LCL)
   d. A torn posterior cruciate ligament (PCL)
   e. A torn anterior cruciate ligament (ACL)

5. A 15-year-old girl comes to the ED for evaluation of a painful right knee. She reports that her right knee "gives out" periodically. She also tells you that she has difficulty straightening the knee occasionally when her knee is partially flexed. On physical examination, there is a mild effusion and a positive Apley compression test. There is no erythema or warmth. She vaguely remembers injuring the knee while playing field hockey last summer. The most likely diagnosis is:

   a. Anterior cruciate ligament (ACL) tear
   b. Patellofemoral pain syndrome
   c. Juvenile rheumatoid arthritis (JRA)
   d. Medial meniscal tear
   e. Chondromalacia patella

6. A 19-year-old boy comes to the ED with a complaint of a swollen right knee. He states that while playing football yesterday, he felt a "pop" in the knee. He was able to ambulate on the extremity after the incident, but over the following 24 hours, the knee swelled up. The LEAST likely diagnosis in this case is:

   a. MCL sprain
   b. Subluxating patella
   c. ACL injury
   d. Osteochondral fracture
   e. Medial meniscus tear

7. A 14-year-old male soccer player reports pain and tenderness over the anterior aspect of his knee. He tells you that the symptoms have been occurring for the past 2 months. He denies acute trauma to the knee. The pain seems worse when he is playing soccer and going up and down stairs. He denies fever, weight loss, or fatigue. He has no prior history of joint pain. He was vacationing on Cape Cod, Massachusetts, 3 months ago. The most likely etiology for this boy's pain is:

a. Neoplasm
b. Patellar bursitis
c. Osteomyelitis
d. Lyme disease
e. Osgood-Schlatter disease

8. A 16-year-old girl comes to the ED because she has been having knee pain for 3 months. She states that the knee pain often occurs immediately after sitting in a movie theatre for 2 hours and resolves after increased mobilization. This history is classic for:

a. Patellofemoral pain syndrome
b. Rheumatoid arthritis
c. Quadriceps muscle sprain
d. Patellar tendonitis
e. Slipped capital femoral epiphysis

9. A 12-year-old girl comes to the ED with nonspecific left knee pain that has been occurring for approximately 1 month. She denies fever, trauma, or other joint involvement. You suspect osteochondritis dissecans (OCD). AP (anterior-posterior) and lateral x-rays are negative for any pathologic lesion. The next step in your attempt to make the diagnosis is:

a. Bone scan
b. MRI
c. Sedimentation rate (ESR)
d. Orthopedic consultation
e. Intercondylar x-rays

10. An obese 13-year-old boy comes to the ED with left knee pain that has been occurring for 7 days. He denies trauma to the knee, swelling, redness, or fever. He states that when he moves his left leg, the left knee hurts. On physical exam, the patient experiences pain with passive range of motion of the hip. There is no point tenderness, erythema, or effusion of the knee. The best treatment for this patient is:

a. Surgery
b. Antibiotics
c. Immobilization
d. NSAIDs (nonsteroidal antiinflammatory drugs)
e. Crutches

ANSWERS

1. a   Because this child is 10 years of age, his physes are still open; thus, this child is likely to have a Salter-Harris I fracture of the distal femoral physis. The injury usually follows significant direct or indirect trauma. The patient has severe pain, refuses to bear weight, and experiences joint and soft-tissue swelling. X-rays may be normal if the injury is a nondisplaced Salter-Harris I fracture. A torn ACL would be unlikely in this child because at this age the physes are often weaker than the ligaments. Radiographs would be abnormal in a child with a patellar fracture, epicondylar, or supracondylar fracture.

2. a   This case describes an ACL tear. An acute tear of the ACL usually involves a rotational force on a fixed foot. The patient often reports the sensation of a "pop." The joint usually swells immediately due to hemarthrosis and has a decreased range of motion. The Lachman test is very sensitive in detecting ACL injuries, but it may be falsely negative soon after the injury, when the knee is swollen and painful. In the ED the treatment for this injury is immobilization and orthopedic follow-up. An MRI will likely be obtained at that time. Arthrocentesis and CBC/blood culture are indicated when there is concern for a septic joint. Emergent orthopedic consultation is not necessary with an isolated ACL tear.

3. a   Patellar dislocation or subluxation occurs as the quadriceps muscles pull along the patellar tendon to extend the knee. If the vastus medialis fibers do not keep the patella in the intercondylar groove, the patella may dislocate laterally. This injury often occurs in gymnasts or dancers. The patient often feels or hears a ripping or popping sensation or sound. A patellar subluxation presents with a history similar to a dislocation, but the patient is in no longer in pain and has a normal physical examination. If this were an ACL or a posterior cruciate ligament (PCL) tear, the knee would be swollen and persistently painful. A Salter-Harris fracture presents with focal tenderness over the fracture, and motion is often painful and limited.

4. e   ACL injuries occur in many scenarios, but they usually involve rotational forces on a fixed foot, as with this football player. The patient often reports the sensation of a "pop," and cannot bear weight im-

mediately after the injury because of pain. A PCL injury is extremely rare and usually results from a direct force on the tibial tubercle, pushing the tibia posteriorly on the femur. The posterior drawer sign will be present. Isolated sprains of the lateral and medial collateral ligaments (LCL and MCL) are usually not associated with significant effusions. MCL sprains occur after a blow to the lateral side of the knee. LCL sprains occur after a blow to the medial side of the knee.

5. d The Apley compression test is positive in patients with injuries to their menisci. The menisci are fibrocartilage pads that act as shock absorbers to the knee joint. The patient with a meniscal injury may report an acute popping sensation and the feeling of the knee "giving out." The patient may more chronically report that the knee suddenly refuses to extend fully, "locking up" and then suddenly "unlocking."

6. a A subluxating patella, meniscal tear, and osteochondral fracture may cause a "popping" sensation. The patellofemoral pain syndrome may be associated with "giving way" of the knee. An MCL sprain is not associated with a "popping" or "giving out" sensation. An ACL tear is possible, although the swelling is often more acute.

7. e Osgood-Schlatter disease typically causes a chronic history of knee pain exacerbated by squatting or jumping. The disease is usually seen in patients between 10 and 15 years of age. The patients have localized tenderness and occasionally swelling over the tibial tubercle. Osteomyelitis is usually associated with fever. Patellar bursitis presents with pain under the patella. A neoplasm is usually visible on x-ray and does not usually present with this history. Lyme arthritis presents as an acute diffusely swollen knee without erythema or area of focal pain.

8. a A patient with patellofemoral pain syndrome classically has pain when sitting for a prolonged time with the knee flexed at 90 degrees. The pain disappears once the patient is ambulatory. The pain may be exacerbated with running, especially going down inclines or stairs. The patient may also have the sensation of the knee "giving out" when descending.

9. e Osteochondritis dissecans (OCD) is the separation of a small portion of the femoral condyle from the overlying cartilage. The patient is usually an adolescent with a 1–4 week history of nonspecific knee pain. Anterior and lateral x-rays may not show the lesion. A tunnel or intercondylar view should be obtained as the next diagnostic test. Laboratory evaluation is unnecessary because there is low suspicion for infection or systemic disease. Orthopedic consult is not necessary in the ED for this patient with knee pain for 1 month. Outpatient orthopedic follow-up is appropriate.

10. a Radiographs of the knee and hips are indicated in this obese child with knee pain. In subacute injuries, inquiry is made about hip or groin pain because the hip and knee share sensory nerves. Legg-Calvé-Perthes disease or a slipped capital femoral epiphysis (SCFE) may cause knee pain. This obese teenager has SCFE. Orthopedic consultation, admission to the hospital with strict bed rest, and operative intervention are necessary.

CHAPTER **40**

Injury—Shoulder

VINCENT J. WANG, M.D.

QUESTIONS

1. A 3-week-old boy comes to the ED with a nontender, left-sided swelling anteriorly, between the neck and acromioclavicular joint. The patient was born 9 pounds, 12 ounces by normal spontaneous vaginal delivery. He has otherwise been well. The mother says that the boy is right-handed. You recommend:

   a. No treatment
   b. A shoulder immobilizer
   c. Manual reduction immediately
   d. Clavicle strap
   e. Filing a child abuse report

2. An 18-year-old boy comes to you after being thrown to the ground during a wrestling match. He complains of right shoulder pain. On examination, he is in severe pain, with his arm internally rotated and slightly abducted. The contour of the affected shoulder is sharp, with a prominent acromion. Treatment includes:

   a. Closed reduction
   b. Shoulder immobilization
   c. Clavicle strap
   d. Operative reduction
   e. Cervical collar

3. A 14-year-old girl is brought to you after being involved in a high-speed motor vehicular collision. She had no LOC, and she is lucid and cooperative. She complains of abdominal pain and left shoulder pain. On palpation of her neck and shoulder, she has no swelling or point tenderness. She has full range of motion. You suspect the following study will make the diagnosis:

   a. Cervical spine radiographs
   b. AP and scapular shoulder radiographs
   c. AP shoulder radiograph with weights
   d. Abdominal CT scan
   e. Chest radiograph

4. A 15-year-old boy complains of right shoulder pain. He was riding his bicycle when he fell onto his right side. On examination, he has diffuse swelling and tenderness over his shoulder. You also note anesthesia over the lateral portion of his upper arm. AP (anterior-posterior) and lateral views of the shoulder reveal no fractures or dislocations. Your next step in management includes:

   a. Obtaining C-spine radiographs
   b. Obtaining AP and lateral views of the humerus
   c. Obtaining an axillary view of the shoulder
   d. Obtaining a fluoroscopic study of the shoulder
   e. Discharging the patient with a sling and analgesics

5. A 4-year-old boy has sustained a left upper extremity injury after falling onto his left side from a slide. He is scared and apprehensive, and he keeps asking to go home. An appropriate approach to his evaluation would be:

   a. Leaving his jacket and shirt on during the examination
   b. Examining the uninjured extremity first
   c. Palpating and examining only the sites that the child identifies as painful
   d. Obtaining the history only from the parents
   e. Obtaining radiographs of the entire extremity

ANSWERS

1. b   Clavicular fractures are the most common fractures in childhood, with more than half occurring before the age of 10 years. The usual scenario is a direct blow to the clavicle or a fall on an outstretched hand. Clavicular fractures also occur commonly during the delivery of a baby. The patient in the scenario was a large baby at birth, who probably had a shoulder dystocia and subsequent left clavicular fracture. The mother's statement that the boy is right-handed is unusual for children less than 1 year of age, and suggests that he may not have used his left hand as readily since birth. The location of the swelling suggests a clavicle fracture. Shoulder immobilization is currently recommended. (Kliegman RM. "Fractures." In: Behrman RE et al., eds. The Fetus and the Neonatal Infant. *Nelson Textbook of Pediatrics,* fifteenth edition. Philadelphia, W.B. Saunders, 1996:469.)

2. a   Shoulder or glenohumeral joint dislocations are rare under 12 years of age, and occur primarily as the skeleton matures. More than 95% of dislocations are anterior, but approximately 5% are posterior. In addition to internal rotation and slight abduction, the contour of the affected shoulder is sharp, with a prominent acromion. Trauma to the axillary nerve and vessels may have been sustained; therefore, sensation over the shoulder and distal pulses should be documented. Treatment involves closed reduction.

3. d   Given her otherwise normal physical examination, shoulder pathology is unlikely. When the spleen is injured, the hemoperitoneum may produce referred pain in the left shoulder (Kehr's sign). This occurs when blood is in contact with the diaphragm. Other sources of referred left-shoulder pain include herniated cervical discs and, rarely, injured myocardium. An abdominal CT scan would be the most helpful diagnostic test.

4. c   When suspecting a shoulder dislocation, an axillary view is imperative to evaluate dislocation of the humeral head. Given his examination and apparent injury to the axillary nerve, the patient has a shoulder dislocation and/or a fracture of the surgical neck of the humerus. Because the AP and lateral shoulder radiographs are normal, the injury must be a shoulder dislocation.

5. b   A 4-year-old child may be anxious and scared, but he may be able to give an accurate history, and he may be able to identify areas of pain. It is important to utilize all sources of information. A thorough examination should be performed, which includes removing his clothes and thoroughly examining both upper extremities. The entire extremity should be examined. The examiner may gain trust and decrease anxiety by examining the uninjured extremity first. Radiographic tests are important, but the physical examination will guide the examiner to appropriate radiographic tests.

CHAPTER 41

Jaundice—Unconjugated Hyperbilirubinemia

JACQUELINE BRYNGIL, M.D.

QUESTIONS

1. You are evaluating an 18-hour-old full-term Caucasian male in the ED for poor breast feeding. You note jaundice to the level of the umbilicus. There is no history of fever. On examination, the infant is well appearing and afebrile. Serum indirect to direct bilirubin is 17.5/0.1 mg/dl. Your most appropriate next step would be:

    a. Advise parent to discontinue breast feeding
    b. Obtain a Type and Coombs and CBC
    c. Perform a sepsis workup with lumbar puncture
    d. Administer IV fluids and antibiotics
    e. Perform an exchange transfusion

2. During your evaluation of a 7-day-old infant (born after 32 weeks gestation) who was brought to the ED unresponsive, you note scleral icterus. The infant was born during a home birth with a midwife and there was no prenatal care performed outside of the home. The mother noted a slight yellowing of the skin but was told that this was "just a little jaundice," not to worry and that it was due to breast feeding. One day prior, the baby was noted to have some twitching of the limbs and face and decreased feeding. On further examination the pupils are fixed and there is no hepatosplenomegaly. Vital signs are HR 110, RR 56, BP 70/palpable, and T 37.1°C rectally. Your most likely finding on further assessment of this infant is:

    a. Subdural hematomas and positive skeletal survey
    b. Gram-positive cocci on Gram stain of the CSF
    c. Mother type O/infant type A blood group
    d. Deficiency of bilirubin glucuronyl transferase
    e. Elevated serum conjugated bilirubin

3. You are evaluating a 10-year-old boy for "yellowing of the skin and eyes" noted by his mother. He has had no symptoms of abdominal pain, fever, vomiting, or lethargy. On physical examination he has no abdominal tenderness or hepatosplenomegaly; however, he appears slightly jaundiced and has scleral icterus. There is no history of travel, he has not taken any drugs recently, and only recalls eating a bean paste at a friend's home several days before. His blood work is most likely to reveal:

    a. A peripheral smear with schistosomes
    b. Bilirubin glucuronyl transferase deficiency
    c. A peripheral smear with spherocytes
    d. Glucose-6-phosphate dehydrogenase deficiency
    e. A peripheral smear with sickled RBCs

4. You are called to evaluate a 10-day-old breast-fed infant for jaundice. There is no history of fever, maternal-fetal blood group discrepancy, or family history of hemolytic disease. Vital signs are T 36.4°C, HR 130, RR 32, and BP 80/palpable. A serum bilirubin panel is 7.5/0.2 mg/dl. Your most appropriate next course of action would be:

    a. Initiate phototherapy and IV hydration
    b. Perform a sepsis workup, including lumbar puncture
    c. Reassure the parents and discharge home
    d. Obtain a peripheral smear for hemolysis
    e. Discontinuation of breast feeding

ANSWERS

1. b   Jaundice in the full-term neonate is not considered physiologic if it occurs in the first 24 hours of life. Obtaining a Type and Coombs', as well as a CBC to look for polycythemia, should be foremost in this infant, because forms of Coombs-positive hemolytic anemias present the most danger to the newborn. Management of this infant should also include phototherapy and hydration. Cessation of breast feeding is not recommended in cases of nonphysiologic jaundice. A sepsis workup should be performed in all ill-appearing infants. An exchange transfusion should be considered if the unconjugated bilirubin rises more than 5 mg/dl in 24 hours, or when levels exceed 25 mg/dl.

2. c   This baby has symptoms of kernicterus, a devastating neurologic disorder caused by elevated unconjugated serum bilirubin, which leads to staining of the basal ganglia and symptoms of encephalopathy. It is more common among preterm infants with isoimmune hemolytic anemias, particularly with ABO hemolytic disease of the newborn. It is likely that this mother did not have blood typing performed after her delivery. Although abused children may present unresponsive, there is nothing to suggest the presence of child abuse in this case. Sepsis is also a consideration in an unresponsive newborn and a lumbar puncture should be considered; however, it is unlikely that the symptoms are the result of meningitis in this case. Although Crigler-Najjar syndrome, which is associated with a deficiency of bilirubin glucuronyl transferase, should be considered as a potential cause of this child's unresponsiveness, it is extremely rare and kernicterus may occur as early as the third day of life. Kernicterus is due to elevated levels of unconjugated, not conjugated, bilirubin.

3. d   This patient is likely to have glucose-6-phosphate dehydrogenase deficiency syndrome, and his hemolysis and subsequent jaundice are likely to have been induced by the bean paste because interaction with fava beans often leads to hemolysis. Other forms of hemolytic anemias (e.g., hereditary spherocytosis and sickle-cell anemia) would have presented earlier. It is unlikely for this patient to have contracted malaria because there was no history of travel. Although there is a mild form of Crigler-Najjar syndrome that can present later in childhood or adolescence, this is rare and unlikely in this child.

4. c   This infant most likely has jaundice associated with breast feeding and requires parental reassurance only. Jaundice associated with breast feeding generally occurs by the seventh day of life and may last until 3 weeks of age. In the absence of other signs or symptoms of concern in this case, performing a sepsis workup, a workup for hemolytic disease, and a liver biopsy would be inappropriate. At a level of 7.5 mg/dl, this infant does not require phototherapy and should be encouraged to continue breast feeding.

CHAPTER 42

Jaundice—Conjugated Hyperbilirubinemia

JACQUELINE BRYNGIL, M.D.

QUESTIONS

1. A 1-month-old infant is brought to the ED for evaluation for decreased feeding. On his examination you note T 37.2°C, HR 140, RR 28, and BP 86/p. You note scleral icterus, jaundice, and abdominal distension. His birth history is unremarkable. Examination of the serum bilirubin reveals the presence of elevated conjugated (direct) bilirubin. All of the following may be likely causes of this child's condition, EXCEPT:

   a. Sepsis
   b. Gilbert's syndrome
   c. Neonatal hepatitis
   d. Alagille syndrome
   e. Biliary atresia

2. You are evaluating a 5-day-old infant in the ED for jaundice. Serum bilirubin levels show a significant elevation in the conjugated (direct) bilirubin. Physical examination reveals hepatomegaly, scattered petechiae, scleral icterus, and microcephaly. Further evaluation of this patient will most likely reveal:

   a. Family history of unusual facial characteristics
   b. Presence of alpha 1-antitrypsin deficiency
   c. Paucity of extrahepatic bile ducts
   d. Positive TORCH screen
   e. Presence of a heart murmur

3. A 14-year-old boy is brought to the ED for two days of vomiting. The patient had recently been camping, and then developed vomiting, abdominal pain, and a low-grade fever. On physical examination the patient is alert and in no distress. You note scleral icterus and tenderness in the right upper quadrant of the abdomen. In addition to an elevated direct bilirubin, laboratory findings most compatible with this patient include:

   a. Positive direct Coombs' test
   b. Decreased glucose
   c. Elevated transaminase levels
   d. Decreased hematocrit
   e. Elevated ammonia

4. A 5-year-old girl is brought to the ED for vomiting, malaise, altered mental status, and jaundice. There is no history of fever. You obtain laboratory studies that indicate an elevated direct bilirubin and elevated transaminase levels. The grandmother informs you that the child has recently eaten some of her garden mushrooms. Your most appropriate management for this patient is:

   a. Administer immunoglobulin to family members
   b. Perform a liver biopsy
   c. Administer IV fluids and discharge to home
   d. Send a serum toxicology screen
   e. Administer IV fluids and admit for supportive care

ANSWERS

1. b Gilbert's syndrome causes unconjugated (indirect) hyperbilirubinemia and does not usually present in infancy. Sepsis, most specifically that caused by *Escherichia coli* endotoxin, is a common and treatable cause of infantile conjugated hyperbilirubinemia, and should always be in the differential diagnosis. Neonatal hepatitis can be idiopathic or infectious and involves injury to the hepatocytes. It typically presents in infants less than 8 weeks of age. Alagille syndrome involves a paucity of intrahepatic bile ducts and is usually familial. Biliary atresia involves abnormalities of the extrahepatic bile ducts, leading to cholestasis. This typically presents early in infancy and is often difficult to distinguish from neonatal hepatitis. Evaluation for many of these conditions also involves liver biopsy.

2. d This patient has symptoms suggestive of a TORCH or STORCH (syphilis, toxoplasmosis, other agents, rubella, CMV, herpes simplex) infection acquired in utero. These infants may also suffer from seizures and irritability. Patients with Alagille syndrome typically have family members with distinctive facial characteristics (i.e., long, thin faces with broad foreheads) and do not present with microcephaly and petechiae. In alpha 1-antitrypsin deficiency, there is no associated microcephaly or petechiae, nor are these findings found in patients with biliary atresia or congestive heart failure.

3. c This patient has symptoms consistent with viral hepatitis, which is the most common cause of direct hyperbilirubinemia, and therefore would be likely to have elevated transaminase levels. It is typically associated with malaise, vomiting, and low-grade fever. An elevated direct Coombs' test is associated with autoimmune hemolytic anemias. These tend to occur primarily in newborns and are characterized by an elevated indirect bilirubin. Hypoglycemia and an indirect hyperbilirubinemia are commonly seen in infants with galactosemia. Hemolytic anemias, which are associated with a decreased hematocrit, generally do not present acutely. In addition, this patient does not appear to have signs of fulminant hepatic failure, which would be associated with coagulopathies and an elevated ammonia level.

4. e It is likely that the cause of this patient's jaundice is a toxic hepatitis, possibly due to mushroom ingestion of the *Amanita* species. Treatment for this condition is supportive and requires inpatient hospitalization. Most toxins do not appear on a serum toxicology screen. Administration of immunoglobulin should be given in cases of infectious hepatitis, most of which are associated with fever. In cases of protracted jaundice, a liver biopsy is often indicated for diagnostic purposes. Given the description of illness of this patient, discharge home from the ED would be inappropriate.

CHAPTER 43

Limp

ROBERT G. FLOOD, M.D.

QUESTIONS

1. A 10-month-old boy is brought to the ED by his parents with a subjective fever for the past 2 days, and has now been refusing to crawl for the past 12 hours. He has had no recent upper respiratory symptoms, and his immunizations are up to date. On physical exam, he is noted to have T 38.9°C, but is in no acute distress. He is holding his right hip in a flexed, abducted, and externally rotated position. Severe discomfort is noted with minimal movement of the right lower extremity. Which of the following would be the most appropriate next step in the management of this patient?

   a. Ibuprofen for 4–7 days
   b. CT scan of the right hip
   c. Arthrocentesis of the right hip
   d. Triple-phase bone scan
   e. MRI of the right hip

2. A 4-year-old boy is brought to the ED by his mother with a limp for the past 24 hours. He has no history of trauma or fever, but he did have an upper respiratory tract infection (URI) that resolved a few days ago. On physical exam, he is noted to be afebrile and nontoxic appearing. He refuses to bear weight on the left leg, but can sit unassisted. Examination of the spine and extremity is normal, except for minimal discomfort upon range of motion of the left hip. Which of the following is the most appropriate management of this patient?

   a. Ibuprofen for 4–7 days
   b. IV antibiotics for 3 weeks
   c. IV antibiotics for 6 weeks
   d. IV antibiotics for 3 days
   e. Acetaminophen for 4–7 days

3. The same patient in Question 2 returns to the ED 3 months later because of continued limp. He has no further pain in his hip or any other joint, and he has no history of fever or rash. The physical exam is normal with the exception of restricted range of motion of his left hip. Which of the following is the most likely cause of his condition?

   a. Chronic sequelae of a septic hip
   b. Aseptic necrosis of the left femoral head
   c. Acute septic arthritis of the left hip
   d. Developmental dysplasia of the left hip
   e. Juvenile rheumatoid arthritis (JRA)

4. A 12-year-old boy is brought into the ED by his father for the evaluation of pain in his right thigh and knee. He has no history of trauma, recent infections, or fever. On physical exam, the patient is noted to be moderately obese but afebrile, and he is in no acute distress. The rest of the physical exam is normal with the exception of the right hip, which has an obligatory external rotation when flexed. Which of the following is the most appropriate management of this patient's condition?

   a. IV antibiotics for 4–6 weeks
   b. Ibuprofen for 4–7 days
   c. Acetaminophen for pain
   d. Urgent operative intervention
   e. Placement of a knee immobilizer

5. A 10-year-old girl is brought into the ED by her father with the complaint of left ankle and foot pain for the past 3 days. She is a competitive tennis player, but has had no recent trauma, fever, or infections. On physical exam, she is noted to afebrile and in no acute distress. The rest of the physical exam is normal with the exception of her left foot, which is noted to have tenderness at the insertion point of her Achilles tendon on the calcaneus. Which of the following is the most likely diagnosis?

a. Acute sprain of the ankle and foot
b. Kohler's disease
c. Juvenile rheumatoid arthritis
d. Osgood-Schlatter disease
e. Sever's disease

ANSWERS

1. c   With a history of fever and pain with range of motion of the hip, a septic joint is the most likely diagnosis. Other supporting evidence of this diagnosis would be an elevated sedimentation rate and a leukocytosis. The definitive diagnosis, however, is made by arthrocentesis of the hip, at which time the synovial fluid may appear purulent with WBC counts of 25,000–100,000/μL, a positive Gram stain (50%), and positive culture (70–80%). Although *H. influenzae*, *S. aureus*, and *S. pneumoniae* have been associated with septic joints, the most likely organism in this immunized patient is *S. aureus*. A triple-phase bone scan may be considered in the evaluation of acute osteomyelitis. A CT scan or MRI may also be helpful in the evaluation of bony tumors and soft tissue collections, respectively; however, these should only be considered in this patient after the diagnosis of a septic hip has definitively been excluded by arthrocentesis. Although nonsteroidal antiinflammatory agents (NSAIDs) may be helpful for analgesia, this therapy alone would be more appropriate for transient synovitis of the hip. (Behrman RE et al., eds. *Nelson Textbook of Pediatrics,* fifteenth edition. Philadelphia: W.B. Saunders, 1996.)

2. a   The patient most likely has transient (toxic) synovitis of the hip. It is characterized by acute onset of pain and limp, often following an upper respiratory tract infection. It occurs predominantly in children between 3 and 8 years of age, and the cause is uncertain. These children are usually ambulatory and the hip is not held in flexion, abduction, or external rotation unless a joint effusion is present. They are usually afebrile or have a low-grade temperature of less than 38 °C. Supporting evidence of transient synovitis may include a normal sedimentation rate and an absence of serum leukocytosis. Treatment includes the use of NSAIDs along with a period of limited activity. Antibiotics have no role in the treatment of transient synovitis, but they would be the appropriate treatment for septic arthritis, as discussed in Question 1.

3. b   The patient most likely has aseptic necrosis of the femoral head, or Legg-Calvé-Perthes disease (LCPD). LCPD typically occurs between the ages of 4 and 8 years, and there is a male predilection, with a 5:1 ratio. The patient may present with an antalgic limp, but the disorder most often is painless and most children stay active. The onset of symptoms is most often insidious, developing over several weeks or months. Examination at the time of diagnosis may only show restricted range of motion with limited hip abduction and medial rotation. Because transient synovitis can present in the similar age group, all patients with suspected transient synovitis of the hip should be followed over the next 3–6 months to exclude the possibility of LCPD. Juvenile rheumatoid arthritis (JRA), and, more specifically, pauciarticular disease type II, may present with a painful hip, but range of motion is usually preserved unless a large effusion is present. (Pauciarticular disease type I generally spares the hips and hip girdle.) In addition, this form of JRA predominantly affects boys older than 8 years of age and accounts for only 10–15% of the patients with JRA. (Behrman RE et al., eds). *Nelson Textbook of Pediatrics,* fifteenth edition. Philadelphia: W.B. Saunders, 1996.)Developmental dysplasia of the hip may not always be diagnosed at birth, but it is not likely in this patient, because he was previously well. A septic joint is unlikely

in this clinical presentation, although chronic inflammatory changes may result following the treatment of a septic joint.

4. d   The patient most likely has slipped capital femoral epiphysis (SCFE), which is the most common hip disorder of adolescence. The condition most commonly occurs during a growth spurt when the growth plate is least resistant to shear stress. It is more common in obese patients, and male patients are affected twice as often as females. The patient typically complains of limp and pain, which may be localized to the hip or knee. Thus, all patients with knee pain should have a thorough evaluation of the hip. The treatment is primarily surgical, with multiple pinning in situ. Antibiotics play no role in the treatment of this disorder, although NSAIDs and acetaminophen may help with pain control postoperatively. Finally, a knee immobilizer would not be helpful in this hip condition.

5. e   The patient most likely has Sever's disease, or apophysitis of the calcaneus at the insertion of the Achilles tendon. This is thought to be an overuse injury, and the patient typically presents with pain and tenderness at the Achilles insertion. Treatment consists of limitation of activities, arch supports or elevation of the heel, and NSAIDs. Heel cord stretching may prevent recurrences, and severe cases may be treated with a short-leg walking cast for 6–8 weeks. Kohler's disease is avascular necrosis of the tarsal navicular that is thought to be caused by repetitive stress to the ossification nucleus, which compromises the blood supply; tenderness is often elicited on the dorsum of the foot near the talonavicular joint. Osgood-Schlatter disease is apophysitis of the tibial tubercle, and is also thought to be an overuse syndrome. Although JRA may present with ankle pain, joint swelling is usually present.

CHAPTER 44

Lymphadenopathy

BEN WILLWERTH, M.D.

QUESTIONS

1. A 4-year-old generally healthy boy is brought to the ED because of a "lump" in front of his right ear. His mother notes that this "lump" has been present for approximately 2 weeks, since the time of a 3-day febrile illness that was accompanied by conjunctivitis. He is currently asymptomatic. His exam reveals a 2 × 1-cm rubbery, nontender preauricular lymph node on the right and a few similarly sized anterior cervical lymph nodes. There is no overlying erythema. No other lymph nodes are identified. There is no hepatosplenomegaly. The most appropriate management at this time is:

   a. Obtaining a monospot
   b. Obtaining a CBC
   c. Obtaining a CXR
   d. Placing a PPD skin test
   e. Outpatient observation

2. A 3-year-old girl is referred to the ED for evaluation of swelling of her neck. She had a URI a week ago, which has now resolved. Today, she was noted to have a fever of 40°C and a swollen neck on one side. On your physical exam, she has a 3 × 4-cm tender hard swelling in her right anterior cervical region with overlying erythema. The most appropriate treatment of this girl's illness at this time is:

   a. Cephalexin
   b. Ampicillin
   c. Cefazolin
   d. Aspiration
   e. Excision

3. A 2-year-old girl is brought to your ED because she has had high fevers for several days and is now irritable. On your physical exam, she is noted to have a diffuse erythrodermal rash, a red tongue, dry, cracking lips, several small (1–2 cm) mildly tender anterior cervical lymph nodes, and conjunctivitis. She was started on amoxicillin 2 days earlier after being diagnosed with otitis media. Recognition of this constellation of symptoms and signs is important so that the following intervention can be instituted:

   a. Administration of intravenous gammaglobulin
   b. Administration of intravenous penicillin
   c. Administration of acyclovir
   d. Performance of a skin biopsy
   e. Discontinuation of amoxicillin

4. A 16-year-old boy comes to the ED because of the persistence of posterior cervical lymph nodes over the past month. He feels well now, but had fever, sore throat, and lethargy approximately 1 month ago. He denies any exposure to cats. There is no family history of a positive PPD. His current exam is normal, other than several enlarged nontender posterior cervical lymph nodes. Monospot tests done at the start and end of his illness 1 month ago were negative. The most likely etiologic agent of this boy's illness is:

   a. *Bartonella henselae*
   b. *Mycobacterium tuberculosis*
   c. Cytomegalovirus (CMV)
   d. *Mycobacterium avium intracellulare*
   e. Epstein–Barr virus

5. A 17-year-old girl comes to your ED because of fever, fatigue, malaise, and diffuse pruritus for the past 3 weeks. She finished an appropriate course of cephalexin for cervical adenitis today. She is currently afebrile and nontoxic. She has a 3 × 4-cm nontender firm lymph node in her cervical region that she states has been slowly enlarging. She has no hepatosplenomegaly or rash. A Monospot and CXR are negative and a CBC with differential is normal. Your most appropriate next step would be:

a. Symptomatic treatment
b. IV cefazolin
c. IV prednisone
d. Oncology consultation
e. Benadryl PO

6. An 8-year-old boy is referred to your ED because of facial swelling. He was well until 1 week ago, when he developed fever and malaise. These symptoms persisted, and he awoke today with a cough and swollen face. On your exam, he has facial edema and distended neck veins. He has cervical, axillary, and inguinal lymphadenopathy. His treatment is likely to involve:

a. Diuretics
b. Radiation therapy
c. Antihistamines
d. Gammaglobulin
e. Antibiotics

ANSWERS

1. e   This child has persistent regional lymphadenopathy as a result of his prior viral illness, which included conjunctivitis. The preauricular nodes drain the conjunctiva, and often enlarge in viral conjunctivitis. It may take 2–3 weeks for this reactive lymphadenopathy to begin to resolve. A Monospot is not indicated because this patient did not have a clinical course consistent with infectious mononucleosis. A CBC could help identify leukemia, which is very unlikely in the absence of constitutional symptoms, generalized lymphadenopathy, or hepatosplenomegaly. A CXR and PPD would help screen for Hodgkin's lymphoma and tuberculosis, but the clinical presentation of this patient is much more consistent with reactive lymphadenopathy than with these systemic illnesses; thus, these tests need not be performed at this time.

2. c   The most common etiologies of lymphadenitis are the bacterial pathogens group A beta-hemolytic *Streptococcus* and *Staphylococcus aureus*. Antimicrobials that are effective in the treatment of these pathogens (e.g., first-generation cephalosporins, including cephalexin and cefazolin) should be used in the initial treatment of lymphadenitis. Because of the large size of the node and fever, IV therapy (cefazolin) is indicated in this case. Ampicillin does not offer adequate *Staphylococcus* coverage for lymphadenitis. Aspiration of an infected lymph node can be helpful diagnostically and therapeutically if the node is fluctuant, which it is not in this case. Surgical excision of an infected lymph node is recommended in suspected atypical *Mycobacterium* lymphadenitis; thus, it is not indicated for this child.

3. a   This child has Kawasaki disease, a rare but important cause of acute cervical lymphadenopathy. This syndrome is often accompanied by several days of fever, a polymorphous truncal rash, mucous membrane involvement, limbal sparing nonexudative conjunctivitis, and extremity edema or erythema. Administration of IV gammaglobulin has been shown to reduce the risk of coronary artery aneurysms, a serious complication of this illness. IV penicillin would treat group A strep-induced scarlet fever, but this child's young age and mucous membrane involvement argue against strep as the etiology of her illness. Acyclovir is indicated early in the course of severe herpes stomatitis (which can lead to lymphadenopathy), but this child's exam is not consistent with herpes stomatitis. The constellation of this child's symptoms and physical findings should lead to the diagnosis of Kawasaki disease; thus, neither a skin biopsy nor discontinuation of the amoxicillin would be indicated.

4. c   This child has chronic cervical adenopathy as a result of his prior infection with cytomegalovirus (CMV). CMV can cause an illness similar to infectious mononucleosis with subsequent chronic adenopathy. Heterophile antibody testing (Monospot) will be negative. *Bartonella henselae* can cause chronic lymphadenopathy, but there is often a history of a scratch by a kitten, with subsequent formation of a papule at the inoculation site and subsequent lymphadenopathy. This adolescent's current lack of symptoms and absence of contact with a person with a positive PPD make *Mycobacterium* tuberculosis an unlikely etiology. Atypical *Mycobacterium* infections (e.g., *Mycobacterium avium intracellulare*)

can cause lymphadenopathy without other symptomatology, but they usually affect children less than 5 years old and usually lead to unilateral lymphadenopathy. Epstein-Barr virus (EBV) should reliably cause a positive Monospot in a boy this age; this boy had two negative Monospot tests.

5. d   This girl's constitutional symptoms, pruritus, and progressive cervical lymphadenopathy suggest an oncologic process, specifically Hodgkin's lymphoma. Thus, oncologic consultation is indicated. Symptomatic treatment of her illness would be inappropriate at this time because her lymphadenopathy has been unresponsive to antibiotics and has been progressive. Cefazolin would be an appropriate antibiotic if bacterial adenitis were suspected, which is not true in this case because the adenopathy has enlarged but is nontender. Steroids should not be given if the suspicion of an oncologic process exists. Benadryl may help control the patient's pruritus, but further diagnostic testing is indicated at this time.

6. b   This child has superior vena cava (SVC) syndrome, most likely from a malignancy with an accompanying anterior mediastinal mass. Because of the accompanying SVC syndrome, the initial treatment of this mass will include mediastinal radiation. The SVC is thin-walled and is encircled by lymph nodes that drain the thoracic cavity. A malignancy (e.g., leukemia or lymphoma) can lead to massive enlargement of these nodes with subsequent obstruction of the SVC. This obstruction leads to facial edema and distended neck veins, as seen in this case, and plethora. Diuretics are not indicated in SVC syndrome because intravascular volume in general is not increased. Anaphylaxis, for which antihistamines are used, could cause facial edema, but would not explain the recent constitutional symptoms or distended neck veins. Kawasaki disease, which responds to gammaglobulin, can lead to fever and diffuse lymphadenopathy, but is accompanied by other signs (e.g., a diffuse rash, conjunctivitis, mucous membrane involvement, and peripheral edema or erythema). Cat-scratch disease, sometimes treated with azithromycin, often leads to fever and malaise, but usually causes regional lymphadenopathy and does not cause facial edema or distended neck veins.

CHAPTER 45

Neck Mass

BEN WILLWERTH, M.D.

QUESTIONS

1. A 2-month-old boy is brought to your ED because of a mass in his neck noted only when he is crying. He has been acting well. As the child cries during your exam, you note a 2 × 3-cm discrete, soft, compressible, non-tender, mobile mass in the left posterior triangle of the baby's neck. There is no overlying skin erythema. You find no other cervical masses. The most appropriate diagnostic test at this time is:

   a. A CBC
   b. Lateral neck films
   c. CT imaging
   d. Aspiration for culture
   e. Biopsy

2. A 4-year-old girl is referred to your ED because of a mass in her neck. Her mother is concerned that this mass represents a malignancy. On exam, you find a 2 × 2-cm soft, nontender, smooth mass in the midline of the anterior neck. There is no overlying erythema. You tell her mother:

   a. This most likely represents a malignancy, and should be biopsied
   b. This most likely represents a malignancy, and imaging should be done
   c. Not to worry, but that the mass should be removed
   d. Not to worry, but that antibiotics should be taken
   e. Not to worry, and that no intervention will be needed

3. A 3-year-old boy is referred to your ED because of a red neck mass. His mother noticed the mass 1 week ago; it has not changed since the time she initially noted it. He has had no fever, URI symptoms, or vomiting. The family owns a dog and a kitten. The mass is firm, mobile, and tender, with overlying erythema. The most appropriate therapy for this patient is:

   a. Observation alone
   b. Amoxicillin/clavulanate
   c. Erythromycin orally
   d. Incision and drainage
   e. Surgical excision

4. A 15-year-old girl comes to the ED because of 3 weeks of nighttime fevers, fatigue, and generalized weakness. During your examination, you note a large, firm, painless, fixed cervical mass. Your initial evaluation of this patient should include all of the following, EXCEPT:

   a. CBC with differential
   b. Heterophile antibody test (Monospot)
   c. CXR
   d. CT imaging
   e. Aspiration

5. A 6-year-old girl is brought by ambulance to your ER following a motor vehicle collision. She was an unrestrained passenger in a high-speed collision, and was thrown from the car. She did not lose consciousness. She is alert and oriented, and complaining of difficulty breathing. On examination, you find the girl to be in moderate respiratory distress, with a crepitant mass in the right lower neck, just above the sternoclavicular joint. The first diagnostic test that you arrange is:

   a. CT imaging of the head
   b. CT imaging of the neck
   c. A CXR
   d. C-spine radiographs
   e. Ultrasonography of the neck mass

ANSWERS

1. c   This child has a cystic hygroma, which is a cystic lymphatic malformation that occurs in the posterior triangle of the neck. These malformations usually are evident at birth, but some are identified only after an injury, upper respiratory infection, or while the child performs a Valsalva maneuver, such as with crying or coughing. CT scan or ultrasonography, in conjunction with the noted history and exam, can establish the diagnosis by determining that the mass is cystic. CT can also delineate the extent of the hygroma. A CBC or biopsy would be helpful if this mass were suggestive of a malignancy (usually a firm, fixed cervical mass). A lateral neck film is helpful if there are signs of airway compromise (tachypnea, stridor) from a neck mass or if there are signs of a retropharyngeal abscess (fever, drooling). Complete excision, not aspiration, is the definitive treatment for cystic hygromas.

2. c   This child has a thyroglossal duct cyst. The definitive therapy for these cysts is surgical excision. Thyroglossal duct cysts are the most common congenital cysts of the neck. They develop along the line of descent of the thyroid gland in the neck. They are usually midline, adjacent to the hyoid bone and diagnosed in children 2–10 years of age. They can become infected, leading to overlying warmth, redness, and, at times, drainage. If this occurs, the infection should be cleared with antibiotics prior to removal of the cyst. The presentation of this child is inconsistent with a malignancy because of the midline location and softness and mobility of the mass.

3. b   The patient in this scenario has lymphadenitis, which is most commonly caused by group A beta-hemolytic *Streptococcus* or *Staphylococcus aureus.* Amoxicillin/clavulanate is appropriate treatment for this infection. If there was no change in this child's condition after a few days of antibiotic therapy, one should consider cat-scratch disease. Cat-scratch disease is caused by *Bartonella henselae,* which can often be found in the saliva of kittens. There is not always a clear history of a scratch from the kitten. Lymphadenopathy from cat-scratch disease is usually a single node that is warm, tender, and indurated with overlying erythema. Titers can be sent to the lab to confirm this diagnosis. Treatment for well-appearing children is observation alone; rifampin, azithromycin, trimethoprim-sulfamethoxazole, and ciprofloxacin have been used with some effectiveness in children with systemic toxicity. Needle aspiration will provide relief in children with tender, suppurative nodes, but it is otherwise unnecessary. Surgical excision is unnecessary and can lead to formation of a draining sinus.

4. e   This adolescent female's clinical presentation is consistent with a malignancy. Neoplastic etiologies for a neck mass in children include Hodgkin's and non–Hodgkin's lymphoma, rhabdomyosarcoma, neuroblastoma, thyroid carcinoma, and nasopharyngeal carcinoma. Initial evaluation of this patient should include a CBC with differential, a heterophile antibody (Monospot test) to exclude mononucleosis, a CXR to look for hilar lymphadenopathy or a mediastinal mass, and a CT of the involved region of the neck to clarify the character and extent of the neck mass. The mass will likely need to be biopsied during a surgical procedure; however, aspiration is not indicated because the mass is unlikely to be an infection and is not fluctuant.

5. c   This girl should have a CXR performed immediately, because of your clinical suspicion of a pneumomediastinum and pneumothorax. Pneumomediastinum may occasionally be detected on physical exam by the presence of a crepitant neck mass. Children with pneumomediastinum must be watched closely, because pneumomediastinum can progress to a pneumothorax, which is likely what occurred in the preceding scenario. CT imaging of the head and neck, and C-spine radiographs may or may not be necessary based on the remainder of this clinical scenario, but they would not be as urgent as the CXR. Ultrasonography of this neck mass is not indicated.

CHAPTER 46

Neck Stiffness

JILL C. POSNER, M.D.

QUESTIONS

1. A 14-year-old boy complains of neck stiffness and pain following his participation in a wrestling match. He maintains his head position rotated to the left. Physical examination shows left sternocleidomastoid muscle (SCM) spasm and tenderness. There are no neurologic deficits. You suspect that:

   a. The patient has inflammatory muscular torticollis
   b. The patient has rotary atlantoaxial subluxation
   c. The patient has a cervical spine fracture
   d. The patient has a spinal cord contusion
   e. The patient has a sternocleidomastoid muscle strain

2. An 8-year-old girl with Down syndrome complains of neck pain and stiffness after tripping on two stairs and falling. She has no injuries except for severe tenderness and spasm of her right sternocleidomastoid. CT scan shows rotation of C-1 on C-2. There are no neurologic deficits. Management includes:

   a. Anti-inflammatory medications only
   b. A soft collar and anti-inflammatory medications
   c. A hard collar and anti-inflammatory medications
   d. Immobilization and cervical traction
   e. A soft collar and diazepam

3. An 8-year-old football player is brought to the ED by EMTs after being tackled. There is a hard collar in place and the patient is immobilized on a spine board. Immediately after the collision he complained of bilateral arm paresthesias, but now reports full remittance. On examination, there are no neurologic deficits. Management may include all of the following, EXCEPT:

   a. Attempt to "clinically clear" his cervical spine
   b. Maintain spinal immobilization
   c. Obtain cervical spine radiographs
   d. Obtain cervical spine MRI
   e. Consider hospital admission

4. A 2-year-old boy is brought to the ED because of a 5-day history of fever and URI symptoms. On physical exam he has mild stridor, is drooling, and has a stiff neck. You should:

   a. Immediately perform a lumbar puncture
   b. Administer nebulized racemic epinephrine
   c. Treat with IM dexamethasone
   d. Obtain a blood culture and treat with oral antibiotics
   e. Obtain a lateral neck radiograph

5. A 12-year-old girl with viral gastroenteritis was prescribed prochlorperazine by her pediatrician 2 days ago to treat her symptoms. She now presents with a severely stiff neck and rotating her head to the left. You immediately:

   a. Administer activated charcoal
   b. Treat with warm compresses and ibuprofen
   c. Administer diphenhydramine
   d. Obtain cervical spine (C-spine) radiographs
   e. Send blood for a CBC and ESR

6. A 9-year-old girl is brought to the ED for fever, neck pain, and neck stiffness. She denies sore throat. On physical examination, her tonsils are normal in size and without exudate, and she has no cervical lymphadenopathy. She has focal tenderness on palpation of her C-4 vertebrae. There are no neurologic deficits. Management includes all of the following, EXCEPT:

   a. C-spine radiographs
   b. Obtain CBC, blood culture, and ESR
   c. Empirical treatment with IV antibiotics
   d. Perform a lumbar puncture
   e. Discharge with ibuprofen and soft cervical collar

7. A 7-year-old boy complains of a 1-month history of headaches and blurred vision. His school performance has been declining despite a move of his seat to the front of the classroom. There is a strong family history of migraine headaches. On examination, you note that he is tilting his head to the left. You suspect:

    a. The patient has migraine headaches
    b. The patient has a brain tumor
    c. The patient has myopia
    d. The patient has school avoidance
    e. The patient has Klippel-Feil syndrome

8. An 8-year-old girl is brought to the ED because of torticollis. She has fever and a sore throat. On examination she has an exudative tonsillitis. You suspect she has inflammatory torticollis. All of the following would support your diagnosis, EXCEPT:

    a. She has palpable sternocleidomastoid tenderness and spasm
    b. Her chin is rotated toward the side of the sternocleidomastoid spasm
    c. She is taking no medications
    d. She has a normal neurologic examination
    e. She has relief with anti-inflammatory medications and warm compresses

ANSWERS

1. **b** Subluxations of the cervical spine are more common than fractures, resulting from both minor and more severe trauma. Rotary atlantoaxial subluxation, the most frequently occurring of these, generally causes both neck pain and stiffness. The patient will position his head rotated toward the side of the spastic, tender, sternocleidomastoid muscle (SCM). In contrast, patients with inflammatory muscular torticollis experience SCM spasm on the side opposite to the direction of head rotation. The open-mouth radiograph generally shows the rotation of C-1 on C-2, with the odontoid located asymmetrically between the lateral masses of C-1. Although the possibility of cervical spine fracture should be considered in all patients with traumatic neck pain, the mechanism of injury makes the diagnosis unlikely in this case. A cord contusion is also unlikely given the patient's normal neurologic examination.

2. **d** Patients with Down syndrome are susceptible to atlantoaxial subluxation due to laxity of the transverse ligament of the atlas. Unlike most cases of atlantoaxial subluxation, in which the transverse ligament usually remains intact, patients with Down syndrome may rupture the ligament, thus compromising the spinal canal. A high index of suspicion should be maintained when caring for these children. If C-spine radiographs are equivocal, a neck CT scan should be performed. The usual treatment with a soft collar and anti-inflammatory medications is generally inadequate in the patient with Down syndrome. Treatment of these children usually involves immobilization and cervical traction. High-dose steroids are a controversial management option in pediatric patients with spinal cord injuries.

3. **a** The patient described in this scenario may have a spinal cord injury without radiographic abnormality (SCIWORA syndrome). Children younger than 8 years of age are most susceptible to SCIWORA, because of the ligamentous laxity and hypermobility of the pediatric cervical spine. Following a traumatic event, children may develop significant neurological symptoms and progressive paralysis, or they may have transient neurological symptoms that remit fully then recur with worsening neurologic abnormalities. Cervical spine immobilization and hospitalization should be seriously considered, even in the patient with transient symptoms.

4. **e** A patient with a retropharyngeal abscess often presents with a stiff neck in addition to other clinical signs (e.g., fever, drooling, and stridor). This infection, occupying the potential space between the posterior pharyngeal wall and the anterior border of the cervical vertebrae, is most commonly due to group A *Streptococcus, Staphylococcus aureus,* and oral anaerobes. It should not be confused with croup, which causes stridor but not drooling and neck stiffness, or with meningitis. The diagnosis is based on the clinical findings as well as a lateral radiograph of the neck that reveals soft-tissue swelling anterior to the cervical vertebral bodies. Treatment consists of IV antibiotics and usually involves surgical drainage.

5. **c** Dystonic reactions can result from certain drugs with dopamine receptor antagonism. Many neuroleptic and antiemetic agents (which this patient was most likely prescribed) can cause acute torticollis when given in regular therapeutic doses. A dystonic reaction is frightening and quite painful for the child who experiences it. Treatment with diphenhydramine 1–2 mg/kg/dose usually provides rapid relief.

6. e   The findings of focal tenderness, posterior neck pain, and fever in this patient warrant a further diagnostic evaluation. Symptomatic treatment only with anti-inflammatory medications and a soft cervical collar would be inadequate, given the possibility that a serious condition may exist. Infections of the spine in children most frequently occur in the thoracic and lumbar areas, although they can involve the cervical spine. Vertebral osteomyelitis, epidural abscess, and discitis may lead to neck stiffness. Localized pain, fever, and an elevation of the erythrocyte sedimentation rate (ESR) usually accompany these infections. Vertebral osteomyelitis and epidural abscess are usually bacterial in origin, with *S. aureus* being the most common pathogen. Infectious discitis is an uncommon condition, usually affecting children younger than 3 years. Because bacterial cultures are commonly negative, the etiology of this process has been debated. Radiographs of the cervical spine may reveal focal abnormalities of the vertebral body, soft tissues, or disk space; however, technetium bone scanning or MRI is generally more helpful in making a diagnosis. A lumbar puncture to exclude the possibility of meningitis should be strongly considered in patients with posterior neck pain and fever.

7. b   Head tilt or torticollis may be a presenting sign of a posterior fossa brain tumor. Head tilt may represent an attempt to correct for visual disturbances, rather than true neck pain. Neck stiffness is thought to result from irritation of the accessory nerve by the cerebellar tonsils trapped in the occipital foramen. A history of paresthesias, weakness, ataxia, change in bowel or bladder function, vomiting, headaches, and decline in school performance should be sought in patients with neck pain or stiffness in order to assess for the possibility of a brain or spinal cord neoplasm. Complete ophthalmologic and neurologic examinations should be performed in all of these patients.

8. b   The direction of head tilt in relation to the affected sternocleidomastoid muscle can be used to differentiate inflammatory torticollis from that caused by atlanto-axial rotary subluxation. In the former, the muscular spasm causes the chin to rotate away from the affected side. In atlantoaxial rotary subluxation, the ipsilateral sternocleidomastoid muscle is attempting to compensate for the C-1–C-2 abnormality. This results in a head tilt toward the affected side.

CHAPTER 47

Odor—Unusual

MICHELE M. BURNS, M.D.

QUESTIONS

1. All of the following are true statements concerning the sense of smell, EXCEPT:

   a. The human nose can discriminate 4000 odors
   b. The sense of smell is more acute in daylight
   c. The acuity of a person's sense of smell is linked to blood cortisol levels
   d. When a child is unable to detect odor, anosmia should be considered
   e. When a child complains of strange odors, temporal lobe epilepsy should be considered

2. The major component of body odor in humans is:

   a. Sebaceous glands
   b. Eccrine glands
   c. Apocrine glands
   d. Secretions from the oropharynx
   e. Flatus

3. A 10-day-old infant is brought to the ED after a seizure. An odor of caramelized sugar is detected. You suspect that the patient may have a defect in:

   a. Insulin activity or lack of insulin
   b. Phenylalanine hydroxylase
   c. Isovaleryl-CoA dehydrogenase
   d. Transport of methionine
   e. Branch-chain ketoacid decarboxylase

4. A toddler is brought in to the ED secondary to the father's concern of halitosis. The child is afebrile, well appearing, well hydrated, and has a normal oropharyngeal exam. Your next step in the evaluation is to:

   a. Send a rapid strep test
   b. Consult dentistry
   c. Determine amount of oral intake
   d. Examine the nose
   e. Obtain a CXR

5. A 15-year-old girl comes to the ED with an odor of the perineum. All are possible diagnoses, EXCEPT:

   a. *Candida* vaginitis
   b. *Trichomonas* vaginitis
   c. Retained foreign body (FB)
   d. *Gardnerella* vaginitis
   e. Urinary tract infection (UTI)

6. An 11-day-old boy is brought in by his mother for concerns of an unusual odor for the past 2 days. Both the mother and child appear to have good hygiene. Your next step is to:

   a. Obtain a further history of an unintentional ingestion
   b. Send serum amino acids and urine organic acids
   c. Examine the baby for a foreign body
   d. Examine the baby for pharyngitis
   e. Examine the baby for omphalitis

7. The following systemic illnesses are correctly paired with the characteristic odor that often accompanies them, EXCEPT:

   a. Hepatic failure: musty, rotten eggs
   b. Schizophrenia: sweet, grapelike odor
   c. Uremia: fishy odor
   d. Malignancy: trenchant odor
   e. Crohn's disease: feculent odor

8. A fruity odor is detected in persons with diabetic ketoacidosis. Ingestion of which of the following toxins also produces this aroma?

   a. Ethanol
   b. Methanol
   c. Isopropyl alcohol
   d. Ethylene glycol
   e. Propylene glycol

9. The following infectious diseases are correctly paired with the characteristic odor that often accompanies them, EXCEPT:

   a. Rubella: sweet grape
   b. Typhoid fever: freshly baked bread
   c. Yellow fever: butcher shop
   d. Scrofula: stale beer
   e. Omphalitis: foul, putrid

10. The following toxic ingestions are correctly paired with the characteristic odor that often accompanies them, EXCEPT:

    a. Methyl salicylate: oil of wintergreen
    b. Camphor: mothballs
    c. Chloral hydrate: pears
    d. Arsenic: violets
    e. Cyanide: bitter almonds

ANSWERS

1. b   The human nose can detect about 4000 odors. The olfactory area extends from the roof of the nasal cavity 10 mm down the septum and superior turbinates bilaterally. It is unknown how the olfactory receptors are stimulated. Smell is more acute in darkness and is thought to be linked to blood cortisol levels. When a child is unable to detect odor, anosmia should be considered. Likewise, when a child complains of strange odors, particularly if others do not appreciate them, then the diagnosis of temporal lobe epilepsy is possible.

2. c   The unique odor emitted from each person is a combination of body secretions and excretions. The apocrine glands, or the sweat glands located in the axillary, areolar, and anal regions, make the most significant contribution to body odor, in that their initially odorless viscous secretions acquire odor with bacterial decomposition. Sebaceous and eccrine sweat glands provide the skin with aromas as well; body odors are also affected by the aromas from the oronasopharynx, respiratory tract, urine, feces, and flatus. Factors such as hygiene, metabolism, toxins, infections, and systemic diseases can affect an individual's body odor. (Junqueira L, et al. *Basic Histology*, fifth edition. Lange Medical Publications, 1986: 410–412.)

3. e   Inborn errors of metabolism are important to diagnose because they are potentially life-threatening. Diabetic ketoacidosis (DKA) would be an unusual diagnosis in the neonatal period and a sweet/fruity odor of acetone is detected on the breath. It is of note that any condition where a marked metabolic acidosis is present will generate this characteristic fruity odor. Phenylketonuria (PKU) is a disorder of amino acid metabolism with a deficiency of phenylalanine dehydroxylase. As a result, there is an accumulation of phenylacetic acid in the sweat and urine that produces the characteristic musty, mousy, horsey, wolflike, barny odor. A deficiency in isovaleryl-Co-A dehydrogenase, or isovaleric acidemia, produces an odor of sweaty feet/socks or ripe cheese. Oasthouse urine disease is secondary to a defective transport of methionine. The unabsorbed methionine is broken down in the GI tract to α-hydroxybutyric acid, and this is responsible for the yeast, celery, malt, or brewery type of odor. Maple syrup urine disease (MSUD) produces the odor of maple syrup, caramelized sugar, or boiled Chinese herbal medication. The metabolic defect lies in the decarboxylation of the ketoacids of the branch-chain amino acids (leucine, isoleucine, and valine). The odor is thought to be related to the accumulation of isoleucine, specifically.

4. d   Toddlers presenting with unusual odors often have retained foreign bodies (FBs) in their ears, nose, vagina, urethra, or rectum. Nasal FBs are particularly common between the ages of 1 and 5 years. Although tonsillitis, strep throat, and dental abscesses can cause halitosis, this patient had a normal oropharyngeal exam. Halitosis is increased in states of poor oral intake, but this child was well hydrated. The next appropriate step, therefore, would be to examine the nose for an FB or, perhaps, even purulent nasal/sinus drainage. Although a CXR would help to assess whether a lung abscess is present, examination of the nose next is more appropriate with an afebrile, well-appearing child.

5. a   Vaginal secretions are combinations of vulvar secretions from glands (i.e., sweat, sebaceous, Bartholin's, and Skene's) transudate through the vaginal wall, exfoliated cells, cervical mucus, endometrial and oviductal fluids, as well as vaginal microorganisms, and menstrual blood. *Candida* vaginitis is odor free, whereas *Gardnerella* vaginitis and *Trichomonas* have "fishy" odors. Retained foreign bodies, such as tampons and diaphragms, produce foul-smelling odors. A UTI caused by urea-splitting bacteria will generate an ammonia-type odor.

6. e   Unusual odors in a neonate indicate neglect, an inborn error of metabolism, or omphalitis. Both the mother and infant appeared to have good hygiene, making neglect unlikely. An inborn error of metabolism is possible, although the odor has only been detected for 2 days. Before pursuing this workup, the next most appropriate step would be to examine the baby for omphalitis. Older children are more likely to present with ingestions, FBs, and pharyngitis as causes of unusual odor.

7. b   Systemic illnesses are often associated with characteristic odors. Hepatic failure produces "fetor hepaticus," or the odor of musty, rotten eggs. Schizophrenic patients typically have a pungent, heavy body odor, and not the sweet, grapelike odor seen in burn patients infected with *Pseudomonas*. Uremia does present with a fishy odor that is secondary to amine production. Persons with malignancy often have a lot of tissue and cellular breakdown plus gas formation that causes a trenchant odor. Finally, the development of gastric fistulae in patients with Crohn's disease can create a feculent odor.

8. c   The fruity odor detected in diabetes ketoacidosis is secondary to ketone production. Isopropyl alcohol is metabolized to acetone (a 3-carbon ketone); thus, patients who present after this ingestion have a similar odor. Methanol and ethylene glycol are metabolized to odorless, toxic metabolites. Ingestion of ethanol gives a characteristic odor that most physicians are comfortable diagnosing. Propylene glycol is metabolized to the odorless metabolites of lactate and pyruvate. (Olsen, K. *Poisoning & Drug Overdose,* third edition. Stamford, CT: Appleton & Lange, 1999:167,197.)

9. a   Rubella's typical odor is that of freshly plucked feathers, whereas diphtheria produces a smell of sweet grapes. Typhoid gives the odor of freshly baked bread, yellow fever that of a butcher shop, and scrofula that of stale beer. Omphalitis presents with a draining, erythematous umbilical area that smells foul and putrid.

10. d   Many toxins have characteristic odors that aid the physician in making the correct diagnosis. This is especially helpful in those cases where the ingestion was not witnessed or the patient presents with altered mental status. For example, ingestion of methyl salicylates creates an oil of wintergreen aroma, camphor smells like mothballs, and chloral hydrate smells like pears. Arsenic ingestions give a garlic odor, as do ingestions of some organophosphates (e.g., parathion, malathion), phosphorous, selenium, and thallium. Turpentine produces a violetlike aroma in the urine. Last, cyanide smells like bitter almonds, although up to 50% of the population can not detect this "bitter-almond" odor. (Olsen, K. *Poisoning & Drug Overdose,* third edition. Stamford, CT: Appleton & Lange, 1999:30.)

CHAPTER **48**

Oligomenorrhea

JEFFREY P. LOUIE, M.D.

QUESTIONS

1. A 16-year-old girl comes to the ED with a chief complaint of "missing her period." She says she is sexually active and that she is 10 days past her normal date of menses. She denies fevers, vaginal discharge, abdominal pain, and dysuria. She does not have a primary care physician. What is the next appropriate step?

   a. Send a urine pregnancy test
   b. Obtain her home address and inform her that a social worker will be contacting her
   c. Complete your physical exam without a pelvic exam and send a serum pregnancy test
   d. Complete your physical exam with a pelvic exam and send a urine pregnancy test
   e. Complete your physical exam and instruct the patient to follow up with the city health department

2. An 18-year-old female patient complains that she has not had her menstrual period in 5 months. She denies sexual activity, abdominal pain, and vaginal discharge. On examination, her vital signs are: HR 45, BP 100/50, and RR 14. She is in no distress, but she is thin, weighing 50 kg. She has no neck or abdominal masses. Her pelvic examination is normal. On closer examination of her mouth, her teeth appear eroded and the examination of her extremities reveals calluses on her fingers. What is your next step?

   a. Obtain serum electrolytes
   b. Send a TSH (thyroid-stimulating hormone) level
   c. No further testing is needed
   d. Obtain a head CT
   e. Send a hemoglobin electrophoresis

3. A 14-year-old girl is brought to the ED by her mother because she has not had a menstrual period in 5 months. The patient states she is not sexually active and started having her periods at age 13. Her mother states that her daughter has gained weight over the last year. Her vital signs are: HR 90, RR 14, and BP 130/60. She is well appearing, but somewhat obese (weight 70 kg). Her neck is supple with no masses. Of significance, her lower abdomen feels firm, but not tender. You immediately:

   a. Explain to the mother that irregular periods are normal in the first 2 years of onset
   b. Send a urine test for HCG (human chorionic gonadotropin)
   c. Obtain abdominal radiographs
   d. Obtain an abdominal ultrasound (U/S)
   e. Prescribe oral contraceptives

4. A fourth-year medical student presents an 18-year-old, obese female patient whose chief complaint is missed menses for 9 weeks. The medical student describes the patient as also having chin hair and a sparse mustache. The rest of the patient's exam is normal. Her urine pregnancy test is negative. The medical student then gives her differential diagnosis. Which of the following answers is NOT correct as a cause for this patient's clinical status?

   a. Congenital adrenal hyperplasia
   b. Turner's syndrome
   c. Polycystic ovary syndrome (PCOS)
   d. Cushing's disease
   e. Hypothyroidism

5. A 15-year-old girl is brought to the ED for a chief complaint of a white discharge from her breasts. Her triage note describes that she has a history of depression. She also admits to being sexually active, but denies vaginal discharge or abdominal pain. She cannot remember her last period. A urine pregnancy test is pending. As you begin to examine this patient, you begin thinking about the differential diagnosis. Which of the following is the most likely to make the diagnosis?

a. Nothing more—the urine pregnancy test is the most important diagnostic test
b. The need for psychiatric and gynecologic evaluation
c. Determining previous and current medication use
d. Sending a prolactin level
e. Sending out for thyroid function studies

ANSWERS

1. d   One must document whether or not the patient is pregnant. A urine pregnancy test (positive at levels greater than 25 mIU/ml) would be quite appropriate in this setting because the patient is already "late" and the expected level of HCG would be about 100 mIU/ml by this time. Performing a pelvic examination is controversial, but in a patient who does not have a primary care physician and has no follow-up, a pelvic examination is warranted to insure normal anatomy, to diagnose cervicitis or pelvic inflammatory disease (PID), if present, and to obtain specimens for chlamydia and gonorrhea cultures. An effort should obviously be made to obtain a follow-up appointment with an appropriate provider.

2. a   The main etiology of this patient's oligomenorrhea is secondary to her chronic malnutrition. Her clinical condition of a slim body, bradycardia, dental erosion, and calluses on her fingers fit the clinical picture of an eating disorder. A full medical exam is now warranted, including an ECG and appropriate labs. A consultation to psychiatry is also required, along with an adolescent and gynecology referral.

3. b   The goal in the evaluation of any patient with oligomenorrhea is the determination of her pregnancy status. This patient is pregnant, and the mass felt in her abdomen is a 20-week uterus. Although periods may be irregular during the first 2 years after menses, 5 months is a long time between periods, and the pregnancy status must still be determined. An obese patient may have polycystic ovary syndrome (PCOS), which is treated with oral contraceptives; however, the pregnancy status *must* be known before starting any contraceptive.

4. b   Congenital adrenal hyperplasia, PCOS, Cushing's disease, and hypothyroidism can all cause oligomenorrhea and hirsutism. Turner's syndrome (karyotype 45,X) patients are normally diagnosed at birth; however, some patients may be diagnosed in adolescence, with a common chief complaint of primary amenorrhea or delayed puberty. Turner's syndrome patients do not normally have problems with hirsutism. In fact, the opposite may be true. These patients may have sparse or absent pubic or axillary hair.

5. c   Given her history of depression, it would be prudent to determine if she is currently taking antidepressants or any other medications. Antidepressants (tricyclic antidepressants, phenothiazines and their derivatives, and reserpine derivatives) are well known to cause galactorrhea secondary to their ability to inhibit the hypothalamic prolactin-inhibiting factor. Other medications can cause galactorrhea by hypothalamic suppression, and include opiates, benzodiazepines, butyrophenones, and methyldopa. Cessation of oral contraceptives can also cause galactorrhea. A pregnancy test is warranted in any female patient who cannot recall or is unsure of her menstrual cycles. Other causes of galactorrhea should be pursued if no medications or breast trauma/stimulation are determined by the interview and include thyroid studies (hypothroidism) and a prolactin level (which would be elevated with a prolactinoma).

CHAPTER 49

Oral Lesions

VINCENT J. WANG, M.D.

QUESTIONS

1. A 2-month-old boy has plaques in his mouth. His mother noticed white spots in his mouth 1 day earlier. He has been feeding without difficulty and has been well. On examination, he is well appearing. He has white plaques on the buccal mucosa and palate. The plaques do not rub off. Appropriate treatment includes:

    a. Nystatin orally
    b. Amoxicillin orally
    c. Acyclovir topically
    d. Hydrogen peroxide mouth rinses
    e. Supportive care only

2. A 4-year-old girl has painful lesions on the lips. She has had fever for 1–2 days and cries when she eats. She has vesicles on the upper and lower lip, the tongue, and the buccal mucosa. There is mild erythema. Her examination is otherwise normal. Treatment includes:

    a. Nystatin orally
    b. Amoxicillin orally
    c. Hydrogen peroxide mouth rinses
    d. Hydrocortisone topically
    e. Supportive care

3. A 6-year-old girl complains of a sore throat. She has had a low-grade fever for 1–2 days and complains of pain when she swallows. On examination, she has a "strawberry"-appearing tongue, palatal petechiae, and moderate tonsillar swelling with exudate and erythema. Treatment includes:

    a. Penicillin orally for 10 days
    b. Ciprofloxin orally for 10 days
    c. Tetracycline orally for 10 days
    d. IV EBV gamma globulin once
    e. Antipyresis only

4. A 17-year-old girl is referred to you because she has oral ulcers, hyperplastic mucosa, and edema of her lips and gums. She has also had abdominal pain over the past 3 months, associated with diarrhea and weight loss. You suspect she has:

    a. Acute necrotizing ulcerative gingivostomatitis (ANUG)
    b. Kawasaki disease
    c. Rhabdomyosarcoma
    d. Crohn's disease
    e. Stevens-Johnson syndrome

5. A 10-year-old boy with a known seizure disorder develops oral lesions. For the past 5 years, he has been taking phenytoin for his seizure disorder. He has 5–10-mm ulcerations of his gingiva and buccal mucosa. The lesions are painful. He has no other mucosal or dermal lesions. His examination is otherwise normal and he is well appearing. Management includes:

    a. Changing his anticonvulsant medication
    b. Penicillin orally for 10 days
    c. Rinsing his mouth with dilute hydrogen peroxide
    d. Nystatin orally for 5 days
    e. No treatment is necessary

ANSWERS

1. a   Candidiasis is a common oral infection in neonates and infants. Patients are typically well appearing and otherwise without symptoms. White plaques may appear on the buccal mucosa, palate, and gingivae, and do not "rub off." Treatment for oral candidiasis is nystatin given orally. If oral candidiasis occurs after infancy, an underlying immune deficiency must be considered. Amoxicillin would be an acceptable therapy for a streptococcal pharyngitis. Acyclovir may be used for herpes stomatitis, which is usually painful and presents with vesicles and ulcers on an erythematous base. Hydrogen peroxide mouth rinses are indicated for acute necrotizing ulcerative gingivitis.

2. e   Herpes stomatitis is a common oral infection that may be recurrent. Classically, vesicles or ulcers will present on the lips and peri-orally, but lesions may occur anywhere in the mouth. Treatment is largely supportive, although some reports suggest that early treatment with acyclovir may be helpful. Hydrocortisone is indicated for inflammatory lesions and is not indicated in this scenario. The other treatments are not indicated (see Question 1).

3. a   Streptococcal pharyngitis is most commonly caused by group A *Streptococcus.* Penicillin orally for 10 days is a standard course of therapy, but bicillin may also be given intramuscularly. Ciprofloxacin is not currently recommended for children. Tetracycline should not be given to children before the age of 12 years. Even though infectious mononucleosis may cause similar symptoms, the patient's symptoms and findings are classic for streptococcal pharyngitis. If necessary, the diagnosis of streptococcal pharyngitis may be confirmed with a rapid antigen assay and throat culture. EBV gamma globulin does not exist.

4. d   Crohn's disease may occur in any portion of the gastrointestinal (GI) tract, including the mouth. Oral lesions may consist of ulcers, polypoid papulous hyperplastic mucosa, and edema of the gingiva, buccal mucosa, and lips. With the other constitutional symptoms, the history strongly suggests Crohn's disease. ANUG may be manifested by tender, bleeding gums with "punched-out" areas secondary to gum loss between the teeth. Kawasaki disease is associated with a strawberry-colored tongue and an erythematous oropharynx, along with a constellation of other symptoms. A rhabdomyosarcoma may develop as a tumorous growth in the oral cavity. Stevens-Johnson syndrome may manifest as erythematous plaques that evolve into vesicles or bullae.

5. e   Aphthous ulcers may present with lesions on the lips, tongue, gingivae, and buccal mucosa. The lesions are painful, but there are no other findings. Treatment is supportive and the lesions resolve spontaneously within 1 week. Phenytoin may produce gingival hyperplasia rather than ulcers. Stevens Johnson syndrome is unlikely, given the long-standing use of phenytoin and the rest of his clinical examination. Oral antibiotics or antifungal agents are not indicated. There is no need for mouth rinses.

CHAPTER 50

Pain—Abdomen

BARBARA M. GARCIA PEÑA, M.D., M.P.H.

QUESTIONS

1. A 2-week-old boy is brought to the ED with a chief complaint of vomiting and what the parents perceive as abdominal pain. The baby has been "crying out" constantly. The vomitus is described as "green." On physical examination, his vital signs are: T 37.8°C, HR 140, RR 40, and BP 90/45. The baby appears unwell and has a taut, distended abdomen. There is no stool in the vault on rectal examination. Plain radiography of the abdomen shows distended loops of bowel with no air visible in sigmoid colon or rectum. Which of the following should be performed next in the evaluation of this patient?

   a. Abdominal CT scan
   b. Abdominal U/S
   c. Upper GI (UGI) series
   d. Barium enema
   e. IV pyelogram (IVP)

2. A 3-year-old girl is brought to the ED with a chief complaint of abdominal pain of 24-hour duration. She has vomited twice (nonbilious, nonbloody). She has had no diarrhea. Her parents inform you that she has been drinking more than usual and that fluids are "passing right through her." She has had no fever. On physical examination, she is afebrile, with HR 150, RR 40, and BP 80/40. She appears listless, moderately dehydrated, and is breathing very deeply. She has diffuse abdominal tenderness, and no distension, masses, or peritoneal signs. Rectal examination is negative for occult blood. Which of the following is the most appropriate first step in diagnosis?

   a. Abdominal x-ray
   b. Bedside glucose level
   c. Air-contrast enema
   d. Abdominal U/S
   e. Abdominal CT

3. A 4-year-old girl is brought to the ED by her father with complaints of abdominal pain, runny nose, and cough. She has had a low-grade fever, but no vomiting or diarrhea. Vital signs are: T 38.2°C, HR 100, RR 40, BP 100/60, and saturated O_2 95%. Cardiac examination is unremarkable. Lungs are clear bilaterally. Her abdominal examination reveals mild tenderness on the right, but no rebound or masses palpated. Rectal exam is normal. Which of the following is the most appropriate next step in the evaluation of this patient?

   a. CXR
   b. Abdominal x-ray
   c. Abdominal U/S
   d. Abdominal CT
   e. Barium enema

4. A 9-year-old boy comes to the ED with abdominal pain of 12-hour duration. He describes the pain as periumbilical. He has vomited once (nonbilious, nonbloody) and has not had diarrhea. He states that he has no appetite. On exam, he is febrile to 38.1°C, with stable vital signs. He is very tender in the right lower quadrant, with associated guarding and rebound tenderness. Rectal exam is nontender and negative for occult blood. Which of the following is the most appropriate next step in management of this patient?

   a. CBC
   b. Abdominal x-ray
   c. Surgical consult
   d. Abdominal U/S
   e. Abdominal CT

5. A 7-year-old boy is brought to the ED with periumbilical abdominal pain. This is his fifth visit to the ED or primary care doctor in 3 months with the same complaint. He has had no vomiting, diarrhea, fever, or weight loss. He has had normal lab tests, abdominal plain films and ultrasound, upper GI series, and abdominal CT in the past. On exam, he is afebrile with stable vital signs. His abdominal examination shows mild midabdominal tenderness without guarding or rebound tenderness. Rectal examination is normal, with stool negative for occult blood. Which of the following is the most appropriate next step in the diagnostic workup of this patient?

a. Repeat CT scan
b. Abdominal MRI
c. Parental reassurance
d. Barium enema
e. CXR

6. A 14-year-old runaway girl comes to the ED with a complaint of right lower quadrant pain. She has not vomited or had diarrhea. She denies sexual activity. Upon examination, vital signs are: T 37.9°C, HR 90, RR 12, BP 100/60. Her abdominal examination reveals mild right lower quadrant tenderness without rebound or guarding. Pelvic examination reveals a friable erythematous cervix with tenderness to palpation. She is tender in the right adnexal area. Rectal examination is normal. Which of the following is the most appropriate treatment option?

a. IV ampicillin and gentamicin
b. IV cefoxitin and IV doxycycline
c. IM ceftriaxone and PO azithromycin
d. PO cefixime and PO azithromycin
e. IM ceftriaxone

7. A 16-year-old boy comes to the ED with severe, sudden-onset right lower quadrant pain that began 1 hour ago. He has vomited twice, but has had no diarrhea. On exam, he is febrile and tachycardic. He is very uncomfortable on the examination table. His abdominal exam demonstrates right lower quadrant tenderness without guarding or rebound. Rectal exam is normal. Which of the following is the most appropriate next step in diagnosis and management?

a. General surgical consultation
b. Obtain abdominal U/S
c. Obtain CT scan
d. Genital examination
e. CBC

8. An 8-year-old girl comes to the ED with diffuse abdominal pain for 12 hours. She has had no fever, vomiting, or diarrhea. On examination, she is afebrile with stable vital signs. Her abdominal examination demonstrates diffuse tenderness without rebound. Rectal exam is negative for occult blood. There is a nonblanching erythematous rash on her thighs. Urinalysis is negative. Which of the following is the most appropriate treatment for this patient?

a. Prednisone
b. Ceftriaxone
c. Laparotomy
d. IV immunoglobulin
e. No treatment

ANSWERS

1. c   This infant's clinical picture is most consistent with malrotation, with possible midgut volvulus. The green "bilious" vomiting suggests obstruction. A UGI series helps to delineate malrotation and is the best imaging modality to aid in the diagnosis. An abdominal CT scan or ultrasound would not be indicated, because it is difficult to evaluate the causes of obstruction using these modalities. A barium enema would be indicted for intussusception and an IVP is indicated if abnormalities of the kidney are suspected.

2. b   This child is presenting with signs and symptoms of DKA. The presence of polydipsia and polyuria in the history in an ill-appearing dehydrated child with signs of acidosis leads one to the diagnosis. The abdominal pain in children with DKA is due to the ketoacidosis. The most appropriate step in diagnosis is the bedside glucose level. A CBC would not lead one to the diagnosis. In addition, a KUB, abdominal U/S, and abdominal CT scan are most likely be normal in a patient with DKA.

3. a   Pneumonia is a common cause of abdominal pain and is the most likely diagnosis in this child presenting with abdominal pain. Her RR is elevated and her O_2 saturation is on the lower end of normal.

4. c   This boy presents with classic history and physical examination for appendicitis. Clinical pathway studies have shown that laboratory and radiographic testing are not indicated in these children. A surgi-

cal consult should be obtained immediately, because the child needs to go to the operating room as expediently as possible.

5. c The syndrome of functional abdominal pain is responsible for more than 80% of outpatient physician visits for abdominal pain. The child's growth and development are normal and the abdominal examination usually shows only mild midabdominal tenderness. Tests such as CBC, U/S, and ESR, as well as radiologic studies, are all normal. Because of the lack of suspicious historical and physical exam findings, no further radiographic testing is needed for this patient. The emergency physician's task is to allay fears of any serious organic illness and should provide an avenue for continued supportive follow-up through referral to the primary physician.

6. b This patient has pelvic inflammatory disease (PID). Although she denied sexual activity, one must assume that pregnancy and sexually transmitted diseases (STDs) are possible. For treatment in this runaway girl (and for the majority of symptomatic adolescent girls), hospitalization is necessary to ensure compliance and teaching. The first-line inpatient regimen for PID is IV cefoxitin and doxycycline to cover for gonococcus and chlamydia, respectively. The antibiotic regimens given in "c" and "d" are appropriate options for outpatient therapy. IV gentamycin can be used for gonorrhea, but ampicillin is not effective therapy for chlamydia.

7. d Sudden-onset lower abdominal pain in an adolescent male should make one think of testicular torsion, which commonly presents with acute abdominal pain as the sole complaint. A thorough genital examination should be performed on all males with abdominal pain. A general surgical consultation, CBC, and ultrasonography or CT scan may be obtained if the patient's genital examination is normal, because appendicitis would also be high on the differential diagnosis.

8. a Henoch-Schönlein purpura (HSP) typically presents with a classic triad of abdominal pain, arthritis, and lower extremity purpuric rash. Renal involvement is also seen in the acute phase in up to 50% of cases. Treatment with prednisone is recommended if the patient is having moderate to severe abdominal pain, to help prevent the surgical gastrointestinal complications associated with HSP. It is also recommended in situations of central nervous system involvement and nephrotic syndrome. In the majority of cases treatment is supportive. NSAIDS can be used for arthralgias. Antibiotics and IV immunoglobulin are not indicated in HSP. Laparotomy may become necessary in rare instances where patients develop intestinal obstruction or perforation, but is not indicated in this situation.

CHAPTER 51

Pain—Back

JOHN J. REEVES, M.D.

QUESTIONS

1. A 16-year-old high school weightlifter reports back pain for 3 months. He denies any specific trauma. A physical exam reveals pain over the lower lumbar spine. Anterior-posterior (AP) and lateral radiographs of the spine are normal. The remainder of his examination, including strength, sensation, deep tendon reflexes, and rectal tone, is normal. What would you obtain next?

   a. Bone scan
   b. Neurosurgery consult
   c. Oblique spine radiographs
   d. Spinal MRI
   e. Spinal CT

2. A 5-year-old female patient is brought to the ED for evaluation of a limp. Her mother reports that 2 weeks ago the child fell from her bunk bed, landing on her back. She appeared to be fine until 5 days ago, when she was noted to have difficulty walking. Other than a slight limp on the right and mild tenderness over the lumbar spine, her examination is unremarkable. What test would be most helpful?

   a. CBC
   b. Spinal MRI
   c. ESR
   d. Radionucleotide bone scan
   e. Plain spine radiograph series

3. An 18-year-old female basketball player, recently emigrated from the Caribbean, comes to the ED with sudden onset of severe back pain located in the midthoracic area. Vital signs are: RR 28, HR 110, BP 85/55, and an O_2 saturation of 100% on room air. Through an interpreter, you discover that the child has a history of a "leaky heart valve." After plain radiographs are obtained, what test would you obtain next?

   a. A cardiac enzyme profile
   b. Hemoglobin electrophoresis
   c. Sickle-cell preparation
   d. Thoracic spine radiographs
   e. Chest CT scan

4. A 10-year-old male patient is seen after a fall from an amusement park ride, which collapsed while he was riding on it. He fell about 20 feet, landing in a seated position. After a thorough trauma evaluation, the child is noted only to have lower back pain and tenderness. Given the likely injury in this patient, what would you expect to see on plain radiographs of the spine?

   a. Herniation of an intervertebral disk
   b. Anterior buckling of a lumbar vertebral body
   c. Fracture of the cartilaginous end-plate of a vertebral body
   d. Fracture of the pars interarticularis
   e. Fracture of a spinous process

5. The mother of a 5-year-old boy complains that her son is incontinent. Although his mother reports that he has been toilet trained since age 2, over the last 2 weeks he has been wetting his bed almost nightly. He has also been having difficulty with daytime bathroom accidents. The mother denies weight loss, urinary frequency, fever, abdominal pain or new psychological stressors in the home environment. What evaluation would be most likely to reveal an abnormality?

   a. Serum glucose
   b. A rectal examination
   c. Urinalysis with culture
   d. An abdominal U/S
   e. A psychological evaluation

ANSWERS

1. **c** Although the child's plain radiographs are normal, the history is very suggestive of a fracture to the pars interarticularis (spondylolysis). This injury is often seen on the oblique radiographs only. Further imaging (e.g., with a bone scan) would be indicated if normal radiographs are seen but the child continues with symptoms of spondylolysis. MRI and neurosurgical consultation should be reserved for children with evidence of spinal cord impingement. Spinal CT can be used to delineate the extent of a suspected fracture, but this is rarely indicated in the initial diagnosis of this injury.

2. **b** The most concerning aspect of this child's history and examination is the delay in the onset of the limp. Although a limp immediately following a fall would more likely suggest a musculoskeletal etiology, this child's limp is more likely secondary to neurologic causes. Other neurological deficits may be seen, but they are not always present. Although all of the diagnoses could cause back pain and a limp, the history of trauma makes an epidural hematoma more likely. A herniated intervertebral disk is a rare diagnosis in a young child, but it would not be impossible. Of the selected tests given, a spinal MRI would be the most sensitive test to diagnose a compression injury from a spinal epidural hematoma.

3. **e** The child is slightly tachycardic and hypotensive and is complaining of upper back pain. These factors and her history of possible valvular heart disease raises the suspicion of Marfan's syndrome and its association with thoracic aortic aneurysm. Failure to quickly pursue this diagnosis could prove fatal. The best test for diagnosis of this rare entity is a thoracic aortogram; however, a properly performed chest CT is also fairly sensitive. Of the given choices, a chest CT would be most helpful. Spondylolysis and spondylolisthesis cause lumbar pain. MI can cause back pain, but it is unlikely in this child. The symptomatology of an MI is also usually less striking. Sickle-cell pain crisis with chest syndrome is possible, but her lack of even mild hypoxia and the presence of other concerning vital signs would make this a less likely cause of her chest symptoms.

4. **b** Falls in the seated position are associated with vertebral compression fractures. The characteristic radiographic findings are anterior buckling or compression of the affected vertebral body. Fractures of the cartilaginous end-plate are normally seen in distraction-type injuries. Spinous process fractures would be unusual in this setting, because they are usually caused by lifting or hyperextension injuries (e.g., the clay shoveler's fracture) or, rarely, from direct trauma. Fracture of the pars interarticularis (spodylolysis) is more common after repetitive minor trauma. A herniated intervertebral disk and muscle strain are often associated with heavy lifting and are generally a disease of older children and adults; these injuries are not seen on a plain radiograph.

5. **b** Incontinence is a common complaint in the pediatric population and is occasionally evaluated in the ED. Although many children with this complaint have psychological causes for their symptoms, more serious pathology should be considered. New-onset, type I diabetes, a UTI, and urologic abnormalities are all possible causes of new-onset bedwetting in a previously toilet-trained child. The lack of other supporting factors for these diagnoses raises the suspicion for spinal cord compression and the need for a more thorough neurologic examination, which includes evaluation of rectal tone.

CHAPTER 52

Pain—Chest

JOHN J. REEVES, M.D.

QUESTIONS

1. A 16-year-old male patient is involved in a high-speed, head-on automobile collision. On arrival to the ED he is noted to be anxious and is complaining of chest pain. Vital signs are: HR 108, RR 28, and BP 116/48. Which study would be most important to obtain next?

   a. Portable CXR
   b. 12-lead ECG, with rhythm strip
   c. Hemoglobin and hematocrit level
   d. CT scan of the chest
   e. Needle thoracentesis

2. A 13-year-old boy comes with his mother to the ED for evaluation of chest pain. He states that he has noted occasional sharp, stabbing pain that occurs intermittently while exercising. The pain only lasts a few seconds and is located in the area below his left nipple. He denies syncope or near syncope, but does think that his heart was going "a little fast" during these periods. Family history includes two grandparents that have recently died from "heart problems." The boy has an unremarkable examination and a normal CXR and 12-lead ECG. What is most appropriate next step at this time?

   a. A cardiac stress test
   b. Echocardiogram
   c. No further evaluation is necessary
   d. Outpatient psychiatric evaluation
   e. 24-hour Holter monitor

3. While working in a Texas ED in August, you are asked to evaluate an 11-year-old girl with a history of asthma who just suffered a syncopal episode. According to the patient's mother, the girl was playing soccer when she was noted to cry out and then to collapse on the field. She regained consciousness within a few minutes after falling. She is currently lying on a stretcher in no acute distress. Her current vital signs are: lying—blood pressure 110/80, HR 80; standing—BP 90/77, HR 90. Her physical examination is unrevealing. What would be the most appropriate next step?

   a. IV fluid administration
   b. Inpatient cardiac monitoring
   c. Brief observation, then discharge home
   d. Urinalysis for myoglobinuria
   e. Treatment with bronchodilator

4. An 18-year-old male patient is brought to the ED after he developed chest pain at a fraternity party. He is currently agitated but oriented and in no acute distress, complaining only of mild chest pain. A quick physical examination reveals tachycardia. A 12-lead ECG would most likely show which of the following?

   a. A corrected QT interval of 460 msec
   b. A HR of 220 bpm and absent p waves
   c. A sawtooth pattern with HR 200 bpm
   d. ST-segment elevation
   e. Low-voltage QRS complexes

5. A 6-year-old girl comes to the ED with mild diffuse chest pain on inspiration. Her mother reports that she has been waking up at night with a bad cough for the past 2 months, but has otherwise been healthy. Physical examination is unremarkable. Which of the following is likely to be abnormal?

 a. An overnight sleep study
 b. A 24-hour Holter monitor
 c. Pulmonary function tests (PFTs)
 d. An oblique "rib view" CXR
 e. A 12-lead ECG

6. A 14-year-old girl is evaluated for chest pain at rest. The patient states that she was at home talking with her mother when she noted onset of chest pain over her left chest and difficulty catching her breath. She denies any prior episodes of chest pain, palpitations, syncope, near-syncope, or exercise-related symptoms. She does report that her grandfather recently passed away from a "heart attack." A physical examination, CXR, and 12-lead ECG are normal. What is the most appropriate next step?

 a. Arrange for a ventilation-perfusion scan
 b. Arrange for a 24-hour Holter monitor
 c. Admit for overnight telemetry monitoring
 d. Reassure the patient that it is unlikely to be a serious problem
 e. Perform a urine screen for drugs of abuse

ANSWERS

1. a   Given the limited information, the boy could have a number of causes for his symptoms. Pneumothorax, hemothorax, aortic rupture, cardiac arrhythmia from cardiac contusion, pulmonary contusion, cardiac tamponade, ruptured esophagus, tracheobronchial disruption, rib fracture, vertebral injury, and simple chest wall contusion can all be caused by a rapid deceleration injury and blunt force trauma. Clearly, a more thorough physical examination would help to narrow the diagnostic possibilities. Of the choices, a CXR will give the most information in the shortest amount of time and will help to direct care further. A chest CT is rarely, if ever, the first test to obtain in a trauma evaluation. The remaining choices would help to evaluate for specific causes of traumatic chest pain, but all will give only limited information.

2. c   Although the boy has a number of concerning "red flags" (e.g., symptoms during exercise and a fast heart rate), one's overall impression is of benign chest pain. The short duration of symptoms and the brief, sharp, inconsistent nature of the symptoms all suggest a benign precordial catch syndrome. This is very common in young healthy teens and adults. Although a CXR and an ECG are probably indicated, findings would presumably be normal. The family history adds no information.

3. b   As with most diagnoses in the ED, the key lies in the history. The child is at risk for dehydration, an asthma attack, and heat stroke, given her history and the fact that she is exercising in what is invariably extremely hot weather. However, the fact that she apparently had pain (revealed by the cry) followed by sudden LOC suggest a sudden cardiac event with possible myocardial ischemia. Although vasovagal stimulation causes syncope by producing bradycardia and hypotension, there is no history for an inciting traumatic or anxiety-producing event. Moderate orthostatic vital sign changes are frequently seen in teenagers and adults and are nonspecific findings. There are no exam findings to suggest an asthma flare-up. It is extremely unlikely that a child would collapse from a severe asthma attack and not be in severe distress after the event. The presence of myoglobin in the urine would not explain her event.

4. d   The given ECG patterns are examples of prolonged QT syndrome, supraventricular tachycardia (SVT), atrial flutter, myocardial ischemia, and pericarditis/myocarditis, all of which can be associated with chest pain. However, this patient presents with agitation that is out of proportion to his physical findings, suggesting a possible drug exposure. Although further evaluation is required, given the limited information, myocardial ischemia/infarction secondary to cocaine abuse should be high on the list. Atrial fibrillation and pericarditis/myocarditis would be unusual in this setting. Prolonged QT syndrome and SVT are possible in this scenario, but his symptoms of agitation would be hard to explain.

5. c   This child has classic symptoms of cough-variant asthma; hence, PFTs would be expected to be abnormal. Evaluation for an arrhythmia with a Holter monitor or ECG is not supported by the history. No

history of trauma was given, making a rib fracture unlikely. An overnight sleep study has no role in evaluation of this patient.

6. d In a previously healthy child, with no symptoms associated with exertion, no evidence of palpitations, syncope, near syncope, and without evidence of cardiac or pulmonary pathology, a CXR and 12-lead ECG are sufficient evaluation. There is no reason to suspect that this child will need further evaluation for a pulmonary embolus or an arrhythmia. A urine drug screen may be indicated in some patients, although the history in this case does not support this suspicion.

CHAPTER **53**

Pain—Dysphagia

VINCENT J. WANG, M.D.

QUESTIONS

1. A 2-day-old girl has had difficulty feeding. She was born full term, without complications. Since birth, she seems to cry often. When she feeds, she sucks for a few seconds, and then stops feeding and begins crying. After crying for several seconds, she can resume feeding. The parents think this is abnormal, but are not sure because they are first-time parents. On examination, the baby has alternating episodes of tachypnea and crying spells. Her lungs are clear, her heart rate (HR) is regular without murmurs, and her abdomen is soft. The diagnosis may be confirmed by:

   a. Obtaining a CXR
   b. Obtaining an abdominal x-ray
   c. Obtaining an ABG
   d. Passing a feeding tube through her nares
   e. Follow up in 2 weeks

2. A 10-year-old boy complains of difficulty swallowing. He admits to having a hamburger-eating contest with one of his friends and says that he won by eating 10 hamburgers in 5 minutes. However, he began complaining of difficulty swallowing after the tenth hamburger. He has not had fever. On examination, he is alert, but has excessive secretions in his mouth. His RR is 16. His oropharynx and lung examinations are normal. Treatment may include:

   a. Recommending meat tenderizer
   b. Immediate intubation
   c. Administering glucagon
   d. Administering glucose and insulin
   e. Performing the Heimlich maneuver

3. A 3-month-old boy has had constipation and difficulty feeding. The constipation began 4 days ago and he has been less active. The mother says that he has not fed as well lately, even though she has been sweetening his formula with honey. On examination, he is afebrile, appears lethargic, and has a weak cry. You note excessive secretions in his mouth. Appropriate treatment may involve:

   a. Application of viscous lidocaine to his oropharynx
   b. Ceftriaxone after blood and urine cultures are obtained
   c. Administration of pralidoxime
   d. Prophylactic intubation
   e. Consultation with a feeding specialist

4. A 3-year-old girl complains of difficulty swallowing. She has had fevers for several days. She complains of a sore throat and difficulty moving her neck. She is alert, but holds her neck straight, preferring not to move her head. She is not drooling. Her Brudzinski's sign is equivocal, but her Kernig's sign is negative. Her oropharynx is erythematous, with large bilateral tonsillar swelling. Her rapid strep test is positive. The next step in treatment includes:

   a. Amoxicillin PO for 10 days
   b. Erythromycin PO for 10 days
   c. Lateral neck x-ray
   d. CXR
   e. Prophylactic intubation

ANSWERS

1. d   Choanal atresia may be partial or complete. If the atresia is partial, the patient may have normal breathing until she has an intercurrent illness that obstructs the nasal passages. Because neonates and infants are obligate nose breathers, choanal atresia will manifest with varying degrees of respiratory distress. Crying relieves the obstructions because the children may then breath through their mouths. Children may have difficulty feeding, because they cannot feed and breathe at the same time. The diagnosis may be confirmed by passing a feeding tube through each naris.

2. c   Esophageal foreign bodies (FBs) usually present acutely. FBs may be food, coins, or any object that a child has swallowed. In this case, the likely FB is hamburger meat. Plain radiographs are unlikely to demonstrate an FB in this case, and the diagnosis may be confirmed with fluoroscopy or with a UGI series. Treatment may involve administration of glucagon because this will enhance peristalsis and potentially move the foreign body. However, treatment with glucagon carries a small risk of esophageal perforation. If the patient is in no distress, a period of observation may be warranted. If the patient is in distress, or if the problem has failed to resolve during observation, FB removal via endoscopy is necessary. There is no role for the administration of meat tenderizer. Intubation is not necessary now, because the respiratory status is not compromised, and this is not a case of epiglottitis. Glucose and insulin are not likely to help. The Heimlich maneuver is indicated in cases of FBs lodged in the airway, rather than the esophagus.

3. d   Botulism is characterized as a descending paralysis. Constipation is often the first symptom, followed by lethargy, a weak cry, poor feeding, drooling, dysphagia, and, eventually, respiratory paralysis. The patient does not require prophylactic intubation now, but will likely require this in the course of the disease. Guillain-Barré syndrome may resemble botulism, but it is less likely in this age group and in this scenario. Treatment with viscous lidocaine may be used for stomatitis infections. Ceftriaxone is indicated for possible bacteremia or sepsis, which may be confused with this diagnosis. Pralidoxime is indicated for organophosphate poisonings, and would be unlikely in this case. Feeding specialist consultation is indicated for less acute disorders of swallowing.

4. c   Retropharyngeal abscess may present with fever and difficulty swallowing. This is a complication of a streptococcal infection that is often preceded by a pharyngitis. The patient may have difficulty moving her neck because of spasm of the associated muscles, but she will not have true meningismus. A pharyngitis may have similar symptoms, but is not likely to have neck pain. A lateral neck film, or a neck CT scan, is therefore necessary to evaluate for this complication.

CHAPTER 54

Pain—Dysuria

VINCENT J. WANG, M.D.

QUESTIONS

1. A 3-year-old boy, recently diagnosed with a URI, complains of pain when voiding. He has not had vomiting or abdominal pain. On examination, his abdomen is soft and he has no tenderness in the costovertebral angle (CVA) area. His joints are normal, without swelling or pain on motion; however, you note conjunctivitis, oral ulcers, and target lesions over his body. You suspect that the underlying condition is:

   a. Reiter's syndrome
   b. Stevens-Johnson syndrome
   c. Kawasaki disease
   d. Cystitis
   e. Pyelonephritis

2. A 4-year-old girl has fever and painful urination. The mother suspects that the new bubble bath she is using has been causing her symptoms. She has not had vaginal discharge. Her vital signs are: T 40°C, HR 130, RR 20, and BP 90/50. She is alert, but uncomfortable. Her abdomen is soft and she has pain when percussing the CVA area. The most likely cause of her symptoms is:

   a. Kidney infection with *Escherichia coli*
   b. Bladder infection with *Staphylococcus aureus*
   c. Vaginal irritation from the bubble bath
   d. Urethral infection with *Neisseria gonorrhoeae*
   e. Local trauma

3. A 6-year-old girl complains of dysuria. Her vital signs are: T 37°C, HR 100, RR 20, and BP 90/50. She is well appearing, her abdomen is soft, and she has no CVA tenderness. Her only physical finding is mild erythema surrounding her urethra. You treat her with:

   a. IV ampicillin and gentamicin
   b. Sitz baths
   c. IM ceftriaxone
   d. IV corticosteroids
   e. Corticosteroids orally

4. A 17-year-old boy complains of dysuria. He is sexually active, but does not use condoms. He complains of discharge from his urethra and pain on voiding. On examination, he has no abdominal pain. His genitalia are normal, without lesions or discharge. Appropriate treatment includes all of the following, EXCEPT:

   a. Urethral cultures
   b. Urine cultures
   c. Hepatitis A (HAV) testing
   d. Abstinence from sexual activity until his partner is evaluated
   e. IM ceftriaxone

5. A 6-year-old girl complains of anal itching and dysuria. She has not had fever or abdominal pain. She is alert, her abdomen is soft, and her anogenital examination is normal, except for mild erythema perianally. Her urinalysis is normal. You recommend:

   a. Trimethoprim-sulfamethoxazole orally
   b. Sitz baths
   c. IM ceftriaxone
   d. Estrogen cream topically
   e. Mebendazole orally

ANSWERS

1. b   Stevens-Johnson syndrome, or erythema multiforme major, is a serious systemic disorder, characterized by involvement of two mucosal surfaces and the skin. (Darmstadt GL, Lane A. Vesiculobullous disorders. In: *Nelson Textbook of Pediatrics,* fifteenth edition. Philadelphia: W.B. Saunders, 1996; 604: 1850–1851.) Dysuria, conjunctivitis, oral lesions, and target lesions may be present. The skin may also become denuded. Reiter's syndrome is characterized by conjunctivitis, arthritis, and urethritis. Kawasaki disease may cause a bilateral limbal-sparing conjunctivitis and the rash may appear similar to erythema multiforme, but oral lesions are typically described as being injected, rather than having oral ulcers. (Schaller JG. Kawasaki disease. In: *Nelson Textbook of Pediatrics,* fifteenth edition. Philadelphia: W.B. Saunders, 1996; 152.2:678–679.) Cystitis and pyelonephritis are acute infections of the urinary tract. These would not be associated with ocular and cutaneous findings.

2. a.   Pyelonephritis is an infection of the urinary tract involving the kidneys. Fever is usually over 39°C, and it is associated with flank pain/tenderness, and dysuria. *E. coli* is a common organism for pyelonephritis and cystitis. Cystitis may or may not have a fever and will often present with isolated suprapubic pain or tenderness. Vulvovaginitis is commonly seen in prepubertal girls, often with a history of bubble-bath use, but vulvovaginitis should not cause fever and flank pain. Urethritis is associated with a urethral discharge and is frequently seen in adolescents. There is no evidence of local trauma causing her symptoms.

3. b   Chemical urethritis may develop because various chemicals irritate the urethral mucosa. Common irritants include detergents, fabric softeners, perfumed soaps, and bubble baths. Patients have minimal or no physical findings and are otherwise well appearing. There is no discharge present on examination. Treatment involves sitz baths as needed and eliminating the source of irritation.

4. c   All of the preceding responses are appropriate except for "c." Testing for HIV, syphilis, and hepatitis B (HBV) are appropriate, but hepatitis A (HAV) is not transmitted via sexual activity, and testing for HAV therefore is not indicated.

5. e   *Enterobius vermicularis* infestation may cause itching in the perianal area, which may spread to the vaginal area in girls. Girls may complain of dysuria, rather than itching. Patients may have mild erythema of the perianal area. Treatment is mebendazole orally.

CHAPTER 55

Pain—Earache

VINCENT J. WANG, M.D.

QUESTIONS

1. A 12-year-old boy complains of ear pain. He was involved in a fight and was hit in the left ear. On examination he is afebrile and has a swollen, boggy, purple pinna. His tympanic membrane is normal. Treatment includes:

   a. Dicloxacillin orally (PO)
   b. Mupirocin topically
   c. Aspiration
   d. Debridement
   e. Warm soaks

2. A 13-year-old girl complains of ear pain. She has 10 earrings placed over the pinna and ear lobe. She has pain, erythema, and swelling of her pinna around a superior earring site. In addition to removal of the earring, treatment includes:

   a. Amoxicillin PO
   b. Dicloxacillin PO
   c. Aspiration
   d. Debridement
   e. Antibiotic/steroid otic suspension

3. A 16-year-old boy complains of ear pain. He notes severe pain of his right ear. On examination, he has a right-sided facial droop and vesicles on the right tympanic membrane. His neurological examination is otherwise normal. Treatment includes:

   a. Amoxicillin PO
   b. Acyclovir PO
   c. Aspiration of the vesicle
   d. Tympanocentesis
   e. Antibiotic/steroid otic suspension

4. A 4-year-old boy complains of ear pain and drainage. He has been swimming in the local lakes this summer. On examination he has a tender right auricle and foul-smelling greenish discharge. The right tympanic membrane is clear. Treatment includes:

   a. Warm soaks
   b. Dicloxacillin PO
   c. Nystatin otic drops
   d. Antibiotic/steroid otic suspension
   e. Admission and parenteral antibiotics

5. An 18-month-old girl is sent home from daycare because of fever and irritability. Her temperature is 38.2°C and her right tympanic membrane is erythematous and bulging. Her canal wall is normal. Appropriate treatment includes:

   a. Penicillin PO 50 mg/kg/day
   b. Cefaclor PO 100 mg/kg/day
   c. Amoxicillin PO 50 mg/kg/day
   d. IM ceftriaxone 50 mg/kg once
   e. Nystatin drops to the affected ear

6. A 10-year-old boy was riding his bicycle when he fell to the side, hitting his head on the ground. He denies loss of consciousness (LOC). He is otherwise well, except for a layer of blood behind his right tympanic membrane. Further management includes:

   a. Treatment with amoxicillin and outpatient follow-up
   b. Obtaining a coagulation profile
   c. Obtaining a head CT scan
   d. Tympanocentesis
   e. Treatment with ibuprofen and outpatient follow-up

7. A 5-year-old boy complains of right-sided ear pain. On examination, his right ear is normal, but you note multiple caries in his mouth. The nerve involved with this referred pain is:

a. Cranial nerve V
b. Cranial nerve VII
c. Cranial nerve IX
d. Cranial nerve X
e. Cervical nerves C2 and C3

ANSWERS

1. c   Sterile aspiration is necessary to avoid pressure necrosis caused by this hematoma of the pinna. After aspiration, a molded pressure dressing is also necessary to prevent a resulting "cauliflower" or "boxer's" ear. Antibiotics are not indicated. There is also no indication for debridement or warm soaks.

2. b   Earrings placed in the pinna are especially prone to infection, as compared with earrings in the earlobe. Treatment includes removal of the earring(s) and administration of an oral antistaphylococcal antibiotic. Dicloxicillin would be adequate. There is no role for aspiration or debridement in this vignette. Antibiotic/steroid otic suspensions are also not indicated.

3. b   Ramsay Hunt syndrome or herpes zoster oticus may be characterized by vesicles on the tympanic membrane, external auditory meatus, and the auricle, after infection of cranial nerves VII and VIII. Patients may also have facial paralysis, vertigo, and hearing loss. Patients may be treated with acyclovir if diagnosed early in the course of the disease; otherwise, treatment is supportive.

4. d   "Swimmer's ear" or otitis externa is characterized by ear pain, foul-smelling discharge, and an erythematous ear canal. Swimming can predispose patients to developing this condition. Treatment involves an otic suspension containing an antibiotic, hydrocortisone, and an acidic medium. The canal can occasionally become so edematous that placement of a wick is necessary to ensure adequate penetration of the drops. Complications of otitis externa include cellulitis. Oral antibiotics may be added, or, if the infection is fulminant, otorhinolaryngology consultation and admission for parenteral antibiotics may be necessary.

5. d   Bacterial otitis media is primarily caused by *S. pneumoniae,* nontypable *H. influenzae,* and *Moraxella catarrhalis.* Ceftriaxone as a single injection is an acceptable alternative to oral antibiotics. Penicillin does not treat the organisms effectively. Cefaclor does not penetrate the inner ear in high enough concentrations to be effective. Current recommendations for amoxicillin dosing are 80–90 mg/kg/day because of resistant *S. pneumoniae.* (Dowell SF, Butler JC, Giebink S, et al. Acute otitis media: management and surveillance in an era of pneumococcal resistance—a report from the drug-resistant *Streptococcus pneumoniae* therapeutic working group. Pediatr Infect Dis J 1999; 18:1–9.) Children at risk for resistant *S. pneumoniae* are children under age 3, children with daycare exposure, or children who have had antibiotic treatment within the past 6 months.

6. c   Hemotympanum may be because of a basilar skull fracture, so a head CT scan is warranted for further evaluation. Other signs consistent with a basilar skull fracture include ecchymoses behind the ear (Battle's sign), periorbital ecchymoses (raccoon eyes), or CSF drainage from the nose or ears.

7. a   Cranial nerve V supplies areas of referred ear pain from dental etiologies and oral mucosal etiologies. Cranial nerve VII pain may be a precursor of a facial palsy or Ramsay Hunt syndrome. Cranial nerve IX supplies the oropharynx, nasopharynx, and posterior third of the tongue; therefore, inflammation of these areas may cause referred ear pain. Inflammation of the tongue, larynx, and trachea may cause referred ear pain via cranial nerve X. Injuries to cervical nerves C2 and C3 may cause referred ear pain to the pinna and mastoid areas.

CHAPTER **56**

Headaches

MARK WALTZMAN, M.D.

QUESTIONS

1. A 7-year-old boy is brought to the ED with a complaint of headache. His father states that the boy has been well until the day before his visit to the ED, when he began to complain of a mild headache. The father attributed his son's pain to the cold weather and poor heat supply to the home, but the headache has since worsened and the boy has had several episodes of vomiting. Both parents state that they have also been suffering from headaches over the past few days. Physical exam is normal. The SINGLE most effective therapy in the ED should be:

   a. IV hydration
   b. Morphine sulfate
   c. 100% O_2
   d. Ibuprofen
   e. Compazine

2. A 5-year-old girl is brought to the ED with a complaint of a severe headache. The mother states that the girl has been well until 1 hour ago, when she began to cry and hold her head. There was no history of trauma. Physical exam is significant for an obviously uncomfortable, crying child. There is a large port wine stain to the right side of the face. The remainder of the evaluation is normal, including a neurologic exam. The most likely diagnosis in this child is:

   a. Migraine headache
   b. Tension headache
   c. Intracranial bleed
   d. Brain tumor
   e. Meningitis

3. A 14-year-old boy is brought to the ED for evaluation of headache. He states that he has been having a frontal headache for the past 2–3 days. The headache is sharp and pounding. There is no history of trauma. Physical exam reveals an alert and oriented boy. Pupils are equal and reactive, with mild pain on lateral movement in the right eye. There is no proptosis. There is no photophobia. Remainder of the exam, including a neurologic exam, is normal. Treatment should consist of:

   a. IV Solu-Medrol
   b. IV Cefotaxime
   c. Oral sumatriptan
   d. Oral prochlorperazine (Compazine)
   e. Morphine sulfate

4. A 15-year-old girl comes to the ED complaining of a headache. She reports a left, frontal headache that has persisted over the past 3 days. No fever has been associated with the headache. Exam is significant for mild left mandibular swelling. The remainder of the exam is normal. Treatment should include which of the following?

   a. Oral amoxicillin
   b. Oral ibuprofen
   c. Oral sumatriptan
   d. IV hydralazine
   e. Clonidine

ANSWERS

1. c   Headaches associated with vascular changes are believed to be caused by vasodilation. Hypoxia is a potent stimulus for cerebral vasodilation. Children with acute hypoxic insult (e.g., carbon monoxide [CO] poisoning) may present with headaches, lethargy, seizures, and coma if severely intoxicated. Treatment for CO poisoning is administration of 100% O_2 to displace CO bound to hemoglobin. The other treatments may help with symptoms, but they will not treat the underlying disease state. Further treatment should include evaluation of the home for the source of the CO (likely a faulty space heater).

2. c   Sudden, severe headaches should raise the suspicion of an acute vascular event (subarachnoid or intracranial bleed). Patients with Sturge-Weber syndrome present with large port wine stains to the face. These patients have higher incidence of AV malformations of the dura. Acute, severe headache in such a patient should raise suspicion of a ruptured AVM. Although migraine headaches may present acutely, they rarely present so abruptly. Headaches due to tension, brain tumor, and meningitis also tend to develop gradually.

3. b   Pain associated with extraocular muscle movement may be elicited with a retroorbital cellulitis or abscess. Diagnosis can be confirmed by CT examination of the orbits. Treatment should consist of antibiotics, and, in some cases, surgical consultation for possible drainage of an abscess. Although opiates and compazine may ameliorate the symptoms, they do not treat the underlying cause. Sumatryptan is useful in the management of migraine headaches.

4. a   Pain from a dental infection or abscess can be referred to the scalp. Findings on physical exam of mandibular swelling should alert the examiner to a possible dental abscess. Treatment consists of antibiotics and referral to a dentist for drainage.

CHAPTER 57

Joint Pain

VINCENT J. WANG, M.D.

QUESTIONS

1. A 14-month-old boy is brought to the ED for fever and a limp. He has had fever for 2 days and a limp for 3 days. He now refuses to walk. He has no other medical problems. On physical examination he has a temperature of 38.7°C. His right leg is externally rotated and flexed at the hip. He refuses to stand on his right leg and cries whenever you move any part of it. His WBC is 10,000 and his ESR is 25 mm/hr. Plain radiographs of his hips are normal. Your management is:

   a. Radiograph of his femur
   b. Hip ultrasound
   c. Admit for IV antibiotics
   d. Abdominal CT scan
   e. Discharge home on ibuprofen

2. A 15-year-old girl complains of right knee pain, fever, and a rash. She says that she had had chills and fever several days ago, but now feels better. Her rash began several days ago as well. She is at the end of her menstrual period, but has not been sexually active for more than 1 month. She denies dysuria or vaginal discharge. Her physical examination reveals mild swelling and erythema of her right knee. She also has crops of vesiculopustules on an erythematous base over her legs. The test with the highest yield for establishing the diagnosis is:

   a. Gram stain of the skin lesions
   b. Gram stain of the synovial fluid
   c. Culture of the synovial fluid
   d. Culture of the blood
   e. Serum VDRL (venereal disease research laboratory)

3. A 5-year-old boy is brought to the ED for knee pain. He has had increasing pain over the past 2 weeks. He has not had fever or a history of trauma. His vital signs are: T 37.4°C, HR 100, RR 20, and BP 110/70. He has no swelling or erythema of his lower extremities. He has full range of motion of his knees, but appears to have decreased range of motion of his left hip. Which of the following tests will be the most helpful?

   a. Complete blood count
   b. Sedimentation rate
   c. Hip radiographs
   d. Hip ultrasound
   e. Antinuclear antibody

4. A 6-year-old girl complains of joint pains. She has had intermittent joint pains of her knees, ankles, elbows, and wrists. She complains of left wrist pain now. Her vital signs are: T 37.6°C, HR 100, RR 20, and BP 95/60. Her examination is notable for mild swelling of her left wrist and pain with motion. You also note a faint erythematous rash on her chest with blanching in the center and a serpiginous border. Her WBC is 14,000, ESR is 25 mm/hr, and her antistreptolysin O titer is positive. Untreated, she might develop:

   a. Purpura on her buttocks
   b. Choreaform movements
   c. Renal failure
   d. Coronary artery aneurysms
   e. Cartilage necrosis

5. You are in Lyme, Connecticut. A 4-year-old boy is brought to the ED for a limp. He had a cough and rhinorrhea 2 weeks ago. He has not had a rash. He had recovered from the flulike symptoms but began having a low-grade fever and right-sided hip pain for 2 days. His vital signs are: T 38.1°C, HR 110, RR 24, and BP 95/50. He is alert and playful, but he has a right-sided limp when he tries to walk. Range of motion of his hip is normal and he has no tenderness. His WBC is 7,500 and his ESR is 5 mm/hr. Plain radiographs of his hips are normal. ELISA (enzyme-linked immunosorbent assay) for Lyme disease is positive. Appropriate ED management is:

   a. Azithromycin PO
   b. IM ceftriaxone
   c. Hip ultrasound
   d. Arthrocentesis
   e. Send Western blot testing

6. An 18-year-old sexually active girl is referred to the ED because of joint pains. She has had fevers to 38.5°C over the past 2 weeks, accompanied by a maculopapular rash. She complains of soreness and swelling of the joints of her hands, but the joint pains seemed to have improved on the day of the visit. On physical examination, she has no swelling of her hands, and only minimal pain on motion of her fingers. You note icterus of her eyes. You diagnose the patient with:

   a. Hepatitis B arthritis
   b. Juvenile rheumatoid arthritis (JRA)
   c. Systemic lupus erythematosus (SLE)
   d. Serum sickness
   e. Poststreptococcal arthritis

7. A 5-year-old boy is referred to the ED because of pallor and joint pains. He has been less active for the past few weeks, and appears more pale than usual. He has also complained of pain of his left elbow. He has not had trauma. His vital signs are: T 37.6°C, HR 130, RR 24, and BP 110/60. He is alert, but pale and weak appearing. His chest is clear to auscultation, his cardiovascular examination is normal, but you palpate a spleen tip approximately 4 cm below the left costal margin. He has diffuse lymphadenopathy. Which of the following tests will most likely make the diagnosis?

   a. ESR
   b. CBC with smear
   c. Elbow radiograph
   d. Antinuclear antibody
   e. Antistreptolysin O titer

8. A 9-year-old girl is brought to the ED because of a rash and joint pains. She complains of feeling tired over the past few weeks. She has had a rash over both of her cheeks for several days, and she says that her wrists and elbows have been sore and occasionally swollen. On examination, you note an erythematous malar rash extending over the bridge of her nose and mild swelling over her wrists, with mild tenderness. Other symptoms found with the diagnosis that you make include all of the following, EXCEPT:

   a. Thrombocytopenia
   b. Renal failure
   c. Pericarditis
   d. Sacroiliitis
   e. Psychosis

ANSWERS

1. b   The diagnosis of septic arthritis should be driven by clinical suspicion. Ancillary testing may aid in the diagnosis, but if the history and physical examination findings are suggestive, the patient will need appropriate imaging and/or intervention for the diagnosis. A hip ultrasound is indicated even though the other tests are normal. Joint effusion, which is likely to be present in this case, can be aspirated and sent for cell counts as well as culture. Arthrotomy and irrigation is indicated if septic arthritis is diagnosed. It is unlikely for a femur fracture to cause these symptoms. Abdominal CT scan would be indicated if the pathology appeared to be suggestive of an appendicitis, which may mimic hip pain. Discharge to home is not appropriate.

2. a   Gonococcal arthritis commonly presents with symptoms as noted in this vignette. The test with the highest yield will be a Gram stain of the skin lesions. Cervical, rectal, or throat cultures may also yield the diagnosis. Gram stain or culture of the synovial fluid may be helpful, but a Gram stain of the skin lesions is more likely to be positive. Likewise, culture of the blood is also often negative. A serum VDRL is not helpful.

3. c   This patient presents with a history and symptoms classic for Legg-Calvé-Perthes disease, which typically develops insidiously over time and affects children between 4 and 8 years of age. He does not have systemic signs suggesting an infectious/inflammatory process; therefore, a CBC and ESR are unlikely to be helpful, as is a hip ultrasound. Antinuclear antibody testing is also unlikely to be helpful, because this presentation is not extremely suggestive of rheumatologic process.

4. b   Acute rheumatic fever (ARF) may cause a migratory polyarthritis and erythema marginatum as described in this vignette. Other major criteria (Jones criteria) for ARF are carditis, subcutaneous nodules, and Sydenham's chorea. The latter criterion manifests as choreaform movements, later in the course of the disease. This patient also has two of the minor Jones criteria—fever and elevated acute phase reactant—as well as evidence of a preceding streptococcal infection. Henoch-Schönlein purpura (HSP) may be associated with joint pains, but this is associated with a purpuric rash. Renal involvement may be associated with HSP. Coronary artery aneurysms are seen with Kawasaki disease. Cartilage necrosis is a complication of septic arthritis, which is not suggested in this vignette.

5. e   ELISA for Lyme disease is notorious for giving false-positive results. A Western blot test is indicated to confirm the diagnosis. His arthritis may be consistent with that of Lyme disease, but this is less likely without antecedent symptoms suggestive of Lyme disease. The clinical scenario describes a patient who probably has toxic synovitis. His pain is also atypical for a bacterial septic arthritis. Appropriate ED management would be to send a confirmatory Western blot test and discharge to home with close follow-up.

6. a   Hepatitis B can cause a polyarthritis of the small joints of the hands. Immune complexes circulate for 1–3 weeks before jaundice develops, and the symptoms are as described in this vignette. The other etiologies are consistent with joint pains, but not with jaundice.

7. b   This patient has systemic findings of acute lymphoblastic leukemia (ALL). Approximately 25% of patients present with bone pain or arthralgias, which are thought to be caused by leukemic infiltration of the bone marrow. An ESR is unlikely to be helpful because it may be elevated, but will not lead to a specific diagnosis. An elbow radiograph will also be unlikely. This patient does not have manifestations of a rheumatoid process or a poststreptococcal arthritis.

8. d   Systemic lupus erythematosus (SLE), the disease described in the vignette, may produce each of the symptoms except for sacroiliitis. Joint involvement in SLE is usually non-erosive, involving the peripheral joints. Sacroiliitis is most commonly seen in type II pauciarticular JRA.

CHAPTER **58**

Pain—Scrotal

VINCENT J. WANG, M.D.

QUESTIONS

1. A 14-year-old boy comes to the ED with right-sided testicular pain. The pain began suddenly approximately 1 hour ago. On examination, he has a swollen and diffusely tender right testicle, which is positionally higher than the other testicle. The cremasteric reflex is absent on the right. Treatment includes:

   a. Trimethoprim–sulfamethoxazole
   b. Azithromycin
   c. Surgical exploration
   d. Ibuprofen
   e. Needle aspiration and evacuation

2. A 10-year-old boy comes to the ED with left-sided testicular pain and abdominal pain for 8 hours. On examination, he has a swollen and erythematous left testicle, with diffuse tenderness, but mild right testicular tenderness as well. Cremasteric reflexes are difficult to elicit. Definitive diagnostic testing at this point includes:

   a. Abdominal radiograph
   b. Abdominal U/S
   c. Abdominal and pelvic CT scan
   d. Testicular U/S
   e. No further testing is required

3. A 10-year-old boy comes to the ED with right-sided testicular pain. He complains of pain for the past day. On examination, he has tenderness over the superior lateral aspect of the testis. There is a blue dot over this site of tenderness. Treatment includes:

   a. Trimethoprim–sulfamethoxazole
   b. Azithromycin
   c. Surgical exploration
   d. Ibuprofen
   e. Needle aspiration and evacuation

4. A 12-year-old boy fell onto the frame of his bicycle. He complains of right-sided scrotal pain. On examination, he has a tense swollen scrotum, especially on the right. He has severe tenderness on the right. Treatment includes:

   a. Cold compresses
   b. Needle aspiration
   c. Surgical exploration
   d. Sitz baths
   e. Observation only

5. A 17-year-old boy comes to the ED with right-sided testicular pain for 5 days. He is not sexually active and he denies discharge. On examination he has mild right-sided scrotal pain and mild swelling. He has mild relief with elevation of his scrotum. His cremasteric reflexes are normal. Treatment should include:

   a. Trimethoprim–sulfamethoxazole
   b. Ceftriaxone
   c. Corticosteroids
   d. Aspiration and evacuation
   e. Surgical exploration

6. A 17-year-old boy with bilateral facial swelling comes to the ED with right lower quadrant abdominal pain. The patient developed fever, malaise, and bilateral cheek swelling 5 days ago. He developed abdominal pain today. On examination, he has significant swelling bilaterally along the angles of the mandible. He has right lower quadrant abdominal pain, but on examination of his scrotum, you note right-sided testicular swelling and tenderness. Treatment includes:

   a. Trimethoprim–sulfamethoxazole
   b. Ceftriaxone
   c. Corticosteroids
   d. Laparotomy
   e. Surgical exploration of the testicle

7. A 2-day-old boy comes to the ED with right-sided scrotal swelling. He was in his usual state of health when the parents noticed the scrotal swelling. On examination, he has right-sided scrotal swelling without tenderness. Both testicles are descended and appear normal. The scrotal sac transilluminates. Treatment includes:

   a. Trimethoprim–sulfamethoxazole
   b. Acetaminophen
   c. Cold compresses
   d. Surgical exploration
   e. Observation and outpatient follow-up

8. A 4-year-old boy comes to the ED with bilateral scrotal swelling. He is otherwise well. He has mild swelling of his scrotum, which is painless. His testicles are normal and nontender. The rest of his examination is normal. His urinalysis is normal. His symptoms are most likely to be caused by:

   a. Kawasaki disease
   b. Nephrotic syndrome
   c. Idiopathic scrotal edema
   d. Testicular torsion
   e. Epididymitis

9. A 1-day-old boy comes to the ED with painless and smooth testicular enlargement. The scrotum is dark, with no erythema or edema. Treatment includes:

   a. Acetaminophen
   b. Trimethoprim–sulfamethoxazole
   c. Orchiopexy
   d. Testiculectomy
   e. Observation

ANSWERS

1. c   Testicular torsion is a urological emergency and is the most common cause of acute painful scrotal swelling in children. Torsion is most common in the newborn period and in early puberty, with two-thirds of patients between 12–18 years of age. The onset of pain is characteristically severe and sudden, and is often associated with abdominal pain, nausea, and vomiting. On examination, the testis has a higher lie than the unaffected testis. The cremasteric reflex is absent on the involved side. There may be erythema over the scrotum. Urinalysis is negative. Trimethoprim–sulfamethoxazole would be appropriate treatment for epididymitis, another common cause of scrotal pain. Azithromycin may be used for certain venereal diseases. Needle aspiration and evacuation is not indicated.

2. d   Definitive testing for scrotal pathology would be a testicular ultrasound. The history and examination point to scrotal pathology; however, the diagnosis is not clearly testicular torsion and, therefore, further testing is required. An abdominal radiograph or ultrasound would not be helpful. An abdominal and pelvic CT scan may or may not include the scrotum and would not provide an adequate assessment of blood flow and function of the testicles. A testicular nuclear perfusion scan with technetium-99 pertechnetate may be an alternative to testicular ultrasound.

3. d   Torsion of the testicular appendage may mimic testicular torsion. This is most common in boys between the ages of 7 and 12 years, and, if examined early, scrotal tenderness may be localized to the superior lateral aspect of the testis. A "blue dot" may be a visible sign of an infarcted appendage. Treatment includes analgesics, scrotal support, and rest. Antibiotics are not indicated. Surgical exploration is required if the diagnosis is not certain. There is no role for needle aspiration and evacuation.

4. c   Scrotal trauma usually results from a straddle injury or a direct blow to the perineum. With minimal trauma, and a normal testis, patients may be managed expectantly. With significant testicular tenderness, however, further evaluation must be performed emergently. A testicular ultrasound may be performed to delineate the injury. Scrotal exploration is indicated for testicular ruptures and large hematoceles that may heal more readily if drained surgically. If there is a testicular laceration, this should also be explored surgically and the associated hematoma should be drained.

5. a   Epididymitis is an inflammation or infection of the epididymis, usually seen in adolescents or adults. The onset of tenderness and swelling is more gradual than it is with torsion of the testis or an appendage. Tenderness may be localized to the epididymis early in the course, but tenderness will spread to the testis and surrounding scrotal wall with time. Prehn's sign (elevation of the scrotum relieves pain in epididymitis) is helpful in adults, but it is not reliable in children. Cremasteric reflexes should be normal. Treatment includes analgesics, sitz baths, scrotal support, and antibiotics (e.g., trimethoprim-sulfamethoxazole or tetracycline). Chlamydia and gonorrhea infections should be considered in a patient with risk factors or with or without urethral discharge.

6. c   Mumps orchitis typically presents 4–6 days after the onset of parotid swelling. Pain may often be referred to the lower abdomen, mimicking appendicitis. Treatment is supportive, but adrenocorticotropic hormone (ACTH) and corticosteroids may provide some relief.

7. e   A hydrocele is a collection of fluid within the tunica vaginalis. The testis appears normal, so this patient has a simple hydrocele. However, if the patient has pain, erythema, or another abnormal finding, the hydrocele may be an accompanying finding with another, more emergent problem. Treatment for a simple hydrocele is observation, because the fluid will usually be reabsorbed by 12–18 months of life.

8. c   Idiopathic scrotal edema is rare and accounts for 2–5% of acute scrotal swelling. A prepubertal boy usually presents with acute, but painless, edema of the scrotum that may extend up onto the abdominal wall. Symptoms may be unilateral or bilateral, and the scrotal skin is occasionally erythematous. The urinalysis is normal. Kawasaki disease is a vasculitis that occasionally presents with scrotal swelling, but this diagnosis is unlikely in the absence of other findings. Nephrotic syndrome may produce scrotal swelling, as well as swelling in other dependent parts of the body; however, the urinalysis would demonstrate proteinuria. Testicular torsion and epididymitis are unlikely in the absence of pain.

9. e   Antenatal testicular torsion probably occurs during the late period of embryonic development, as the testis is descending into the scrotum. Patients have painless and smooth testicular enlargement. The scrotal sac appears dark in color. Previous treatment has been surgical exploration, but current practice is to observe these children. The torsed testis is usually resorbed within 4–6 months.

CHAPTER 59

Pallor

ROBERT L. CLOUTIER, M.D.

QUESTIONS

1. A 14-month-old boy is brought to the ED by his mother because of pallor. She states she is here at the urging of his visiting grandmother, who last saw the child 6 months ago. The grandmother believes that the child is paler than when she saw him on her last visit. The child is otherwise well appearing and playful, without a significant past medical history. Of the following, the most likely diagnosis is:

   a. Iron-deficiency anemia
   b. Transient erythroblastopenia of childhood (TEC)
   c. Vitamin B12 deficiency
   d. Spherocytosis
   e. Diamond-Blackfan syndrome

2. A 2-month-old boy is brought to the ED at the request of his pediatrician for evaluation of pallor and marginal feeding for the last 2 weeks. The infant was born at 38 weeks and has had no previous history of illness. The patient has lab results from the office, which are as follows: WBC 10,200, Hgb 7.2 g/dl, platelets 233,000, MCV (mean corpuscular volume) is 67 fl and the reticulocyte count is 1%. On physical exam there is no organomegaly noted on the abdominal exam. What is the next step in diagnosis?

   a. Iron studies
   b. Bone marrow examination
   c. Hemoglobin electrophoresis
   d. Fibrinogen level
   e. Lead level

3. In carefully considering the differential diagnosis, the reason the above patient could not be suffering from a hemoglobinopathy at this time is:

   a. Fetal hemoglobin levels are protective
   b. The infant must have hepatomegaly on abdominal exam
   c. Hemoglobinopathies are primarily found in patients of Mediterranean descent
   d. The infant would be near death if he had not been previously diagnosed
   e. Thalassemia can be diagnosed only after 3 months of age

4. You receive a phone referral to the ED from a physician who would like to have a patient evaluated for pallor and anemia. The physician states that he has been attempting to treat a 3-year-old boy's anemia with supplemental iron but has noticed only a worsening of his pallor and anemia. You discuss the possibility of a wide range of conditions that could be responsible for this. These include all of the following EXCEPT:

   a. Ulcerative colitis
   b. Juvenile rheumatoid arthritis (JRA)
   c. Hyperthyroidism
   d. Subacute bacterial endocarditis
   e. Addison's disease

5. As you now evaluate the patient from the preceding question, you order lab studies. Which test will help you most in differentiating a chronic inflammatory process from iron-deficiency anemia?

   a. Transferrin levels
   b. Total iron-binding capacity
   c. Serum iron
   d. Peripheral smear
   e. MCV

6. A 2-year-old girl is brought to the ED by her parents because of pallor. The parents have noticed that the child has become increasingly pale over the last 3–4 days. Upon physical examination you notice a quiet, pale child, with an HR of 100 and a BP of 95/45. You notice the child has three strawberry-colored hemangiomas on the scalp, each approximately 1–2 cm in diameter. She also has a bruit over the abdomen. What is the most likely cause of this patient's pallor?

a. Microangiopathic hemolytic anemia
b. Iron-deficiency anemia
c. Hereditary spherocytosis
d. Autoimmune hemolytic anemia
e. Diamond-Blackfan syndrome

7. A 6-month-old Cambodian boy is brought to the ED with pallor. The parents state the child has been well until the previous 4 weeks, when they have noticed increasing pallor and lethargy. The infant was born at 32 weeks, but had been healthy up to this point. He is formula fed and has had no dietary changes. Your physical exam reveals an enlarged liver 1cm below the costal margin. Which pair of tests would you order to aid you most in the diagnosis?

a. MCV and reticulocyte count
b. Serum iron and total iron-binding capacity
c. MCV and serum lead levels
d. Total iron-binding capacity and transferrin level
e. Solubility testing and reticulocyte count

ANSWERS

1. a Nutritional anemias are the most common causes of pallor, with children less than 2 years of age being affected most frequently. It is during this time that dietary intake may be inadequate to keep pace with a rapidly increasing RBC mass. Premature infants are more likely to be affected than term infants, since their iron stores at birth will be smaller. The initially smaller iron stores, in addition to a more accelerated rate of red cell growth, leads to an earlier appearance of symptoms in these infants, usually at around 6 months of age. Term infants are rarely affected before the age of 10–12 months.

2. b The hypoplastic and aplastic anemias include Diamond-Blackfan syndrome, Fanconi's anemia, transient erythroblastopenia of childhood (TEC) and acquired aplastic anemias. The acquired aplastic anemias are usually caused by medications or chemicals. The aplastic anemias may also herald the presence of a malignancy. This particular child is suffering from Diamond-Blackfan syndrome, which is a congenital hypoplastic anemia, usually noticed in the first few months of life. It affects primarily RBCs, with WBCs being affected 10% of the time. Thrombocytopenia is exceedingly rare. On presentation the anemia can be severe. The RBCs appear normocytic or macrocytic and the reticulocyte count is low. Diagnosis hinges on an examination of the bone marrow for absence of erythrocyte precursors. Fanconi's anemia affects all cell lines and is accompanied by anatomic abnormalities that include microcephaly, strabismus, small stature, mental retardation, and abnormalities of the thumbs and radii. Hyper- or hypopigmentation may also accompany this syndrome. TEC is an acquired, self-limited hypoplastic anemia that usually follows a viral illness. These patients tend to have a normal MCV at the time of diagnosis but a reduced reticulocyte count and a negative Coombs' test. WBCs may be moderately decreased, but platelets are spared. When patients are less than 6 months old, this disorder may be difficult to distinguish from Diamond-Blackfan syndrome. Spontaneous recovery is the hallmark that generally allows distinction between the two.

3. a The hemoglobinopathies represent disorders of heme synthesis; these include the sideroblastic anemias and the thalassemia syndromes. Sideroblastic anemias are either inherited or acquired and are characterized by poor iron use within the developing RBC. Serum iron and ferritin levels are consequently markedly elevated. Such abnormal iron utilization accounts for the pathologic finding of ringed sideroblasts in the bone marrow. In the thalassemias there is defective synthesis of the beta-globin portion of the heme molecule. Patients with thalassemia major (beta-thalassemia) will become symptomatic between 6–12 months of age, when functional adult hemoglobin (Hgb A) is not produced to replace declining fetal hemoglobin levels. Fetal hemoglobin is protective. Although patients of Mediterranean descent are frequently implicated in thalassemia disorders, children of Pakistani, Southeast Asian, Chinese, and Indian descent are also frequently diagnosed. Since this child is so young, the finding of hepatomegaly would be important for other causes of pallor, most likely secondary to a hemolytic process but not because of a hemoglobinopathy.

4. e   With the exception of Addison's disease, the other diagnoses are capable of causing pallor and anemia. The anemias caused by these disorders rarely represent true emergencies unless compounded by a primary hematologic disorder. Usually the anemias are microcytic or normocytic, and are consistent with impaired iron use. This concept may be useful in evaluating a patient with a poorly understood cause of anemia who may have a previously undiagnosed nonhematologic systemic disease.

5. b   A low iron-binding capacity will distinguish iron-deficiency anemia from that caused by a chronic inflammatory disease. The serum iron should also be reduced, but this will not be a distinguishing factor from iron-deficiency anemia.

6. a   Disorders of blood flow may result in increased RBC destruction, and a microangiopathic anemia. Physical examination of the skin may be the only means of detecting the origin of this consumptive coagulopathy with RBC destruction. It is the profuse web of vessels within the hemangioma itself that traps red cells and leads to their destruction. Rarely is this source of microangiopathic anemia an emergency, unless the thrombocytopenia caused by the underlying disease itself becomes responsible for chronic blood loss. For example, with hemolytic uremic syndrome (HUS), in addition to the microangiopathic anemia caused by abnormal fibrin deposition, there is an additional and more significant underlying hemolytic process that is more likely to account for life-threatening anemia.

7. a   This child is suffering from thalassemia and is presenting as his fetal hemoglobin levels are falling without adequate replacement by Hgb A. In the thalassemias the reticulocyte count tends to be elevated and the MCV low. The most recognizable features of thalassemia are the gross appearance of the cells on peripheral smear. The cells appear to be of various sizes and display a central pallor that extends outward to the cell membrane. In addition, there is evidence of active erythropoiesis, with nucleated red cells, basophilic stippling, and polychromasia. In patients with HbS beta-thalassemia, the changes noted above are not as severe. There are, instead, microcytic cells that have less variability in morphology. Target cells are common and sickled forms may or may not be present.

CHAPTER 60

Polydipsia

DOMINIC CHALUT, M.D.

QUESTIONS

1. A 1-year-old girl is referred to the ED for hypernatremic (Na: 163 mmol/L) dehydration. The parents have noted polydipsia over the last month. You suspect excessive water renal loss. What will help you differentiate between diabetes insipidus and nephrogenic diabetes insipidus?

   a. IV administration of normal saline (NS) bolus
   b. Administration of intranasal desmopressin acetate
   c. Administration of a diuretic
   d. Water deprivation
   e. Performing a head CT scan

2. You see a 10-year-old boy with a history of polydipsia and polyuria. He has had polydipsia and polyuria for several weeks now. However, he never awakes at night with those symptoms. This fact is suggestive of:

   a. Diabetes mellitus
   b. UTI
   c. Diabetes insipidus (ADH-deficient)
   d. Nephrogenic diabetes insipidus
   e. Psychogenic polydipsia

3. A 4-year-old boy who had a resection of a pituitary adenoma presents with polyuria. He is otherwise well. He has not had fever or dysuria. What is the most likely diagnosis?

   a. Nephrogenic diabetes insipidus
   b. UTI
   c. Psychogenic polydipsia
   d. Diabetes insipidus (ADH-deficient)
   e. Diabetes mellitus

4. A 2-year-old girl is brought to the ED because of a 2-week history of polydipsia and polyuria. She has lost weight over the past few weeks, despite a vigorous appetite. On physical exam she looks dehydrated. Your most likely diagnosis is:

   a. Psychogenic polydipsia
   b. Diabetes mellitus
   c. UTI
   d. Hypokalemia
   e. Hypothyroidism

5. A 10-year-old child with sickle-cell anemia is brought to the ED because of a long history of mild polydipsia. The child is well hydrated and afebrile. How is the polydipsia caused?

   a. Increased insensible water loss
   b. Limited ability to concentrate the urine
   c. Glycosuria
   d. Reduced intravascular volume
   e. Decreased sensitivity to antidiuretic hormone (ADH)

ANSWERS

1. b   Patients with ADH-deficient diabetes insipidus should respond to the exogenous hormone analogue. Nephrogenic diabetes insipidus will still have excessive renal water loss despite ADH therapy. The water-deprivation test is dangerous, because it may precipitate hypernatremia and rapid weight loss. The bolus of normal saline will not alter the renal water loss in both conditions. Finally, the head CT is not discriminative.

2. e A history of nocturnal polydipsia and polyuria is helpful, because most children with psychogenic polydipsia do not awaken in the middle of the night for fluids or urination.

3. d ADH is produced by the posterior pituitary gland. After the resection of a pituitary adenoma, deficiency in ADH is common, causing an inability of the renal collecting tubules to reabsorb the water. In nephrogenic diabetes insipidus, the collecting tubules are resistant to ADH stimulation. UTI, diabetes mellitus, and psychogenic polydipsia are not specifically associated with pituitary surgery.

4. b Prominent symptoms of diabetes mellitus include weight loss, polyuria, polyphagia, and polydipsia. Psychogenic polydipsia is diagnosed when the ingestion of water is excessive (i.e., when there is no clinical dehydration). UTI will usually present with a history of fever. Hypokalemia and hypothyroidism are usually not associated with dehydration.

5. b The chronic sickling of cells in the medulla of the kidney results in a limited ability to concentrate urine and mild polydipsia.

CHAPTER 61

Rash—Eczematous

KAREN DALE GRUSKIN, M.D.

QUESTIONS

1. A 2-week-old infant is brought to the ED with a rash of the scalp consisting of greasy yellow scales. Choose the correct statement:

   a. Based on age alone, the diagnosis is most likely to be atopic dermatitis

   b. A similar-appearing rash may be seen in the diaper area

   c. Before prescribing medical treatment for the rash, scrapings for fungal culture should be obtained

   d. Therapy of choice is a tar-based shampoo daily for 1 week

   e. Therapy of choice is a 7-day course of oral antibiotics

2. A mother brings her 1-year-old boy with a history of chronic otitis media to have his ear examined and for evaluation of a diaper rash. The mother states that the child almost always has an ear infection and a diaper rash. He has been on multiple courses of oral antibiotics for the otitis and topical preparations for the diaper rash. Most recently, her primary care physician prescribed an oral antifungal agent with no response. On physical exam the patient has a draining otitis media and some small areas of erythematous rash, mostly in the creases of the leg folds. You note a few satellite lesions. The most appropriate next step in management would be:

   a. Continuing the clotrimazole for another week

   b. A routine culture

   c. A punch skin biopsy

   d. A CBC

   e. A stronger topical steroid cream

3. A mother brings in her 8-year-old son because of an exquisitely tender erythematous rash. The boy has a history of a seizure disorder but has otherwise been well. The rash covers almost all surfaces of his body; a few blisters are noted as well as some areas of exfoliation. Vital signs are: T 38.2°C, HR 110, RR 20, and BP 103/72. The child's exam is otherwise unremarkable. Which of the following statements is true?

   a. An underlying immunodeficiency is rarely associated with this disorder

   b. The patient's phenytoin should be empirically continued

   c. This illness rarely leads to significant morbidity or mortality

   d. Secondary infections are common and may lead to scarring

   e. This child should be managed as an outpatient

4. A 10-year-old boy is brought to the ED with dry, erythematous patches on his cheeks, arms, and legs, of 2 weeks' duration. He is an afebrile, well-appearing, happy child. His mother is most concerned about the child's constant scratching of the rash. Which of the following statements is true?

   a. This disorder is not associated with a genetic predisposition

   b. Topical antifungal medication is appropriate therapy

   c. This child probably presented for the first time with similar symptoms at some point within the last year

   d. If pruritus is severe, initial therapy should include an oral steroid

   e. Low-dose topical steroids is appropriate therapy

5. A 6-year-old child with severe atopic dermatitis has large areas that appear vesiculopustular. His mother states that these lesions began to appear approximately 24 hours ago and have increased in size. Approximately 70% of his body is covered with vesicles; T is 39°C. Which of the following statements describes the best initial management of this patient?

   a. Admit the patient for IV antibiotics, pending bacterial blood culture results
   b. Obtain a scraping for bacterial and viral culture, then await further results prior to initiating therapy
   c. Increase the strength of the patient's current topical steroid cream
   d. Begin therapy with acyclovir, pending further studies
   e. Obtain bacterial blood cultures and begin oral antibiotic therapy

6. A blond, fair-skinned adolescent hiker comes to the ED for evaluation of a diffuse erythematous rash over his face and neck. The rash developed during the last 4 hours while he was hiking in the mountains on a hot sunny day. He insists that he applied a SPF 15 sunscreen 30 minutes before beginning his hike. You recommend:

   a. Cold compresses for a first-degree sunburn
   b. Ibuprofen for pain of a second-degree sunburn
   c. Change to a different sunscreen
   d. That the same sunscreen be reapplied every 2 hours while outdoors
   e. A topical 1% steroid cream

7. A 4-year-old girl is brought to the ED by her father, 2 days after they have returned from their first camping trip, for evaluation of a rash covering her face and inner right wrist. Linear streaks are noted. Her eyes are almost swollen shut. Choose the true statement:

   a. This is a hypersensitivity reaction
   b. The rash cannot be due to poison ivy because it took 2 days to evolve
   c. There is no effective therapy
   d. Areas of linear vesicular eruption are not associated with this disorder
   e. This disorder is contagious

8. The 4-year-old from Question 7 returns to the ED 2 days after finishing a 5-day course of oral steroids. Her father informs you that the rash improved and almost disappeared but has now returned. You counsel the father that his daughter needs:

   a. A 2-week course of topical steroids
   b. 5 more days of oral steroids at the same strength
   c. 5 more days of topical steroids
   d. No further treatment
   e. A 2-week course of tapering oral steroids

9. An 11-year-old girl is brought to you for evaluation of an area of alopecia on her scalp. You note a 4 × 4 cm area with broken hairs. The best initial recommendation would be:

   a. A 3-week course of topical antifungal cream if the area fluoresces under Wood's light examination
   b. A 3-week course of oral griseofluvin if the area fluoresces under Wood's light examination
   c. A 4–8-week course of oral griseofulvin
   d. A 4–8-week course of topical antifungal cream
   e. Referral to a dermatologist

10. A mother brings her 3-year-old son for evaluation of a diffuse pruritic papular rash. On physical exam, you note lesions on his palms, wrists, flexures of his elbows, and belt-line. You recommend permethrin 5% cream for all members of the family, to be applied from the neck down, as well as washing of bedding, stuffed animals, towels, and clothes. The patient returns to the ED 1 week later complaining of continued pruritus in spite of visible improvement of lesions. You recommend:

   a. Diphenlyhramine every 6–8 hours as needed
   b. 1 application of gamma benzene hexachloride (lindane)
   c. A repeat application of permethrin 5% cream
   d. A potent topical steroid cream b.i.d. (twice a day)
   e. A skin biopsy

ANSWERS

1. b   Seborrhic dermatitis of the scalp, also known as cradle cap, is a very commonly seen rash in newborns. It is characterized by nonpruritic, erythematous, greasy, yellow to salmon-colored plaques in areas of the body that have high concentrations of sebaceous glands. The rash is commonly first seen during the first 2–12 weeks of age, on the scalp and/or diaper area, disappearing around the first birthday. Approximately 10% of infants with seborrhic dermatitis will have a recurrence after the onset of puberty. The diagnosis is usually made clinically. Therapy is frequent shampooing with an antiseborrheic shampoo containing sulfur and salicylic acid and gentle scrubbing of the scales. Atopic dermatitis usually has a slightly older age of onset and less commonly affects the scalp and diaper areas only.

2. c   This scenario describes a classical presentation of Letterer-Siwe disease or infantile Langerhans' cell histiocytosis. 80% of patients with Letterer-Siwe disease have cutaneous involvement, often as the initial presenting complaint. When seen in the diaper area, the rash often resembles and is mistaken for candidiasis; however, no response is seen to classical candidiasis therapies. Repeated episodes of otitis media or chronic draining ears, unresponsive to usual symptomatic treatment and antibiotics, are another common manifestation of Letterer-Siwe disease. The diagnostic test of choice is a punch skin biopsy, because the presence of cells of the monocyte lineage containing the characteristic electron microscopic findings of Langerhans' cells is pathognomonic for the disease.

3. d   This patient is presenting with an exfoliative dermatitis/erythroderma or toxic epidermal necrolysis (TEN), which is a generalized inflammatory condition of the skin. The term is commonly applied to any generalized exfoliative process independent of etiology; when severe, the necrolysis may be potentially life threatening in the acute phase. Common etiologies include: drug reactions, viral infections, bacterial antigen exposure, severe combined immunodeficiency (SCID), HIV, and graft-versus-host disease. The skin is typically erythematous and exquisitely sensitive to touch. Blisters may be present and large areas can be denuded with gentle rubbing (positive Nikolsky's sign). Morbidity and mortality can be as high as 25–75% and is caused by temperature instability, fluid losses, high-output heart failure, and sepsis. Therapy is primarily supportive, with early treatment of bacterial superinfection. Secondary infections are common and may lead to permanent scarring.

4. e   Persons affected with atopic dermatitis usually have a positive family history for atopic dermatitis and/or allergic rhinitis, hay fever, or asthma. Of patients with atopic dermatitis, 90% develop symptoms by 5 years of age, with 50–75% showing symptoms before 6 months of age. Initial therapy should consist of emollients and topical steroids. Oral steroids are almost never indicated.

5. d   Children with severe atopic dermatitis are at risk for developing eczema herpeticum, a diffuse cutaneous herpetic infection. Culture, Tzanck test, or one of the newer monoclonal antibody tests can verify the diagnosis. Acyclovir has been shown to decrease severity as well as hasten improvement. The decision to treat orally versus intravenously is based on clinical severity, with medication started as soon as possible. Children with atopic dermatitis are also at risk for bacterial superinfection; however, they usually do not present with diffuse vesiculopustular lesions; the typical presentation is an impetiginous rash with areas of crusting.

6. c   Although a sunburn is not a bad guess for the diagnosis of this rash, the proper diagnosis is a photosensitivity reaction to a sunscreen containing para-aminobenzoic acid (PABA). Photosensitivity reactions usually begin upon exposure to the sun, with the rash developing over 2–6 hours. Sunburns usually begin later and evolve more slowly than photosensitivity reactions. PABA is a common offending agent and PABA sunscreens are now commercially available over the counter. Management includes removal and then avoidance of offending agent and minimizing exposure to natural light until the rash is resolved.

7. a   The poison ivy plant is one of the most common causes of *Rhus* dermatitis. The rash is due to a delayed hypersensitivity reaction to an oleoresin found in the leaves, roots, or twigs of the plant. Prior sensitization is necessary for rash development, but the plant is ubiquituous (even found on vacant city lots), so contact can easily occur in nonwooded areas and go undetected. *Rhus* dermatitis can also develop after exposure to resin-carrying clothing. The rash usually develops over 1–3 days, although it can be seen within the first 8 hours of contact in highly sensitized individuals. Areas of linear vesicular eruption are a clue to diagnosis but not one of exclusion. Facial involvement characteristically lacks the linearity of the rash often found elsewhere. Steroids are an effective therapy.

8. e   Topical steroid therapy is somewhat useful for mild cases of *Rhus* dermatitis; however, for more serious cases and those involving the face, oral steroids are the best choice. When prescribing oral steroids for *Rhus* dermatitis, doses in the range of 0.5–1 mg/kg/day with a 2-week tapering course should be used. If oral steroids are stopped abruptly, recrudescence of the rash may occur.

9. c   This patient has a typical lesion of tinea capitis. Some patients will have a large, boggy area called a kerion, which represents an exaggerated host response to a fungal infection. Although some forms of tinea will fluoresce when exposed to ultraviolet light from a Wood's lamp, not all do. *Trichophyton tonsurans* does not fluoresce and is currently a common etiological agent for tinea capitis. Topical antifun-

gal agents do not generally reach the hair bulb and are therefore ineffective in the therapy of tinea capitis. Griseofluvin is the oral agent of choice and often needs to be continued for more than 4 weeks. Ideally, griseofluvin should be continued for 2 weeks after fungal cultures are negative. Many adverse side affects, including granulocytopenia, have been reported with griseofulvin. It is recommended to follow CBCs routinely on patients prescribed griseofluvin.

10. a   The pruritus associated with a scabies infection often will persist after the parasite has been eliminated. This is thought to be due to an autosensitization. An antihistamine for symptomatic relief is the best first option for a child who after 1 week has improvement/resolution of lesions but persistent itching.

CHAPTER 62

Rash—Maculopapular

KAREN DALE GRUSKIN, M.D.

QUESTIONS

1. A 6-year-old girl, whose family recently immigrated to Texas from Mexico, is brought to the ED for evaluation of a diffuse maculopapular rash. The child is febrile to 40.3°C and ill appearing. Choose the LEAST likely diagnosis:

   a. Rubella
   b. Rubeola
   c. Rocky Mountain spotted fever
   d. Kawasaki syndrome
   e. Erythema multiforme (EM)

2. A 9-year-old boy is brought to the ED for evaluation of a maculopapular rash. The rash consists of diffuse macules with central clearing. There are some areas of confluence and some areas of raised lesions. The child also has mouth sores. Choose the LEAST likely cause of this reaction:

   a. Trimethoprim/sulfasoxazole
   b. Herpes simplex
   c. *Streptococcus pneumoniae*
   d. Phenytoin
   e. *Mycoplasma pneumoniae*

3. A 4-year-old girl is brought to the ED for evaluation. She has been febrile for 2 weeks and has erythematous lips. The parents state that she had conjunctivitis, treated with eye ointment for 5 days, and an associated fine papular rash that is now gone. On physical exam she is ill appearing, irritable, has an injected oropharynx, and a large left cervical node. Appropriate management includes:

   a. IV immunoglobulin and low-dose aspirin
   b. Low-dose aspirin alone
   c. High-dose steroids and high-dose aspirin
   d. IV immunoglobulin and high-dose aspirin
   e. High-dose steroids and low-dose aspirin

4. A 3-year-old boy is brought to the ED for evaluation of fever and rash. The child was well until 3 days ago, when he developed fever, cough, and scleral injection. The rash began last night on the face and seems to be spreading down to the trunk. The rash is made up of reddish macules. The child is febrile to 39.2°C and has conjunctivitis and rhinorrhea. Which of the following can most simply diagnose this disorder?

   a. Tzanck smear
   b. Oropharygeal findings
   c. Involvement of the palms and soles
   d. Response to immunoglobulin therapy
   e. Skin biopsy

5. A 17-year-old college freshman is brought to the ED after returning from spring break with a rash. He states he has had 3–4 days of fever, headache, and myalgias. The rash started yesterday and is now on his wrists and ankles. The patient is ill appearing, with the following vital signs: T 39.4°C, RR 24, HR 140, and BP 130/77. The rash consists of erythematous macules with scattered petechiae. Proper management includes:

   a. Penicillin
   b. Ceftriaxone
   c. Acyclovir
   d. Doxycycline
   e. Immunoglobulin

6. A mother brings in her 8-year-old daughter for evaluation of pruritic vesicles on her fingers. On exam the child has lesions on her tonsillar pillars and small vesicles on the lateral margins of her fingers. T is 38.1°C. The most likely etiology of the rash is:

   a. Parvovirus B19
   b. Epstein-Barr virus
   c. Human herpes virus 6 (HHV-6)
   d. Rubella virus
   e. Coxsackie A16

7. A pregnant mother brings her daughter in to the ED for evaluation of a rash. The child has erythematous cheeks and a lacey, maculopapular rash over her arms and trunk. She is otherwise well appearing. You counsel the mother to:

   a. Avoid touching the child
   b. Treat the rash with oatmeal baths
   c. See her obstetrician
   d. Keep her daughter home from daycare until the rash resolves
   e. Give diphenylhydramine for itching

8. A 5-year-old boy is brought to you with a diffuse, sand-papery rash. On physical exam he is febrile, has tender anterior cervical lymph nodes, and has an erythematous injected oropharynx with exudate. The best management option is:

   a. 10-day course of trimethoprim-sulfamethoxazole
   b. IM procaine penicillin
   c. IM benzathine penicillin
   d. 10-day course of tetracycline
   e. 5-day course of amoxicillin

9. You are asked to see an 11-year-old boy with multiple small, discrete oval macules scattered over the trunk. The lesions appear to be flaking. The child is afebrile and otherwise well appearing. The lesions have been present for 2–3 weeks and he has not had a similar rash in the past. Uninvolved skin is normal in appearance. The most likely diagnosis is:

   a. Guttate psoriasis
   b. Pityriasis rosea
   c. Eczema
   d. Contact dermatitis
   e. Papular acrodermatitis

10. A 13-year-old girl comes to you for evaluation of diffuse, hypopigmented macules scattered over her upper back. The macules first appeared after she had spent the day in the sun. She is afebrile and otherwise well. Appropriate management would be:

    a. Topical steroid cream
    b. Oral steroids
    c. Selenium sulfide shampoo
    d. Permethrin 5% topical cream
    e. Tar shampoo

ANSWERS

1. a   All of the disorders listed are associated with maculopapular rashes, although rubella (German measles) is usually a mild disease that is not associated with a fever. The other disorders listed can all cause potentially life-threatening illnesses.

2. c   Erythema multiforme (EM) in children most commonly results from an immune-mediated acute hypersensitivity reaction following exposure to a sensitizing antigen that is a drug, food, or infectious organism. Trimethoprim/sulfasoxazole and phenytoin are among the most common drug causes. Nuts, berries, and shellfish are the most common food offenders. Herpes simplex and *M. pneumoniae* are the most common infectious offenders. *S. pneumoniae* is not a common cause of EM.

3. d   The patient in this scenario is exhibiting four of the five features of Kawasaki disease. Kawasaki disease is a clinical diagnosis based on an unremitting fever of at least 5 days duration and four of the five following features: 1) rash; 2) nonexudative bulbar conjunctivitis with limbal sparing; 3) red cracked lips, strawberry tongue, and erythematous oropharynx; 4) erythema, swelling, and/or induration of peripheral extremities; and 5) a solitary unilateral enlarged (greater than 1.5 cm diameter) cervical lymph node. Children are commonly irritable and/or ill appearing. Initial therapy of choice is intravenous immunoglobulin and high-dose aspirin (80–100 mg/kg/day). The aspirin dose is usually decreased after the fever has subsided. Therapy is most beneficial when started within 10 days of onset of illness, but should not be withheld for patients presenting after this time.

4. b   This patient is exhibiting features of measles (rubeola). The rash usually follows 2–3 days after a prodrome of fever, coryza, and conjunctivitis. The rash typically begins as reddish maculopapules on the scalp and face and spreads downwards, becoming confluent cephalically as it spreads. Koplik's spots are pathognomonic for the disease and can be seen from 12–24 hours before the onset of the exanthem until the full-blown exanthem erupts. Most typically, these spots appear on the buccal mucosa opposite the molars, as pinpoint white lesions on an erythematous base. Measles virus can be cultured, but is technically difficult and slow. Measles can also be diagnosed by comparing acute and convalescent serum samples for measles antibodies. Therapy is primarily supportive, although vitamin A is now recommended in some instances.

5. d   The patient has Rocky Mountain spotted fever (RMSF). It is not uncommon for a victim to be unaware of a tick bite; hence, one must have a high index of suspicion for this disorder in any patient presenting with a hemorrhagic rash beginning on the wrists and/or ankles. Laboratory tests can show a normal WBC but low sodium (Na) and platelets. Therapy with doxycycline or chloramphenicol is highly effective and is usually curative when given early in the course of disease. RMSF is associated with a fatality rate of 5% with antimicrobial treatment and 13–40% without such therapy.

6. e   The classic exanthem of Coxsackie A16 infection, also appropriately called hand-foot-mouth disease, is common and easily recognized. Small crescent- or football-shaped vesicles can be found in the oropharynx and on the skin. Skin lesions are most commonly located on the dorsal and lateral aspects of fingers, hands, and feet but may develop elsewhere. Skin lesions may be pruritic or mildly tender.

7. c   This child is exhibiting the classic "slapped-cheek" appearance of erythema infectiosum (fifth disease). Of little medical significance in an otherwise healthy child, erythema infectiosum can cause aplastic crises in patients with sickle cell anemia as well as fetal anemia, congestive heart failure and hydrops. Pregnant women exposed to parvovirus B19 should be referred to their obstetricians to discuss risks to the fetus. The rash is typically asymptomatic and would not require therapy for pruritis. The disease is spread by respiratory droplets and not by direct contact with the rash. Patients are usually not contagious by the time the rash appears.

8. c   Scarlet fever is caused by phage–infected group A *Streptococcus*. Appropriate therapy consists of a minimum of 10 days of appropriate antibiotic or IM benzathine penicillin. Appropriate antibiotics include penicillin, amoxicillin, ampicillin, erythromycin, and first-generation cephalosporins. Tetracyclines and sulfonamides should not be used. Single-dose ceftriaxone does not provide an adequate duration of therapy.

9. a   About one-third of cases of psoriasis begin during childhood. The guttate form is characterized by multiple small, discrete round to oval macules with a loosely adherent scale. Lesions are most common on the trunk.

10. c   Tinea versicolor gets its name from variable coloration of affected skin. In the summer months lesions appear hypopigmented compared to unaffected skin because the causative agent, *Pityrosporum oribulare*, blocks the normal tanning of sun-exposed skin. In the winter affected areas are relatively darker than unaffected skin because of a mild erythematous reaction. Treatment consists of selenium sulfide shampoos weekly for 3 weeks and then monthly for 3 months. Another therapeutic option is a course of a topical or oral antifungal agent.

CHAPTER 63

Papular Lesions

KAREN DALE GRUSKIN, M.D.

QUESTIONS

1. A 6-year-old child comes to the ED for the evaluation of a group of "bumps" on the left cheek. The child's mother had first noticed them a few months ago and was not particularly concerned about the bumps until a friend told her that they should be removed immediately. On physical exam there are 3 1–2 mm firm white papules with central white cores that fill the entire papule. Initial management includes:

   a. Nightly adhesive taping for 1 month
   b. Piercing, with gentle expression of pus from lesions
   c. Surgical removal
   d. No therapy
   e. Topical antifungal cream

2. A 3-year-old girl is brought to the ED for the evaluation of a small red lesion on her left shoulder, which her mother first noticed a few weeks ago. The nonblanching lesion has been bleeding frequently due to the rubbing of the child's bathing-suit strap. Which of the following is the most likely diagnosis?

   a. Strawberry hemangioma
   b. Pyogenic granuloma
   c. Spitz nevus
   d. Juvenile xanthogranuloma
   e. Mastocyoma

3. A 2-year-old child comes to the ED with a flesh-colored papule 1.5 cm in diameter, with a surrounding rim of erythema. You suspect the diagnosis is a mastocytoma. To confirm your suspicions you should:

   a. Scratch the papular lesion gently with a tongue blade to determine if urtication occurs (Darier's sign)
   b. Search for evidence of autoinoculation in scratch lines (pseudo-Koebner's phenomenon)
   c. Search for additional lesions in a linear pattern (Koebner's phenomenon)
   d. Obtain a CBC with differential, looking for an elevated eosinophilic count
   e. Obtain a family history

4. You are evaluating a 12-year-old boy with small, flat-topped papules, linearly arranged on the long axis of his arm. The boy is unaware of how long they have been present and denies any pruritis. These lesions are most likely due to:

   a. Papilloma virus
   b. Autoimmune reaction
   c. Unknown etiology
   d. Histamine release
   e. Herpes virus

5. A 6-year-old girl comes to the ED with a 0.25 cm flesh-colored solitary papule on her face. She has no other skin lesions and the rest of her exam is unremarkable. Based on the color of the lesion, which of the following is the least likely diagnosis?

   a. Spitz nevus
   b. Pyogenic granuloma
   c. Flat wart
   d. Mastocytoma
   e. Juvenile xanthomas

6. An 8-year-old boy is brought to the ER by his father, who noted an erythematous round lesion 3 cm in diameter, with no scale and central clearing on his left shin. His primary care physician prescribed a 3-week course of lotrimin, with no improvement of the lesion. Which of the following statements is correct?

   a. The etiology is an idiosyncratic response to infection
   b. The advancing border of the lesion would not be firm on palpation
   c. A potassium hydroxide test would be negative
   d. A second course of clotrimazole would be beneficial
   e. An oral course of griseofluvin would be the next therapy of choice

ANSWERS

1. d   The clue to the diagnosis of these lesions are the central white cores that fill the entire surface of the papules. Milia are mostly commonly seen in the newborn period due to the retention of keratinous and sebaceous material in follicular openings; however, they may occur in an older patient, especially after dermal trauma. Widespread milia beyond the newborn period are associated with hereditary trichodysplasia or the oral-facial-digital syndrome type I. Unless associated with a syndrome, milia will usually resolve spontaneously.

2. b   All the lesions listed in the answer to this question may appear as a red lesion; however, a pyogenic granuloma is most consistent with the presenting symptomatology. Hemangiomas may bleed with minor trauma as they involute; however, they usually are first noticed within the first few months of life and grow in size during the first 2 years. A spitz nevus has a red, smooth, dome-shaped surface that usually does not bleed. A juvenile xanthogranuloma may appear suddenly and appear red in color but usually will not bleed. Additionally, when blanched, a juvenile xanthogranuloma will usually appear yellow. Pyogenic granulomas are classically small red lesions with a crusted granular surface that often bleed after minor trauma.

3. a   The hallmark of a positive Darier's sign is usually enough to clinch the diagnosis of a solitary mastocytoma. Mastocytomas are lesions of unclear etiology made up of mast cells. A positive reaction/ Darier's sign is due to histamine-induced erythema, swelling, and urtication, secondary to scratching and subsequent degranulation of these mast cells. Although there are familial reports of mastocytoma, the overwhelming majority of patients have no familial association; therefore, a family history would not be helpful in confirming the diagnosis.

4. c   Lichen striatus is an asymptomatic eruption of unknown etiology that usually resolves spontaneously within a 2-year time period.

5. c   Flat warts are usually flesh colored. Spitz nevus and pyogenic granulomas are red lesions; juvenile xanthomas and mastocytomas can present with a red coloration.

6. c   Granuloma annulare can easily be confused with tinea corporis; however, the distinguishing physical finding is the lack of scale in a granuloma annulare. The lesion may begin as a small papule that clears centrally as the margin advances or as a group of papules arranged in a ringlike configuration. The lesions are most commonly found in areas of frequent minor trauma such as the shins. There is no medical therapy for these lesions and most of them will resolve spontaneously over a 2-year period. A potassium hydroxide test will aid in the diagnosis of a yeast (*Candida*) infection. Treatment for tinea corporis would have been lotrimin; such unnecessary therapy is often prescribed when the improper diagnosis is made. Griseofulvin is the therapy of choice for tinea capitis.

CHAPTER 64

Rash—Papulosquamous Lesions

KAREN DALE GRUSKIN, M.D.

QUESTIONS

1. A sexually active 15-year-old male patient comes to the ED with a diffuse papulosquamous rash over his chest. Lesions are reddish brown, varying in size from a few millimeters to 1 cm in diameter. The lesions are generally discrete and are symmetrically distributed following the lines of cleavage on the back. Which of the following clinical clues is most useful in differentiating the two most likely diagnoses?

   a. Lack of pruritus
   b. Involvement of palms
   c. Mucous membrane lesions
   d. Rash pattern
   e. Sex of the patient

2. A mother describes a single oval lesion on the flank of her 14-year-old son, persisting for 2 weeks. He now has a diffuse, papulosquamous rash consisting of small (1 cm) oval lesions that cover his entire back. Your management would be:

   a. Oral griseofulvin
   b. Topical ketoconazole
   c. No therapy
   d. Oral steroids
   e. Tar shampoo

3. A 13-year-old boy is brought in for evaluation of follicular papules on the backs of his fingers, sides of his neck, and extensor surfaces of his elbows and knees. He also has fine scaling of his scalp and areas of his trunk have salmon-colored plaques. His palms and soles are thickened. You correctly make the diagnosis of:

   a. Pityriasis alba
   b. Pityriasis rosea
   c. Pityriasis versicolor
   d. Pityriasis rubra pilaris
   e. Guttate psoriasis

4. All of the following statements regarding psoriasis are true EXCEPT:

   a. No therapy is beneficial
   b. The rash most commonly involves the scalp, perineum, and extensor surfaces of the body
   c. When a scale is removed, pinpoint bleeding may occur
   d. Small, pitted nails may be associated with the disease
   e. The severity of the rash waxes and wanes

5. A family brings you their recently adopted 10-month-old daughter. She is very thin and has a rash and chronic diarrhea. All stool cultures have been negative, as have multiple searches for ova and parasites. The rash is most prominent around her mouth and on her fingers and toes. The rash resembles psoriasis, with both eroded and crusted areas. The parents are at their wit's end and are requesting a second opinion. You recommend:

   a. An empiric trial of antibiotics
   b. A lab test
   c. A fungal culture
   d. An empiric trial of topical steroids
   e. Skin biopsy

ANSWERS

1. c   Pityriasis rosea and secondary syphilis are often confused and one must carefully consider the diagnosis of syphilis in any sexually active adolescent presenting with a diffuse papulosquamous rash. Both entities tend to be nonpruritic and affect both sexes. Pityriasis occasionally, but not commonly, involves the palms. Only secondary syphilis routinely has mucous membrane lesions as a disease manifestation. These lesions can be found on almost any mucosal surface and consist of painless, slightly raised, grayish/white plaques with areas of central erosions.

2. c   A herald patch is seen in approximately 80% of children with pityriasis rosea. Another clue to the diagnosis is a distribution of the lesions along the dermatomes in the shape of a "Christmas tree," although this finding is not always present. The disorder is a benign, self-limiting condition thought to be of viral etiology. The initial herald patch may be confused with tinea corporis and the diffuse stage may be confused with secondary syphilis, drug eruption, Mucha-Habermann disease, seborrheic dermatitis, nummular eczema, and psoriasis. No therapy is necessary. If itching is present, it may be treated with oral antihistamines or some topical 0.5% steroid cream.

3. d   The scenario describes many of the features of childhood onset of pityriasis rubra pilaris. The exact etiology of this disease is unknown, but is felt to be due to a disorder of keratinization. The onset of the disease may be gradual, beginning in the scalp and spreading to involve the face and fingers. Acuminate follicular papules with keratotic plugs occur on the dorsum of the fingers, side of the neck, and extensors of the extremities. The skin is generally salmon-colored and scaling (giving a "plucked-chicken" appearance). The condition responds to vitamin A and its derivatives.

4. a   Psoriasis is a chronic papulosquamous disease that makes up 4% of all skin disorders encountered in children. There is a predisposition for involvement of scalp, perineum, and extensor surfaces of the body, particularly the elbows and knees. The rash of psoriasis commonly has a silvery scale, which causes pinpoint areas of bleeding when removed (Auspitz sign). Therapy with topical agents, including steroids, tar derivatives, emollients, and ultraviolet light, helps to slow the turnover rate of the epidermis.

5. b   Acrodermatitis enteropathica is caused by a zinc deficiency. The disease is characterized by skin rash, diarrhea, and alopecia. The rash is most prominent on the face and extremities. Plasma zinc levels are usually under 50 μg/dl. The hereditary form usually presents at around 9 months of age.

CHAPTER 65

Rash—Purpura

VINCENT J. WANG, M.D.

QUESTIONS

1. A 5-year-old boy is brought to the ED because of bruising. The child's teacher filed a report because she saw bruising on his lower legs. The mother reports that the child had 1 nosebleed previously, when he was younger. On examination, he is alert and in NAD. He has 4–5 ecchymoses in various stages of healing on his shins and knees. His examination is otherwise normal. Treatment includes:

   a. Obtaining a skeletal survey
   b. Sending a CBC
   c. Sending a PT/PTT
   d. IM Vitamin K
   e. No treatment is necessary

2. A 2-year-old girl is brought to the ED because of fever and a rash. She has had fever for the past 2–3 days and she has been more tired appearing. She lives in California and has no prior medical problems. She has not traveled elsewhere and has no history of tick bites. Her vital signs are: T 39°C, HR 160, RR 24, and BP 70/40. She is lethargic. Her physical examination is notable for numerous petechiae and purpura on her arms and legs. Her distal extremities are cool and mottled. Appropriate treatment over the course of the disease may include:

   a. Corticosteroids IV
   b. Penicillin IV
   c. Doxycycline IV
   d. Acyclovir IV
   e. Supportive therapy only

3. A 4-year-old boy is brought to the ED for a rash. He began having a rash on his lower legs several days ago. It has now spread to his buttocks and lower back. He has not had fever, although he does complain of lower extremity joint pain, and pain when he walks. On examination, he has purpuric lesions on the posterior aspects of his legs and on his buttocks. He has mild swelling of his ankles bilaterally. Which of the following laboratory findings are most likely to be seen with this disease?

   a. PTT 70
   b. PT 18
   c. Platelet count 5000
   d. Urinalysis: 10 RBCs
   e. Rheumatoid factor positive

4. A 3-year-old girl is brought to the ED because of epistaxis. She has never had epistaxis before today. She is otherwise well. Her vital signs are: T 37°C, HR 110, RR 20, and BP 95/60. She has epistaxis from the right nares. She has a dark red, bullous lesion, 0.5 cm in diameter, on her upper gum. She also has purpuric lesions on her legs. Her laboratory tests are: WBC 14,500, hct 35, platelets 5000. You are contemplating corticosteroid therapy. Which of the following tests should be performed?

   a. Hemoglobin electrophoresis
   b. Bone marrow biopsy
   c. Blood culture
   d. CXR
   e. Serum ACTH level

5. A 3-year-old boy complains of joint pain and swelling. The parents report that he fell from the bed, onto his right arm. They say that he seems to bruise more easily, and has occasionally had joint swelling. However, since multiple maternal uncles have had similar problems, they have not been concerned up to this point. On physical examination, he is afebrile and has moderate swelling of his right elbow, but only mild tenderness. The site is not erythematous or warm. His radiographs are normal. Which of the following laboratory findings would be consistent with this disease?

   a. WBCs 18,000
   b. PT 18
   c. Platelet count 5000
   d. PTT 40
   e. Hemoglobin 8

6. A 2-year-old girl had ingested rat poison last week, and now presents with a rash. She was evaluated at an ED immediately after the ingestion, but had a normal PT, PTT, and CBC. She has now developed a purpuric rash over her arms and legs. Her vital signs are: T 37.6°C, HR 120, RR 24, and BP 85/45. She is alert and interactive. Her respiratory, cardiac, and abdominal examinations are normal. She does have multiple areas of purpura over her arms and legs. Treatment at this point should be:

a. Activated charcoal
b. Hemodialysis
c. Vitamin K
d. Platelet transfusion
e. Calcium chloride

ANSWERS

1. e The history and physical examination are consistent with normal activity for an active child. An occasional episode of epistaxis is not usually associated with a significant bleeding dyscrasia, and ecchymoses on the shins are compatible with normal activity for a young child. More frequent epistaxis or frequent bruising at other sites are more concerning, and would warrant a hematological evaluation. Ecchymoses found at sites not likely to be traumatized, i.e. the back, abdomen, or chest, especially if found in various stages of healing, may be concerning for nonaccidental trauma. Treatment with vitamin K is indicated for newborns and patients with this nutritional deficiency.

2. b Meningococcemia is a cause of purpura and fever that must not be overlooked. It may be rapidly fulminant and should be treated promptly. Even though resistance exists, most meningococcal isolates are sensitive to penicillin. A broad-spectrum antibiotic should be given initially, but may be changed to penicillin once sensitivities are back. Corticosteroid therapy has been shown to be helpful for meningitis caused by *Haemofluous influenzae,* but not to *Neisseria meningitidis.* Doxycycline would be the treatment of choice for Rocky Mountain spotted fever; however, this patient is not in an area where the disease is endemic and there is no history of tick bites that would suggest this diagnosis. Varicella may occasionally cause purpura fulminans, but this diagnosis is not consistent with her history and findings.

3. d Henoch-Schönlein purpura (HSP) is a vasculitis that typically manifests with findings as described in this scenario, but may also have upper extremity involvement, gastrointestinal involvement, and renal involvement. The WBC count is usually normal but may be elevated; the coagulation profile is normal; the platelet count is normal; and antinuclear antibody (ANA) and rheumatoid factors are negative. However, with renal involvement, the urinalysis may reveal RBC, WBC, casts and protein.

4. b Idiopathic thrombocytopenic purpura (ITP) may occasionally be indistinguishable from the presentation of acute leukemia or aplastic anemia. A bone marrow biopsy may be performed to assess megakaryocyte production and to confirm the diagnosis. This is especially important if treatment with corticosteroids is being considered, since this treatment will potentially obscure the diagnosis of acute leukemia.

5. d The diagnosis of hemophilia should be considered in any patient who has prolonged bleeding, purpura, or hemarthroses after minor trauma, especially with a significant family history. Hemophilia is associated with a prolonged PTT but a normal PT. In addition, the WBC, platelet count, and hemoglobin levels should be normal.

6. c Toxic ingestion of rat poison, which contains warfarin, may cause purpura. The initial evaluation of the patient who ingests rat poison is unlikely to reveal laboratory abnormalities. However, days later, when the warfarin has taken effect, the patient will have an abnormal PT. The hemoglobin may also be low, secondary to bleeding. Administration of vitamin K is indicated to inhibit this reversible process. If bleeding is significant, fresh frozen plasma (FFP) may be indicated. There is no role for activated charcoal for an ingestion that has occurred days ago. Hemodialysis is not necessary when there is a treatment as effective as vitamin K and FFP. Platelet transfusion and calcium chloride are not indicated.

CHAPTER 66

Rash—Urticaria

KAREN DALE GRUSKIN, M.D.

QUESTIONS

1. A 12-year-old patient comes to the ED for evaluation of a swollen face and rash. The symptoms developed suddenly while the child was sitting in class. The swelling of the face includes the eyes and lips. The rash is pruritic, with waxing and waning areas of white palpable centers with surrounding erythema. The child has been previously well, with no similar symptoms in the past. The child is taking no medications and has no known food allergies. This disorder:

    a. Represents a type II sensitivity reaction
    b. Can be associated with an acute viral illness
    c. Is not associated with a genetic predisposition
    d. Is usually associated with a clear precipitating factor
    e. Is not associated with chronic systemic disease

2. A 7-year-old child who has just been stung by a bee is brought to the ED with facial swelling, wheezing, and shortness of breath. O_2 saturation is 93% on room air. RR is 40, labored with auditory stridor. The best initial management should include all of the following EXCEPT:

    a. Oxygen
    b. Epinephrine
    c. Diphenyhydramine
    d. Methylprednisolone
    e. Intubation

3. A 15-year-old homeless male patient comes to the ED complaining of fevers, arthralgias, and urticarial rash, persisting for 2 weeks. He has been living on the streets and using IV drugs for the past year. He is not ill appearing, with normal vital signs and no fever. He has diffuse urticarial lesions on his trunk and extremities. The test most likely to confirm his diagnosis is:

    a. Bacterial blood culture
    b. Rapid plasma reagin (RPR)
    c. Hepatitis screen
    d. Rheumatoid factor
    e. Serum IgE level

4. A 10-year-old child with chronic urticaria that has not responded to diphenylhydramine or hydroxyzine is referred to you for further management recommendations. She is uncomfortable because of pruritus, but has normal vital signs and an otherwise unremarkable exam. She is allergic to steroids. Choose the best next management option:

    a. Daily long-acting epinephrine injection
    b. Oral cimetidine
    c. Oral danazol
    d. Albuterol nebulization therapy
    e. IV immunoglobulin therapy

ANSWERS

1. b   This patient is exhibiting signs and symptoms of acute urticaria and angioedema due to a type I or type III hypersensitivity reaction. Inciting factors are multiple and include: viral illnesses, especially hepatitis and mononucleosis; bacterial infections; systemic diseases, especially JRA, lymphoma, and SLE; heat or cold contact; minor trauma; and, medications, especially opiates, radiologic contrast dyes, aspirin, NSAIDs, and ACE inhibitors. Genetic factors are important in several relatively rare causes including hereditary angioedema, familial cold, and localized heat urticaria. Idiopathic urticaria/angioedema is the most common form and is a diagnosis of exclusion.

2. e   This patient is exhibiting a Hymenoptera reaction with concerning respiratory symptomatology, as evidenced by the decreased O_2 saturation, stridor, and tachypnea. These symptoms are due to airway

edema and can rapidly worsen if acute interventions are not made. All the listed answers are correct except intubation. It would be most appropriate to administer oxygen, give subcutaneous epinephrine, IV/IM diphenylhydramine, and await effect. Methylprednisolone, although not providing an immediate effect, may be given to suppress the appearance of new urticarial lesions. Intubation is rarely necessary, but is an option if respiratory status worsens and the patient does not respond to initial medical therapy.

3. c   When urticaria is observed in a patient with arthralgia and fever of unknown origin, it should alert the physician to the possibility of hepatitis B virus. This patient is at high risk for hepatitis because of his IV drug abuse and social situation. It may be appropriate to send an RPR empirically in any adolescent in this type of social situation; however, the described symptoms are not typical of syphilis. He is currently afebrile and has had fevers for 2 weeks, making a bacterial sepsis unlikely. Urticaria can be seen in a patient with JRA, but this presentation is more consistent with possible hepatitis. An IgE level would not be helpful in making the diagnosis.

4. b   Cimetidine is an H_2 blocker that may alleviate the pruritus seen in this patient with chronic urticaria. Histamine response is mediated through both H_1 and H_2 receptors. Both diphenylhydramine and hydoxyzine act on H_1 receptors. Danazol is a synthetic steroid and is the drug of choice for patient with severe hereditary angioedema. Epinephrine injections are most useful as initial therapy, but given the drug's short duration of action and painful mode of administration, it has no role in chronic therapy. Albuterol may be useful in a patient with urticaria and wheezing, but this patient has no respiratory symptoms. Immunoglobulin has no role in the treatment of urticaria.

CHAPTER 67

Rash—Vesicobullous

KAREN DALE GRUSKIN, M.D.

QUESTIONS

1. A 4-year-old child is brought to the ED with a vesicobullous rash, which her mother first noted 3 days prior to presentation. The lesions are grouped together in a 2 × 5 cm crescent on the right upper back. The child's grandmother had a similar rash 2 weeks ago. You counsel the mother that:

   a. The child has herpes zoster, she did not contract it from her grandmother, and the rash will most likely heal more slowly than her grandmother's rash
   b. The child has herpes zoster; she did contract it from her grandmother, and the rash will most likely heal faster than her grandmother's rash
   c. The child has varicella; she did not contract it from her grandmother, and the rash will most likely heal faster than her grandmother's rash
   d. The child has varicella; she did contract it from her grandmother, and the rash will most likely heal faster than her grandmother's rash
   e. The child has herpes zoster; she did not contract it from her grandmother, and the rash will most likely heal faster than her grandmother's rash

2. A 10-year-old girl is brought to the ED with vesiculobullous lesions on the tip of her nose and injected sclera. The lesions developed a few days after the child had been complaining that her nose hurt. There are approximately 6 lesions that appear to be in a bandlike distribution. The best initial management would include:

   a. Obtain fluid from the vesicle for immunofluorescent monoclonal antibody testing and give zoster immunoglobulin while awaiting results
   b. Obtain a scraping of the base of the vesicle for immunofluorescent monoclonal antibody testing and, if findings are positive for varicella-zoster virus (VZV), start ophthalmic steroid drops
   c. Obtain a scraping of the base of the vesicle for immunofluorescent monoclonal antibody testing and, if positive for varicella-zoster virus, refer the patient to an ophthalmologist within the next 24 hours

   d. Obtain fluid from the vesicle for immunofluorescent monoclonal antibody testing and, if positive for varicella-zoster virus, refer the patient to an ophthalmologist within the next 24 hours
   e. Obtain fluid from the vesicle for immunofluorescent monoclonal antibody testing, start oral acyclovir, and emergently refer patient to an ophthalmologist

3. A two-year-old girl is brought to the ED on the day after her birthday party, for evaluation of 0.25 cm bullae on the dorsal surface of her second to fourth toes bilaterally. The bullae are mildly tender on palpation and are filled with clear fluid. She has never had similar blisters in the past. Her mother has no idea how they could have developed. Proper management would include placing a bulky dressing and:

   a. A consult with social services
   b. Recommendation that shoes are checked for correct sizing
   c. Further questioning on child's past medical history
   d. Referral to department of social services
   e. Referral to a dermatologist, should symptoms reoccur

4. A 5-year-old girl with leukemia is brought to the ED with a diffuse, vesiculobullous rash with areas of excoriation. Some of the lesions appear to be tear-shaped vesicles on an erythematous base. The child is somewhat ill appearing, with vital signs of T 38.6°C, HR 130, RR 20, and BP 100/76. It is expected that she is neutropenic, based on the timing of her last course of chemotherapy. Which of the following would be the most appropriate next step in management?

   a. Administer IV acyclovir
   b. Administer varicella immunoglobulin and IV antibiotics
   c. Administer IV acyclovir and IV antibiotics
   d. Administer IV acyclovir, varicella immunoglobulin, and IV antibiotics
   e. Administer varicella immunoglobulin and varicella vaccine

5. A mother brings her 10-month-old child to the ED for evaluation of a rash that appears to be spreading. The child is well appearing, with T 38.3°C and scattered pruritic vesicles on the nape of the neck, upper back, and arms. Which of the following statements is true?

   a. The child may return to daycare immediately
   b. The child may return to daycare on the sixth day after the onset of the rash
   c. The child may return to daycare immediately if all lesions are covered
   d. The child may return to daycare 1 day after no new lesions erupt
   e. The child may return to daycare on the third day after the onset of the rash

ANSWERS

1. e   Herpes zoster is caused by the reactivation of a herpes virus that has lain dormant in a dorsal root ganglion of a patient with a history of previous varicella infection. Herpes zoster is not contracted by direct contact with an infected individual. Herpes zoster is more common in older patients but can occur at any age. Younger patients tend to have less serious infections, with quicker resolution of the rash. In the elderly, the rash can take up to 5 weeks to heal, but in children it usually resolves over 1–2 weeks.

2. c   Varicella-zoster (VZV) lesions on the tip of the nose indicate involvement of the nasociliary nerve and possible ocular involvement. When in doubt of the diagnosis, scrapings of the base of a lesion, not fluid, should be obtained for rapid immunofluorescent staining. Herpes lesions can also cause ocular symptoms, but associated vesicles are usually located periorbitally. Ocular involvement stemming from either etiology dictates early but not emergent referral to an ophthalmologist. Acyclovir is not recommended for routine use in patients with herpes zoster but should be considered in patients with ophthalmic disease or underlying disorders that put the patient at risk for disseminated infection.

3. b   Blisters on the bilateral feet of a young child should always raise the possibility of an inflicted burn because of immersion in hot water; however; an inflicted injury would not only involve the dorsum of the toes. The blisters described in this scenario most likely represent friction blisters from new shoes.

4. c   Immunosuppression resulting from chemotherapy for leukemia puts this patient at high risk and warrants IV acyclovir for probable disseminated varicella. Given the patient's ill appearance and probable neutropenia, IV antibiotics should also be initiated after appropriate cultures are obtained. Scraping of the base of the lesions should also be obtained to confirm the diagnosis of varicella-zoster virus (VZV) and not herpes simplex virus (HSV), because the two can be easily confused clinically, although HSV is less likely to present with a diffuse rash. Bacterial superinfection of varicella lesions is common.

5. b   A child with varicella may return to daycare on the sixth day after the onset of the rash or sooner, if all lesions are crusted.

CHAPTER 68

Respiratory Distress

VINCENT J. WANG, M.D.

QUESTIONS

1. A 2-year-old girl is brought to the ED by her parents for difficulty breathing. She has been well until this evening, when she began having cough and fever. She developed difficulty breathing within the past hour. On examination, her vital signs are: T 39.5°C, HR 140, RR 28, and BP 100/60. She sits leaning forward, and refuses to drink from her "sippy" cup. She is somewhat lethargic in appearance, with subcostal and suprasternal retractions as well as audible stridor. Immediate treatment includes:

   a. CBC and blood culture, then ceftriaxone
   b. Nebulized racemic epinephrine
   c. Nebulized albuterol
   d. Endotracheal intubation
   e. Subcutaneous (SC) epinephrine

2. A 3-year-old boy complains of difficulty breathing. He has had cough and rhinorrhea for 2–3 days, accompanied by fevers of 38–39°C. Today, he developed a barky cough and began breathing more rapidly. On examination, his vital signs are: T 38.5°C, HR 120, RR 28, and BP 105/60. He is stridulous at rest, in moderate respiratory distress. He has no rales or wheezing on auscultation of his chest. Immediate treatment includes:

   a. Nebulized levalbuterol
   b. Nebulized racemic epinephrine
   c. SC epinephrine
   d. Endotracheal intubation
   e. Nebulized albuterol

3. A 16-year-old girl is brought to the ED after being involved in a high-speed motor vehicular accident. On examination, her vital signs are: T 37°C, HR 150, RR 40, and BP 90/50. She has jugular venous distension, her trachea is shifted leftward, and the right side of her chest has decreased breath sounds. Immediate treatment includes:

   a. Needle thoracostomy
   b. Needle cricothyrotomy
   c. Rapid-sequence intubation
   d. Securing vascular access
   e. Obtaining a CXR

4. A 1-week-old boy is brought to the ED for difficulty breathing. He was born without complications. He has been breathing rapidly since birth, and seems "uncomfortable" according to the parents. These symptoms seem worse with feeding. Shortly after crying, he seems to be better, but he begins to breathe rapidly again afterwards. Diagnosis may be made by:

   a. Obtaining a CXR
   b. Obtaining a lateral neck radiograph
   c. Pulse oximetry
   d. Passing a nasogastric tube through the nares
   e. Airway fluoroscopy

5. A 6-month-old girl has difficulty breathing. She has been well until 1 week ago, when her eyes seemed to be more "droopy," according to the parents. Also, she has less stools than normal. The parents believe in natural foods, and have added natural sweeteners to her diet. On examination, she is alert, but has a bilateral ptosis. Her vital signs are: T 37.5°C, HR 120, RR 20, and BP 90/50. Her breath sounds are clear and symmetric, but her respiratory efforts seem diminished. Her O$_2$ saturation (measured by pulse oximeter reading) is 100%. You should:

   a. Obtain blood, urine, and CSF cultures and discharge to home with follow-up tomorrow
   b. Obtain blood, urine, and CSF cultures, give ceftriaxone, and discharge to home with follow-up tomorrow
   c. Obtain blood, urine, and CSF cultures and admit for IV antibiotics
   d. Admit for observation
   e. Discharge to home with follow-up tomorrow

6. A 3-year-old boy is brought to the ED because of fast breathing. His aunt had given him oil of wintergreen this afternoon, but the parents say that he had never choked or gagged. On examination, he is alert and rambunctious. His vital signs are: T 37°C, HR 110, RR 44, and BP 90/50. O$_2$ saturation is 95%. His lungs are clear and symmetric. His heart is normal and his abdomen is soft. Treatment includes:

   a. IV administration of midazolam
   b. IV administration of sodium bicarbonate (NaHCO$_3$)
   c. Nebulized albuterol treatments
   d. Obtaining a CXR
   e. Obtaining inspiratory and expiratory CXRs

7. A 2-month-old girl is brought to the ED because of difficulty breathing. She has had cough and rhinorrhea for the past 2 days. She has no other medical problems. Which of the following signs suggest respiratory muscle fatigue?

   a. Respiratory rate (RR) of 30
   b. RR of 50
   c. Intercostal retractions
   d. Thoracoabdominal dissociation
   e. Nasal flaring

ANSWERS

1. d Epiglottitis is rare now that immunization against *Haemophilus influenzae* type B is common. However, epiglottitis may still occur, especially among recent immigrants or those who have not received their vaccinations. Immediate treatment includes securing the airway. Attempts at performing blood tests or administering antibiotics should be deferred until the airway can be protected. The other treatments may be used for croup, asthma, or allergic reactions, respectively.

2. b Croup is a viral laryngotracheobronchitis and is the most common cause of upper airway obstruction in children between 3 months and 3 years of age. Treatment for mild cases of croup is supportive. Patients with more significant symptoms (i.e. stridor while agitated but not at rest) may benefit from dexamethasone PO/IM. Patients who have significant respiratory distress (i.e. stridor at rest) should receive racemic epinephrine and should be observed. Epinephrine SC is indicated for allergic reactions. Intubation should be considered if the croup progresses to respiratory failure, which is not the case here. Nebulized albuterol or levalbuterol should be used for asthmatic exacerbations.

3. a Tension pneumothorax is a life-threatening emergency, requiring needle thoracostomy followed by chest-tube placement. Needle cricothyrotomy is indicated in patients with upper airway obstruction that are not able to be intubated. Rapid-sequence intubation is indicated for respiratory failure, and may be indicated in this patient, but not initially. Securing vascular access is not an immediate priority.

Obtaining a CXR would confirm the diagnosis, but treatment is the priority in this case, and should not be delayed for a radiograph.

4. d   Choanal atresia may be partial or complete. Infants are obligate nose breathers and therefore will have difficulty breathing with this condition. Infants may have difficulty feeding, and often find relief when crying, because they breathe through their mouths when they cry. The diagnosis may be made by passing a nasogastric feeding tube through each nares.

5. d   Infant botulism may cause respiratory difficulty and may initially be mistaken for sepsis. Botulism spores may be found in unpasteurized products, such as honey or canned products. Initially, patients may have a descending paralysis, eventually involving the respiratory muscles. Patients should be admitted for observation. If early in the course, botulism antitoxin may be given. Many patients will require mechanical ventilatory support.

6. b   Oil of wintergreen has a large amount of aspirin as one of its active ingredients. This patient likely has a metabolic acidosis and is compensating with rapid respirations, producing a respiratory alkalosis. Treatment for aspirin toxicity involves administration of sodium bicarbonate and supportive care.

7. d   Thoracoabdominal dissociation occurs when the abdomen protrudes and the chest collapses during inspiration. This is a common sign of respiratory muscle fatigue and is also known as respiratory alternans, or paradoxical breathing. A RR of 30 is normal for a 2-month-old infant. A RR of 50, nasal flaring, or use of intercostal muscles for respiration suggest mild respiratory distress, but not necessarily fatigue.

CHAPTER 69

The Septic-Appearing Infant

ROBERT L. CLOUTIER, M.D.

QUESTIONS

1. A 3-month-old boy is brought to the ED appearing lethargic. The infant has had 5–10 episodes of diarrhea per day and poor feeding for the last 3 days. There has been no fever. The infant has an unremarkable perinatal and past medical history. Vital signs are: T 37.8°C, HR 165, RR 40, and BP 90/45. Which of the following statements regarding this patient's condition is true?

   a. An afebrile patient is rarely septic
   b. Fever is a good indicator of sepsis
   c. Septic infants in this age group are hypothermic
   d. Fever is an inaccurate indicator of sepsis
   e. Lethargy is the most accurate indicator of sepsis

2. A 2-week-old infant is brought to the ED for lethargy. While in the ED, the patient has a seizure and becomes apneic. Endotracheal intubation is performed and IV access established. IV ampicillin and gentamicin are administered. The electrolytes are as follows: Na 130 mEq/l, K 3.9 mEq/l, Cl 96 mEq/l, and CO_2 14 mEq/l. A lumbar puncture is attempted but appears traumatic, with the following results: RBCs 40,000 per hpf, WBCs 85 per hpf. The seizure stops after an appropriate dose of midazolam. Which of the following should be administered?

   a. 3% NaCl
   b. Hydrocortisone
   c. Acyclovir
   d. Sodium bicarbonate ($NaHCO_3$)
   e. Vancomycin

3. An 8-week-old boy is brought to the ED with a history of 1 week of violent coughing. The parents have noticed the coughing is worse at night. Their concern was raised tonight, when the boy stopped breathing for approximately 12–15 seconds after one of the coughing spells. During this time he was noted to have perioral cyanosis. The infant is up to date on immunizations. Physical examination is unremarkable, and pulse oximetry shows an O_2 saturation of 98% on room air. The CXR is negative and the CBC is as follows: WBCs 14,100 (differential 67%, neutrophils 23%), hemoglobin 11.5 mg/dl, and platelets 231,000. What would be the next step?

   a. 12-lead ECG
   b. Sepsis evaluation
   c. Admit and start erythromycin
   d. Admit and start IV ampicillin
   e. Home apnea monitor

4. A 3-week-old infant is brought to the ED with extreme irritability. On physical examination you note a diffuse maculopapular rash, hepatosplenomegaly, and an extremely tender left lower extremity. The accompanying x-ray shows periosteal elevation of the left tibia. The most likely diagnosis for this infant is:

   a. Congenital syphilis
   b. Congenital rubella
   c. Toxoplasmosis
   d. Varicella
   e. Osteomyelitis

5. A 4-day-old girl is brought to the ED appearing lethargic and in respiratory distress. She has been feeding poorly since birth and is often seemingly "out of breath," according to the parents. On physical exam, her breathing appears extremely labored and the extremities cool and mottled. There is a gallop rhythm noted on auscultation. The femoral pulses are very weak but equal. The vital signs are: HR 166, RR 80, and BP 70/32 in the right upper extremity; O_2 saturation is 89% on 100% oxygen. Which of the following is the least likely cause of her symptoms?

   a. Coarctation of the aorta
   b. Transposition of the great vessels
   c. Hypoplastic left heart syndrome
   d. Critical aortic stenosis
   e. Interrupted aortic arch

6. A 5-week-old infant with no significant perinatal medical history is brought to the ED with lethargy and a fever of 39.0°C. The parents state that the fever has been episodic over the last 2 days and that the child has not been feeding as well since then, particularly during episodes of fever. The infant is crying but consolable. RR is 72; BP is 86/52. The HR on the monitor is 240 with an absence of P waves. What is the next step in management?

   a. IV adenosine
   b. Syncronized cardioversion
   c. Carotid massage
   d. IV verapamil
   e. Echocardiogram

7. A 6-day-old girl is brought to the ED by the parents, who report that she has been a lethargic infant. According to the parents, the child has been vomiting all night and was extremely irritable yesterday. The child was born at home and had no prenatal care. The fingerstick glucose level on arrival is 35. The parents state the child has not been a very good eater since birth. Of note on physical exam, the genitalia appear to have an enlarged clitoris with local hair growth. Which of the following lab abnormalities would you expect?

   a. Elevated 17 hydroxy-progesterone
   b. Increased serum sodium
   c. Increased serum aldosterone
   d. Decreased serum potassium
   e. Increased serum cortisol

8. An 18-month-old boy is brought to the ED. He appears lethargic, fatigued, and dehydrated. He has been suffering from diarrhea and vomiting for the last 3–4 days. The mother notes he has often been sick since birth and has never been a very vigorous eater. In addition, she states that the patient had meconium plug syndrome as an infant. Nonetheless, she has never seen him this sick in the past. The vital signs are: T 38.5°C, HR 150, RR 32, and BP 85/34; O_2 saturation is 99% on room air. Other than dry mucous membranes, the physical examination is unremarkable. Electrolyte values are: Na 131 mEq/l, K 2.2 mEq/l, Cl 96 mEq/l, CO_2 17mEq/l, BUN 25 mg/dl, Cr 0.5 mg/dl, and glucose 90 mg/dl. The ammonia level is 75 µg/dl. The most likely diagnosis is:

   a. A urea cycle disorder
   b. Adrenal hyperplasia
   c. Cystic fibrosis
   d. Malabsorption syndrome
   e. Inflammatory bowel disease

ANSWERS

1. d Fever alone is indeed a very inaccurate indicator of sepsis. In combination with other symptoms (e.g., vomiting, diarrhea, lethargy, and anorexia) it may become more important. In the patient less than 2 months of age, hypothermia tends to be more common but not ubiquitous. In summary, remember there is no foolproof indicator of sepsis—the truly septic child is generally represented by a constellation of signs and symptoms which will include those listed above.

2. c Herpes simplex virus (HSV) tends to manifest itself as encephalitis between days 7–21 of life and therefore should be kept in mind. In neonates presenting with fever without historical suspicion of HSV and without physical exam evidence of HSV infection, one could be justified in withholding empiric acyclovir treatment. In the ill-appearing neonate, however, acyclovir should be strongly considered, especially in the setting of lethargy and seizures. A maternal history of HSV and the classic skin, eye, and mucous membrane findings of HSV infection may not be present in cases of herpes encephalitis. Hypertonic saline is used in cases of seizures secondary to significant hyponatremia (usually less than 120–125 mEq/l). Hydrocortisone would be of use in congenital adrenal hyperplasia; affected patients

are usually hyperkalemic. Vancomycin does not need to be added to the antibiotic regimen for this patient, and sodium bicarbonate therapy is not indicated with this degree of acidosis.

3. c   This patient's presentation is consistent with pertussis. Although pertussis is associated with older patients, infants are susceptible to the disease and may suffer very significant sequelae—apnea, seizures, and death have been reported. Lymphocytosis is variable among the infant population, as is the presence of the "shaggy right heart border" on CXR. The characteristic "whoop" of pertussis is very common within the neonatal population. Patients should be admitted for supportive care. Erythromycin started at this stage is not likely to improve the boy's symptoms but will decrease the transmissibility of the disease.

4. a   Congenital syphilis is the most likely diagnosis in this case. It tends to present in the first 4 weeks of life with extreme irritability, pallor, jaundice, hepatosplenomegaly, edema, and painful limbs. A maculopapular rash is also possible, along with radiographic findings that underlie tender bones (periosteitis) and joints.

5. b   This patient has some form of ductal-dependent congenital heart lesion that is now becoming critical as the ductus arteriosus begins to close and prevents shunting of blood from the pulmonary to the systemic side. Ductal-dependent lesions include transposition of the great vessels, coarctation of the aorta, interrupted aortic arch, critical aortic stenosis, and hypoplastic left heart syndrome. Transposition of the great arteries, however, presents with severe hypoxemia that is usually present in the immediate newborn period. In the severe forms of the other diseases listed, patients present in shock sometime in the first few days to weeks of life, when the ductus arteriosus closes, preventing forward flow of blood to the systemic circulation. With coarctation, please keep in mind that the presence of equal femoral pulses does not rule out coarctation, especially with the scenario just depicted above; although pulses may indeed be equal, they may simply be equally weak.

6. a   This patient is in SVT, most likely triggered by the fever. SVT is idiopathic 50% of the time; is caused by drugs, fever, or infection 20% of the time; and is associated with congenital heart disease 20% of the time. Given that fever may be a precipitant, it is understandable that the condition is often mistaken for sepsis. The physical exam is key to the diagnosis: HR is commonly 250–300. The optimal treatment for this particular patient involves immediate intervention with a 1 mg/kg dose of adenosine, administered rapid IV push. The dose may be repeated. This patient is not hemodynamically unstable enough to warrant immediate synchronized cardioversion with 0.5–1 joule/kg. Verapamil is useful in older patients with SVT, but is strictly contraindicated in children less than 2 years of age (it has been reported to cause sudden death). Lastly, carotid massage is not indicated in children.

7. a   This patient has a classic presentation for congenital adrenal hyperplasia. You would expect her 17-hydroxy progesterone and potassium levels to be increased, and her serum sodium, cortisol, and aldosterone levels to be decreased. The disease emanates from a defect in 17 alpha hydroxylase in the steroid synthesis pathway. The increase in virilizing hormones leads to the "masculinization" of female genitalia on physical exam. Deficiencies of cortisol and aldosterone cause hypoglycemia and the sodium/potassium abnormalities, respectively.

8. c   This patient with a history of chronic illness, meconium plug syndrome, and hypoelectrolytemia is very likely to be suffering from cystic fibrosis and warrants admission for evaluation and treatment. Children with urea cycle defects have much more severe elevations of serum ammonia. Adrenal hyperplasia is associated with hyperkalemia in the salt-wasting form of the disease. Malabsorption syndromes usually begin earlier in infancy; inflammatory bowel disease usually presents later in childhood.

CHAPTER 70

Seizures

VINCENT W. CHIANG, M.D.

QUESTIONS

1. A 14-month-old boy presents to you in the ED for evaluation. The patient began to cry when his mother took a stuffed animal away from him. After a short period of vigorous crying, the patient appeared to stop breathing during exhalation. He became blue around the lips, became limp, and then lost consciousness. Within 30 seconds, the patient awoke and is now completely asymptomatic. Upon questioning, the mother states that this has happened twice in the past since the patient was 10 months old. Based on the history, your next step would be to:

   a. Reassure the mother
   b. Give IV fosphenytoin
   c. Obtain a CT scan of the head
   d. Request a neurology consult
   e. Send urine for toxicologic screen

2. A 9-month-old girl presents in the ED actively seizing. The patient has been in her usual state of health until 2 days ago, when she developed watery, green diarrhea. The patient has been unable to tolerate anything PO except water during her illness. IV access is obtained, laboratory studies are sent, and a dose of lorazepam is given, without effect. The studies reveal electrolyte levels of Na 121, K 4.0, Cl 101, CO_2 9, and glucose 180. Your next treatment is administration of:

   a. Phenobarbital
   b. Fosphenytoin
   c. NaCl
   d. $NaHCO_3$
   e. Insulin

3. A 14-year-old boy presents in the ED in status epilepticus. The patient has a known seizure disorder and has been seizing for over 40 minutes. All of the following are possible complications of his prolonged seizure activity EXCEPT:

   a. Hyperthermia
   b. Hyperglycemia
   c. Hypoglycemia
   d. Hypercarbia
   e. Hypernatremia

4. A 20-month-old girl presents in the ED with a seizure. The patient was in her usual state of health when she began to have a generalized tonic-clonic seizure. The parents called 911, and by the time the EMTs arrived (in less than 5 minutes), the patient had stopped seizing. Upon arrival to the ED, the patient is alert and nontoxic appearing. Vital signs on arrival are: T 40.3°C, HR 120, RR 26, and BP 96/54. The patient has a normal neurologic examination, and no source of fever can be identified. Your workup in the ED would include:

   a. A neurology consult
   b. A CT scan of the head
   c. An EEG
   d. Blood and urine cultures
   e. A lumbar puncture

5. A 1-year-old boy is brought into the ED in status epilepticus. His mother found him seizing in his crib and immediately called 911. Ambulance personnel arrived within minutes and noted him to still be actively seizing. During the transport to the hospital, the patient has received 3 appropriate doses of IV lorazepam. He is still seizing upon arrival to the ED. An appropriate next step would be:

   a. 5 mg/kg IV phenytoin in NS over 5 min
   b. 20 mg/kg IV phenytoin in NS over 5 min
   c. 10 mg/kg IV phenytoin in D5W over 10 min
   d. 20 mg/kg IV phenytoin in NS over 30 min
   e. 20 mg/kg IV phenytoin in D5W over 20 min

ANSWERS

1. a   The patient presents with a classic history for cyanotic breath-holding spells, which are commonly mistaken for seizure activity. They occur in about 4–5% of all children. Breath-holding spells typically present between the ages of 6–18 months and disappear by age 5 years. There are two types—cyanotic and pallid. Cyanotic breath-holding spells are more common. There is usually some initiating event that triggers the episode (pain, fear, agitation), followed by an episode of crying, an interruption of breathing during exhalation, and cyanosis, ending with limpness and transient unconsciousness. The patients usually recover immediately and there is no postictal period. The diagnosis is made on the history alone and the prognosis is excellent.

2. c   The patient has laboratory studies consistent with hyponatremic dehydration. Seizures due to metabolic derangements are often refractory to anticonvulsant therapy until the electrolyte imbalance or other abnormality is corrected. Hypoglycemia, hyponatremia, hypocalcemia, and hypomagnesemia are all associated with seizures. Mild acidosis and hyperglycemia typically do not cause seizures.

3. e   A number of systemic alterations can occur as a result of seizure activity. A massive sympathetic discharge can lead to tachycardia, hypertension, and hyperglycemia. Failure of adequate ventilation can lead to hypoxia, hypercarbia, and respiratory acidosis. Prolonged skeletal muscle activity can lead to lactic acidosis, rhabdomyolysis, hyperkalemia, hyperthermia, and hypoglycemia. Disorders of sodium (hypo- or hypernatremia) are usually a cause, not a result, of seizure activity.

4. d   The patient has had a simple febrile seizure. If the history is consistent with a simple febrile seizure, the patient has a normal neurologic examination, and has no stigmata of a CNS infection, further evaluation for the cause of the seizure is not necessary. The evaluation, however, should focus on the possible etiology of the fever. It should be noted that the typical signs of CNS infection (i.e., meningitis) may be absent in patients less than 12–18 months of age and a low threshold to obtain a lumbar puncture should be maintained.

5. d   Phenytoin is an excellent second-line agent for the treatment of seizures. The loading dose is 10–20 mg/kg. There are two major limitations in its administration: First, it must be administered slowly (no faster than 1 mg/kg/min) due to its possible cardiac effects. Second, it cannot be given in solutions containing dextrose. Fosphenytoin was created to overcome these limitations. It is a prodrug whose active metabolite is phenytoin. The drug is dosed in phenytoin equivalents (PE), it can be given up to 150 mg PE/minute, and it can be given in dextrose-containing solutions.

CHAPTER 71

Sore Throat

CYNTHIA R. JACOBSTEIN, M.D.

QUESTIONS

1. A 3-year-old girl comes to the ED with a history of fever and decreased movement of her neck. She has had limited oral intake on the day of presentation and is more irritable than normal, according to her parents. She is fully immunized. Vital signs are: T 39.2°C, RR 30, O_2 saturation (measured by pulse oximetry) is 98% on room air. She is fussy but consolable while sitting on her mother's lap, leaning slightly forward without drooling or stridor. A quick look at her pharynx reveals mild erythema without exudate or asymmetry. Which of the following tests will be most helpful?

   a. Blood culture
   b. CBC and differential
   c. Heterophile antibody test
   d. Lateral neck radiograph
   e. AP airway radiograph

2. A 15-month-old boy is brought to the ED with a history of fever for 2 days and a rash on his hands. His mother reports he has had decreased oral intake with relatively normal urine output. On exam, the child has a temperature of 38.6°C. He is slightly cranky but easily consolable and in no acute distress. His mucous membranes are moist, and there are multiple vesicles visible in his posterior pharynx. He has vesicles on the palms of his hands. What therapy will you recommend?

   a. IM ceftriaxone
   b. Oral penicillin
   c. Symptomatic treatment only
   d. Oral acyclovir
   e. Oral clindamycin

3. A 6-year-old girl is brought to the ED with complaints of fever and sore throat for 2 days. She has also had a 3-day history of cough and rhinorrhea. She continues to drink fluid well and denies any other complaints. On exam, T is 38.0°C, and HR, RR, and BP are normal. She is interactive and well appearing. Her mucous membranes are moist; she has mild tonsillar hypertrophy but no exudate. You also note mild submandibular lymphadenopathy. A rapid group A strep antigen test is negative. You should:

   a. Start oral penicillin, pending throat culture results
   b. Perform heterophile antibody test
   c. Order a CBC with differential
   d. Start oral prednisone
   e. Begin symptomatic treatment, pending throat culture results

4. A 12-year-old boy comes to the ED with the chief complaint of sore throat for 3–4 days. He has had some low-grade fever and decreased oral intake. His mother reports that his voice sounds funny to her. He has no snoring or difficulty breathing. On examination, he is febrile and the tonsils appear erythematous; the left tonsil appears much larger than the right and the group A strep antigen test is positive. Which of the following would be MOST appropriate?

   a. Admit for IV clindamycin
   b. Discharge patient on oral penicillin
   c. Administer IM dexamethasone, followed by oral penicillin
   d. Needle aspiration, followed by IV antibiotics
   e. Symptomatic therapy only, pending results of a heterophile antibody test

ANSWERS

1. d The presentation is suggestive of retropharyngeal abscess or epiglottitis. The child is young, with a high fever, mild toxicity, and the suggestion of respiratory distress. The immunization history makes epiglottitis less likely. A lateral neck x-ray provides information about the size of the prevertebral soft tissue space (which is enlarged in retropharyngeal abscess) and the epiglottis (which is enlarged in epiglottitis). The child may need to be accompanied by a physician and/or respiratory therapist during the x-ray if the respiratory distress is severe. Although a blood culture and CBC may be included in the workup, they will most likely provide supportive rather than diagnostic information. Lack of tonsillar hypertrophy makes Epstein-Barr virus infection less likely; in addition the Monospot has low sensitivity in children less than 5 years. An AP airway film will contribute little, if any, further information to the patient's care.

2. c The illness described is typical for Coxsackie virus infection, given the posterior pharyngeal and palmar vesicles. Vesicles on the soles of the feet would complete the classic hand-foot-mouth syndrome, but are not necessary to make this clinical diagnosis. This illness is self-limiting and requires no specific antimicrobial treatment, but adequate hydration and fever and pain control are indicated.

3. e The most likely diagnosis is infectious pharyngitis, with etiologies including viral or group A *Streptococcus* (GABHS). The presence of URI symptoms makes a viral etiology more likely. However, GABHS cannot be completely ruled out, even in the setting of a negative rapid antigen test. Thus, it would be prudent to test for GABHS by throat culture rather than simply initiating a course of antibiotics that may not be indicated. Additional laboratory studies are not necessary at this point, and the child's hydration status (as evidenced both by history and physical exam) does not warrant IV fluid therapy.

4. d The most likely diagnoses, given the history of sore throat in an older child/teen who has voice changes, are peritonsillar cellulitis/abscess or marked tonsillar hypertrophy (e.g., from Epstein-Barr virus infection). Physical exam makes the diagnosis of peritonsillar cellulitis/abscess by the presence of asymmetry and bulging of one side of the posterior aspect of the soft palate, usually with deviation of the uvula away from the affected side. The treatment of a peritonsillar abscess includes drainage and antibiotics, generally delivered via the IV route. The organisms that are typically present in peritonsillar abscesses include group A *Streptococcus* and anaerobes. *Staphylococcus aureus* may also be found in this infection. Typical findings of mononucleosis include bilateral tonsillar enlargement with exudate and posterior cervical adenopathy, with or without hepatosplenomegaly.

CHAPTER 72

Stridor

SUJIT SHARMA, M.D.

QUESTIONS

1. A 4-year-old boy is brought to the ED by his mother for breathing difficulty and fever for the past 3 days. On exam he is drooling and appears slightly lethargic. His vital signs are: T 39.2°C, HR 136, RR 32, and BP 108/64. Pulse oximetry shows an O_2 saturation of 96% on room air. You note inspiratory stridor. Lateral neck films show widening of the prevertebral space. Which of the following would be most appropriate?

   a. Intubation in the OR
   b. IV antibiotics
   c. IV epinephrine
   d. Inhaled racemic epinephrine
   e. IM steroids

2. A 3-year-old girl with a history of asthma is brought to the ED by her parents for a barking cough and breathing difficulty. The mother notes that the patient has had a runny nose and congestion for the past 2 days, and that she has been drooling more than usual. On exam she has a temperature of 38.6°C. You note inspiratory stridor while she is crying, but not at rest. Which of the following is most appropriate?

   a. Inhaled racemic epinephrine
   b. Inhaled steroid
   c. IM steroid
   d. IV epinephrine
   e. Inhaled albuterol

3. A 13-month-old girl is brought in by her mother for breathing difficulty. She states that 4 hours ago her child began having "noisy" breathing, as well as some coughing. She has been otherwise well, with no prior cold symptoms or fever. On exam she is afebrile, with an RR of 52. You note inspiratory and expiratory stridor, with mild subcostal retractions. Pulse oximetry shows an O_2 saturation of 93% on room air. Which of the following is most likely to be helpful for this patient?

   a. Epinephrine
   b. Albuterol
   c. Endotracheal intubation
   d. Antibiotics
   e. Bronchoscopy

4. A 7-year-old girl is brought to the ED in severe respiratory distress. Her mother says that she has had severe abdominal pain over the past 2 days, for which she was evaluated earlier that morning. At that time the mother was told that the girl was suffering from gastritis. She did not have any vomiting or fever associated with this illness and is otherwise healthy. On exam she is afebrile and appears to be in severe respiratory distress. You note inspiratory stridor as well as some facial edema. Pulse oximetry shows an O_2 saturation of 88% on room air. Which of the following is the most likely cause of her symptoms?

   a. Viral infection of her upper airway
   b. Bacterial tracheitis
   c. Aspiration of a foreign body
   d. Complement component deficiency
   e. Allergic reaction

5. A 1-month-old boy is brought in to the ED by his mother with a complaint of "noisy" breathing over the past 5 days. The patient was a full-term baby with no medical problems and is otherwise thriving well. He has had no recent fever, nasal congestion, or cough. The mother notes that his breathing is more labored while he is lying on his back and quieter while he is prone. On examination the patient appears alert. He is afebrile, but you note inspiratory stridor with subcostal retractions while he is supine. His RR is 48 and pulse oximetry shows an O_2 saturation of 96% on room air. Which of the following would be most appropriate?

   a. Inhaled racemic epinephrine
   b. IM dexamethasone
   c. Immediate endotracheal intubation
   d. Laryngoscopy in the ED
   e. Reassurance and outpatient follow-up

ANSWERS

1. **b** This patient has a retropharyngeal abscess. The symptoms are usually less acute than in patients with epiglottitis. Increase in the prevertebral space on lateral neck x-ray is diagnostic. Group A *Streptococcus* is the usual culprit, along with anaerobic organisms, and occasionally *Staphylococcus aureus*. IV antibiotics should be started immediately, most likely to be followed by surgical drainage.

2. **c** This patient has croup. If one were to perform x-rays of the neck, subglottic narrowing ("steeple sign") might be seen. Inhaled racemic epinephrine should be reserved for patients with stridor at rest. IM steroid (dexamethasone) has been shown to be of benefit in those treated as outpatients. One might also opt to treat this patient symptomatically.

3. **e** The history of acute onset of breathing difficulty without other symptoms to suggest infectious etiology in a patient of this age should make one strongly suspect foreign body aspiration. The quality of the stridor can help to identify the anatomic location. In this case, biphasic stridor indicates the obstruction is both extra- and intrathoracic. This patient appears to be in mild distress and hypoxic. Although supportive measures such as supplemental oxygen should be started right away, definitive therapy via direct visualization (bronchoscopy) should be done as soon as possible.

4. **d** This patient has a deficiency of C1 esterase inhibitor, also known as hereditary angioedema. Abdominal pain or cramping can be an initial complaint, secondary to inflammation/edema of the intestinal wall in these patients. The attacks are brought on during times of stress and usually present in late childhood or adolescence. Definitive therapy involves administration of purified C1 esterase inhibitor, which has limited availability.

5. **e** This patient has congenital stridor, most likely caused by laryngomalacia. Although most cases present soon after birth, symptoms may not appear until the second month of life. Significant airway obstruction can occur in severe cases. In this case, the patient is in no distress and improves with positioning. No immediate therapy is needed in the ED. Reassurance to the parents that the condition will improve as the child's airway structures become more developed is adequate. Follow-up with the primary care physician is important, so that the condition can be monitored with consideration of otolaryngology evaluation if the symptoms worsen or do not resolve over time.

CHAPTER 73

Syncope

VINCENT J. WANG, M.D.

QUESTIONS

1. A 14-year-old boy was brought to the ED after fainting. The patient collapsed in church after standing for a prolonged period. Bystanders report that he collapsed for just a few seconds. In the ED, his HR is 70 and his BP is 120/75. There are no orthostatic changes. On examination, he is now alert and cooperative. His neurologic and cardiovascular examinations are normal. Diagnostic evaluation should include:

   a. ECG
   b. Echocardiogram
   c. Tilt-table testing
   d. Urine toxicology screen
   e. No testing

2. A 9-year-old girl is brought to the ED after a brief syncopal episode. The patient was running around in her backyard when she suddenly collapsed. She awoke after several seconds, and appeared to be back to baseline almost immediately. Which of the following cardiac diseases could have precipitated the syncopal episode?

   a. Primary AV block
   b. Truncus arteriosus
   c. Prolonged QT syndrome
   d. Patent ductus arteriosus (PDA)
   e. Situs inversus

3. A 3-year-old boy was crying after not getting the toy of his choice. His mother states that he began holding his breath, turned pale, and then had a brief syncopal episode. He has never had a previous episode and he has been otherwise healthy. He presents to you in the ED, playful and interactive, in no acute distress. Appropriate management at this point would include:

   a. Schedule an outpatient EEG
   b. Obtain a CXR
   c. Perform a urinalysis
   d. Reassure and counsel the mother
   e. Obtain an echocardiogram

4. A 17-year-old girl comes to your ED after having a syncopal episode at school. She says it was her turn to speak in the school play. She got up to speak, but felt lightheaded and then fainted. She admits to sexual activity, but she says she had a normal period last month. She normally has heavy bleeding. No one else in the play had fainted. Her physical examination is normal. All of the following screening tests are indicated, EXCEPT:

   a. ECG
   b. Hematocrit
   c. Orthostatic vital signs
   d. Urine pregnancy screen
   e. Carboxyhemoglobin level

5. A 10-year-old boy comes to the ED after fainting. He says he felt like his chest was pounding, and then witnesses saw him collapse. He was unconscious for approximately 10 seconds. On examination, he is alert and well appearing. His HR is 80 and his BP is 100/60. His cardiac examination is normal. His ECG reveals a QRS duration of 0.08 seconds, a P-R interval of 0.15 seconds, and a QTc (corrected QT) interval of 0.6 seconds. This patient is:

   a. At risk for "torsades de pointes"
   b. At risk for supraventricular tachycardia (SVT)
   c. At risk for atrial fibrillation
   d. At risk for right to left cardiac shunting
   e. Not at risk for cardiac disease; his ECG shows normal intervals

6. A 15-year-old girl with a history of anxiety comes to the ED after fainting. She reports that she was about to give an oral presentation and began breathing quickly. She says she "passed out for an hour," but witnesses say that the episode lasted only a few seconds. Her vital signs and physical examination are normal. Her syncope is most likely due to:

a. Hypoglycemia
b. Hyperventilation
c. Cardiac causes
d. Vasovagal mechanisms
e. Toxin ingestion

7. A 3-year-old boy comes to you after a fainting episode. He has been otherwise well, until today, when he appeared to be more sleepy. His grandmother has been visiting for the past week, and says that he was playing with her medications. She says she takes thioridazine (Mellaril), trimethoprim-sulfamethoxazole (Bactrim), lorazepam (Ativan), levothyroxine (Synthroid), and iron. On examination, he is lethargic and ataxic. He has dry flushed skin, dry mucous membranes, tachycardia, hyperthermia, and decreased bowel sounds. His ECG reveals "torsades de pointes." He is likely to be symptomatic from ingestion of:

a. Thioridazine (Mellaril)
b. Trimethoprim-sulfamethoxazole (Bactrim)
c. Lorazepam (Ativan)
d. Levothyroxine (Synthroid)
e. Iron

ANSWERS

1. a   Vasovagal syncope is the most common cause of syncope in children, accounting for 50% of childhood syncope. Even though this patient presents with a classic history for vasovagal syncope, an ECG is still recommended. The ECG is noninvasive and relatively inexpensive. Cardiac disorders such as prolonged QT syndrome, Wolff-Parkinson-White (WPW) syndrome, and heart block may be detected by ECG. An echocardiogram is indicated when structural heart disease is thought to be the cause of syncope. However, with a normal cardiac examination, this is unlikely. Tilt-table testing is controversial, and if used, it should be reserved for patients with recurrent, unexplained syncope. Urine toxicology screening should be performed if indicated. The author also recommends a pregnancy screening in all adolescent girls with syncope.

2. c   Any cardiac disease that potentially disrupts blood flow to the brain may cause syncope. Severe aortic or pulmonic stenosis, tetralogy of Fallot, or pulmonary hypertension without shunting may cause syncope, especially after exertion. Mitral valve orifice obstruction from an atrial myxoma may rarely cause syncope. Several arrhythmias may also cause syncope: complete AV block with Stokes-Adams attacks, sick sinus syndrome, paroxysmal ventricular tachycardia, and prolonged QT syndrome can cause a disruption of cerebral blood flow. AV block does not cause a disruption in blood flow. Truncus arteriosus, patent ductus arteriosus (PDA), and situs inversus are not associated with syncope.

3. d   The patient in this vignette had a breath-holding spell. Given his emotional upset and the progression of his symptoms, this would be the most likely diagnosis. Treatment involves reassuring the mother and counseling her about what to expect with these episodes. An EEG would be warranted in a patient with a history and symptoms consistent with seizure activity. If he had multiple episodes, this might be warranted. With no other symptoms, a CXR and urinalysis are unnecessary. An echocardiogram would be indicated if the patient's symptoms suggested structural cardiac disease, but this is not the case.

4. e   A carboxyhemoglobin level should be sent if the history suggests a potential carbon monoxide (CO) poisoning (e.g., if the patient was in a confined room or if others were symptomatic). This does not appear to be the case. As discussed, an ECG is indicated in all patients with syncope. The author also recommends a pregnancy screen in all adolescent female patients. A hematocrit is reasonable, given her menstrual history. Orthostatic vital signs are helpful to diagnose orthostatic syncope, which is also a possible cause.

5. a   A QTc interval of 0.6 seconds is abnormal, and therefore this patient has prolonged QT syndrome. Patients with prolonged QT syndrome are at risk for developing "torsades de pointes," a malignant form

of ventricular tachycardia. Patients with WPW are at risk for supraventricular tachycardia. Right to left shunting can occur with structural heart disease, but not with an isolated prolonged QT syndrome.

6. b Hyperventilation may cause cerebral vasoconstriction in response to self-induced hypocapnia. This may cause a true syncopal episode, as the brain becomes hypoperfused. Given the history, the other etiologies are not likely.

7. a Mellaril, or thioridazine, is a phenothiazine (piperidine group) antipsychotic medication that can be associated with syncope. (Burns M. "The Antipsychotic Drugs." *Clinical Management of Poisoning and Drug Overdose,* third edition, pp 628–641.)Manifestations of piperidine phenothiazine overdose include CNS effects such as lethargy, slurred speech, ataxia, and coma; peripheral anticholinergic stigmata; and cardiovascular toxicity, including "torsades de pointes." The other medications do not produce this combination of symptoms.

CHAPTER 74

Tachycardia/Palpitations

SUJIT SHARMA, M.D.

QUESTIONS

1. A previously healthy 18-month-old girl is brought into the ED by her mother for concerns of a fast heart rate that she noticed while holding her. The child currently has a URI, for which her parents have been administering an over-the-counter cold preparation. On examination she is afebrile, with a HR of 240. She appears alert and happy, with a blood pressure of 98/48. Which of the following would be the most appropriate choice for management?

   a. Discontinue cold medication
   b. Synchronized cardioversion
   c. Apply ocular pressure
   d. Administer IV adenosine
   e. Administer IV propranolol

2. A 13-year-old girl is brought to the ED after feeling faint at school. She states that she felt "palpitations" in her chest when it happened. Although she has a history of anxiety, she takes no medications and denies any drug ingestion. A 12-lead ECG is performed, showing sinus rhythm and the following intervals: RR 0.64 sec; QT 0.3 sec; P-R interval 0.16 sec; QRS 0.07 sec. The remainder of her examination is normal. Which of the following is most appropriate?

   a. Reassurance only
   b. Administer IV lidocaine
   c. Immediate cardiology consultation
   d. Echocardiography
   e. Administer IV propanolol

3. A 14-year-old boy comes to the ED stating that he felt his heart "skip a beat" while lying down. He is otherwise healthy and has an unremarkable physical examination. The rhythm strip below is recorded while he is being monitored:

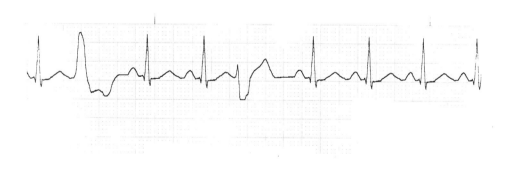

Which of the following would be the most appropriate next steps in management?

   a. Call for a cardiology consultation
   b. Repeat the ECG after exercise
   c. Obtain an emergent echocardiogram
   d. Administer IV lidocaine
   e. Administer IV digoxin

4. A 4-year-old boy is being monitored after sedation with fentanyl and midazolam for reduction of a fractured radius. The nurse brings you a recording of an "irregular" heartbeat, as shown below:

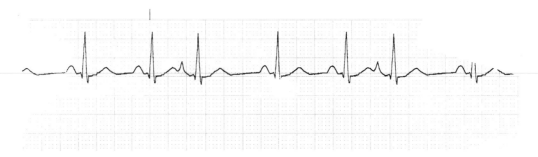

The patient has a BP of 104/62 and is waking up appropriately. He has otherwise been well and has a normal physical examination. Which of the following interventions is most appropriate?

a. No intervention needed
b. Administer IV naloxone
c. Administer IV atropine
d. Administer IV flumazenil
e. Cardiology consultation

5. An 18-month-old boy is brought to the ED by his father because the boy has appeared lethargic over the past 2 hours. The child has been otherwise well and has an unremarkable past medical history. On further questioning, the father does recall the child playing earlier in the day with a bottle of medication that possibly contained capsules the father used to take for depression. On examination the patient is slightly lethargic, with a weak pulse. He is afebrile, with a BP of 92/46 and O_2 saturation of 95% on room air. The rhythm strip is shown below:

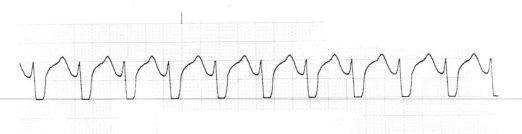

Treatment for this patient should include:

a. Administer IV propranolol
b. Defibrillation
c. Administer IV sodium bicarbonate ($NaHCO_3$)
d. Administer IV diltiazem
e. Administer IV adenosine

ANSWERS

1. d Most over-the-counter cold preparations contain sympathomimetic agents that can incite tachyarrhythmias. In this case, a history of ingestion of these agents, along with the HR of 240, points to SVT as the diagnosis. A rhythm strip and ECG would confirm this suspicion. This patient appears hemodynamically stable, so synchronized cardioversion is not urgently required. Vagal maneuvers can be attempted before pharmacological intervention; however, elicitation of the diving-seal reflex via application of ice to the face is the most widely accepted modality. In most instances, pharmacological intervention is necessary, with adenosine being the drug of choice.

2. a The intervals measured on this patient's ECG are within normal limits, including the QTc interval, which comes out to approximately 0.38 seconds (normal less than 0.45 seconds). No other evidence of arrhythmias or predisposition to arrhythmias exists for this patient, so treatment and further investigation is not necessary. Anxiety is known to produce the feeling of palpitations, and further history may elicit emotional arousal surrounding the event.

3. b Unifocal premature ventricular contractions (PVCs) can account for complaints of "skipped" or "missed" heartbeats. If in otherwise well patients, the PVCs disappear with exercise, and the patient has an otherwise unremarkable history and physical examination, these events do not require further evaluation or treatment.

4. a This rhythm strip shows occasional premature atrial contractions (PACs). PACs are the most common dysrhythmia of childhood and in an otherwise healthy child do not require further investigation or treatment. A 12-lead ECG may be performed to ensure normal findings, but will most likely be normal.

5. c This child's rhythm strip shows ventricular tachycardia. The history points to ingestion of the father's medication as the most likely cause of this. Tricyclic antidepressants are known to cause wide complex tachycardias, including ventricular tachycardia and fibrillation. Alkalinization with sodium bicarbonate to counteract the toxic effects of the medication should be attempted first. Synchronized cardioversion rather than defibrillation would be the other modality of treatment. The other medications listed are not indicated in the treatment ventricular tachycardia.

CHAPTER 75

Urinary Frequency in Childhood

VINCENT J. WANG, M.D.

QUESTIONS

1. A 12-year-old girl complains of abdominal pain and urinary frequency. She has had fever to 38.1°C, abdominal pain, and vomiting for 1–2 days. She complains of voiding more frequently than normal. On examination, she is alert, but uncomfortable. She has diffuse abdominal pain, with greater tenderness on the right during rectal examination. Her urinalysis shows 5–10 WBCs per hpf. Your next step in diagnosis includes:

   a. Renal DMSA scan
   b. Voiding cystourethrogram (VCUG)
   c. Abdominal CT scan
   d. Abdominal radiograph
   e. Urinary pregnancy screen

2. A 3-year-old girl is brought to the ED because of urinary frequency. She complains of abdominal pain as well. On examination, her T is 37.9°C. Her abdomen is soft and nontender. Her genitourinary examination is normal. Her urinalysis shows 10–15 WBCs per hpf; 5–10 RBCs per hpf; and a specific gravity (SG) of 1.020. A urine culture has been sent. Your next step in management includes:

   a. Renal ultrasonography
   b. Abdominal CT scan
   c. Pelvic ultrasonography
   d. Outpatient treatment with sitz baths
   e. Oral trimethoprim-sulfamethoxazole

3. A 5-year-old boy has been voiding more frequently. The parents report that he seems to strain when he voids, and that he voids small quantities at a time. On examination, he is afebrile and his abdomen is soft and nontender. His urinalysis shows 0–1 WBCs per hpf, 5–10 RBCs per hpf, and an SG of 1.015. Your next step in management includes:

   a. Renal CT scan
   b. Pelvic ultrasonography
   c. Retrograde urethrogram
   d. Follow-up urinalysis in a few days
   e. Referral to a psychologist

4. A 16-year-old female patient complains of urinary frequency. She says she feels bloated and has had urinary frequency for the past month. She denies abdominal pain, fever, or vaginal bleeding. She says she has been sexually active, but her partners have used condoms. On examination, she is obese, but her abdomen is nontender. Her pelvic examination is normal. Her urinalysis shows 0–1 WBCs per hpf, 0–1 RBCs per hpf, and an SG of 1.020. In consideration of likely diagnoses, you must perform which of the following tests?

   a. Urine culture
   b. Urine pregnancy screen
   c. Urine calcium level
   d. CT of abdomen and pelvis
   e. Psychological evaluation

5. An 8-year-old boy complains of urinary frequency and abdominal pain. He has had frequent, small bowel movements and frequent voiding. He has not had fever or vomiting. On examination, his abdomen is slightly distended, nontender, with multiple soft masses palpable throughout his abdomen. The likely etiology of his urinary frequency is:

   a. Cystitis
   b. Neuroblastoma
   c. Wilm's tumor
   d. Constipation
   e. Teratoma

6. A 2-week-old boy is brought to the ED because his diapers seem to be constantly soaked with urine. He has been voiding frequently since birth. He has also had episodes of vomiting. On examination, his vital signs are: T 36.5°C, HR 160, RR 28, and BP 85/50. His eyes are sunken and his mucous membranes are dry. His glans penis appears small, and is almost covered by his scrotal sac. You would expect the following set of serum electrolytes:

   a. Na 123, K 3.4, Cl 90, HCO_3 16
   b. Na 125, K 6.0, Cl 92, HCO_3 14
   c. Na 152, K 3.5, Cl 120, HCO_3 18
   d. Na 150, K 5.3, Cl 95, HCO_3 28
   e. Na 140, K 4.8, Cl 110, HCO_3 12

7. A 14-year-old girl complains of polyuria and polydipsia. She was diagnosed with Letterer-Siwe disease several years ago. She says she feels the need to drink frequently, and urinates nearly every hour. She does not awaken at night to void. Her urine SG is 1.020, and her urinalysis is otherwise normal. You suspect she has:

   a. Cystitis
   b. Diabetes mellitus
   c. Diabetes insipidus
   d. Psychogenic water drinking
   e. Extraordinary urinary frequency syndrome

ANSWERS

1. c   Urinary frequency may be a symptom of a pelvic appendicitis or an appendiceal abscess. Her symptoms may be attributed to cystitis, but given the localized tenderness during rectal examination, further evaluation for appendicitis is warranted. Renal DMSA scan and VCUG are warranted in some children with urinary tract infections (UTIs), and are not necessary for the initial evaluation of cystitis, if at all, in this older child. An abdominal radiograph is unlikely to be helpful, especially because the location of the appendicitis may be pelvic. Pregnancy as the cause of symptoms would be unlikely in this case.

2. e   UTIs are a common cause of urinary frequency, because the inflammation from infection decreases bladder capacity. Further radiologic imaging is not necessary during the initial visit, but the patient should have a renal U/S and VCUG at a later time. Vulvovaginitis is also a common cause of urinary frequency, but the urinalysis is usually absent of pyuria.

3. b   This patient has symptoms suggestive of a partial urethral obstruction. Whereas a retrograde urethrogram will demonstrate an interruption of urethral flow, it may not demonstrate a partial obstruction. Pelvic ultrasonography or CT scan would be the best tests to further delineate this problem. However, a renal CT scan is helpful for intrinsic renal pathology, but is not helpful in this scenario. In an asymptomatic child with a urinalysis suspicious for a UTI, a repeat urinalysis in a few days would be warranted. Psychogenic urinary frequency is a diagnosis of exclusion, and does not usually cause such symptoms.

4. b   The possibility of pregnancy as a cause of urinary frequency in a sexually active adolescent female must never be overlooked. Even with proper condom use, pregnancy is still a possibility. A UTI is unlikely, given a normal urinalysis and the history of symptoms for 1 month. Hypercalciuria may cause urinary frequency associated with dysuria. The urinalysis may demonstrate hematuria and/or crystal-

luria. However, hypercalciuria is rare, and other diagnoses should be considered first. Although a CT of the abdomen and pelvis would evaluate for potential abdominal masses, a urine pregnancy screen is indicated prior to this study. Also, the most likely abdominal mass is a gravid uterus. Psychogenic pain is a diagnosis of exclusion, and may be considered if the other etiologies are ruled out.

5. d   Constipation is frequently associated with urinary tract dysfunction. Even though neuroblastoma and teratoma may be abdominal masses causing extrinsic compression of the bladder, this patient's history is typical for constipation. Wilm's tumor, if large enough, may also cause extrinsic compression of the bladder. A UTI is unlikely, given the boy's signs and symptoms.

6. b   Salt-losing patients with congenital adrenal hyperplasia (CAH) may demonstrate the findings as noted in the vignette. A female will have virilization of her genitalia, while a male will be normal. Serum electrolytes may demonstrate hyponatremia, hyperkalemia, and a metabolic acidosis because of dehydration. Pyloric stenosis may occasionally be mistaken for CAH, but this diagnosis would be unlikely in a patient with urinary frequency and the associated genitalia findings.

7. d   Patients with histiocytosis are at risk for central diabetes insipidus, but they should have polyuria and polydipsia in the context of a dilute urine, because of a deficiency of antidiuretic hormone (ADH). In addition, the history of the absence of symptoms at night suggest a psychogenic cause to the symptoms. Diabetes mellitus, likewise, is unlikely in the absence of nighttime symptoms and also in the presence of a normal urinalysis. Cystitis does not cause polydipsia. The extraordinary urinary frequency syndrome is a recently described entity in younger children, thought to be psychogenic in origin. Pollakiuria (urinary frequency) is present, but polydipsia and polyuria are absent.

CHAPTER **76**

Vaginal Bleeding

JACQUELINE BRYNGIL, M.D.

QUESTIONS

1. You are examining a 6-year-old girl brought in by her mother with a complaint of vaginal bleeding. Her vital signs are: T 37.5°C, HR 92, RR 18, and BP 110/65. On examination you note that she is Tanner stage I for both breasts and pubic hair. She has no bruising or signs of external vaginal trauma. Your next most appropriate step in evaluating this child would be:

    a. Speculum examination in the ED
    b. Visual inspection in the knee-chest position
    c. Examination under anesthesia in the OR
    d. Social services consultation
    e. Obtaining FSH/LH (follicle-stimulating hormone/luteinizing hormone) levels

2. A 3-year-old African-American girl is brought to the ED with a chief complaint of vaginal bleeding. Your examination reveals the presence of a purple, doughnut-shaped mass protruding from the anterior aspect of the labia majora. The most appropriate management of this patient would be:

    a. Surgical resection
    b. Order sitz baths and estrogen cream
    c. Obtain a CBC with smear
    d. Apply hydrocortisone cream
    e. Refer for biopsy

3. You are called in to the ED to see a 13-year-old girl with an HR of 100, BP 110/60, and slight pallor. She states that her period has lasted for 10 days, and she has gone through at least 5 pads per day since its onset. The bleeding is painless. She reports that her periods began last year and occur every 2–3 months. Her symptoms are most likely the result of:

    a. Thrombocytopenia
    b. Pregnancy
    c. Anovulation
    d. Polycystic ovary syndrome (PCOS)
    e. von Willebrand's disease

4. The same patient (see Question 3) has a hematocrit of 20 mg/dl and her platelet count is 160 × 10⁹/l. Your most appropriate next step in her management would be:

    a. Transfuse with 2 units of type-specific packed RBCs
    b. Administer conjugated estrogens IV
    c. Administer cefixime and azithromycin PO
    d. Transfuse with 6 units of platelets
    e. Administer a combined estrogen-progestin tablet PO

5. You are evaluating a 17-year-old female patient who complains of lower abdominal pain. She states that she has a history of irregular menses and that she has been experiencing heavier-than-normal vaginal bleeding for the past 2 days. Her vital signs are: T 37.1°C, HR 130, RR 18, and BP 90/50. On physical examination, she is slightly pale. Her pelvic examination reveals vaginal bleeding with a closed os. There is no uterine enlargement. You cannot appreciate adnexal masses. A urine HCG is positive. Your next most appropriate management of this patient is:

    a. Administration of estrogen-progestin tablet PO
    b. Immediate laparoscopic exploration by gynecology
    c. Transvaginal U/S in the ED
    d. Surgical consultation for laparotomy
    e. Reassurance and outpatient follow-up

ANSWERS

1. b   Visual inspection of the vaginal vault with the patient in the knee-chest position is the next appropriate examination for this child. If the source of the bleeding is not visualized, then a speculum examination under anesthesia (either procedural sedation or general anesthesia) would be warranted. A speculum examination in the ED in a virginal, unsedated child is inappropriate, as would be a social service consultation without evidence of abuse. As this child is at the appropriate Tanner stage for her age and shows no other signs of precocious puberty, a laboratory evaluation at this time would not be necessary.

2. b   Sitz baths, along with topical estrogen cream, is the preferred initial management of urethral prolapse. Urethral prolapse is characterized by the presence of a red to purple doughnut-shaped mass that is often accompanied by symptoms of bleeding and urinary retention. It occurs most commonly in young African-American girls. If the prolapse fails to recede after conservative measures have been tried, surgical excision with re-anastomosis may be necessary. This is not a tumor and evaluation for this is unnecessary. Hydrocortisone cream is ineffective in treating this condition.

3. c   Dysfunctional uterine bleeding (DUB) is irregular, prolonged, or excessive menstrual bleeding associated with anovulation and unrelated to pregnancy. In this patient, with her history of irregular menses prior to this event, it is likely that her cycles are still anovulatory. Although DUB is the most likely cause of her symptoms, other etiologies of prolonged bleeding must be considered. Bleeding disorders, such as thrombocytopenia and von Willebrand's disease; endocrine disorders, such as polycystic ovary syndrome; and pelvic diseases caused by chlamydia or gonorrhea should be considered if associated signs are noted.

4. e   Management of DUB consists of stopping the bleeding, changing the state of the endometrium from proliferative to secretory, and controlling the sloughing. This is best accomplished with a combination of estrogen, which supports the endometrium and acutely stops the bleeding, and progestin, which induces the secretory state. Antibiotics should also be administered if pelvic inflammatory disease (PID) is diagnosed; however, in this case there is no evidence to support infection in the patient. Transfusion may be necessary if the patient is hemodynamically unstable, but this is not the case. This patient is not thrombocytopenic, and there is no reason to suspect that her platelets are dysfunctional; therefore, a platelet transfusion is also unnecessary. IV estrogen is rarely indicated; however, it may be necessary in cases of severe or prolonged bleeding.

5. c   Bleeding associated with pregnancy is not normal and should be further evaluated. This patient may have a ruptured ectopic pregnancy or a threatened abortion. Diagnosis of these conditions is best achieved via ultrasonography. This patient is also showing signs of early hemodynamic compromise, so fluid resuscitation is also an important part of this patient's management. Depending on the outcome of the ultrasonographic evaluation, a laparoscopic exploration or laparotomy may be necessary to treat a ruptured ectopic pregnancy. There is no role for estrogen-progestin tablet therapy in this case.

CHAPTER 77

Vaginal Discharge

JACQUELINE BRYNGIL, M.D.

QUESTIONS

1. During examination of a 1-month-old girl for a rash, you note a thin, yellowish vaginal discharge. The infant is afebrile and has no external signs of vaginal trauma or irritation. The mother states that she was on "some medication" for a sexually acquired infection at the time of the patient's vaginal delivery. Your most appropriate management of this patient is:

   a. Culture of discharge and metronidazole
   b. Counseling of parent on perineal hygiene
   c. Culture of discharge and IM ceftriaxone
   d. Social services consultation
   e. Gynecological examination with cultures under sedation

2. You are examining a 3-year-old girl brought in to the ED by the parents because of vaginal odor and intermittently bloody discharge. On her examination she is well appearing. She is Tanner stage I. You note some nonbloody vaginal discharge and are aware of the presence of a foul smell at the introitus. Rectal examination of the patient is normal. The patient is afebrile. On visual inspection of the perineum you are most likely to note:

   a. Vaginal trauma
   b. Urethral prolapse
   c. Flat warts
   d. Accelerated Tanner staging
   e. A vaginal foreign body

3. A 15-year-old girl complains of vaginal itching persisting for several months. She has been treated repeatedly with topical antifungals without improvement. Further questioning reveals that she has never experienced vaginal discharge, but has occasionally noted scant blood on her undergarments. On examination, you note vulvar hypopigmentation. She has never had sexual relations. This patient can be most successfully treated with:

   a. PO fluconazole
   b. Topical hydrocortisone
   c. Oral contraceptives
   d. Topical lindane
   e. PO mebendazole

4. You are examining a 17-year-old girl for a complaint of vaginal discharge. She states that she is sexually active and uses oral contraceptive pills as her only form of birth control. Her discharge has been foul smelling and thin but is not pruritic. She has no complaint of abdominal pain. You would expect which of the following to be true about her condition?

   a. Treatment of choice is IM ceftriaxone
   b. Wet prep will show motile flagellates
   c. Vaginal pH will be about 3.0
   d. Amine-like odor with suspension in 10% potassium hydroxide
   e. Treatment of choice is PO fluconazole

5. A 3-week-old girl is brought in by her mother for a mucoid vaginal discharge. The infant's vital signs are: T 37.4°C (rectally), HR 120, RR 26, and BP 80/45. The mother has a history of treatment for a sexually transmitted disease (STD) at the time of her delivery. On examination, you note a thin, clear, odorless discharge from the vagina. The patient is alert and easily consoled. Your most appropriate next step in management of this patient is:

   a. Perform a full sepsis workup, including cultures of blood, urine, and CSF
   b. Culture of the vaginal discharge and discharge home
   c. Culture of the vaginal discharge and IV ampicillin
   d. Culture of the vaginal discharge and topical nystatin
   e. Urologic consultation for evaluation

ANSWERS

1. **a**   Trichomonal vaginitis may be seen in infants up to 8 weeks of age who have acquired the infection perinatally through an infected mother. These patients are generally asymptomatic except for the discharge. Culture of the discharge reveals flagellated trichomonads. The treatment of choice is metronidazole for 7 days. Discharge associated with gonococcal infections is usually thick or purulent. Although poor perineal hygiene often presents with vaginal secretions, it usually is associated with irritation of the perineum and, in older patients, pruritis. Unless gonococcus is cultured or the patient has obvious signs of perineal trauma, social services does not need to be contacted in this case. A full gynecological examination should be reserved for cases where evidence of perineal trauma exists.

2. **e**   In many instances, the presence of a vaginal foreign body (FB) cannot be detected on rectal examination, as most are composed of toilet tissue. The FB typically is easily visible on visual inspection in the knee-chest position. Symptoms include a foul odor and sometimes a bloody discharge from the vagina. Although vaginal bleeding may signal vaginal trauma, it would be unlikely with a malodorous discharge. Flat warts are not associated with discharge, nor is urethral prolapse. Accelerated Tanner staging can be seen in premature adrenarche; however, the discharge is generally not foul smelling.

3. **b**   This patient suffers from lichen sclerosus, a chronic dermatitis characterized by superficial telangiectases that occasionally bleed after excoriation, and atrophic skin changes. This skin condition is responsive to topical steroids and hormone creams. PO fluconazole, a common treatment of vulvovaginal candidiasis, would not be helpful. Oral contraceptives, despite their hormone content, are not effective in helping the atrophic tissue mature. Topical lindane is used to treat pubic lice and PO mebendazole is the treatment of choice for pinworms. Although pubic lice and pinworms would produce perineal itching, this patient does not have other characteristic symptoms to lead to those diagnoses.

4. **d**   The symptoms this patient is exhibiting are seen most often with bacterial vaginosis, particularly *Gardnerella* vaginitis, with a discharge that emits a fishy or amine-like odor when suspended in 10% potassium hydroxide solution. IM ceftriaxone is the treatment of choice for *N. gonorrhea*. Motile flagellates are associated with trichomoniasis, which typically presents with a pruritic, frothy discharge. In bacterial vaginosis, the vaginal pH is typically above 4.5. PO fluconazole is one of the recommended treatments for vaginal candidiasis, which typically presents with pruritic, cheesy discharge.

5. **b**   The infant described has physiologic leukorrhea, which is typically seen in infants ages 2–3 weeks of age and is normal. The appropriate management is supportive and the discharge should be cultured, if present, to rule out other etiologies. There are no indications that this infant is septic; therefore, a full sepsis workup would be inappropriate. IV ampicillin should be given if the child has a culture positive for *N. gonorrhea*; however, there is no treatment required for physiologic leukorrhea. Topical nystatin, the treatment of vulvovaginal candidiasis, would not be necessary. Should the discharge persist or should the patient develop signs of sepsis, a urologic consultation would be warranted to rule out genitourinary malformations.

CHAPTER **78**

Vomiting

RON L. KAPLAN, M.D.

QUESTIONS

1. A 3-week-old girl is brought to the ED with vomiting since the first week of life. Her formula has been changed twice, with no improvement. Birth history and perinatal course were unremarkable. She has effortless spitting up shortly after feeding, with milky material dribbling from her mouth. Her birth weight was 7 pounds, 2 ounces and she now weighs 8 pounds. Her physical exam is unremarkable. What is the next appropriate step?

   a. Abdominal x-rays
   b. pH probe
   c. Barium swallow
   d. Start cisapride
   e. Reassurance

2. A 5-week-old boy is brought to the ED with persistent vomiting. He started spitting up around 2 weeks ago, but the vomiting is now projectile, nonbloody, and nonbilious. The vomiting occurs shortly after feeding and does not improve with oral rehydration solution. He has no fever and no diarrhea. Over the last few days he has become less active with decreased urine output. Which study is likely to confirm a diagnosis?

   a. Abdominal x-rays
   b. Abdominal U/S
   c. pH probe
   d. Air contrast enema
   e. Abdominal CT

3. Which of the following laboratory values would be expected for the patient in Question 2? (All values are in mEq/l.)

	Sodium (Na)	Potassium (K)	Chloride (Cl)	CO_2
a.	130	5.9	105	20
b.	155	3.8	118	16
c.	137	2.9	94	28
d.	140	3.0	114	14
e.	138	4.8	96	22

4. A 1-year-old girl is brought to the ED with intermittent vomiting and episodes of irritability with apparent abdominal discomfort. She has no fevers. Her abdomen appears somewhat tender, with no palpable masses. Electrolytes and urinalysis are normal. Stool is heme positive. Abdominal x-rays appear normal. What would be the most appropriate next step?

   a. Air contrast enema
   b. Abdominal U/S
   c. Abdominal CT
   d. Upper GI series
   e. No further tests

5. An 18-month-old girl is brought to the ED with vomiting, fever to 39°C, and fussiness for 2 days. She has had no diarrhea. There is no significant past medical history, and her history and physical are otherwise unremarkable. Which test is most likely to reveal a specific diagnosis?

   a. *H. pylori* serology
   b. Abdominal x-rays
   c. Ammonia level
   d. Abdominal U/S
   e. Urinalysis

6. A 4-year-old boy is brought to the ED with the sudden onset of intermittent abdominal pain and vomiting with streaks of blood. He has no fever or diarrhea. He has been well previously, with no significant past medical history. His mother denies known exposures to potential toxins or foreign bodies, but admits that she has not been able to watch him as closely because she has a new baby at home. Which study is most likely to suggest a diagnosis?

   a. Abdominal x-rays
   b. Air contrast enema
   c. Urine toxicology screen
   d. Liver function tests
   e. Head CT scan

ANSWERS

1. e   Gastroesophageal reflux is very common in infants in this age group. These children have effortless spitting up, with milky material dribbling from the mouth shortly after feeding. The history and physical exam are otherwise unremarkable. This infant appears well and has had appropriate weight gain (½ to 1 ounce per day after the first week). Radiographic evaluation of this patient is not indicated in the ED. In the infant with a more severe presentation, reflux may be evaluated by barium swallow or pH probe. Medications should not be initiated in the ED without appropriate evaluation and discussion with the primary care provider.

2. b   This child has the classic presentation for pyloric stenosis. It is most common in male infants 4–6 weeks of age. Spitting up progresses to projectile vomiting, with subsequent dehydration. The olive-shaped mass is often difficult to palpate. Ultrasound reveals the hypertrophied pylorus and is the diagnostic procedure of choice in most centers. Barium swallow can also confirm the diagnosis and is used in centers without experience in interpreting pyloric ultrasounds.

3. c   Because of protracted vomiting, infants with pyloric stenosis often develop a hypochloremic, hypokalemic metabolic alkalosis. Electrolyte abnormalities should be corrected prior to surgery.

4. a   The presence of blood in the stool, along with the history of intermittent pain and vomiting in a child of this age, is strongly suggestive of intussusception. A mass is often not palpable on abdominal exam and is sometimes more easily appreciated on bimanual rectal and abdominal exams. This diagnosis should be considered regardless of findings on x-rays, which may be normal. On occasion, plain films of the abdomen may reveal paucity of gas in the right upper quadrant or a mass effect. Air contrast or barium enema is the diagnostic procedure of choice, and it is most often successful in reducing the intussusception.

5. e   Vomiting is a common finding in children with infections outside of the gastrointestinal (GI) tract, such as urinary tract infections (UTIs) and otitis media. UTI should be considered in this situation. The role of *Helicobacter pylori* and peptic ulcer disease in children is unclear. Hyperammonemia may be seen with inborn errors of metabolism that may present with vomiting.

6. a   Vomiting may result from a number of ingestions, particularly iron, lead, theophylline, and aspirin. This should be considered in the child with vomiting without a clear etiology. This patient presents with the hemorrhagic gastritis associated with iron ingestion. Iron is a common medication, and the fact that a new baby is present in the home suggests the possibility that the mother has prenatal vitamin and iron supplements available. Abdominal x-rays can be useful in demonstrating the presence of the radiopaque pills in the GI tract.

CHAPTER 79

Weakness/Flaccid Paralysis

KAREN DULL, M.D.

QUESTIONS

1. A 12-year-old, previously healthy girl comes into the ED complaining of weakness of both of her legs, and associated incontinence. She had fever and malaise 1 week ago. She has had a sensation of paresthesias (pins and needles) in her lower extremities for the last 3 days. Examination is significant for a temperature of 38.9°C and a decreased ability to move her lower extremities. She is able to feel a pinprick above her umbilicus, but not below it. She has no focal back tenderness. Immediate initial management should include:

   a. IV dexamethasone
   b. Emergent CT of the spine
   c. Nerve conduction studies
   d. IV antibiotics
   e. Lumbar puncture

2. A 9-month-old, previously healthy boy comes into the ED with difficulty breathing. His parents have also noted that he drools a lot. He does not crawl or sit up yet, but he smiles and lifts his head while in a prone position. On physical exam he is an alert infant lying on his back who makes and keeps eye contact with you as you move around the room. Vital signs are: HR 140, RR 48, and BP 95/55. His exam has labored respirations, tongue fasciculations, and global hypotonia. You are not able to elicit any tendon reflexes or a gag reflex. He will reach for objects, but he has difficulty holding on to them. Electrolytes and CPK (creatine phosphokinase) are within normal limits. This patient is most likely to have a disorder of the:

   a. Central nervous system (CNS)
   b. Anterior horn cell
   c. Peripheral nerves
   d. Neuromuscular junction
   e. Muscle fibers

3. The diagnosis for the patient in Question 2 can be made by:

   a. MRI of the spinal cord
   b. CT of the head
   c. Clinical exam only
   d. Muscle biopsy
   e. Challenge with edrophonium

4. A 5-year-old girl comes into the ED with weakness in her lower extremities, which (her parents state) began as pain in her lower legs 2 weeks ago. She had negative x-rays 1 week ago. She has refused to walk since yesterday, when she complained of a "scratchy" feeling in her ankles; today, she reports that she also has the same symptoms in her knees. On physical exam she is afebrile and her vital signs are normal. Her exam is significant for absent patellar reflexes and marked weakness of the flexors and extensors of her ankles, which improves as you move proximally. On examination of the CSF, you would expect to see:

   a. Pleocytosis, elevated protein, normal glucose
   b. Absent pleocytosis, normal protein, elevated glucose
   c. Absent pleocytosis, elevated protein, low glucose
   d. Pleocytosis, low protein, normal glucose
   e. Absent pleocytosis, elevated protein, normal glucose

5. A 3-month-old girl who is breast fed is brought to the ED with constipation and poor feeding persisting for 1 week. On exam you note that the infant appears tired. She is afebrile, with normal vital signs. She is drooling and does not make eye contact with you. When you examine her eyes more closely, you note that her pupils are dilated and respond poorly to light. The rest of her exam is significant for generalized hypotonia. When you tickle her foot, she cries with a very weak cry. Her deep tendon reflexes are 1+ throughout. As part of your treatment, you consider:

   a. IV immunoglobulin
   b. Acyclovir
   c. Endotracheal intubation
   d. Gentamicin
   e. Antitoxin

6. A 16-year-old girl comes into the ED, unable to move her legs shortly after running a race at her track meet. On exam she is very anxious but her sensory exam is normal. You start her on maintenance IV fluids, with D5 ½ NS with 20 mEq of KCl per liter, and order an MRI. While awaiting the MRI, she gets her strength back and begins to move her legs. The most likely cause of her symptoms is:

   a. Hypovolemia
   b. Hypoglycemia
   c. Hyponatremia
   d. Hypokalemia
   e. Conversion reaction

7. An 8-year-old boy comes into the ED with weakness and dizziness persisting for the last 6 hours. His mother found him in the garage, acting confused. He has had no recent illnesses. His vital signs are: HR 50, RR 36, and BP 124/69. On exam you note that he is sweating, with generalized weakness and some intermittent muscle twitches. His pupils are 2 mm and reactive. He has wheezing in both lung fields, although his mother states he has had no previous asthma. Treatment includes:

   a. Narcan
   b. Atropine
   c. Glucocorticoids
   d. Epinephrine
   e. Hemodialysis

ANSWERS

1. a   Transverse myelitis affects the spinal cord, producing weakness and sensory dysfunction. It commonly follows a viral illness. The MRI may show focal spinal cord widening, but transverse myelitis is a diagnosis of exclusion. The differential diagnosis includes epidural or subdural abscess, extradural or intradural tumors, and spinal arteriovenous malformations (AVM). Early transverse myelitis can be similar to Guillain-Barré syndrome, but in Guillain-Barré syndrome, bowel and bladder function are commonly preserved until later in the disease. High-dose corticosteroids should be begun until cord compression by a mass lesion is ruled out. Possible spinal cord compression is best evaluated using MRI, not CT.

2. b   Werdnig-Hoffman disease is a disease of the anterior horn cell that presents with gradual weakness of the proximal muscles. It is marked by fasciculations and early prominent loss of reflexes. The disease gradually progresses to respiratory insufficiency.

3. d   The diagnosis of Werdnig-Hoffman disease is usually made by muscle biopsy. The biopsy shows a characteristic immature denervation that is distinct from normal mature muscle. Sural nerve biopsy may show mild neuropathic changes.

4. e   Guillain-Barré syndrome is a postinfectious demyelinating polyneuropathy that generally presents as ascending symmetrical weakness over a period of days to weeks. It usually begins in the legs and moves proximally. *Campylobacter jejuni* has been shown to be associated with the disease. The protein level in the CSF is usually doubled; the CSF glucose and cell count are normal.

5. c Botulism affects the neuromuscular junction. It occurs when an infant ingests *Clostridium* spores. It has traditionally been associated with honey, which has a high concentration of spores. Breast feeding is also associated with botulism; this seems to be related to the changes in the gut flora. Botulism is characterized by global muscle weakness, constipation, and mydriasis. The sensory exam is normal. The diagnosis is usually made on the basis of history and physical exam. The CSF may show an normal glucose, increased protein concentration, and no pleocytosis. An EMG will show a characteristic brief, low-amplitude, overabundant motor reaction potentials. The diagnosis is confirmed by demonstrating the presence of *C. botulinum* in the stool.

6. d Hypokalemic periodic paralysis presents as sudden paralysis that may involve all the extremities, usually after a large carbohydrate load or during rest following strenuous exercise. Improvement of paralysis usually occurs after IV potassium (KCl) has been administered.

7. b Organophosphates are commonly found in pesticides that irreversibly phosphorylate acetylcholinesterase, allowing acetylcholine accumulation, which causes muscarinic (salivation, lacrimation, urination, and gastrointestinal cramping) and nicotinic effects (weakness, sweating, muscle twitching, tremors, and paralysis). The management includes careful decontamination to avoid pesticide exposure of medical personnel, along with administration of atropine and pralidoxime. Atropine should be given in a dose of 0.05–0.1 mg/kg to children and 2–5 mg/kg for adolescents and adults. The dose may need to be repeated.

CHAPTER 80

Wheezing

VINCENT J. WANG, M.D.

QUESTIONS

1. A 5-month-old girl is brought to the ED with wheezing. Her parents report that she has had cough, rhinorrhea, and a low-grade fever for several days. She attends daycare, where many other children have similar symptoms. She is alert and interactive, but with an RR of 60. Her pulse oximetry shows an O_2 saturation of 93% on room air. Her most likely diagnosis is:

   a. Anaphylaxis
   b. Foreign body aspiration
   c. Bronchiolitis
   d. Asthma
   e. Congestive heart failure (CHF)

2. A 2-year-old boy with severe gastroesophageal reflux and developmental delay is brought to the ED by his mother because he has been breathing faster than usual. He has had cough for several days and has a low-grade fever. On examination, he has an RR of 36 and has minimal intercostal retractions. He has wheezing in the right upper lobe. His pulse oximetry shows an O_2 saturation of 99% on room air. Treatment includes:

   a. SC epinephrine
   b. Intubation and assisted ventilation
   c. Nebulized albuterol
   d. Amoxicillin
   e. IV furosemide

3. A 4-year-old boy was eating peanuts at a baseball game when he suddenly developed wheezing. He presents in the ED in moderate distress, with swelling of his lips and tongue. He has diffuse wheezing. Appropriate treatment at this time includes:

   a. SC epinephrine
   b. Intubation and assisted ventilation
   c. Nebulized albuterol
   d. Amoxicillin orally
   e. IV furosemide

4. A 1-year-old girl was eating at home when she suddenly developed coughing and choking. She is brought to the ED, where on examination you note asymmetrical breath sounds and wheezing in the right chest. Helpful tests include all of the following, EXCEPT:

   a. Inspiratory and expiratory CXRs
   b. Soft tissue neck radiographs
   c. Bilateral decubitus CXRs
   d. Bronchoscopy
   e. Airway fluoroscopy

5. A 3-month-old boy has had difficulty breathing. The patient is brought to the ED by his aunt, who is not sure of his history, but says that he takes some kind of medicine daily. He has had cough for several days. On examination, he is small for age and in moderate distress. His HR is 180 and his RR is 55. He has diffuse wheezing on auscultation of his chest, and you think you hear a murmur. He is diaphoretic and his abdomen is distended, with his liver edge palpable 3 cm below his right costal margin. Treatment includes:

   a. SC epinephrine
   b. Intubation and assisted ventilation
   c. Nebulized albuterol
   d. Amoxicillin orally
   e. IV furosemide

6. A 2-year-old white (Caucasian) boy has cough and wheezing. He has had multiple URIs in the past and the mother says he has frequent oily stools. On examination, he is small for age and in mild distress. The most helpful diagnostic test is:

   a. CT of the chest
   b. CXR
   c. Sweat testing
   d. Echocardiogram
   e. Bronchoscopy

7. A 5-year-old girl complains of recurrent coughing and wheezing. She has had multiple episodes in the past. She has also had atopic dermatitis and a history of sinusitis. She developed symptoms currently, when the weather changed. She is alert, well nourished, and well developed. She has an RR of 30, with minimal intercostal retractions. The most likely diagnosis can be made by:

a. Clinical history and examination
b. CXR
c. Sweat testing
d. Echocardiogram
e. Bronchoscopy

ANSWERS

1. c The patient has bronchiolitis, an acute viral infection of the lower respiratory tract. Treatment is largely supportive. Adequate hydration and feeding may be compromised as a result of the respiratory illness. Treatment may include IV hydration and administration of oxygen for hypoxia. Nebulized albuterol or racemic epinephrine treatments may also be helpful. The other choices are common causes of respiratory distress and wheezing, but given the history, bronchiolitis would be the most likely diagnosis.

2. d Pulmonary aspiration may occur in patients with neuromuscular disorders or developmental delay. Patients often have a history of recurrent aspiration of gastric contents, with associated aspiration pneumonia. The patient is in minimal distress; therefore, oral antibiotic therapy for pneumonia would be appropriate.

3. a Anaphylaxis typically presents with an acute onset of respiratory distress, accompanied by urticaria and other signs of capillary leakage phenomena. The patient in this scenario probably has an allergy to peanuts. Given his respiratory distress and oropharyngeal swelling, subcutaneous epinephrine is indicated immediately.

4. b Soft tissue neck films are diagnostically helpful for obstruction of the upper airway, such as epiglottitis or croup, but are not helpful in this scenario. The sudden onset of symptoms in the given scenario, without fever, upper respiratory symptoms, and anaphylactic symptoms, strongly suggests a foreign body aspiration. Foreign body aspiration typically occurs in toddlers, but may occasionally occur in older infants. In addition, this patient's physical examination confirms the diagnosis. Each of the tests except soft tissue neck radiographs will aid in the diagnosis. Bronchoscopy will confirm the diagnosis, as well as treat the problem.

5. e The patient has signs and symptoms suggestive of congestive heart failure (CHF). The history suggests that he has a chronic condition, and his symptoms are consistent with this diagnosis. CHF is an uncommon cause of wheezing in childhood. Other signs and symptoms of CHF include cyanosis, heart murmurs, poor perfusion, abnormal pulses, and distended neck veins. Judicious use of furosemide is indicated.

6. c Cystic fibrosis is the most common life-threatening recessive genetic trait among patients of Caucasian ethnicity, and is characterized by recurrent respiratory infections, failure to thrive, and malabsorption. Sweat testing or DNA testing may be used to confirm the diagnosis. CT scanning of the chest would help diagnose extrinsic causes of wheezing, such as mediastinal tumors, enlarged lymph nodes, or other congenital structural anomalies. A CXR would help diagnose pneumonia, foreign body aspirations, and bronchiolitis. An echocardiogram would evaluate cardiac disease; bronchoscopy would delineate any structural anomalies and detect foreign body aspiration.

7. a Asthma is the most common cause of wheezing in children older than 1 year. It is characterized by recurrent episodes of wheezing and/or coughing, often precipitated by environmental allergens, weather changes, and exercise. Patients with asthma often have other atopic disease, such as sinusitis, atopic dermatitis, conjunctivitis, and allergic rhinitis. With this history, further testing is not necessary, but some would obtain a CXR to rule out other causes of wheezing. Nevertheless, the diagnosis of asthma is made by history and physical examination.

CHAPTER 81

Weight Loss

VINCENT J. WANG, M.D.

QUESTIONS

1. You are evaluating an infant in the ED because of concerns of the parents that the infant is not gaining appropriate weight. Which of the following patients demonstrates normal growth and behavior?

   a. A 4-week-old boy who has forceful vomiting, worsening over 1 week
   b. A 1-week-old boy who weighs less than his birth weight
   c. A 4-week-old girl who becomes diaphoretic during feeds
   d. A 3-week-old boy who has a weak sucking reflex
   e. A 4-week-old girl who has malodorous loose stools

2. A 2-month-old girl is referred to you in the ED for poor feeding since birth. She is thin and small for age, with head circumference, length, and weight below the fifth percentile. Helpful diagnostic testing includes:

   a. Bone marrow biopsy
   b. Skeletal series
   c. Social work consult
   d. Serum chemistries
   e. Sweat testing

3. A 12-year-old boy complains of fatigue and weight loss. His mother reports that he has had less energy over the past few weeks. He has been anorexic and has lost approximately 4–5 kg. On examination, his HR is 90 bpm and his BP is 85/50. You notice hyperpigmentation of his genitalia and his nipples. Treatment includes:

   a. IV administration of ceftriaxone
   b. IV administration of dopamine
   c. Dietary counseling
   d. IV administration of hydrocortisone
   e. Testing pancreatic enzymes

4. A 14-year-old girl complains of intermittent abdominal pain for many months. She has had loose stools and a 5-kg weight loss. She also complains of joint pains. Helpful diagnostic testing includes:

   a. Abdominal U/S
   b. Pelvic U/S
   c. Urinalysis
   d. Erythrocyte sedimentation rate (ESR)
   e. Arthrocentesis

ANSWERS

1. b   Infants lose weight after birth, but typically regain their birth weight by 10–14 days of life. While some spitting up may be because of feeding techniques, projectile vomiting is abnormal and suggests that the patient may have pyloric stenosis. Congenital heart disease or pulmonary disease will often cause infants to sweat or tire during feedings. The sucking reflex is an inborn reflex in all children, and therefore, weak or poor sucking is abnormal and may suggest a neuromuscular or neurologic disease. The stooling patterns of children may vary, but a history of malodorous loose stools, in the setting of failure to thrive, suggests malabsorption in the GI tract.

2. d   Patients who present with abnormalities of all three growth parameters may have genetic, metabolic, or neurologic etiologies for their growth delay. Serum chemistries may reveal an underlying metabolic disorder. A bone marrow biopsy would help diagnose a hematologic or oncologic process, which is unlikely to cause tri-parameter growth delay in an infant. Skeletal dysplasias may cause proportional length and weight decreases, but would be unlikely to cause changes in head circumference. Thus, a skeletal series is unlikely to be helpful. A social work consult to determine if the patient is being deprived or neglected is helpful in a patient with a subnormal weight, when other diagnoses have been excluded. Even with severe deprivation, the infant's length may not be affected. Sweat testing for the diagnosis of cystic fibrosis is helpful in patients who present with poor weight gain, but it would be rare that cystic fibrosis causes length and head circumference changes.

3. d   Addison's disease will typically present with the gradual onset of symptoms as described. Hyperpigmentation may also involve the axilla, umbilicus, and joints. Administration of IV fluids and hydrocortisone are indicated, before the patient develops an adrenal crisis. Given the constellation of symptoms, sepsis is unlikely, and there is no indication for antibiotics at this time. Dopamine is not indicated for the low BP. Although anorexia nervosa may present with chronic fatigue, dehydration, and low BP, the other symptoms do not support this diagnosis, and therefore dietary counseling will not be helpful. Cystic fibrosis would also be unlikely in this scenario; therefore, testing pancreatic enzymes is not indicated.

4. d   Inflammatory bowel disease may cause chronic abdominal pain, diarrhea, and weight loss. Arthritis and rash may be associated as well. An elevated ESR may aid the diagnosis, but endoscopy will provide the definitive diagnosis. Abdominal or pelvic ultrasound will be helpful to evaluate an appendicitis, an abdominal mass, or pelvic pathology. A UTI may present with persistent abdominal pain, but the other symptoms suggest that this is not the likely etiology. Arthrocentesis of the affected joints is unlikely to reveal a diagnosis, since most joint fluid specimens will be normal.

Medical Emergencies

CHAPTER 82

Cardiac Emergencies

SUJIT SHARMA, M.D.

QUESTIONS

1. The parents of a 2-month-old girl note that she is breathing rapidly. Her HR is 170 and RR is 52. Lungs are clear to auscultation, and a systolic murmur is heard. The liver edge is palpable 3 cm below the right costal margin. Which of the following conditions is the most UNLIKELY cause of her symptoms?

   a. Ventricular septal defect (VSD)
   b. Atrial septal defect (ASD)
   c. Patent ductus arteriosus (PDA)
   d. Anomalous left coronary artery
   e. Atrioventricular (AV) canal defect

2. The parents of a 3-month-old boy complain that he is breathing fast and has not been gaining weight. His RR is 68 with a HR of 180. He is slightly pale and has an O_2 saturation of 93% on room air. You note a systolic murmur on cardiac auscultation and a liver edge 4 cm below the costal margin. Which of the following conditions is the patient most likely to be suffering from?

   a. VSD
   b. Transposition of the great arteries
   c. Pulmonary atresia
   d. Cystic fibrosis
   e. Tetralogy of Fallot

3. A 2-month-old boy presents with tachypnea, poor feeding, and lethargy. His HR is 160 and BP is 85/60 in upper and lower extremities. No murmur is heard. Which of the following conditions is the most likely cause of his symptoms?

   a. Anomalous left coronary artery
   b. VSD
   c. ASD
   d. Congenital heart block
   e. Coarctation of the aorta

4. A 3-month-old girl presents to the ED with a history of poor feeding and respiratory difficulty, which has been getting worse over the past 2–3 weeks. HR is 168; RR is 72, with grunting. The liver is 3 cm below the right costal margin and you hear a systolic heart murmur. Which of the following is most likely to worsen the patient's condition?

   a. Elevate head and chest
   b. Administer O_2
   c. Furosemide (Lasix)
   d. IV 20 ml/kg NS bolus
   e. Digoxin

5. A 5-day-old girl is brought to the ED appearing lethargic and pale. Vital signs are: T 37.2°C, HR 186, RR 72 (labored), and BP 48/palpable. Capillary refill time is greater than 4 seconds and no rash is noted. An emergent portable CXR shows cardiomegaly. Which of the following should you administer?

   a. Dopamine
   b. Dobutamine
   c. Prostaglandin
   d. Furosemide
   e. Epinephrine

6. A 1-month-old boy, born to a mother with systemic lupus erythematosus (SLE), comes to the ED with tachypnea, grunting respirations, and hepatomegaly. He has an HR of 36, and a BP of 82/43. Which of the following should be administered?

   a. Digoxin
   b. Propranolol
   c. Theophylline
   d. Atropine
   e. Isoproterenol

7. A 10-month-old boy is brought to the ED with a history of being irritable through the night. His parents report that he has become more pale and lethargic over the past few hours. On presentation in the ED he appears difficult to arouse. His skin is mottled, with poor perfusion. The HR is 240; BP is 60/palpable. Which of the following should be the initial intervention for this patient?

   a. Carotid massage
   b. IV lidocaine
   c. IV verapamil
   d. Synchronized cardioversion
   e. IV digoxin

8. A 5-year-old boy with a history of a fast heart rate is evaluated in the ED for fever and cough and is diagnosed with a URI. His mother is interested in using over-the-counter cold medications for symptomatic relief. What advice do you give?

   a. Oral medications with a combination of antihistamine and sympathomimetic agents are safe to use
   b. Oral medications with only pure antihistamine effect should be used
   c. Oral medications with only pure sympathomimetic effect should be used
   d. Neo-Synephrine nose drops should be used
   e. None of these medications should be used

9. A 10-year-old girl with a history of Tetralogy of Fallot repair as an infant comes in to ED with complaints of palpitations. She is well perfused and has a normal BP. Her lead II rhythm strip is shown below:

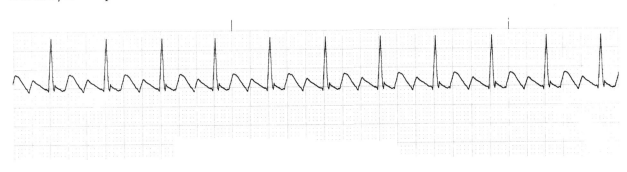

Which of the following therapies should be used initially for treatment of this condition?

   a. Adenosine
   b. Procainamide
   c. Diltiazem
   d. Cardioversion
   e. Digoxin

10. An 11-year-old girl presents to the ED in sustained wide complex tachycardia with an HR of 150. Her BP is 95/55 and capillary refill time is 2 seconds. Which of the following would have NO role as first- or second-line therapy?

   a. IV procainamide
   b. IV lidocaine
   c. Cardioversion
   d. IV propranolol
   e. IV amiodarone

11. Serum electrolytes on a 2-year-old girl presenting with DKA reveal the following values: Na 129 mEq/l, K 6.9 mEq/L, Cl 97 mEq/L, CO_2 8 mEq/L, BUN 18 mg/dL, Cr 0.9 mg/dL, and glucose 421 mg/dL. Which of the following findings are likely to appear first on the ECG?

   a. Increase in PR interval
   b. Peaked T waves
   c. Decrease in P wave amplitude
   d. Widening of QRS complex
   e. Increase in P wave duration

12. A 14-year-old boy with asthma and a history of depression is believed to have had a syncopal episode at school. A 12-lead ECG performed in the ED shows sinus rhythm with the following rates and intervals: HR 100, RR 0.64 sec, QRS 0.08 sec, QT 0.4 sec, and PR 0.12 sec. Which of the following is the most likely cause of this patient's problem?

    a. Hypercalcemia
    b. Amitriptyline
    c. Albuterol
    d. Theophylline
    e. Ipratoprium bromide

13. A previously healthy 13-year-old boy presents to the ED with complaints of chest pain and shortness of breath. Other than a recent URI, his medical history is unremarkable. He is afebrile, with an HR of 116 and a BP of 94/60. Breath sounds are present throughout the chest, but his heart sounds seem distant. Which of the following will be MOST helpful in determining the clinical severity of the disease process?

    a. CXR
    b. ABG
    c. Measurement of pulsus paradoxus
    d. 12-lead ECG
    e. Determination of pulsus alterans

14. A previously healthy 14-year-old boy presents with complaints of chest pain for 2 days. He just recovered from a "flulike" illness last week. He is afebrile, with normal vital signs. His pulsus paradoxus measurement is less than 10 mmHg. A continuous friction rub is heard on cardiac auscultation. All of the following are possible findings on ancillary studies, EXCEPT:

    a. Diminished precordial voltage on ECG
    b. Elevation of ST segments on ECG
    c. Normal cardiac silhouette on CXR
    d. Diffuse T wave inversions on ECG
    e. Clear lung fields by CXR

15. A 9-year-old with a history of ASD presents with fever for 3 weeks. On physical exam a heart murmur is heard and you note subungual hemorrhages. Total peripheral WBC count is 21,000/mm³, with a platelet count of 98,000/mm³. Which of the following bacterial pathogens is the most likely cause of these findings?

    a. *Streptococcus pneumoniae*
    b. *Streptococcus viridans*
    c. *Enterococcus faecalis*
    d. *Staphylococcus aureus*
    e. *Staphylococcus epidermidis*

16. A 15-month-old boy with a history of congenital heart disease presents to the ED acutely cyanotic, crying, and irritable. Initial interventions, including positioning, oxygen administration, and IM morphine sulphate produce no improvement. In considering further measures, which of the following would be contraindicated?

    a. IV fluid bolus
    b. IV propranolol
    c. IV verapamil
    d. IV sodium bicarbonate (NaHCO₃)
    e. IV phenylephrine

17. A 7-year-old girl comes to the ED with complaints of fever and joint pain for the past 4 days. On examination you note a holosystolic heart murmur, heard best at the apex, as well as swelling of the left knee and ankle. Which of the following statements regarding her illness are true?

    a. Joint effusions do not occur
    b. Polyarthritis is frequently found
    c. Joint involvement is typically static
    d. Smaller joints are typically involved
    e. The fevers are usually high grade

ANSWERS

1. b All of the above-named conditions in Question 1 may present with clinical manifestations of congestive heart failure (CHF). VSD, ASD, PDA, and AV canal defects all cause CHF by left to right shunting and subsequent volume overload. However, ASD does not typically present until after 6 months of age. Coronary artery anomalies (e.g., anomalous left coronary artery) cause CHF via ischemia to the ventricular myocardium, and typically will present in the first 6 months of life.

2. a Tetralogy of Fallot, pulmonary atresia, and transposition of the great arteries are cyanotic cardiac diseases associated with right to left shunting of blood within the heart, causing cyanosis, not CHF. Cystic fibrosis is unlikely in this patient, because his respiratory problems are due to CHF. A VSD would cause the signs and symptoms noted in this patient via left to right shunting of blood and subsequent volume overload. This takes place after the immediate newborn period, when pulmonary vascular resis-

tance drops enough to allow for increased flow to the lungs. Other conditions causing left to right shunting that may also present in the first three months of life include AV canal defects as well as patent ductus arteriosus (PDA). Extracardiac shunting of blood via AV malformations should also be kept in mind.

3. a Cardiac output depends on four main components: heart rate, preload, afterload, and contractility. An anomalous left coronary artery arises from the pulmonary artery rather than the aorta. Myocardial contractility will be primarily impaired, secondary to ischemic damage to the ventricular myocardium. This is apparent on the 12-lead ECG. Although septal defects are much more common congenital abnormalities causing heart failure via increases in preload, you would expect to auscultate a murmur on examination. Coarctation of the aorta can present with signs of heart failure as well, via increasing afterload; however, one would expect differential blood pressures between the upper and lower extremities, as well as diminished femoral pulses. Patients with congenital heart block can develop signs of heart failure due to severe bradycardia, but the HR will usually be below 60.

4. d Supportive measures in initial management of patients in CHF, such as positioning and O_2 administration are easily initiated. Further therapy includes medications aimed at correcting some of the underlying problems, such as furosemide (Lasix) and digoxin. Bolusing a patient in CHF with large amounts of IV fluids is contraindicated, however, because this is likely to worsen the volume-overload state already present.

5. c These constellation of findings in a 5-day-old infant are consistent with cardiogenic shock related to closing of the ductus arteriosus. Disease states in which cardiac output from the left side of the heart is impeded (i.e., critical aortic stenosis) depend on a patent ductus arteriosus to allow blood to flow to the aorta from the pulmonary artery. These patients will therefore present rather acutely with cardiogenic shock when the ductus arteriosus closes, usually within the first two weeks of life. Other conditions one would expect to present similarly are hypoplastic left heart syndrome, interrupted aortic arch, and severe coarctation of the aorta. This patient has a ductal-dependent lesion, so keeping the ductus arteriosus patent with prostaglandin E_1 (PGE_1) is critical to his immediate survival. Other supportive medications such as pressor agents and diuretics may be needed in the event that the heart has sustained significant damage; however, starting PGE_1 would be the priority.

6. e The history and presentation in this case are consistent with congenital heart block as the cause of this patient's bradycardia. In particular, infants born to mothers with SLE may develop heart block. As with sinus bradycardia in infants, assuring adequate ventilation and oxygenation and treatment of acidosis are crucial initial steps in the management of heart block. Specific to the treatment of complete/congenital heart block, pharmacologic intervention should include isoproterenol and/or epinephrine, followed by temporary pacing. Although atropine is indicated in the treatment of sinus bradycardia, it is not helpful in the treatment of congenital heart block. Propranolol and digoxin should not be used in the treatment of heart block.

7. d This patient is presenting in shock. The history and presentation support the diagnosis of SVT as the cause. Although vagal maneuvers or IV adenosine should be used as initial interventions in patients presenting with mild to moderate CHF secondary to SVT, patients presenting with severe CHF and shock require immediate attention. Although adenosine can be used in these instances if it is immediately available, synchronized cardioversion should be performed as soon as possible (assuming that the ABC's—airway, breathing, and circulation—have been attended to). Lidocaine is not indicated in the treatment of SVT. Verapamil is contraindicated in infants less than 1 year of age. IV digoxin is a secondary treatment for critical SVT in the acute setting and is the drug of choice for chronic treatment of AV nodal reentrant SVT in children.

8. b The sympathomimetic amines in many of the over-the-counter cold preparations can provoke an episode of SVT and therefore should not be used in patients with a history compatible with SVT. Agents with pure antihistaminic effect (i.e. diphenhydramine), are safe for use in these patients, however, as are pure cough-suppressant agents.

9. e Stable patients presenting in atrial flutter, as in this case, or fibrillation, should initially be converted chemically with digoxin for the first 24 hours. Procainamide is the second-line choice if there is no re-

sponse to digoxin. Synchronized cardioversion would be the next step if the patient still had not converted to a sinus rhythm, or if there were any signs of decompensation. Adenosine will slow down the AV block, but will usually not work to correct the arrhythmia. Diltiazem is not indicated.

10. d   Treatment of ventricular tachycardia depends on the clinical status of the patient at the time of diagnosis. In the stable patient, pharmacological intervention, usually starting with lidocaine, can be used, as can amiodarone or procainamide. Synchronized cardioversion should be the initial intervention if there are any clinical signs of cardiac decompensation. IV propranolol is not used in the treatment of ventricular tachycardia.

11. b   Hyperkalemia would be the most concerning electrolyte abnormality in this patient in regards to possible arrhythmia. Peaking of the T waves are the first ECG finding in hyperkalemia and can be seen with concentrations of 5–6 mEq/l. Widening of the QRS usually takes place above 6 meq/l; decreases in the p wave amplitude/duration and PR-interval prolongation take place above levels of 7 meq/l.

12. b   This patient has a corrected QT interval (QTc) of 0.5 sec, which is significantly prolonged. The condition can be congenital or acquired, as in this case. Many drugs can cause a prolongation of the QT interval; however, of the drugs listed, amitriptyline is the one most likely to cause QT prolongation. Hypercalcemia will cause shortening of the QT interval, whereas hypocalcemia will cause prolongation.

13. c   This patient has clinical signs of pericardial effusion secondary to pericarditis, and therefore should be assessed immediately for signs of tamponade. Although there may be distension of the neck veins, enlargement of the cardiac shadow on CXR, or nonspecific ECG changes, these signs will not illuminate the degree of limitation to cardiac output as will testing for pulsus paradoxus.

14. a   This patient's presentation is consistent with acute pericarditis. The finding of a friction rub on auscultation is not only indicative of inflammation, but also indicates that there is not significant fluid accumulation. Decrease in precordial voltages on ECG and an increase in the cardiac silhouette are findings directly related to the accumulation of pericardial fluid, and therefore should not be seen in this patient. ST-segment elevations and T wave inversions are findings related to pericarditis without significant fluid accumulation, as are clear lung fields on CXR.

15. b   This patient has findings very suggestive of infective endocarditis. *Streptococcus viridans* most commonly enters the bloodstream during oral (dental) procedures, and is therefore most commonly seen in patients with underlying congenital heart disease. *Staphylococcus aureus* is also commonly isolated, usually in patients with structurally normal hearts and in those with postoperative congenital heart disease.

16. c   Medical interventions for the treatment of cyanotic (hypoxemic) spells are aimed at increasing systemic vascular resistance (by administering phenylephrine) and increasing pulmonary blood flow (via fluid bolus) as a means to decrease right to left shunting. Propranolol and sodium bicarbonate appear to help in breaking part of the vicious circle of infundibular spasm and acidosis. Verapamil is an agent that directly decreases systemic vascular tone and would thereby worsen right to left shunting. It can also cause profound hypotension in infants and its use is therefore contraindicated in children less than 3 years of age.

17. b   This patient presents with signs very suggestive of acute rheumatic fever (ARF). Murmurs indicative of mitral insufficiency (apical systolic murmur) or aortic insufficiency (diastolic decrescendo murmur) should make one very suspicious of acute carditis. Polyarthritis is the most common of the major Jones criteria, followed by carditis. Actual joint inflammation should be noted on exam. ARF is typically a migratory polyarthritis involving the larger joints of the upper and lower extremities. Fevers in ARF are typically low grade and not associated with chills or rigors.

CHAPTER 83

Neurologic Emergencies

JOYCE SOPRANO, M.D.

QUESTIONS

1. A 17-month-old boy is brought to the ED for evaluation of possible recurrent seizures. His parents report that several times the patient turned blue while crying, became stiff, then "passed out" and became limp, with twitching of his arms and legs. After awakening he returned to his previous activity. His physical examination is normal. The most appropriate initial management is:

   a. Reassure parents and discharge home
   b. Obtain serum sodium and calcium levels
   c. Obtain a head CT scan
   d. Obtain an EEG
   e. Obtain a neurologic consultation

2. A 10-month-old girl is rushed to the ED after a seizure. While taking a nap, the patient was found with her eyes rolled back and shaking of all four extremities. The episode lasted 2–3 minutes. Other than a slight cold for the past 2 days, the patient has been well up to this point. On arrival to the ED, the patient is sleepy but arouses to painful stimuli. She has a T of 40°C. Other than generalized hypotonia, her neurologic examination is nonfocal. The workup should include:

   a. No further tests
   b. Lumbar puncture
   c. EEG, lumbar puncture
   d. WBC count, blood culture, lumbar puncture
   e. Head CT scan, blood culture, lumbar puncture

3. A previously healthy 15-year-old male is brought to the ED after a seizure. While at school he developed drooping of his right face and shaking of his right arm that quickly spread to generalized tonic-clonic activity. The episode lasted less than 5 minutes, and was followed by a brief period of sleepiness and weakness of his right arm. On physical examination, he is alert and oriented. His vital signs and physical examination are normal. The most appropriate management is:

   a. Schedule outpatient EEG and discharge
   b. Start carbamazepine PO and discharge
   c. Start phenytoin IV and admit
   d. Obtain emergent EEG
   e. Obtain emergent head CT scan

4. A 7-year-old girl with a long-standing seizure disorder is brought to the ED by ambulance in status epilepticus. She developed sustained generalized tonic-clonic seizure activity 30 minutes prior to arrival. Ambulance personnel were unable to obtain IV access and gave no anticonvulsant medications prior to arrival. The patient is maintained on phenytoin and carbamazepine. On arrival to the ED, her vital signs are stable, but she is having continued generalized tonic-clonic activity. You are unable to obtain IV access. The most appropriate management is:

   a. Lorazepam 0.1 mg/kg IM, repeated as needed
   b. Diazepam 1.0 mg/kg rectally (PR), followed by IM lorazepam 0.1 mg/kg
   c. Diazepam 0.5 mg/kg PR, followed by IM fosphenytoin 10 mg/kg
   d. Diazepam 0.5 mg/kg PR, followed by IM phenobarbital 10 mg/kg
   e. Paraldehyde 0.3 mg/kg PR, followed by IM fosphenytoin 10 mg/kg

5. A 3-year-old girl is referred for altered mental status. She had a low-grade fever and cold symptoms for several days, then developed a severe headache, ataxia, and increasing lethargy on the day of admission. On physical examination she is difficult to arouse. T is 39.2°C, HR 120, RR 24, and BP 94/56. She has no rash, her neck is supple, and her pupils are equal and reactive. Her reflexes are brisk and she has ankle clonus. After obtaining IV access and sending routine blood tests, the most appropriate next step is:

   a. Give normal saline (NS) 20 cc/kg IV bolus
   b. Perform a lumbar puncture
   c. Give ceftriaxone and acyclovir IV
   d. Obtain an emergent head CT scan
   e. Obtain an emergent EEG

6. A 5-day-old infant is referred to the ED for irritability for 24 hours. He is the full-term product of an uncomplicated pregnancy, born by vaginal delivery without complications. Although his mother had a history of genital herpes, she had no active lesions at the time of delivery. On physical examination, the baby is afebrile, irritable, and has no rash or mucous membrane lesions. His peripheral WBC count is 12,000. Lumbar puncture is traumatic, yielding a cell count of 40,000 RBCs per high-power field (hpf) and 62 WBCs per hpf. Blood and CSF cultures are pending. The most appropriate management is:

   a. Discharge home and await culture results
   b. Give ceftriaxone IM and discharge home
   c. Give ampicillin and gentamicin IV and admit
   d. Give acyclovir IV and admit
   e. Give ampicillin, gentamicin, and acyclovir IV and admit

7. A 14-year-old girl complains of a severe headache persisting for 12 hours. She describes the headache as throbbing and localized to the right frontal area. She has taken acetaminophen without relief. She has had similar headaches in the past, but none this severe. On physical examination, the patient is afebrile and has normal vital signs. Her optic discs are sharp and her neck is supple. The most appropriate management is:

   a. Obtain an emergent head CT scan
   b. Perform a lumbar puncture to measure opening pressure
   c. Administer propranolol PO
   d. Administer ketorolac IM
   e. Administer acetazolamide PO

8. A 12-year-old girl is brought to the ED with left-sided weakness. While at school she became nauseated, vomited once, and developed weakness of her left arm. There is no history of trauma or recent illness. On physical examination, she is afebrile and her vital signs are normal. She is alert, has slight dysarthria, a left facial droop, and weakness of the left arm. She has a II/VI systolic murmur. The most appropriate initial step is:

   a. Obtain an ECG
   b. Obtain an echocardiogram
   c. Obtain a head CT scan
   d. Obtain a brain MRI
   e. Administer heparin IV

9. A 4-year-old boy is referred to the ED with fever and refusal to walk. He has had a low-grade fever, intermittent nausea and vomiting, and nonspecific abdominal pain for several days. He refused to walk on the morning of admission. On physical examination, he is irritable, with a temperature of 38.4°C. He has a supple neck, a soft abdomen, and diffuse tenderness of the lower thoracic spine. He has decreased strength and sensation of the legs, 4+ patellar reflexes, and ankle clonus. Initial management should be to:

   a. Perform a lumbar puncture
   b. Administer broad-spectrum antibiotics IV
   c. Obtain thoracic spine plain radiographs
   d. Obtain an emergent spine CT scan
   e. Obtain an emergent spine MRI

10. A 13-year-old girl is seen in the ED for leg weakness and difficulty urinating. She reports that over the past several days she has had tingling of her legs, and now feels too weak to walk. She has been unable to urinate for the past several hours. She has had no fever, but had a URI 1 week ago. On physical examination, she is afebrile and well appearing. The strength and sensation in her legs are markedly decreased, and she has decreased sensation on her lower abdomen. Lower extremity reflexes are brisk. She has poor rectal tone and a palpable distended bladder on abdominal exam. Treatment of this condition might include:

   a. Plasmapheresis
   b. Interferon
   c. Supportive care
   d. Surgical drainage
   e. Neostigmine

11. A 7-year-old girl is brought to the ED because she is unable to walk. She reports that several days ago she had tingling of her feet. She now complains that her feet feel numb and she is having difficulty walking. Other than slight vomiting and diarrhea 10 days ago, she has been well. On physical examination she is afebrile and well appearing. She has decreased strength and sensation of the legs from the knees distally. She has absent patellar and ankle reflexes. Her rectal tone is normal. The most important initial management is:

    a. Perform a lumbar puncture
    b. Perform nerve conduction velocities
    c. Perform electromyography
    d. Obtain a spine MRI
    e. Perform a Tensilon test

12. A 6-month-old infant is brought to the ED with lethargy. His parents report that he has been constipated and feeding poorly for the past 2 days, and today has become increasingly lethargic. On physical examination he is afebrile, with normal vital signs. He has a poor suck, generalized hypotonia, and absent reflexes. Your evaluation is most likely to reveal:

    a. Hypokalemia
    b. CSF pleocytosis
    c. Positive Tensilon test
    d. Positive stool culture
    e. Abnormal head CT scan

13. A 3-year-old boy is brought to the ED with difficulty walking. His parents report that he awoke that morning with mild unsteadiness that worsened throughout the day, such that he is now refusing to walk. Other than chickenpox (varicella) 2 weeks ago, he has been well until today. On physical examination, he is afebrile and well appearing. He has mild truncal unsteadiness and an ataxic gait. The strength in his lower extremities is normal. The most likely additional finding is:

    a. A large mass in the posterior fossa on head CT scan
    b. Mild elevations of CSF lymphocytes and protein
    c. An elevated blood ethanol level
    d. Acute otitis media
    e. Absent ankle reflexes

14. A 6-year-old girl is rushed to the ED because her mother thinks she is having seizures. She reports that her daughter has had a worsening jerking of the face and hands over the past 4 days. At first the mother thought this was a nervous habit. The patient has been well other than a slight sore throat 2 months ago and nasal congestion 1 week ago. On physical examination the patient is afebrile, alert, and well appearing. She has involuntary jerking of the face and hands, mild hypotonia, and normal reflexes. The most appropriate initial management of this patient is:

    a. Administer diphenhydramine IV
    b. Administer lorazepam IV
    c. Administer carbamazepine PO
    d. Obtain a 12-lead ECG
    e. Obtain an EEG

15. An 11-year-old boy complains of blurry left-sided vision that has been worsening over the past 2 days. He has pain of the left eye as well, but no headache or vomiting. On physical examination, he is afebrile, with HR 80 and BP 100/60. His visual acuity in the left eye is markedly decreased, and his left optic disc margins are blurred. His left pupil dilates after swinging the flashlight from the right eye to the left. The remainder of his exam is normal. The most appropriate management is:

    a. Recommend treatment for multiple sclerosis (MS)
    b. Obtain an emergent head CT scan
    c. Start acetazolamide PO
    d. Start broad-spectrum antibiotics IV
    e. Start prednisone PO

ANSWERS

1. a   This patient is having cyanotic breath-holding spells, which can often be mistaken for seizures. The classic history and lack of a postictal period differentiate this condition from seizures. The family should be reassured that the episodes, though recurrent, will resolve prior to age 4–5 years. Further testing is not necessary when the diagnosis of breath-holding spells is clear.

2. d   This patient had a simple febrile seizure (single generalized seizure lasting less than 15 minutes). Frequently the patient develops the seizure at the onset of a high fever. Lumbar puncture is recommended in patients less than 12 months old, in any case of suspected meningitis, and when the febrile

seizure is complex. Head CT scan and EEG are not recommended in the workup of simple febrile seizures. The source of the fever should be evaluated based on the age of the patient and height of the fever. In this patient, WBC count and blood culture should be obtained to exclude occult bacteremia. Obtaining serum calcium, magnesium, and phosphorus are not indicated in this setting.

3. e Head CT scan is indicated in the emergency management of any seizure with focal features to exclude trauma or structural abnormalities. EEG is not recommended in the emergency management of most seizures but should be scheduled as an outpatient study. Anticonvulsant medications are generally not indicated after a single uncomplicated, nonfebrile seizure until results of the EEG are known.

4. c Benzodiazepines are the first drug of choice for the treatment of status epilepticus. In the absence of IV access, diazepam can be given rectally at a dose of 0.5–1.0 mg/kg. Since the duration of action is less than 30 minutes, additional anticonvulsant medication is needed to prevent seizure recurrence. Since the patient is chronically on phenytoin, the second drug of choice in this case is fosphenytoin, which, unlike phenytoin, can be given IM. The initial dose of fosphenytoin should be 5–10 mg/kg until the patient's serum phenytoin level is obtained. Lorazepam cannot be used IM, and rectal paraldehyde is recommended only when other agents are ineffective.

5. b This clinical scenario is most consistent with encephalitis or meningitis. Since the patient has no signs of increased intracranial pressure (ICP), lumbar puncture should be performed prior to head CT scan. Antibiotics and antiviral medications should be started after CSF is obtained. Head CT and EEG may be required, depending on the CSF results and clinical course. As long as vital signs are stable, large IV fluid boluses should be avoided in any patient with altered mental status, to avoid possible increases in cerebral edema.

6. e Even though the patient's mother had no active herpes lesions at the time of delivery, viral shedding can still occur, putting the infant at risk of developing herpes infection. Herpes encephalitis in infants can occur with and without mucocutaneous manifestations. Symptoms range from slight fever and irritability to fulminant coma and death. Bacterial meningitis can cause similar symptoms in infants. Since the CSF is uninterpretable in this case, the infant must be treated presumptively for both bacterial meningitis and herpes encephalitis, pending results of CSF culture.

7. d This patient suffers from common migraines, which often can be treated successfully with ketorolac IM. Propranolol is indicated for the chronic suppression of migraines, not the acute management. Head CT scan is not necessary in a patient with a history of similar episodes and a nonfocal neurologic exam. Idiopathic intracranial hypertension (IIH) is unlikely in this patient without papilledema, thus measurement of opening pressure is not indicated. Acetazolamide is indicated for the treatment of IIH, not migraine.

8. c This patient has a neurologic deficit that may be due to a cerebrovascular accident (CVA) in the right middle cerebral artery distribution. Head CT scan should be done initially to exclude a hemorrhagic process; MRI should then be obtained if no hemorrhage is seen. ECG and echocardiogram should be obtained to determine a possible etiology of embolic stroke. Heparin has not been tested for the treatment of stroke in children, and should not be part of the initial management.

9. e This clinical scenario is suggestive of an infectious spinal cord process, such as an epidural abscess or transverse myelitis. Diagnosis is made by spine MRI, which should be obtained emergently. Plain radiographs of the spine are indicated if there is a history of trauma. Spine CT scan is not sufficient to evaluate compressive and demyelinating lesions of the spinal cord. Antibiotics may be indicated by the findings of spine MRI, but are not recommended in the initial management of this patient. Lumbar puncture is contraindicated in cases of possible spinal cord compression.

10. c The lower extremity motor and sensory deficit, together with poor rectal tone and urinary retention, are symptoms of a spinal cord disorder. The spastic weakness seen in spinal cord disorders may initially be preceded by flaccid weakness. Transverse myelitis often follows a mild viral infection, as in this case. Treatment is supportive care only, because corticosteroids have not been shown to improve outcome. Patients with epidural abscess usually have a fever and are more ill appearing. Guillain-Barré syndrome is a disease of the peripheral nerves that causes a lower motor neuron deficit with flaccid paralysis and is usually treated by plasmapheresis. Transverse myelitis may be the first manifestation of multiple sclerosis (MS); however, the diagnosis of MS would not be made at this stage. After a diagnosis of MS has

been made, many patients are started on treatment with interferons. Myasthenia gravis is a disorder of the neuromuscular junction that does not cause sensory loss. It is most often treated with neostigmine.

11. **a**   This patient with peripheral neuropathy of the lower extremities that has been worsening over several days most likely has Guillain-Barré syndrome. The diagnosis of Guillain-Barré syndrome is made by performing a lumbar puncture for CSF analysis, which shows elevated protein but normal glucose and WBC count in most cases. Although nerve conduction velocities and electromyography may support the diagnosis, they are not indicated in the initial management of this patient. Spine MRI is not indicated in conditions of peripheral nerve dysfunction. A Tensilon test is performed to diagnose myasthenia gravis, a disorder of the neuromuscular junction in which there is no deficit of the sensory nerves.

12. **d**   This clinical scenario is consistent with infantile botulism. The diagnosis is confirmed with isolation of the *Clostridium botulinum* toxin or organism from the stool. Hypokalemic periodic paralysis is seen in young adults. CSF pleocytosis is not seen in infantile botulism, and this afebrile infant is unlikely to have meningitis. Infantile myasthenia gravis, which is diagnosed by a positive Tensilon test, is extremely rare and would be expected to present with muscular weakness that improves with rest. Head CT is likely to be normal in disorders of the lower motor neuron.

13. **b**   This clinical scenario is most consistent with acute cerebellar ataxia, or postinfection cerebellitis, which commonly follows 1–2 weeks after primary varicella infection. The CSF in this disorder generally shows mild elevations in lymphocytes and protein. Patients with posterior fossa tumors would be expected to have other signs of increased intracranial pressure (ICP) on physical exam, and would be expected to have symptoms progressing over several days to weeks. Ethanol intoxication would be expected to cause sedation as well as ataxia. Although otitis media could cause slight unsteadiness, labyrinthitis with this degree of ataxia is unusual in young children. Reflexes are normal in acute cerebellar ataxia.

14. **d**   This patient likely has Sydenham's chorea, seen most often following a streptococcal infection. Because patients with this disorder have a high incidence of rheumatic fever, an ECG should be obtained in the initial workup. Acute dystonic reactions, seen after exposure to antidopaminergic drugs, typically cause sustained muscle contractions of the neck and trunk and are treated with diphenhydramine. Since the movements are typically bilateral and there is no alteration of consciousness, seizure is unlikely; thus anticonvulsant medications and EEG are not indicated at this time.

15. **e**   This patient with unilateral papilledema and visual deficit has optic neuritis. Prednisone may shorten the course of symptoms. When the papilledema is unilateral and there are no other signs of increased ICP, head CT scan is not indicated. Antibiotics are not used in this inflammatory condition. Acetazolamide is indicated for the treatment of pseudotumor cerebri, which results in bilateral papilledema and headaches. Although papilledema may be the initial symptom of multiple sclerosis in 20% of cases, the diagnosis would not be made at this stage.

CHAPTER **84**

Infectious Diseases

STEPHEN PORTER, M.D.

QUESTIONS

1. You are seeing an 8-month-old boy in the ED. He has a temperature of 41°C rectally but is otherwise well. Which of the following is true?

   a. The peripheral WBC in the absence of a blood culture is adequate prior to initiating antibiotic therapy
   b. An ESR reliably distinguishes bacteremic children from those with viral infection
   c. The Yale Observation Scale (YOS) is predictive of an at-risk group in need of empirical antibiotics
   d. The child's response to antipyresis can guide assessment of risk for bacteremia
   e. The extreme height of fever combined with an elevated WBC indicates a higher risk for bacteremia

2. A 13-month-old girl has had fever for 3 days. The fever has been as high as 38.6°C. She is happy and interactive. On examination, she has fluid behind both tympanic membranes, with minimal erythema. No other source is identified clinically. Which of the following combinations of laboratory tests is appropriate?

   a. Blood culture and CBC
   b. CBC alone
   c. Blood culture, CBC, culture and analysis of catheterized urine, and CSF culture and cell count
   d. Urine for UA and culture by bladder catheterization
   e. CXR

3. A 23-month-old girl is brought back to the ED for reevaluation after a blood culture drawn from the day prior is shown to have Gram-positive cocci in pairs. The only other tests at her first visit were a CBC (WBC 17,200) and UA (normal). Her temperature is now 39°C. A dose of IM ceftriaxone was given empirically 26 hours ago. Her treatment should include all of the following EXCEPT:

   a. A lumbar puncture
   b. Repeat blood culture
   c. Oral penicillin
   d. CXR
   e. Acetaminophen

4. Early empirical antibiotic therapy is indicated for which of the following patients, who are all febrile to 38.6°C, with appropriate vital signs for their given age?

   a. An 8-year-old asthmatic who had a short course of prednisone 1 week ago
   b. A 7-month-old who was born at 26 weeks gestational age and who is on monthly IV immunoglobulin for RSV prophylaxis
   c. A 5-year-old in induction phase of chemotherapy for leukemia
   d. A native-born 4-month-old child whose sibling has sickle-cell disease (homozygous SCD)
   e. A 23-month-old who gets frequent URIs

5. A 4-year-old girl is brought to the ED for lethargy. The parents state that she was well until 18 hours previously, when she became febrile and was more difficult to arouse. She is lethargic in appearance and her vital signs are: T 39.8°C, HR 190, RR 40, and BP 85/40. Which of the following interventions is the LEAST important?

   a. CBC, PT/PTT, and blood culture
   b. IM antibiotics if the first two IV attempts are unsuccessful
   c. Fluid resuscitation with normal saline (NS) IV
   d. Administration of acetaminophen rectally
   e. Oxygen

6. It is August. A 2-month-old child has had a fever for 1 day. On arrival to triage, the patient's T is 38.8°C. A lumbar puncture reveals a CSF WBC of 50/hpf (70% neutrophils), RBC 40/hpf, protein 80 mg/dl, and glucose 40 mg/dl. These findings are best described by which of the following statements?

   a. Consistent with enteroviral meningitis
   b. Consistent with meningitis from *S. pneumoniae*
   c. Consistent with herpetic meningoencephalitis
   d. Consistent with either a viral or bacterial source
   e. None of the above

7. Age-specific incidence rates have been established for the risk of meningitis caused by bacterial organisms. Which of the following incidence rates (listed in order of decreasing incidence) is correct for the age given?

    a. 2-week-old infant: *S. pneumoniae* > group B *Streptococcus* (GBS) > *Listeria monocytogenes* > *Neisseria meningitidis*

    b. 2-month-old infant: *S. pneumoniae* > GBS > *N. meningitidis* > *H. influenzae*

    c. 3-year-old infant: *N. meningitidis* > GBS > *S. pneumoniae* > *H. influenzae*

    d. 3-week-old infant: GBS > *S. pneumoniae* > *L. monocytogenes* > *E. coli*

    e. 5-month-old infant: *S. pneumoniae* > *N. meningitidis* > GBS > *H. influenzae*

8. A 2-year-old boy is brought to the ED for fever, throat pain, and parental concern that his neck seems "stiff." All of the following could cause these symptoms EXCEPT:

    a. Sinusitis
    b. Cervical adenitis
    c. Pneumonia
    d. Pharyngitis
    e. Retropharyngeal abscess

9. A lumbar puncture is most strongly indicated for a patient who presents with which of the following scenarios?

    a. An 8-day-old infant with a temperature of 37.8°C
    b. A 5-month-old infant with a brief generalized tonic-clonic episode and a temperature on arrival of 38.6°C
    c. A 4½-month-old infant with a fever to 40°C, well-appearing and without clinical signs of infection
    d. A 3-year-old child with a ventriculoperitoneal (VP) shunt who has a T of 38.6°C and throat and neck pain, along with enlarged erythematous tonsils, palatal petechiae, and tender adenopathy at the angle of the jaw
    e. None of the above

10. You are treating a 3-month-old girl who was transferred from another hospital with history of fever, irritability, and a lumbar puncture that showed 50 RBC and 2000 WBC per hpf, with a predominance of neutrophils. Her initial serum electrolytes included a sodium (Na) value of 141. Now, 8 hours after the initial dose of antibiotics, she has a generalized seizure. All of the following interventions have a potential role in the ED EXCEPT:

    a. D10 IV
    b. Oxygen
    c. CT scan
    d. 3% NaCl IV
    e. Fluid restriction

11. You are treating a 5-month-old girl who has had fever, vomiting, and lethargy. Her CSF evaluation showed 20 RBC and 1200 WBC per hpf with 80% neutrophils and Gram-positive cocci in pairs on Gram stain. She was given IV ampicillin 50 mg/kg at another hospital 6 hours ago. Which of the following combinations of medications is most appropriate?

    a. Ceftriaxone and dexamethasone
    b. Ceftriaxone and acyclovir
    c. Ceftriaxone and vancomycin
    d. Ceftriaxone, vancomycin, and dexamethasone
    e. Chloramphenicol

12. A 7-year-old boy comes to the ED in the month of July because of fever and nuchal rigidity in the context of several days of viral symptoms. He looks well overall. There are no concerns for his hydration status. His CSF findings include 700 WBCs/hpf, 40 RBCs/hpf, protein 80 mg/dl, and glucose 50 mg/dl. The differential includes 40% neutrophils, 50% lymphocytes, and 10% monocytes. Further interpretation of his clinical picture would be augmented by knowledge of all of the following EXCEPT:

    a. Family contacts with tuberculosis (TB)
    b. Regional epidemiology of *Borrelia burgdorferi* (Lyme disease)
    c. Immune status
    d. Recent antibiotic use
    e. Resistance profile of the flora in the patient's nasopharyngeal (NP) secretions

13. A 15-year-old girl complains of sore throat and fever. On examination, she is alert and in no acute distress. She has moderate tonsillar hypertrophy with exudates and erythema. Which one of the following organisms is the most likely causative agent for typical bacterial pharyngitis in this patient?

    a. *H. influenzae*
    b. *Mycoplasma pneumoniae*
    c. *Neisseria gonorrhoeae*
    d. *Klebsiella pneumoniae*
    e. *Mycoplasma catarrhalis*

14. You are contemplating the correct therapy for a 9-month-old infant who has a T of 38.6°C, fussiness, URI symptoms and a right tympanic membrane notable for erythema, distortion of landmarks, and decreased mobility. Which one of the following should have the LEAST impact on your decision process?

    a. Previous antibiotic use
    b. Daycare attendance
    c. Resistance pattern of pneumococci in your area
    d. Previous otitis media diagnoses
    e. Data from a CBC

15. An 18-month-old child has a temperature of 38.1°C, recent history of congestion and rhinorrhea, and parental concern that she "still has a fever." Her temperature at initial diagnosis 4 days ago was 39.4°C; in the last 24 hours her fever peaked at 38.3°C. Her examination is significant for bilateral TMs notable for dullness, decreased mobility, and a retracted appearance on otoscopic exam. The child is currently being treated with amoxicillin 60 mg/kg/day, and is on day 4 of therapy. Which one of the following is the appropriate treatment regimen for this child, given the above data?

    a. Add hydroxyzine orally every 8 hours (q8h)
    b. Change to cefpodoxime b.i.d.
    c. No change in therapy
    d. Give ceftriaxone IM (single dose)
    e. Add pseudoephedrine orally q8h

16. A 23-month-old child has ear pain and drainage from the left canal. The parents are quite upset, because she just had an ear infection 3 weeks ago that they were told was "cured" at a 2-week follow-up visit. On exam, her left ear is tender to touch and has purulent drainage obscuring the canal. Which of the following is inconsistent with your likely diagnosis?

    a. Tenderness of the external ear
    b. Presence of fever
    c. Bacteria on Gram stain of drainage
    d. No history of swimming
    e. Itching as the initial symptom

17. A 3-year-old has a history of 1 week of ongoing purulent nasal discharge and fever in excess of 38.5°C for the last 3 days. He appears otherwise well. Which of the following is most appropriate for his diagnosis?

    a. CBC
    b. Gram stain of nasal secretions
    c. Sinus x-ray
    d. Transillumination of his sinuses
    e. Antral puncture

18. A 2-year-old boy has a history of swelling on the right side of his neck and complaints of pain. On exam he has a 4 cm tender lymph node that is mobile. There is some erythema to the skin overlying the node. All of the following measures are true statements, EXCEPT:

    a. PPD placement is indicated
    b. The lack of fever is consistent with his likely diagnosis
    c. Complications from this infection are rare
    d. Aspiration of a fluctuant node provides useful data
    e. Tetracycline orally is indicated

19. CT scan is most strongly indicated for the diagnosis of which of the following conditions?

    a. Retropharyngeal abscess
    b. Epiglottitis
    c. Sinusitis
    d. Lateral pharyngeal abscess
    e. Peritonsillar abscess

20. Compared to a child with epiglottitis, the patient with croup usually can be described as which of the following?

    a. Older
    b. More febrile
    c. Drooling more
    d. Coughing more
    e. None of the above

21. You are treating a 26-month-old girl who manifests stridor at rest in the setting of 2 days of URI symptoms and fevers to 38.5°C. Your management of her case should include which of the following?

    a. Lateral and AP radiographs of the neck
    b. CBC
    c. Dexamethasone therapy
    d. Albuterol nebulization
    e. O_2 mist by nasal cannula

22. An 11-month-old girl has a history of fever to 39.4°C and respiratory distress. Her parents report some decrease in her PO intake and one episode of emesis. Her RR is 50, with subcostal retractions. Her breath sounds are coarse, with some decreased aeration at the right base. No overt rales are heard. Her pulse oximetry reading shows an O_2 saturation of 92% on room air. Radiographs of her chest demonstrate a small pleural effusion on the right with a lower lobe consolidation. Which of the following is true?

    a. *S. pneumoniae* is the most likely pathogen
    b. The patient may be treated with oral amoxicillin
    c. Dehydration is a potential complication
    d. Thoracentesis is indicated
    e. There is no utility for blood cultures

23. A 10-week-old boy has a temperature to 38.2°C, cough, and a parental report of "breathing hard." On exam his RR is 50, with intermittent subcostal retractions. His O_2 saturation is 94% on room air. Auscultory findings include diffuse, coarse rales but no wheezing. CXR shows diffuse patchy atelectasis with hyperinflation. Which of the following pathogens is the most likely cause of his symptoms?

    a. *S. pneumoniae*
    b. GBS (group B *Streptococcus*)
    c. Chlamydia
    d. Varicella
    e. Measles

24. A 7-year-old boy complains of cough and fever. He has been ill for 4 days. On presentation in the ED his T is 38.5°C, his RR is 28 without retractions, and a pulse oximetry reading of O_2 saturation on room air is 96%. Rales are appreciated in both bases posteriorly. Which of the following is true?

   a. Bullous myringitis supports presumptive therapy with erythromycin

   b. A normal WBC count argues against pneumonia

   c. Lobar consolidation is inconsistent with *Mycoplasma* as the etiology

   d. Rash in conjunction with this clinical picture strongly argues for a viral etiology

   e. A cold agglutinin titer of more than 32 is diagnostic for mycoplasmal infection

25. A 4-month-old girl has had rhinorrhea, cough, and fevers to 38.2°C over the last few days. On examination, she has a RR of 50 with intercostal retractions, and a coarse expiratory noise is heard throughout her chest. Her pulse oximetry reading shows an O_2 saturation of 98% on room air. What additional data is most relevant to her care?

   a. Serum WBC

   b. UA

   c. Fluid intake and urine output history

   d. Exposure history regarding TB

   e. Quality of cough reported by parent

26. A 6-month-old boy with a history of cough, rhinorrhea, and wheezing arrives in the ED for evaluation. He is in moderate distress, with a RR of 70, intercostal and subcostal retractions, and an O_2 saturation of 91% on room air. His lung exam is notable for diffuse, coarse wheezing on expiration, without focal rales. Which of the following management strategies is correct?

   a. Methylprednisolone

   b. Racemic epinephrine nebulizer

   c. Albuterol syrup

   d. Ribavirin

   e. Chest physiotherapy

27. A 5-month-old girl has had a history of rhinorrhea and cough over the last 2 weeks. Her parents are concerned because she is coughing so hard that she cannot drink well. She does occasionally vomit after these episodes. She is afebrile and has a RR of 34 at present. Her exam is notable for subconjunctival hemorrhages OU (in both eyes), but is otherwise unremarkable. Her chest is clear to auscultation. Which of the following is true?

   a. A normal WBC is reassuring

   b. The CXR is diagnostic

   c. Respiratory arrest from airway obstruction is a potential complication

   d. Culture of NP secretions has the highest yield to identify the pathogen

   e. A child abuse consult is indicated

28. Referring to the case described in Question 27; which of the following statements are true?

   a. Observation at home is adequate

   b. Chemoprophylaxis for exposed contacts can be deferred if they have completed a series of four vaccinations for DPT (diphtheria, pertussis, and tetanus)

   c. Bacterial superinfection is responsible for few fatalities for disease

   d. 7 days of erythromycin will be sufficient for treatment

   e. Seizures are a potential complication of this scenario

29. An 11-month-old infant has had fever, cough, and occasional emesis over the last few days. On exam, T is 39.5°C, RR is 40, and the pulse oximetry reading shows an O_2 saturation of 93% on room air. His CXR is notable for a lobar consolidation with a small effusion. Hilar prominence is also noted on the plain film. Which of the following is true?

   a. A Mantoux reaction of greater than 5 mm would be diagnostic

   b. Oral amoxicillin provides adequate initial antimicrobial coverage

   b. CNS infection responds well to therapy

   c. Isoniazid should be initiated while awaiting test results

   d. A negative Mantoux reaction excludes TB from the differential

30. It is April in Boston. A 19-month-old girl presents with a history of 2 days of diarrhea (nonbloody) and a few intermittent episodes of emesis. There have been 12 loose stools today. Other children at daycare have had similar symptoms. On exam, her vital signs are T 38.4°C, HR 150, RR 30, and BP 100/60. The abdomen is benign on palpation. The rectal exam yields heme-positive stool. Which of the following is true?

   a. The vital signs would indicate a need for IV hydration

   b. Hematochezia excludes rotavirus as a diagnostic possibility

   c. Fever suggests a bacterial etiology

   d. The stool frequency indicates dehydration

   e. A return to normal stool frequency may take weeks

31. A 2-year-old boy has had a fever to 38.2°C and emesis and diarrhea over 2 days. On exam, his HR is 140, his RR is 36; he is tired appearing, with a soft abdomen. Appropriate management includes which of the following?

   a. Obtaining a CBC

   b. Kaolin-pectin (Kaopectate)

   c. Loperamide

   d. Obtaining a serum bicarbonate level

   e. Oral rehydration

32. An 18-month-old boy has had fever, abdominal pain, and diarrhea. The temperature by report has been as high as 39.5°C at home. His parents have noted an increased number of loose, bloody stools. On exam, his abdomen is nontender, without organomegaly. His CBC is notable for a WBC of 14,000 with a differential of 50% neutrophils, 20% bands, 10% lymphocytes. Potential complications of the likely organism causing his clinical picture include all of the following EXCEPT:

    a. Dehydration
    b. Seizure
    c. UTI
    d. Colonic perforation
    e. Bacteremia

33. All of the following children have histories of diarrhea with heme-positive stools found on rectal exam. Which one of the scenarios provides the strongest indication for admission to the hospital?

    a. A 6-month-old infant with a T of 38.3°C
    b. An 18-month-old child with initial HR of 140 and T of 39°C, who, after IV fluid therapy, is smiling and tolerating liquids
    c. A 3-year-old child with a serum bicarbonate level of 16
    d. An 11-month-old infant with known Hgb SS disease (sickle-cell anemia) who has a temperature of 38.4°C
    e. A 2-year-old child with a T to 40°C and a WBC of 20,000, with a left shift

34. A 6-year-old girl who recently completed a 10-day course of amoxicillin for otitis media has had abdominal pain and loose, watery stools. She has been having diarrhea for 1 week. Her parents have noted occasional blood in her stool. On examination, her vital signs are: T 38.2°C, HR 100, RR 18, and BP 95/60. Her abdomen is diffusely tender, but without peritoneal signs. Her urinalysis (UA) results are: SG 1.010, WBC 0–1, RBC 0–1; UA is otherwise negative. Her stool (produced in the ED) is frankly bloody. Additional tests should include which of the following?

    a. Blood culture
    b. *Clostridium difficile* toxin
    c. Rotavirus antigen testing
    d. Blood chemistry profile, including serum electrolytes
    e. Urine culture

35. You are evaluating a 4-year-old with a complaint of a rash and sores to his face. He has 2–3 small bullous lesions with a few scratched-open macular lesions around his nose that are crusted over. There is minimal erythema to the surrounding skin. No other infectious foci are identified on his exam. He is afebrile. Appropriate management would include:

    a. Sending a wound culture
    b. Obtaining a CBC
    c. Sending a UA
    d. Prescribing mupirocin
    e. Warm-water cleansing

36. A 2-year-old girl is brought to the ED because of a swollen right cheek. There is no history of a skin wound at the current site of the redness. She was noted to be febrile at home (to 39°C) earlier in the day, but here in the ED she has a T of 38°C 3 hours after receiving ibuprofen. Her cheek is warm to touch, red, and tender. Her dentition is normal, without evidence for caries. Appropriate management includes which of the following?

    a. Oral amoxicillin/clavulanic acid
    b. Oral cephalexin
    c. CBC, blood culture, and IV ampicillin/clavulanate
    d. IV ceftriaxone with reevaluation the next day
    e. Warm compresses

37. An 8-year-old boy is referred for evaluation of his chickenpox. He is currently at day 5 of eruption and has had much pruritus and has scratched open many of his sores. Today his fever, which on earlier days peaked at 38.5°C, went up to 39.5°C, and he had one episode of emesis. His vitals signs are T 39°C, HR 130, RR 28, and BP 110/50. He has a few new vesicular lesions and many scratched-open areas. His right arm, in particular, is swollen; is warm to the touch and quite tender along the lateral aspect. His range of motion is somewhat limited by pain. Appropriate management includes all the following EXCEPT:

    a. IV NS 20 ml/kg
    b. Surgical consultation if no improvement within 24 hours
    c. IV penicillin G 125,000 units/kg/dose
    d. Blood culture
    e. Elevation of extremity

38. A 7-year-old girl complains of limping for a few days, vague pain in her left hip area, and fever today. On arrival her temperature is 38.6°C. No infectious etiology is identified on her head, eyes, ears, nose, and throat (HEENT) or chest examination. Her range of motion (ROM) of her left hip is notable for marked tenderness with internal and external rotation, although she can flex her hip somewhat. She is unwilling to bear weight on her left leg. Which of the following tests provides reassurance, if findings are normal, to exclude septic arthritis?

    a. CBC
    b. Blood culture
    c. Plain radiograph of her hip
    d. ESR
    e. None of the above

39. A 10-month-old girl has had 2 days of tactile fevers at home and persistent fussiness. The parents state that their usual maneuvers to comfort the baby "just don't work." She has had one or two episodes of emesis today. On exam she has a T 39.5°C, HR 150, RR 44, and BP 90/50. She is fussy during the exam and is difficult to console. Her abdomen is soft. Your pulmonary exam is limited by her crying. No extremity erythema or joint swelling is appreciated. Her right leg is notable for being held in extension when her left leg is flexed when crying. Her cry intensifies when she is picked up. Appropriate evaluation may include all of the following EXCEPT:

    a. Lumbar puncture
    b. Urine culture
    c. Skeletal survey
    d. Blood culture
    e. Ultrasound (U/S) of right hip

40. Parents of a 20-month-old boy report a change in the toddler's usual gait for 5–6 days and fever for the last 3 days. He is febrile to 39°C and has tenderness over his lower left thigh. On exam, he is able to move his legs through ROM but definitely walks favoring his left leg. His ESR is 30. What plain radiographic finding will be most likely on a lower extremity x-ray, given his clinical history and exam?

    a. Lytic lesion
    b. Obscuration of deep muscle tissue planes
    c. Periosteal elevation
    d. Foreign body
    e. None of the above

41. A 15-year-old boy complains of dysuria and a purulent discharge from his penis. There are no lesions evident externally on his genitalia. There is no inguinal adenopathy. His genitourinary (GU) exam is otherwise unremarkable. He admits to being sexually active. The choice of cefixime 400 mg PO and azithromycin 1 g PO will leave which relevant and important pathogen untreated?

    a. *Chlamydia trachomatis*
    b. *Molluscum* species
    c. *Treponema pallidum*
    d. *N. gonorrhoeae*
    e. *Trichomonas vaginalis*

42. The microbiology lab at your institution called regarding a urine culture sent on a 3-year-old girl seen in the ED 36 hours ago. She had a history of intermittent dysuria and an initial UA positive (1+) for leukocyte esterase, negative for nitrite, and with a centrifuged urine microscopy of 5–10 WBCs/hpf. She was afebrile at presentation in the ED. The culture (from a clean catch) is growing 1000 Gram-negative rods. The patient was not treated empirically with antibiotics. A phone call to the parents establishes that the patient has remained afebrile. The most appropriate next step is:

    a. Amoxicillin PO
    b. Urine catheterization for repeat culture
    c. Repeat clean-catch urine specimen for culture
    d. IV ceftriaxone
    e. Observation and clinical follow-up within 1 week

43. Factors related to risk of UTI include all of the following EXCEPT:

    a. Age
    b. Gender
    c. Urinary tract anomalies
    d. Height of fever
    e. Race

44. A urinalysis was sent on an 18-month-old girl with a clinical history of fever to 38.3°C and intermittent vomiting. Her examination was unremarkable. The UA dipstick was 1+ for leukocyte esterase and nitrite positive. The sensitivity of these data for a true UTI is:

    a. 100% sensitive
    b. 80% sensitive
    c. 60% sensitive
    d. 40% sensitive
    e. 20% sensitive

45. A 3-year-old girl is in the ED for evaluation of vaginal discharge. She verbalizes discomfort with her genital area but has not disclosed a history for abuse. On exam the child has a small ulcer at the posterior fourchette and no discharge. Her hymen is unremarkable. UA by dipstick is negative. Vaginal wall bacterial culture is pending. Additional testing which will direct ED therapy at this visit include which of the following?

    a. RPR (rapid plasma reagin) test
    b. HIV (human immunodeficiency virus) serology
    c. Gram stain
    d. Tzanck smear
    e. None of above

46. A 2-year-old boy has had fever and sore throat. He has been ill for 4 days. On exam he has a temperature of 39°C with otherwise normal vital signs for age. He is able to swallow, although he states that "it hurts." His HEENT exam is notable for patchy, exudative pharyngitis, with anterior and posterior adenopathy. His neck is supple. His abdomen is without splenomegaly. His rapid strep result is negative. The heterophil-antibody (Monospot) test is pending. This test:

    a. Has a 90% chance of being positive
    b. If positive, has a 50% chance of being a false positive
    c. If negative, is definitive at excluding Epstein-Barr virus (EBV) as pathogen
    d. If positive, requires confirmation with specific serologic assays
    e. If positive, provides conclusive evidence of disease

47. It is December in Philadelphia. An 18-year-old male patient complains of high fever and lethargy. He has been ill for 5–6 days; he initially had temperatures to 39°C and cough. His mother noticed that his eyes were red and watery. A rash was noted on his face area and has now spread to his body. His mother had noted a white patch on the inside of his mouth 2 days ago. On exam his temperature is 38.9°C and he is ill appearing. He is alert, but not oriented. His HR is 110 and his RR 30. His HEENT exam is notable for mild conjunctivitis. His oral mucosa is slightly red but otherwise normal. He does have a maculopapular rash on his extremities. His neurological exam is nonfocal except for his mental status change. His disorientation does not resolve with a return to normal temperature. Which one of the following is true?

    a. His risk of mortality is 15%
    b. Sinusitis is the most common bacterial complication of this disease
    c. The portal of entry for this disease is the GI tract
    d. The lack of oral mucosa pathology is inconsistent with the diagnosis
    e. Leukopenia would be an unexpected finding

48. You are seeing a 17-year-old female patient with complaints of being tired, having an intermittent cough, and red eyes. A rash started yesterday in her neck and face, and today has spread to her trunk. Her last menstrual period (LMP) was 2 months ago. On exam she has a T of 38.3°C with otherwise normal vital signs. Her HEENT exam is notable for mild conjunctivitis in both eyes (OU) and a small, discrete, pink/red maculopapular rash on her face, neck, and trunk. She does have some slightly tender adenopathy to her posterior cervical chain. Her lungs are clear to auscultation. A pregnancy test is positive. Her diagnostic evaluation should include which of the following?

    a. Liver function tests
    b. Measles titer
    c. Rubella titer
    d. Varicella titer
    e. CXR

49. Each of the following patients is well appearing at day 2 of illness, with a cutaneous eruption consistent with varicella and a fever to 38.5°C. Oral acyclovir should be most strongly considered for which of the following?

    a. A 3-year-old child with a history of bronchiolitis in infancy, currently on no medications
    b. An 8-year-old child who takes inhaled corticosteroids for asthma, with a hospitalization 1 year ago
    c. A 13-month-old, otherwise healthy infant
    d. A 7-month-old, otherwise healthy infant
    e. A 19-year-old female patient who is in her third month of pregnancy

50. An 11-week-old boy is brought to the ED because of poor feeding and parental concern that he seems weak. On exam he is afebrile, with a RR 30 and an O_2 saturation (by pulse oximetry) of 97% on room air. His HEENT exam is notable for slight ptosis of the right eye. He sucks poorly on your finger. His reflexes are diminished symmetrically and his tone is poor. Management of his case should include which of the following?

    a. Ampicillin and gentamicin
    b. Head CT
    c. IV D25 (25% dextrose)
    d. Measurement of negative inspiratory force
    e. EEG

51. A 7-year-old boy complains of a history of malaise, fever, and now a rash. He recently returned from a camping vacation with his family. He is now in day 4 of illness. On exam he has a T of 38.6°C, HR 120, and RR 26. His HEENT exam is notable for mild conjunctivitis with periorbital edema and a normal oropharynx. A spleen tip is palpable. His skin exam is notable for a red maculopapular rash on his distal extremities that is hemorrhagic at the ankles. Which of the following would be INCONSISTENT with the likely diagnosis?

    a. Hyponatremia
    b. Thrombocytopenia
    c. Leukopenia
    d. A history of vomiting
    e. Seizure activity

52. A 3-year-old girl has had rash and fever. A physical examination finding of petechiae on the extremities could be consistent with infection from all of the following organisms EXCEPT:

    a. *Rickettsia rickettsii*
    b. *N. meningitidis*
    c. *Ehrlichia chaffeensis*
    d. *B. burgdorferi*
    e. HIV

53. A 7-year-old boy complains of a swollen right underarm. There are no family pets, although he has been playing with the neighbors' litter of kittens. He has had minor cuts and bruises over an active summer but no other health issues until he reported soreness in his axillae a few days ago. He is afebrile. On examination his axillae are notable for several 3 cm tender lymph nodes that are nonfluctuant. No peripheral evidence for infection or trauma is noted other than a resolving ecchymosis at his olecranon. You management should include which one of the following:

    a. Aspiration of nodes
    b. Extremity x-ray
    c. Ciprofloxacin PO
    d. Amoxicillin PO
    e. Azithromycin PO

ANSWERS

1. e   Lee and Harper (1998) published data which showed, in the postinfluenza era, that height of fever in combination with elevated WBC can identify a risk group for bacteremia [~10% incidence] (Lee GM, Harper MB. Risk of bacteremia for febrile young children in the post-*Haemophilus influenzae* type b era. Arch Pediatr Adolesc Med 1998;152:624–628.) (See Table 84.2 of *Textbook of Pediatric Emergency Medicine,* fourth edition). No utility has been shown for ESR, the YOS, or response to acetaminophen for identification of individual patients who are at risk from occult bacteremia. For the diagnosis of occult bacteremia, the bacteremia must be documented. Answer "a" is incorrect, because the WBC assists only with risk stratification, not with definitive diagnosis.

2. d   Many authors in recent years have documented a significant rate of UTIs in febrile infants and toddlers. For a toddler in diapers, a catheterized specimen is necessary for culture. The height of the toddler's fever does not meet criteria for occult bacteremia risk. In the absence of a history or physical exam findings to raise concern for pneumonia, a CXR is less imperative than examination of the urine.

3. c   Use of penicillin in a child who remains febrile despite a dose of ceftriaxone 26 hours prior and who is documented to have an organism likely to be *S. pneumoniae* in her blood is incorrect. This child requires a full sepsis evaluation and likely will be admitted to the hospital. The sepsis evaluation should include a repeat culture, and most practitioners would advocate for completion of a lumbar puncture to document any presence of CNS infection. A CXR may identify a pulmonary site of infection not appreciated by auscultation. Acetaminophen will assist with defervescence.

4. c   A child in induction phase for leukemia is considered at increased risk for sepsis; thus, early antibiotic therapy is indicated. A short course of steroids for an asthmatic flare is not considered immunosuppressive to the extent that empirical antibiotics are necessary. Certainly, the 7-month-old former premature infant deserves a careful exam for sources of infection, but the RSV prophylaxis does not in and of itself demand antimicrobial coverage for the given temperature. The 4-month-old infant who has a homozygous sibling with HbSS disease is at potential risk for infection if he or she were also homozy-

gous; however, if the child was born in the U.S., neonatal screening programs include HbSS in most states. If this is not true for a given state, or if the child was foreign born, then empirical coverage may be indicated as formal testing for HbSS disease is undertaken. A child with a history of frequent viral illnesses does not need empirical antibiotic coverage for a temperature of 38.6°C.

5. d This child is in septic shock. Airway and circulatory support take precedence, with prompt administration of antibiotics also an imperative. Acetaminophen is the least important action of the given choices. Some may argue that administration of antibiotics without fluid support may result in further lysis of bacteria and worsening of an already tenuous hemodynamic state. However, this is rare and should not delay antibiotics as other access avenues are attempted (either intraosseous or femoral).

6. d This infant does have evidence for meningitis, given the elevated WBC in the CSF. The WBC number alone cannot be relied upon to differentiate bacterial from viral meningitis, although many textbooks (including this one) provide a table of usual ranges (see Table 84.6 in *Textbook of Pediatric Emergency Medicine*, fourth edition). This child deserves empirical antibiotic coverage and admission to the hospital until bacterial cultures of the CSF provide the definitive answer. Given the time of year, an enteroviral pathogen is a likely suspect and may prove the causative agent. Without knowledge of increased RBCs in the CSF, herpetic meningitis is much less likely.

7. e In a child between the ages of 1 month and 23 months, *S. pneumoniae* is the most common bacterial pathogen for meningitis. It is followed in decreasing incidence by *N. meningitidis*, GBS, and *H. influenzae* (see Table 84.7 in *Textbook of Pediatric Emergency Medicine*, fourth edition). *S. pneumoniae* is less commonly found in infants who are less than 1 month of age, whereas *E. coli*, GBS, and *Listeria* are all more significant pathogens. In infants over 1 month of age, *N. meningitidis* is found more commonly than GBS as a cause of meningitis.

8. a Clinical conditions other than meningitis can cause meningeal irritation and elicit complaints of a "stiff neck." Sinusitis has not been shown to elicit neck pain in and of itself. The four remaining diagnoses have all been associated with neck pain and meningismus.

9. b Simple febrile seizures are a benign event in the majority of infants and children between the ages of 6 months and 5 years. However, the workup of a simple febrile seizure for a child less than 6 months of age (some experts would say 12 months of age) must include a lumbar puncture to rule out meningitis as a cause. An otherwise well 8-day-old infant with a temperature of 37.8°C does not empirically require a lumbar puncture unless other historical or clinical data demand it. The highly febrile 4½ month-old infant is at risk of bacteremia, but the clinical exam will guide the need for lumbar puncture. A 3-year-old child with a history of indwelling VP shunt and an exam highly suggestive of streptococcal pharyngitis may be treated for strep if otherwise well.

10. e Potential complications from bacterial meningitis include seizures. Fluid restriction may be implemented as part of this patient's ICU or inpatient care but will not alter ED events. Fluid administration in the ED should be guided by vital signs and perfusion status. A CT scan would evaluate the potential for subdural effusion or empyema, but these are not common in the first hours/days of therapy in bacterial meningitis. Etiology of the seizure event can include hypoglycemia or hyponatremia caused by SIADH. Seizure-associated apnea may occur. IV glucose is indicated in the presence of hypoglycemia. Oxygen administration for any active seizure with airway management is appropriate. Depending on the relative change in the patients' hemodynamic status and follow-up sodium value, 3% NaCl or NS may be indicated for therapy.

11. c Ceftriaxone is indicated as a broad-spectrum agent with efficacy against all common organisms for meningitis in this age range. Vancomycin adds specific coverage for resistant *S. pneumoniae* organisms, and is therefore indicated, along with a third-generation cephalosporin, for initial empiric treatment of suspected pneumococcal meningitis until culture and sensitivity results are available. Dexamethasone is not indicated for two reasons: lack of data showing a clear benefit in the setting of likely *S. pneumoniae* meningitis; and the time interval since initial antibiotic administration (more than 6 hours). Chloramphenicol, though effective, is not the first-choice agent, given its side-effect profile. Acyclovir is an often-debated addition to therapy in meningitis; there are no clear indications for its use in otherwise uncomplicated meningitis with a documented bacterial source.

12. **e** Knowledge of the patient's NP flora and the resistance profile of the bacteria has no bearing in this case. An otherwise well 7-year-old child, who has mid-range pleocytosis in his CSF has a broad differential for possible etiologies that include TB, Lyme disease, and partially treated bacterial meningitis. The list of "pertinent negatives" in his history should include factors affecting immunocompetence.

13. **c** Only three organisms have a well-defined role in bacterial pharyngitis, one of which is the correct answer here—*N. gonorrhoeae*. *M. pneumoniae* is a cause of pharyngitis, but the question focused on bacterial causation.

14. **e** The CBC does not impact decision making in this setting. Treatment of OM does require consideration of patient age, daycare attendance, recent antibiotic use, and previous OM courses and how they responded to specific antimicrobials. If available, resistance patterns for pneumococci may be of value.

15. **c** The clinical scenario as presented is typical for a resolving illness, and the fever pattern and current otoscopic findings do not mandate any change in therapy. Antihistamines and/or decongestants have no proven efficacy in the treatment of OM. Although cefpodoxime and ceftriaxone are both recommended as alternatives to amoxicillin, the clinical course does not demand different antimicrobial treatment at this time.

16. **b** The likely diagnosis is otitis externa, in which fever is uncommon. In a young child, the lack of history for swimming does not exclude the diagnoses of otitis externa. Itching is a common initial symptom of this diagnosis. Tenderness of the external ear and drainage are also common for otitis externa.

17. **c** The likely diagnosis is acute sinusitis. Sinus x-rays are abnormal in almost every child with sinusitis and, as such, may be viewed as sensitive but not specific as an adjunctive test. CBC data is not helpful in screening for this condition. Gram stain of nasal secretions is not indicated. A minority of patients have asymmetry on transillumination of their sinuses. Antral puncture is reserved for severe disease, immunocompromised hosts, or persistent illness despite adequate oral therapy.

18. **e** Oral tetracycline is contraindicated in children under 8 years of age, given its effect on maturing dentition. Cephalexin would the first-line agent of choice. Screening with PPD placement is reasonable. Lack of fever is not uncommon in cervical adenitis. Complications are not uncommon in this condition. If fluctuant, a node may be amenable to aspiration, which could yield a definitive microorganism.

19. **d** A lateral pharyngeal abscess requires confirmation with CT imaging. Retropharyngeal abscess is often found first by lateral neck plain films and may be confirmed with further CT imaging. Epiglottitis is a diagnosis made clinically in conjunction with plain films. Sinusitis does not require imaging for diagnosis. Peritonsillar abscess is also a clinical diagnosis.

20. **d** Croup classically presents with more coughing by history than does epiglottis (see Table 84.14 of *Textbook of Pediatric Emergency Medicine*, fourth edition). The other answers, older age and drooling, are more typical of epiglottis. Fever can be seen in both conditions, and no specific temperature range differentiates the conditions. Respiratory distress will vary, depending on the severity of the subglottic pathophysiology in croup.

21. **c** Dexamethasone is indicated as therapy in mild to moderate croup. Mist therapy may also be helpful regardless of the child's O_2 saturation, although delivery of mist should not occur via nasal cannula. AP and lateral films are not necessary to diagnose croup. As a recognizable viral syndrome, croup does not require CBC data for diagnosis. Albuterol is not indicated for treatment of croup in the absence of associated bronchospasm.

22. **c** The age of this child (i.e., less than 12 months) and the presence of effusion make *S. pneumoniae* less likely and *S. aureus* more likely in this scenario. Certainly, admission to the hospital is warranted. Dehydration is a potential complication in pneumonia. Thoracentesis is indicated if the fluid layers out and will improve outcome. Blood cultures may yield the causative organism, and may be positive in 50% of cases if the pneumonia is caused by *S. pneumoniae*.

23. **c** *Chlamydia pneumoniae* is the correct answer, given the low-grade fever and the auscultory and x-ray findings. Pneumococcal pneumonia is classically a round pneumonia on x-ray. Varicella could cause a pneumonitis, but the absence of rash makes it unlikely. GBS is less likely to present as a respiratory process primarily at this age. Measles without other URI and rash stigmata is unlikely.

24. a *M. pneumoniae* is the likely causative agent. Bullous myringitis is a common finding in the setting of pneumonia caused by *M. pneumoniae*. A normal WBC is not unusual in the setting of mycoplasmal pneumonia. Findings on x-ray can vary with *Mycoplasma* and may include lobar processes. Cold agglutinin titers can be elevated from many different viral and bacterial sources. Rash is also a very nonspecific finding.

25. c Dehydration is an important complication of bronchiolitis, the most likely clinical diagnosis in this scenario. Quantity of the infant's oral intake and frequency of urine output will inform the issue of current risk for dehydration. The WBC data will not likely alter management for this child. TB exposure history and historical data regarding quality of cough are less likely to be directly relevant to management strategy in the given scenario.

26. b A trial with a nebulized solution of racemic epinephrine is the most appropriate answer. Although both albuterol via nebulization and racemic epinephrine nebulization are not universally accepted as efficacious, they do have some support within the literature for their use. Methylprednisolone (Solu-Medrol) is not indicated in the management of classic bronchiolitis. Albuterol in syrup form has no efficacy in treatment of bronchiolitis. Ribavirin is reserved for use in severe bronchiolitis from RSV. Data supporting chest physiotherapy in bronchiolitis is lacking.

27. c The clinical scenario describes an evolving course of pertussis; as such, answer "c" is most appropriate. Respiratory arrest from obstructed airway is a potential complication. A normal WBC does not rule out pertussis. CXR findings of a right shaggy heart border are suggestive, but a clear CXR is more often the rule. Fluorescent Ab testing of nasopharyngeal (NP) secretions has a higher yield of positive results than does culturing the material. Subconjunctival hemorrhages from pronounced coughing spells are not surprising and do not indicate abuse in this scenario as described.

28. e Seizures are a potential complication of pertussis. Infants under 6 months of age for whom the clinical suspicion of pertussis is high should be admitted to the hospital. All household contacts, regardless of immunization status, should receive chemoprophylaxis. Bacterial superinfection in the setting of pertussis is responsible for the majority of fatalities from this disease. Correct treatment of pertussis includes antibiotics for a full 14 days.

29. a A Mantoux reaction greater than 5mm would be diagnostic, given the CXR findings and the given clinical data. Oral amoxicillin in the setting of a lobar pneumonia with effusion does not adequately treat *S. aureus*. CNS infection in the setting of TB does not carry a good prognosis. Isolation if TB is suspected is appropriate. Single coverage is not recommended if active disease is suspected. A negative Mantoux reaction does not remove TB from the differential.

30. e This clinical scenario is typical for an infection from rotavirus. Microscopic pathology in the GI mucosal layer may persist for up to 8 weeks post-rotavirus infection. Clinically, this correlates with a slow return to normal stooling pattern that parents should be counseled to expect. The vital signs as listed do not demonstrate extreme tachycardia or hypotension such that oral hydration cannot be attempted. Rotavirus can be associated with blood in the stool. Fever is not an infrequent finding in rotaviral infections. The diagnosis of dehydration is a clinical one that is independent of the absolute stool frequency.

31. e Oral rehydration is appropriate for mild dehydration from viral gastroenteritis. A CBC and/or electrolytes are not indicated in this scenario. Kaopectate and loperamide are not recommended for the treatment of emesis and diarrhea in gastroenteritis.

32. c The high fevers, bloody stool, and elevated band count all point to *Shigella* as a possible agent in this scenario. Dehydration, seizure, colonic perforation, and bacteremia (although rare) are all known complications of *Shigella* infection. UTI is not specifically associated with a *Shigella* infestation.

33. d The combination of age, sickle-cell history, fever, and concern for salmonella as an etiologic agent mandates admission to the hospital and coverage with IV antibiotics. Current clinical exam and response to therapy will guide the other case scenarios and all may be eligible for outpatient care and follow-up.

34. b The history of antibiotic use and new bloody diarrhea raises concern for *Clostridium difficile* as the pathogen in this scenario. Diagnosis rests on detection of antigen in the stool. A blood culture, rotavirus

antigen testing, and blood chemistry profile have no specific indications in the scenario as given. A urine culture is unlikely to be positive in light of a negative UA and her symptoms.

35. d   Mupirocin is indicated for the treatment of localized uncomplicated bullous impetigo. The location and appearance of these lesions are typical for this diagnosis. Neither wound culture nor CBC are necessary to guide care. Sending a UA to screen for glomerulonephritis (a known complication of certain strains of streptococci) at this point in care is not indicated.

36. c   This child has risk factors for bacteremia that preceded her cellulitis: facial location, spontaneous cellulitis without preceding wound, and age. She should receive IV antibiotics directed at likely pathogens, including *S. aureus, S. pyogenes,* and less commonly *H. influenzae* or *S. pneumoniae,* and be admitted to the hospital for observation. Oral antibiotics can be appropriate for nonfacial cellulitis in children who are afebrile and otherwise well. Warm compresses alone are insufficient for treatment of facial cellulitis.

37. b   Early surgical consultation is imperative for this child. Necrotizing fasciitis, a known complication of varicella, is high on the list of differential diagnoses. Operative exploration as well as incision and drainage may be necessary. Fluid support, blood cultures, and antibiotics (penicillin and/or clindamycin) are certainly appropriate in this scenario. Extremity elevation is not incorrect, although as an intervention it is modest compared to the need for surgical exploration and formal debridement.

38. e   None of the given answers can exclude the diagnosis of septic arthritis. Clinical suspicion for the diagnosis should prompt plain radiographs, CBC, and ESR data collection. Even if these data are normal, a high clinical suspicion should prompt ultrasound examination for fluid within the hip joint and, if it is present, aspiration should be considered for the acquisition of cell count and cultures.

39. c   Skeletal survey is the least appropriate of the given tests. In a fussy infant who is highly febrile, consideration for meningitis, UTI, and bacteremia are paramount. In addition, the exam was notable for the right leg being held in extension, which raises concern for the possibility of a septic hip. Ultrasound of that hip should be performed to evaluate this condition.

40. b   The history, exam, and laboratory data are consistent with the diagnosis of osteomyelitis. Plain films are often normal early in the disease, but subtle changes can be appreciated beginning day 3–4 of illness. The earliest radiographic finding is a shift of the radiolucent deep muscle plane away from the bone. This child is about 5–6 days into his illness and obscuration of the deep muscle planes around the femur would be consistent with his time course. Lytic lesions and periosteal elevation are late findings (after day 10 of illness).

41. c   Syphilis in the incubating stage may not be noted on physical exam. Treatment with cefixime and azithromycin would cover chlamydia and gonorrhea adequately. IM penicillin, no longer used as first-line therapy for *N. gonorrhoeae,* would cover incubating *T. pallidum.* Screening for syphilis with a RPR is recommended for sexually active adolescents. It is important to note that this screening test will not pick up all incubating cases of syphilis and further outpatient follow-up is indicated for all sexually active adolescents.

42. c   A clean-catch urine culture that grows less than 10^5 of a single organism should be followed up with a repeat culture if clinical suspicion for infection persists. Low-grade bacterial colonization of the urethral tract does not in and of itself mandate antimicrobial treatment. Pain or fever consistent with evolving infection, as well the results of cultures, should guide clinical decision making. A child who can provide an adequate clean-catch specimen does not empirically need a catheterized specimen.

43. d   Age, gender, known urinary tract anomalies, and race have all been postulated as risk factors for UTI, according to recent publications. Height of fever as an independent risk factor has not been shown as a specific predictor for UTI.

44. b   Published data by Shaw and colleagues from Philadelphia has shown the dipstick for either leukocyte esterase or nitrite to have a sensitivity of approximately 80% for the detection of UTI. (Shaw KN, Gorelick M, McGowan KL, et al. Prevalence of urinary tract infection in febrile young children in the emergency department. Pediatrics 1998;102:16e.) Other researchers have advocated for the use of an

"enhanced" UA that requires laboratory personnel to examine an uncentrifuged urine sample for pyuria and bacteriuria; this does have improved sensitivity but is less specific and more costly.

45. d   The Tzanck smear, if positive, will determine the etiology of this lesion and guide therapy. RPR and HIV testing, though informative, will not alter the course of ED therapy with results in a same-day time frame. Certainly a viral culture is necessary for medico-legal confirmation of the lesion's etiology. An empiric Gram stain when there is no discharge is unlikely to yield evidence for specific organisms. Culture for gonococcus and chlamydia would be an arguable option, but is not listed here.

46. e   The heterophil-antibody test (Monospot) has known characteristics. Its sensitivity is not uniform across all ages: Only about 50% of children less than 4 years of age with EBV infection will have high enough titers to give a positive heterophil-antibody test result. However, with a clinical picture suggestive of EBV infection, most clinicians will take a positive heterophil-antibody test as confirmation of their diagnosis. The false positive rate is less than 10%. Additional serologic testing is indicated only if the heterophil-antibody test is negative and formal confirmation of EBV as the pathologic agent is desired.

47. a   This teenager has a history and exam consistent with measles and the development of measles encephalopathy. Mortality risk from measles encephalopathy is high—approximately 15%. Measles is transmitted via the respiratory tract with a resultant viremia and spread to the reticuloendothelial system. Koplik's spots may disappear as the rash progresses inferiorly along the trunk. Purulent otitis media is the most common bacterial complication. Leukopenia is common with uncomplicated measles.

48. c   Rash in a pregnant teenager must include rubella on the differential unless the patient's rubella titers are known. Rubella is a difficult clinical diagnosis to make. Serologic confirmation is imperative in the pregnant patient without known titer results. The clinical history and exam here are not consistent with measles or varicella. Liver function tests and CXR are not indicated in the given scenario.

49. b   The patient on inhaled corticosteroids for asthma should definitely be given acyclovir for a varicella eruption. The other cases in infancy and early childhood do not require this therapy. A teenager with varicella should receive acyclovir, but the additional issue of pregnancy makes the prescription of the medication less clear.

50. d   The clinical concern in this infant includes botulism. Vigilance for onset of respiratory failure is imperative. Gentamicin is contraindicated, because the aminoglycoside may exacerbate the neurologic symptoms. A measurement of negative inspiratory force will inform the infant's ventilation status and may be used to screen for need of intubation and mechanical ventilation. If a dextrose dipstick demonstrated hypoglycemia, an IV bolus of D25 would be indicated; however, empirical use of glucose is not warranted.

51. c   Rocky Mountain spotted fever is the likely diagnosis here. A normal or increased WBC is usual in RMSF. Vomiting is common in this illness. Laboratory data consistent with hyponatremia and/or thrombocytopenia have all been well described. Seizures are a known complication of RMSF, especially in the comatose child.

52. d   A petechial rash in the setting of fever prompts many visits to the pediatric ED. The only infectious agent not commonly associated with petechiae is *B. burgdorferi*, which classically gives an annular erythematous ("bulls-eye"-type) rash as a primary manifestation of infection.

53. e   Cat-scratch disease can be difficult to diagnose and rests largely on clinical history and examination. Azithromycin has been shown to decrease the amount and duration of adenopathy. An extremity x-ray is not indicated without history of trauma, or specific physical examination findings concerning for bony injury, or high concern for ongoing osteomyelitis. Ciprofloxacin is not approved for use in school-age children. Amoxicillin has not been shown to be effective in this clinical situation. Aspiration of the node is not indicated unless it is fluctuant.

CHAPTER **85**

Human Immunodeficiency Virus Infection

CYNTHIA R. JACOBSTEIN, M.D.

QUESTIONS

1. Of the following clinical presentations, the one which is least likely to raise suspicion for the possibility of human immunodeficiency virus (HIV) infection is:

   a. A 2-year-old child with failure to thrive and developmental delay
   b. A 7-month-old infant with generalized adenopathy and hepatosplenomegaly
   c. A 4-year old child with recurrent parotitis
   d. A 4-month old infant with a second episode of oral thrush
   e. A 9-month old infant with a second episode of bacteremia

2. A 30-month-old boy who has been diagnosed with HIV infection comes to the ED with the chief complaint of fever to 40°C rectally for 1 day. He has otherwise been well. His physical exam is unremarkable, other than a temperature of 39.6°C. His evaluation in the ED should include:

   a. An ESR
   b. A blood culture
   c. An LDH level
   d. A CD-4 count
   e. A sputum culture

3. A 4-month-old girl with HIV infection is brought to the ED with fever and respiratory distress. Her temperature is 39°C. Her RR is 70; O_2 saturation is 92% on room air. She has diffuse wheezing. Lab studies include an LDH of 800 IU, and a CXR that shows hyperinflation. Initial management should include:

   a. Hospitalization for treatment
   b. Triple drug therapy for tuberculosis (TB)
   c. Emergent bronchoalveolar lavage
   d. IV trimethoprim-sulfamethoxazole
   e. IV cefotaxime

4. A 4-year-old boy with HIV infection comes to the ED with a 2-day history of fever and cough. He is taking oral liquids well and continues to be very active. He has never had a documented opportunistic infection, and his family is compliant with his care. On exam, he has a T of 38.7°C orally, RR of 24, and an O_2 saturation of 98% on room air. His breath sounds are slightly decreased at the right base. A CXR reveals a right lower lobe infiltrate but is otherwise unremarkable. Management of this patient should include:

   a. Emergent bronchoalveolar lavage
   b. Admission for treatment of presumptive *Pneumocystis carinii* pneumonia (PCP)
   c. Admission for treatment of pulmonary tuberculosis
   d. Admit and observe for possible deterioration
   e. Discharge home on oral antibiotics

5. A 4-year-old girl with HIV infection is brought to the ED with a 1-week history of cough without fever. On exam, she is afebrile, with RR of 30 and an O_2 saturation of 95% on room air. Her breath sounds are clear and she has mild clubbing. The most likely findings on her CXR are:

   a. Normal radiographic findings
   b. Diffuse nodular pattern
   c. Focal infiltrate in the right lower lobe
   d. Diffuse interstitial pattern
   e. Bronchiectasis

6. A 3-year-old boy with HIV infection is brought to the ED with a 2-day history of bloody diarrhea. His caretaker reports decreased oral intake and no urine output since the previous evening. On exam, he has a temperature of 39°C orally and a pulse of 140. He is cranky, his lips are dry, and his mucous membranes are tacky. His abdomen is soft and nontender, with hyperactive bowel sounds. Capillary refill time is 2 seconds. Management of this patient should include blood culture, stool for viral and bacterial cultures, and:

   a. PO trial in the ED with discharge if successful
   b. Discharge home with follow-up in 24 hours
   c. Admission for IV hydration and observation
   d. Admission for IV hydration and IV antibiotics
   e. Admission for IV hydration and diagnostic colonoscopy

7. A 6-year-old girl with HIV infection is brought to the ED following exposure to a child with varicella infection at school on the day prior to presentation. Her caretaker is unaware of any past history of varicella infection. She is afebrile and has a normal physical exam. ED management should include:

   a. Administer IV acyclovir
   b. Start oral acyclovir
   c. Administer IV immunoglobulin
   d. Administer varicella-zoster immunoglobulin (VZIG)
   e. No specific medical therapy is warranted at this time

8. A 2-year-old girl with HIV infection is brought in by her mother because of concerns about her gait. Her mother reports that the child has seemed more unsteady on her feet in the last 24 hours. Brief review of her developmental history reveals that she has been losing milestones over the last 6 months. Her mother denies any history of fever, URI symptoms, trauma, or ingestion. On exam, the child has a temperature of 38.5°C rectally. She is irritable but consolable. She refuses to walk and clings to her mother. A head CT is ordered and is normal. The next management step should be:

   a. Neurology consult
   b. Lumbar puncture
   c. A CD-4 count
   d. Electroencephalogram (EEG)
   e. Emergent MRI

9. A 7-year-old boy with HIV infection comes to the ED with a 12-hour history of severe abdominal pain and nonbilious, nonbloody emesis. He has had no fever. Lab studies reveal 5–10 RBCs per high-power field (hpf) on urinalysis and a normal lipase level. Of the medications listed below, the one most likely to be responsible for his presentation is:

   a. Zidovudine (AZT)
   b. Didanosine (ddI)
   c. Stavudine (d4T)
   d. Indinavir (Crixivan)
   e. Trimethoprim-sulfamethoxazole

ANSWERS

1. d   Common clinical findings in children with HIV infection include failure to thrive, lymphadenopathy, and hepatosplenomegaly. A number of other findings may be seen as well, including recurrent parotitis, recurrent bacterial infections, and chronic diarrhea. Oral thrush is also seen in patients with HIV infection. However, this finding in a young infant is a common pediatric problem and by itself is not likely to represent HIV infection.

2. b   HIV-infected children are at risk for the same febrile illnesses as are children who are not infected with HIV. However, they have a greater incidence of bacteremia than uninfected children do. Therefore, in an otherwise well-appearing HIV-infected child with a significant fever, a blood culture is indicated in the evaluation.

3. d   The presentation is highly suggestive of *Pneumocystis carinii* pneumonia (PCP). This is the most common serious opportunistic infection in children infected with HIV and often presents between 2 and 6 months. Infants with PCP have fever, tachypnea, and rhonchi or wheezes. The oxygen saturation may be low and the LDH is often quite elevated. The typical findings on CXR include a diffuse interstitial pattern, but one can also see patchy infiltrates, hyperinflation, or even a normal chest film. If PCP infection is suspected in the HIV-infected child who is ill with respiratory infection, treatment with IV trimethoprim-sulfamethoxazole should begin as soon as possible and should not wait for further diagnostic evaluation. Bronchoalveolar lavage (in the setting of PCP infection) will be positive 3–4 days following the start of therapy. Although corticosteroids are used in severe cases of PCP, they are not generally considered an emergency medication.

4. e   The patient most likely has bacterial pneumonia caused by one of the same organisms that cause pneumonia in children without HIV infection (i.e., *Streptococcus pneumoniae, Hemophilus influenzae,* group A *Streptococcus,* and *Moraxella catarrhalis*). Given that he is well appearing, with minimal respiratory symptoms and has a history that suggests that close follow-up is possible, outpatient therapy with oral antibiotics may be considered. The presentation is not suggestive for either PCP or tuberculosis. If admission is desired, he should be treated with antibiotics rather than just observed.

5. b   The patient described in this scenario most likely has lymphocytic interstitial pneumonitis (LIP). This condition is thought to be caused by a lymphoproliferative response to the DNA of Epstein-Barr virus. Unlike infection with PCP, LIP has a more insidious onset. Patients with LIP generally do not have fever unless they have developed secondary infection. They may have mild tachypnea and hypoxia. The CXR shows a diffuse nodular pattern, sometimes with widening of the mediastinum and hilum. A focal infiltrate is more suggestive of bacterial pneumonia; a diffuse interstitial pattern is typical in PCP. Bronchiectasis may be seen late in the course of LIP.

6. d   The child in this scenario is ill appearing and dehydrated, thus warranting admission and IV hydration. In addition, the fever and bloody stools raise the concern of bacteremia with *Salmonella.* Thus, parenteral antibiotics should be started pending culture results. Etiologies of infectious diarrhea in HIV-infected children include the same organisms that cause these illnesses in immunocompetent children (i.e., bacteria such as *Salmonella, Shigella, Yersinia, Campylobacter, E. coli,* and *C. difficile;* viruses such as rotavirus). In addition, parasitic (e.g., *Giardia, Cryptosporidium, microsporidium*), mycobacterial, and other viral (e.g., CMV) etiologies should be considered in the HIV-positive child with diarrhea.

7. d   The HIV-infected patient who has varicella exposure but is asymptomatic should be treated with IM varicella-zoster immunoglobulin (VZIG) if the child presents within 96 hours of exposure. Those HIV-positive children who present with clinical manifestations of varicella infection should be treated with IV acyclovir, because infection may be severe in the immunocompromised host. Children with local zoster may be treated on an outpatient basis with oral acyclovir as long as close follow-up is ensured.

8. b   Although encephalopathy is a common finding in children infected with HIV, the presence of fever in this child should prompt the emergency physician to rule out an infectious cause of the acute neurologic change. This includes performing a lumbar puncture. A CT scan of the brain should strongly be considered prior to lumbar puncture if there are neurologic changes, to rule out the presence of a focal CNS lesion such as an abscess.

9. d   The drugs used in the treatment of HIV infection have many side effects, including rash, nausea, diarrhea, anemia, granulocytopenia, peripheral neuropathy, headache, and fatigue. The emergency physician should have some familiarity with these side effects, as they may be the cause of visits to the ED. Several of the medications cause pancreatitis, including the nucleoside reverse transcriptase inhibitors didanosine (ddI), stavudine (d4T), and zalcitibine (ddC). The nucleoside reverse transcriptase inhibitor zidovudine (AZT) causes anemia, granulocytopenia, nausea and vomiting, but does not generally cause pancreatitis. Indinavir (Crixivan), a protease inhibitor, is known to cause nephrolithiasis, the most likely diagnosis in the scenario presented (abdominal pain, vomiting, microscopic hematuria).

CHAPTER 86

Renal and Electrolyte Emergencies

SUJIT SHARMA, M.D.

QUESTIONS

1. A 6-year-old boy is being admitted to the hospital from the ED for observation. He is afebrile and is to remain NPO (no oral intake) during his stay. He weighs 25 kg. His total fluid requirement over the next 24 hours is closest to:

   a. 1500 ml
   b. 1600 ml
   c. 1700 ml
   d. 1800 ml
   e. 1900 ml

The following case applies to questions 2–4: An 8-month-old boy is brought to the ED for vomiting and diarrhea persisting for the past 4 days. Over the previous 24 hours he has become more listless and has not been tolerating oral fluids. On examination the infant is crying but consolable, and nontoxic appearing. Vital signs are: T 37.6°C, HR 164, RR 36, and BP 96/54. His skin and mucosa appear dry. The remainder of the physical examination is unremarkable. His urine specific gravity (SG) is 1.028. Results of serum electrolytes show: Na 136 mEq/l, K 4.0 mEq/l, Cl 90 mEq/l, and HCO_3 12 mEq/l. The BUN is 32 mg/dl. His mother tells you that her son weighed 6 kg at his last primary care visit 1 week ago. He weighs 5.4 kg today.

2. How much fluid should this patient receive over the first 8 hours of his admission?

   a. 300 ml
   b. 400 ml
   c. 500 ml
   d. 600 ml
   e. 700 ml

3. The sodium (Na) requirement for this patient during the first 8 hours would be:

   a. 65 mEq
   b. 50 mEq
   c. 40 mEq
   d. 30 mEq
   e. 20 mEq

4. If the sodium level for this patient were 128 mEq/l, his total sodium deficit would be:

   a. 75 mEq
   b. 65 mEq
   c. 50 mEq
   d. 40 mEq
   e. 30 mEq

5. A 4-month-old boy is brought to the ED by his mother, who states that he has been listless and irritable for the past few hours. She states that he has had loose stools for the past 3 days. Concerned that formula would worsen his condition, she has been administering herbal tea by mouth, which he seemed to enjoy. The patient begins to have a generalized tonic-clonic seizure in the ED, which does not respond to an appropriate dose of IV lorazepam. Which of the following should be administered?

   a. Phenobarbital
   b. Repeat lorazepam
   c. Methylene blue
   d. Hypertonic saline
   e. Furosemide

Questions 6 and 7: A 9-month-old girl is brought to the ED for diarrhea persisting over the past 4 days. Her mother has been feeding her a homemade boiled rice broth solution, with salt added. Today, she has had decreased intake by mouth (PO), as well as some vomiting. On examination the patient appears sleepy and listless; she is not interested in feeding. Her vital signs are: T 36.8°C, HR 168, RR 36, and BP 94/62. Mucous membranes are dry, but the skin turgor appears normal. She weighs 6.3 kg now, but according to her mother, she weighed 7 kg last week at the pediatrician's office. Serum electrolyte levels are: Na 165 mEq/l, K 4.4 mEq/l, Cl 124 mEq/l, and HCO_3 10 mEq/l.

6. Which of the following should be started initially?

   a. IV furosemide 1 mg/kg
   b. IV normal saline (NS) 20 ml/kg
   c. IV D5 W 20 ml/kg
   d. IV D5 NS at twice maintenance
   e. IV D5 ½ NS 20 ml/kg

7. The free water deficit for this patient is closest to:

   a. 700 ml
   b. 560 ml
   c. 500 ml
   d. 420 ml
   e. 300 ml

8. An 8-day-old boy is brought into the ED for seizures. The mother notes that he appeared well until 2 hours ago, when he became fussy and inconsolable. There is no history of fever, vomiting, or diarrhea. He is still actively seizing after one dose of IV lorazepam. Results of serum electrolytes are: Na 130 mEq/l, K 6.4 mEq/l, Cl 99 mEq/l, HCO_3 14 mEq/l, BUN 8 mg/dl, Cr 0.3 mg/dl, Ca 5.9 mEq/l, and Ph 8.4 mEq/l. Which of the following should be administered?

   a. Phenobarbital
   b. Repeat lorazepam
   c. Sodium bicarbonate ($NaHCO_3$)
   d. Calcium gluconate
   e. 3% sodium chloride (NaCl)

9. A 14-year-old boy is brought to the ED for fever, rash, and decreased activity. On exam, you note the patient to be lethargic, with diffuse purpura and petechiae. His vital signs are: T 39.2°C, HR 120, RR 24, and BP 98/64. His O_2 saturation is 94% on room air. The patient is placed on supplemental oxygen and an IV is inserted. Labs are ordered and an ABG shows the following: pH 7.15, pCO_2 36, pO_2 204, and HCO_3 8. Which of the following most accurately describes the patient's acid-base status?

   a. Respiratory acidosis
   b. Metabolic acidosis
   c. Metabolic and respiratory acidosis
   d. Metabolic acidosis with respiratory alkalosis
   e. Respiratory acidosis with metabolic alkalosis

10. A 4-year-old boy is brought to the ED for complaints of worsening abdominal pain over the past 2 days associated with vomiting and low grade fevers. He has had no diarrhea and has had a decrease in appetite. Past medical history is unremarkable; however, his mother notes that he is currently being treated for new-onset allergies, which have caused puffiness to his eyes. On exam, the patient appears to be in slight pain and has the following vital signs: T 38.6°C, HR 118, RR 32, and BP 102/68. His eyes do appear slightly swollen, and his abdomen is slightly distended and diffusely tender to palpation, with rebound tenderness elicited. The remainder of the exam is unremarkable. CBC shows a WBC of 19,000 (74% neutrophils). The urine appears normal in color, and has 5 WBCs/hpf; dipstick is 3+ for protein and the urine is negative for blood. Which of the following would be most important for treatment of this patient?

    a. IV antibiotics
    b. Operative intervention
    c. IV methylprednisilone
    d. IV furosemide
    e. IV fluid therapy

11. A 5-year-old boy with nephrotic syndrome is brought to the ED for increased fatigue and intermittent abdominal pain over the past 3 days. His mother states that he has become less active over the past 3 days and has gained approximately 8 pounds, despite salt and fluid restriction. He is currently taking prednisone. He has had no vomiting, diarrhea, or fever. On exam, he appears tired, with the following vital signs: T 37.2°C, HR 124, RR 42, and BP 102/60. He has generalized edema with abdominal distension and mild tenderness; breath sounds are diminished at both lung bases. Which of the following would be most appropriate for this patient?

    a. Fluid restriction
    b. IV furosemide
    c. IV antibiotics
    d. IV NS 20 ml/kg
    e. IV albumin and furosemide

12. A 7-year-old boy comes to the ED with complaints of headache and malaise over the past 2 days. He has had no fever, vomiting, or diarrhea. His mother notes that his urine began to appear dark in color yesterday, and that he has had minimal urine output today. His past medical history is unremarkable, other than a sore throat he had approximately 2 weeks ago. His vital signs are: T 36.8°C, HR 108, RR 28, and BP 172/105. Which of the following should you administer?

    a. Hydralazine
    b. Furosemide
    c. Nitroprusside
    d. Labetalol
    e. Phentolamine

13. Initial bloodwork for the patient in Question 12 reveals the following: hematocrit (hct) 30%, platelets 420,000, Na 129 mEq/l, K 7.2 mEq/l, Cl 103 mEq/l, HCO$_3$ 13 mEq/l, BUN 48 mg/dl, Cr 2.4 mg/dl, Ca 8.9 mEq/l, Mg 1.8 mEq/l, and phosphorus 4.2 mEq/l. Which of the following should be administered first?

    a. 3% sodium chloride (NaCl)
    b. Calcium gluconate
    c. Furosemide
    d. Sodium bicarbonate (NaHCO$_3$)
    e. Glucose and insulin

14. A 4-year-old boy is brought to the ED for diarrhea that has been persisting for 1 week. His mother has noted the presence of small amounts of blood in the stool over the past 2 days. She is concerned that her son now appears lethargic and that he is no longer urinating, despite adequate oral intake. He has had no fever, vomiting, or abdominal pain. On exam, you note a pale-appearing child with the following vital signs: T 37.3°C, HR 84, RR 36, and BP 144/86. The remainder of the exam is unremarkable. Urinalysis reveals 3+ protein and 40–50 RBCs/hpf, as well as red cell casts. Which of the following would be most helpful in making a diagnosis?

    a. Serum IgA levels
    b. Peripheral blood smear
    c. Nuclear renal scan
    d. Renal biopsy
    e. BUN and creatinine

15. A 3-year-old girl is brought to the ED for intermittent abdominal pain and limping over the past 2 days. She has not had any fever, vomiting, or diarrhea. Her mother does not recall any recent illnesses. On examination, you note a well-appearing child with stable vital signs. Her physical examination is normal except for a nonblanching erythematous rash on both lower extremities. Urinalysis reveals 5–10 RBCs/hpf, but is otherwise normal. Treatment should include:

    a. Prednisone
    b. Ceftriaxone
    c. Salicylates
    d. IV immunoglobulin
    e. Observation

ANSWERS

1. b   When applying the guidelines for fluid requirements (as outlined in Chapter 86 of *Textbook of Pediatric Emergency Medicine,* fourth edition), a total fluid requirement of 1700 cc will be needed for this patient as maintenance over a 24-hour period. Although caloric expenditure is more accurate in determining fluid requirements, the incremental changes in fluid requirements based on weight are more widely used.

2. c   This patient has 10% dehydration, based on the change in his weight. The fluid deficit is 600 ml. Half of this (300 ml) should be replaced in the first 8 hours. His maintenance requirement during those 8 hours would be 200 ml (a third of his daily requirement). This would make his total fluid requirement during those 8 hours 500 ml.

3. d   This patient has isotonic dehydration with a normal sodium level. Despite the current serum electrolyte levels, this patient does have a sodium deficit that must be added to his maintenance needs. The sodium deficit for this patient comes out to approximately 50 mEq. (Please see Chapter 86 of *Textbook of Pediatric Emergency Medicine,* fourth edition, for calculation of deficits.) As with the fluid replacement, half of the deficit (25 mEq) should be replaced in the first 8 hours. His maintenance requirement for sodium is 12–18 mEq per day, and therefore, 4–6 mEq over the first 8 hours. The patient's total sodium needs in the first 8 hours therefore would come to approximately 30 mEq.

4. a   In this situation of hypotonic dehydration, the calculation of the sodium deficit and maintenance requirements is the same as in the case of isotonic dehydration (Question 3). However, added to this requirement would be the extra sodium this patient will need to bring the level up from 128 mEq/l to 135

mEq/l, as in the example given in Chapter 86 of *Textbook of Pediatric Emergency Medicine* (fourth edition). Using an "ideal" sodium level of 135 mEq/l and a "healthy" body weight of 6 kg for this patient, a total of 25 mEq would be needed [(135 − 128) × 6 × 0.6]. Added to the preexisting isotonic sodium deficit of 50 mEq (as in the previous case), a total sodium deficit of 75 mEq exists. The replacement of these fluids can be given in the same fashion as for isotonic dehydration.

5. d Hyponatremia is one of the most common causes for seizures in infants less than 6 months of age. In the face of dilute oral feedings, the immature kidneys of young infants are unable to maintain normal sodium levels. Although one would usually want to confirm the serum sodium level, waiting for the level to return could delay treatment. In this case, the detailed history alone would tip one off to the diagnosis. Repeated doses of antiepileptics are unlikely to resolve the seizure, and increase the likelihood of respiratory compromise. Hypertonic saline (3% NaCl) contains 0.5 mEq of sodium per cc (ml). When given acutely in a dose of 5 ml/kg, the serum level of sodium will be elevated by approximately 4 mEq/l.

6. b This patient has hypertonic/hypernatremic dehydration. Despite having preservation of the extracellular fluid space, she is starting to become rather symptomatically dehydrated. The initial IV fluid bolus should always be with isotonic saline in cases of severe dehydration or shock. Hypotonic fluids may follow the initial fluid bolus. This should be done slowly, however, over a 2-day period, because overly rapid correction of the serum sodium can cause cerebral edema.

7. b This patient has an overall fluid deficit of 700 ml based on the decrease in weight. The free water deficit is 4 ml/kg for every 1 mEq/l of serum sodium greater than 145 mEq/l [(165 − 145) × 4 ml/kg × 7 kg = 560 ml].

8. d This child is having a hypocalcemic seizure, most likely secondary to hypoparathyroidism, because he has hyperphosphatemia as well. Although his sodium level is slightly low, a level of 130 mEq/l is not low enough to cause seizures. The potassium level is most likely increased secondary to metabolic acidosis, which can be seen with convulsions. Treatment of the seizure should address the underlying cause, therefore calcium gluconate should be administered. This should be done under cardiac monitoring.

9. c This patient appears to be in septic shock, most likely due to meningococcemia. He obviously has hemodynamic compromise, which would cause the metabolic acidosis. Adequate respiratory compensation for this degree of metabolic acidosis should be in the range of 20 + 2. This adaptive response to metabolic acidosis is predicted by the following formula: $P_{CO_2} = 1.5 \times [HCO_3] + 8 + 2$. This patient has a P_{CO_2} of 36 and therefore has inadequate respiratory compensation; his acid-base status is best described as metabolic and respiratory acidosis.

10. a This patient most likely has nephrotic syndrome complicated by bacterial peritonitis. When presenting for the first time, as in this patient, this infectious complication can often mimic a surgical abdomen. The findings of edema (which often begin with periorbital swelling) along with proteinuria should alert one to the diagnosis of nephrotic syndrome. A paracentesis would be the diagnostic study of choice for this patient in order to analyze the fluid and obtain a sample for culture. Although this patient may eventually benefit from steroid therapy for the underlying condition, acute management requires the initiation of IV antibiotics to treat the peritonitis.

11. e This patient is having an acute exacerbation of nephrosis despite concurrent steroid therapy. Aside from obvious weight gain and generalized edema, these patients can present with abdominal pain secondary to mucosal edema, as well as respiratory embarrassment due to massive ascites. This patient appears to have both. Therapy should therefore center around removing some of this excess fluid by increasing the intravascular oncotic pressure, followed by diuresis once the fluid has entered the vascular space. Diuretics alone or fluid restriction would worsen the intravascular volume depletion that presently exists. In the face of significant intravascular volume depletion without complications related to massive edema, restoration of intravascular volume with IV normal saline (20 ml/kg) would be appropriate.

12. a This patient is presenting with hypertension due to acute renal failure (most likely poststreptococcal glomerulonephritis). This would be considered a hypertensive emergency because he has severe hypertension with target organ disease. Optimal antihypertensive agents would have rapid onset of action,

such as hydralazine, diazoxide, or nifedipine. Sodium nitroprusside would be contraindicated because the risk of thiocyanate and cyanide toxicity are increased in patients with renal insufficiency. Labetalol has a rapid onset of action but can cause hyperkalemia secondary to beta blockade; therefore, it would be contraindicated in the setting of acute renal failure. Phentolamine is used almost exclusively for catecholamine crisis. Even though this patient's hypertension is related to volume overload, and will eventually benefit from diuretic therapy, furosemide would not be the initial drug of choice in this situation.

13. b   This patient has significant hyperkalemia, a known complication of acute renal failure. A 12-lead ECG should be performed immediately in these situations to assess for cardiac effects of the increased potassium level (peaked T waves, increase in the PR interval, increase in QRS duration). Initial treatment should be with calcium, so as to protect and stabilize the myocardium. Subsequent therapy with bicarbonate or insulin/glucose will act to transfer potassium into the cells acutely, thereby decreasing serum toxicity. The hyponatremia that is noted is caused by dilution from volume overload and need not be addressed at this time.

14. b   This patient is presenting with symptoms consistent with hemolytic uremic syndrome (HUS), the most common cause of acute renal failure in young children. Evidence of acute renal failure is present at many levels: history of decreasing urine output despite adequate intake, examination revealing hypertension, and urinalysis showing signs of nephritis. Although serum BUN and creatinine would help to confirm renal insufficiency, peripheral blood smear will confirm the presence of the other features of HUS—microangiopathic hemolytic anemia and thrombocytopenia. The cornerstone of treatment is early recognition and supportive therapy.

15. e   This patient has Henoch-Schönlein purpura (HSP). The illness is caused by vasculitis of small blood vessels, which gives rise to abdominal pain, arthritis, and purpura. Renal involvement (glomerulonephritis) is common; it does appear to be present in this patient, in the form of microscopic hematuria. IgA levels are often elevated. Arthritis is usually migratory, involving large joints. Abdominal pain can be severe and can be complicated by surgical problems such as intussusception or intestinal perforation. There is no specific therapy for HSP except for the use of corticosteroids in selected cases of severe abdominal pain or severe arthritis.

CHAPTER **87**

Hematologic Emergencies

ROBERT L. CLOUTIER, M.D.

QUESTIONS

1. A 3-year-old boy is brought to the ED by the EMTs following a major motor vehicle accident. He was an unrestrained passenger and did lose consciousness. The patient has suffered an open left femur fracture. His vital signs are: HR 170, BP 85/40, and RR 20, with an O_2 saturation of 100% on room air. He is awake and crying but follows simple commands. Which of the following statements regarding treatment for this patient is TRUE?

   a. Uncross-matched type O-negative blood should be infused immediately
   b. The patient's resuscitation should proceed with only crystalloid and colloid fluids
   c. The patient should be resuscitated with crystalloid and colloid fluids until blood is appropriately cross-matched and a fully compatible unit is made available
   d. The patient should be resuscitated with crystalloid and colloid fluids until an appropriate unit of group- and Rh-specific blood has been made available for immediate infusion
   e. Maintain the initially cross-matched blood in the blood bank for 24 hours and release it for other use after that time if the patient doesn't need it

2. A 2-year-old girl is brought to the ED. The parents are concerned with the child's skin color and dark-colored urine. She is ill appearing, with the following vital signs: HR 120, BP 110/40, and RR 20. The patient's sclera are icteric, her breath sounds are clear, and the abdomen is soft, without hepatosplenomegaly. A bedside urine dipstick is positive for blood and early lab work reveals a Hgb of 3.1, a reticulocyte count of 9%, and a positive Coombs' test. Management strategies for this child should include:

   a. Immediate RBC transfusion with O-negative blood
   b. Transfusion of whole blood
   c. Immediate transfusion with an appropriately cross-matched donor
   d. 2 mg/kg/day of prednisone or equivalent parenteral steroid preparation
   e. Immediate transfusion with group- and Rh-specific blood in addition to steroid therapy

3. An 18-month-old African-American boy is brought to the ED because of pallor, malaise, fever, and icterus. There have been ill contacts among his siblings within the past 3 days. The child has no family history or past medical history indicative of bleeding or clotting problems. It would be important to inquire about exposure to all of following substances as potential causes of the patient's condition EXCEPT:

   a. Naphthalene
   b. Salicylates
   c. Sulfa antibiotics
   d. NSAIDs
   e. Acetaminophen

4. A 9-month-old boy is referred to the ED because of pallor, icterus, tachycardia, a Hgb of 6.2 g/dl, and a negative Coombs' test. The parents report that the child has no past medical or surgical history. However, they state that the child completed a 10-day course of an unknown antibiotic (a white liquid) 3 days ago. The most probable diagnosis is:

   a. Autoimmune hemolytic anemia
   b. Nonimmune hemolytic anemia
   c. Acute lymphocytic leukemia (ALL)
   d. Transient erythrocytopenia of childhood (TEC)
   e. Diamond-Blackfan syndrome

5. An 8-month-old African-American boy is brought to the ED because of irritability and swelling of his hands and feet. He is afebrile and noted to have mild swelling and tenderness of both hands and feet on physical examination. Which of the following diagnostic studies is the MOST appropriate?

   a. Hgb electrophoresis
   b. Peripheral smear
   c. Solubility testing (sickle prep)
   d. Bone scan
   e. Skeletal survey

6. A well-appearing 2-year-old boy with Hemoglobin SS (Hgb SS) disease is brought to the ED because of a 3-day history of cough and rhinorrhea. The patient remained afebrile until this morning, when the mother measured a rectal temperature of 39.1°C. Select the most accurate statement regarding the clinical significance of fever in this patient:

   a. This patient is within the age range of greatest risk for sepsis in sickle-cell disease (SCD) patients
   b. Potential causes of sepsis in this patient include *H. influenzae* and *Pseudomonas aeruginosa*
   c. Fever is irrelevant since the patient's splenic activity is not significantly compromised
   d. Life-threatening sepsis is less likely than if this patient had Hgb SC disease
   e. Close follow-up and outpatient management with amoxicillin is appropriate in the nontoxic-appearing patient

7. A 4-year-old African-American boy is brought to the ED by his father, who states the child has SCD and has been complaining of right hip pain and fever for 4 days. The child is presently nonweight bearing and is holding the leg in a "frog-leg" position. The father states that this pain is very unlike the child's usual crisis pain, both in terms of location and severity. The joint is warm, tender, and swollen, with a marked decrease in range of motion. Which of the following studies will be most helpful for differentiating joint infection from bone infarction?

   a. MRI with gallium
   b. Unenhanced CT scan
   c. 99m Tc bone scan/marrow scan
   d. Plain x-ray with frog-leg views
   e. Radio-labeled WBC scan

8. An ill-appearing 6-year-old boy with Hgb SC disease comes to the ED with the following vital signs: T 37°C, HR 140, BP 75/30, and RR 32 with 100% O$_2$ saturation. The mother states that the patient began complaining of left upper quadrant (LUQ) pain 3 hours ago. Within the last hour the child became increasingly ill, which prompted his mother to call an ambulance. On exam, he has LUQ tenderness, with an enlarged and hardened spleen. Treatment should include which of the following?

   a. Exchange transfusion
   b. Abdominal CT scan
   c. Ceftriaxone IV
   d. 2–10 cc/kg of blood
   e. morphine sulfate IV, titrated to effect

9. A 6-month-old girl is brought to the ED because of a sallow complexion and lethargy. The child has apparently been feeding normally but nonetheless fails to thrive. Her physical examination is notable for splenomegaly. The CBC shows: WBC 10.4, Hgb 5.6, platelets 245, MCV 66, and reticulocyte count of 1.1%. Treatment should include which of the following?

   a. Ferrous sulfate
   b. Folic acid
   c. Transfusion
   d. Vitamin B12
   e. No treatment

10. A 5-month-old African-American boy has vomiting. The mother states the child has had repeated vomiting and diarrhea over the last 2 days. On physical examination, he is cyanotic, tachypneic, and lethargic. His respiratory and cardiac examinations are otherwise normal. His O$_2$ saturation on room air is 98%. Immediate treatment includes:

    a. Methylene blue
    b. Desferoxamine
    c. Exchange transfusion
    d. Sodium bicarbonate
    e. Furosemide

11. A 2-year-old boy has methemoglobinemia. The appropriate first-line agent is given IV over 5 minutes and is repeated 1 hour later without apparent clinical improvement. Given the failure of this agent to resolve the patient's symptoms, which of the following management options is best?

    a. Massive transfusion
    b. IV ascorbic acid
    c. Fresh frozen plasma (FFP)
    d. Salt-poor albumin
    e. IV intrinsic factor

12. A 3-year-old boy is brought to the ED after falling down three steps inside his house. According to the parents, the child hit his head, but there was no loss of consciousness (LOC) and he was ambulatory at the scene. Three weeks ago the child was diagnosed with idiopathic thrombocytopenic purpura (ITP). His platelet count last week was 95,000. On physical examination, you notice an abrasion on the left elbow that has stopped bleeding spontaneously and a 4-cm left frontoparietal contusion. Otherwise the patient has a Glasgow Coma Scale (GCS) of 15 and the rest of his physical examination is unremarkable. Your management strategy should include:

   a. Close observation for 4–6 hours and discharge with close follow-up
   b. Head CT scan followed by admission for IV gamma globulin
   c. Discharge with PO prednisone if the head CT is negative
   d. Admission for platelet transfusion and IV gamma globulin
   e. Admission for administration of red cell D-antigen antibody

13. A 1-month-old boy with a history of Factor VIII deficiency is brought to the ED after falling from a standing height onto a carpeted floor. The patient had no LOC and is playful and appropriate in the ED. He is without evidence of trauma. According to the parents the child has approximately 5% Factor VIII activity. His management should proceed as follows:

   a. Immediate CT of the head following 100% factor correction with cryoprecipitate
   b. A 50% factor correction with cryoprecipitate followed by discharge for home observation
   c. Home observation with explicit parental instructions for head injury and close follow-up
   d. CT of the head, home observation, and factor correction q12h for 3 days
   e. 100% factor correction with FFP and follow-up with a hematology consult in the morning

14. A 4-year-old boy with a history of Wiskott-Aldrich syndrome is brought to the ED with a fever of 39.4°C. Important considerations in the treatment of this patient include:

   a. The incidence of sepsis in these patients is less than in postsplenectomy patients
   b. Patients with this syndrome suffer severe infections by a wider variety of organisms than do splenectomized patients
   c. The risk of mortality from sepsis is approximately 50%-80% in these patients
   d. E. coli represents 50% of sepsis cases in this patient population
   e. Having received vaccination against encapsulated organisms this child has no increased risk of sepsis

15. A 12-year-old boy with a history of von Willebrand's disease Type 1 is brought to the ED after tripping going up a set of stairs and striking both knees. The patient denies other trauma but points out the significant swelling in both his knees since the event. A TRUE statement regarding the treatment of this patient is:

   a. DDAVP would be the agent of choice in terms of effectiveness and safety
   b. DDAVP is the agent of choice in all patients with hemophilia and von Willebrand's disease
   c. The proper dose of DDAVP is 0.3 μg/kg IV push over 30 minutes
   d. The only significant side effect of DDAVP is facial flushing
   e. DDAVP is used only if a test dose has been administered previously to assess for individual response

16. A 7-year-old girl with Factor VIII deficiency (1% activity) is brought to the ED following a 10-foot fall from a patio deck; there was no LOC. The patient has a GCS of 15 and has significant swelling over both knees and her left elbow. You have administered enough Factor VIII for a 100% correction. Over the ED course, the patient's mental status deteriorates. All of the following are management options EXCEPT:

   a. Porcine Factor VIII
   b. DDAVP
   c. Activated Factor IX concentrates
   d. Plasmapheresis
   e. 2-volume exchange transfusion

17. A 7-month-old breast-fed baby boy is brought to the ED after experiencing a focal left-sided seizure. The dextrose stick is 89 mg/dl. The seizure resolves shortly after arrival in the ED, but the child maintains a right-sided gaze preference and has a prolonged postictal period. His lab values are notable for the following: Na 140 mEq/l; K 5.0 mEq/l; Cl 110 mEq/l; HCO_3 16 mEq/l; Ca 9.0 mEq/l; Mg 2.0 mEq/l; Ph 4.5 mEq/l. The CT is positive for radiolucencies consistent with ischemia. The patient is admitted to the Pediatric Intensive Care Unit (PICU) for further evaluation. Which set of etiologies encompasses the MOST LIKELY causes of this event?

   a. Factor VIII deficiency, sepsis, CNS neoplasm
   b. Factor IX deficiency, hyponatremia, CNS neoplasm
   c. Protein S or C deficiency, sepsis
   d. Protein S or C deficiency, hyponatremia
   e. Factor VIII deficiency, protein S or C deficiency

ANSWERS

1. c Trauma is one of the leading causes of death in children and must be acted upon in a swift and decisive manner. With regards to transfusion therapy, the risk-benefit ratio of exposing a patient with relatively stable vital signs to marginally compatible blood, or the possibility of contracting an infectious disease through transfusion must be carefully weighed. In this vignette, the patient is in hypovolemic shock without signs of immediately life-threatening hemorrhage. Under these circumstances, the patient warrants initial volume resuscitation with crystalloid and colloid fluids, followed by optimally compatible blood as needed. Should the need for blood arise in the face of worsening hypovolemic shock or a slowly falling hemoglobin, group- and Rh type-specific but uncross-matched blood may be used.

2. d The patient is suffering from autoimmune hemolytic anemia (AIHA). This can be a very insidious disease with a fulminant presentation, including the sudden onset of pallor, jaundice, and dark urine, with a positive Coombs' test. Although a reticulocytosis is often present in these patients, occasionally they experience prolonged reticulocytopenias. The urinalysis samples will be qualitatively positive for blood without evidence of red cells on the microscopic examination. This is due to the presence of free hemoglobin in the urine from hemolyzed cells. These children require aggressive management but not necessarily with transfused blood products. Though fluid therapy may be indicated, the cornerstones of treatment are prednisone and/or gamma globulin. In many instances the use of these agents will obviate the need for packed RBCs. The existence of known, as well as unknown, antibodies in the patient's bloodstream make the selection of a "compatible unit" extremely difficult, to the extent that transfusion should be reserved for only the most dire circumstances of life-threatening hypoxia or cardiac collapse.

3. e This patient has glucose 6 phosphate dehydrogenase deficiency (G6PD), an X-linked enzymatic disorder resulting in hemolysis of RBCs when affected patients are exposed to oxidative stresses. G6PD is the enzyme required for the production of glutathione via the recycling of NADPH as a cofactor. The list of medications and other agents capable of causing this type of hemolysis is large but does not include acetaminophen.

4. b The patient is suffering from nonimmune hemolytic anemia. The disorder is most often caused by agents directly damaging the surface of RBCs. This disorder may present in similar fashion to AIHA but should be considered strongly in patients with a negative Coombs' test. Treatment consists of removal of the offending agent; transfusions are required only with cases of life-threatening hypoxia, cardiac compromise, or a Hgb level of less than 3 g/dl. Commonly implicated agents include sulfasalizine, naphthalene, and nitrofurantoin. Other causes of nonhemolytic anemia include malaria, certain protozoans, and many Gram-positive and Gram-negative organisms.

5. c This child may be presenting with sickle-cell disease (SCD) for the first time in the ED. The patient is afebrile and therefore a provisional diagnosis of a hemoglobinopathy may have a significant effect on patient disposition. Solubility testing represents the most time effective method of making a provisional diagnosis of SCD. Solubility testing fails to distinguish between those with sickle-cell trait and those with actual disease; therefore, the test must be followed up with a confirmatory test such as hemoglobin electrophoresis. Electrophoresis testing is more time intensive and is not conducive to a rapid turn-around time in the ED. Peripheral smears are notoriously unreliable because a given smear sample may be devoid of "sickled" cells.

6. a The age of greatest risk for sepsis in the patient with sickle-cell disease is between the ages of 6 months and 3 years, when protective antibody formation and splenic activity are limited. The organisms most often implicated are *Streptococcus pneumoniae* and *H. influenzae* in young children; *E. coli* and *Salmonella* are often implicated in older children. Rates of life-threatening sepsis are comparable between patients with Hgb SC disease and Hgb SS disease; however, mortality is lower in those with Hgb SC disease. The diminution of splenic activity in SCD patients begins at a very early age and should never be discounted as an important factor in the treatment of these patients. Their risk of sepsis is several hundredfold greater than in the general population. Lastly, amoxicillin alone is not an appropriate antibiotic choice for this patient.

7. c In the patient with SCD the distinction between bone infarction, septic arthritis, osteomyelitis, and a vaso-occlusive pain crisis may be subtle. Important indicators of intra-articular pathology in this pa-

tient include: 1) fever; 2) pain that is different from other pain crises in both severity and location; 3) a decreased range of motion, along with tenderness and swelling of the joint; and 4) a joint that is warm to the touch and is held in the "frog-leg" position. The best diagnostic aid in this case is a 99mTc-diphosphonate bone scan with a concurrent 99mTc-sulfur colloid marrow scan. This is especially true for patients whose symptoms have persisted for less than 3 days. In the case of a bone infarction, the bone scan should be normal, with a decreased bone marrow uptake; with bone infection, the findings should be the opposite (increased bone uptake and normal bone marrow). Other modalities listed (e.g., MRI and labeled WBC scans) have yet to prove their usefulness definitively.

8. d   This patient is suffering from a splenic sequestration crisis resulting in rapid volume depletion. This complication of SCD requires vascularized splenic tissue and therefore most commonly occurs in patients under the age of 5; however, it may occur at a later age in patients with Hgb SC or beta-thalassemia. The key to this diagnosis is usually an enlarged and hardened spleen noted on physical examination. This represents a true emergency requiring aggressive management. Once recognized, these patients should be given large amounts of IV fluid or albumin to restore intravascular volume. In addition, many patients require a modest transfusion of packed RBCs (2–10 ml/kg) to address tissue hypoxia. Whole blood transfusions have been noted to address both issues of volume and hypoxia simultaneously.

9. c   Thalassemia is characterized by organomegaly and microcytic hypochromic, nucleated RBCs, in a patient with a normal dietary history. Iron deficiency anemia tends to be characterized by hypochromic, rarely nucleated RBCs on peripheral smear, in patients with abnormal dietary histories and no organomegaly. This particular child will likely require transfusion and be dependent on transfusions for life. This child does not suffer from a nutritional anemia or pernicious anemia; therefore, vitamin B12, ferrous sulfate, and folic acid are not recommended.

10. a   This patient is suffering from methemoglobinemia. Methemoglobinemia results from a relative imbalance between hemoglobin and methemoglobin, with iron being more in its ferric rather than its normal ferrous state. Abnormal genetic forms of methemoglobin reductase or relatively immature enzymatic systems common among infants play important roles in precipitating the disease in the context of oxidant stresses. Clinically, this particular patient has a methemoglobin level corresponding to 30–50%. This patient will have a normal O_2 saturation because the pulse oximeter will record saturated hemoglobin only and not the methemoglobin as part of its saturation equation. Methylene blue is widely recognized as the treatment for methemoglobinemia. However, methylene blue may cause an oxidant stress in and of itself, which could be poorly tolerated by a patient with a defective hexosemonophosphate shunt (i.e., G6PD).

11. b   In such a case, 500 mg oral ascorbic acid *may* help alleviate the cyanosis and hypoxia associated with methemoglobinemia. Should this fail, exchange transfusion or hyperbaric oxygen may be required for patients with more severe symptoms.

12. a   This is a highly controversial subject and few hard rules have been established. However it must be kept in mind that intracranial hemorrhage is the leading cause of death in patients with ITP. With minor head trauma, close observation is one of the cornerstones of treatment. The difficulty arises in determining which patients require IV gamma globulin. For this patient, who is not displaying acute signs of increased intracranial pressure, the risk/benefit ratio of steroids or gamma globulin is dubious. This patient is neurologically asymptomatic, without significant ecchymosis or petechiae. Head trauma patients with ITP who exhibit no neurologic signs or symptoms could be further risk stratified by checking their platelet count, because patients with platelet counts above 50,000 rarely bleed intracranially. This patient could be observed for 4–6 hours in the ED and discharged with close follow-up.

13. c   The management of the moderate hemophiliac with minor trauma is difficult and controversial. Patients with moderate hemophilia must be risk stratified in a manner that takes into account their bleeding history and the type of trauma suffered. A CT scan may be helpful in locating sites of intracranial bleeding requiring intervention. It should not, however, be the sole method of determining whether or not replacement factor should be used. With this particular case, the trauma was mild and the patient suffers from relatively mild to moderate hemophilia, with at least 5% clotting factor activity. Therefore, a CT scan is not entirely indicated in this instance. A CT can never replace vigilant observation for signs of late-onset intracranial hemorrhage. Nevertheless, one could make a strong argument for at least a CT

scan in this patient and observation in the hospital. The risk of such an aggressive approach in these patients is the reluctance of parents to bring their child to the ED for every minor trauma, especially if they will be forced to sit through a prolonged evaluation. The second-line risk involves the drawbacks inherent to repeated treatments with blood products such as Factor VIII.

14. c   Mortality rates from sepsis have ranged from 50–80%. The organisms most frequently encountered include *S. pneumoniae, N. meningitidis, H. influenzae,* and *E. coli.* Pneumococcal infections account for approximately 50% of the episodes of sepsis. With patients who have hematologic disorders of immunologic origin or other gaps in host defense (i.e., AIHA or Wiskott-Aldrich syndrome), the rates of sepsis are extremely high. Immunization against encapsulated organisms reduces the incidence of sepsis but does not eliminate it and should not alter management.

15. c   DDAVP acts by increasing levels of Factor VIII coagulant activity, von Willebrand's antigen, and ristocetin cofactor threefold in most subjects. This makes DDAVP an ideal treatment in lieu of blood products option in patients with mild hemophilia and von Willebrand's type 1. However, DDAVP has not been proven to work in all patients. Preferably, patients should receive a test dose of DDAVP while they are in good health, to assess its activity before they might need it for actual treatment. Side effects of DDAVP include facial flushing, headache, hypertension, and water retention. The water retention has led to reports of hyponatremic seizures. The correct dose of DDAVP is 0.3 micrograms (μg) per kg, given as a slow IV push over 30 minutes. DDAVP is ineffective in patients with severe Factor VIII deficiency and von Willebrand's type 3. Lastly, caution must be exercised with DDAVP because it may aggravate thrombocytopenia in patients with the rare von Willebrand's type 2B.

16. b   This patient has an inhibitor and therefore requires an alternative therapy to deal with her now-developing intracranial hemorrhage. Porcine Factor VIII has been advocated by many, since it has been shown that 75% of patients with inhibitors do not have antibodies that cross-react with porcine factor concentrates. Activated Factor IX concentrates are useful in the patient who has extremely high titers of inhibitor that render any type of Factor VIII trial useless. Plasmapheresis and 2-volume exchange transfusions are attempts to reduce the inhibitor burden such that the factor concentrates will be partially effective. However, one must be prepared to perform this with each administration of Factor, because 50% of IgG antibodies are tissue bound and will eventually return to the circulation after the exchange transfusion.

17. c   This patient most likely has either a protein S or C deficiency. However, sepsis must remain a serious consideration in the differential diagnosis. The most dreaded complication of this disease is an intracranial ischemic event with concurrent purpura fulminans, which may also occur with certain forms of sepsis. This patient should be treated aggressively with heparin if it is learned that there is a family history of a thrombotic disease. This patient cannot have hemophilia, because CT findings are consistent with ischemia but not with hemorrhage (remember, Protein C and S deficiency represent hypercoagulable disorders). Hyponatremia is extremely unlikely in a breast-fed infant, because there is no formula to mix improperly, and the measured level of sodium is normal. The CT findings show no mass effect and therefore reduce the likelihood of a CNS neoplasm.

CHAPTER 88

Toxicology Emergencies

MICHELE M. BURNS, M.D.

QUESTIONS

1. Characteristics of a prototypical toxicology patient less than 5 years of age would be:

   a. Reason for ingestion was intentional
   b. Choice of a substance with poor palatability
   c. Gender of child likely to be male
   d. Choice of a psychopharmacologic drug
   e. Choice of a substance with a childproof cap

2. A 3-year-old boy comes to the ED with seizures. The EMTs report that they obtained a rapid glucose test of 30 mg/dl. Ingestion of all of the following agents is possible EXCEPT:

   a. Ethanol
   b. Caffeine
   c. Propranolol
   d. Pepto-Bismol (bismuth and salicylates)
   e. Glipizide

3. An adolescent patient with a history of depression is brought to the ED with lethargy and pinpoint pupils. The bedside glucose test is normal. An antidote to consider is:

   a. Flumazenil
   b. Pyridoxine (vitamin B6)
   c. Benzodiazepine
   d. Naloxone
   e. Glucose

4. In Question 3 above, the patient could have ingested all of the following agents EXCEPT:

   a. Paregoric
   b. Theophylline
   c. Cough/cold preparations
   d. Propoxyphene
   e. Clonidine

5. A 16-year-old boy is being evaluated for altered mental status. Physical exam is unrevealing, other than the presence of lethargy and poor response to verbal and tactile stimuli. His blood chemistry profile shows the following results: Na 140 mEq/l, K 4.6 mEq/l, Cl 110 mEq/l, HCO$_3$ 6 mEq/l, BUN 6 mg/dl, Cr 0.5 mg/dl, glucose 100 mg/dl, and a measured serum osmolarity of 290 mOsm/l. The best antidote of choice is:

   a. Folic acid
   b. Fomepizole (4-MP)
   c. Vitamin B1
   d. Vitamin B6
   e. Dialysis

6. A 2-year-old boy is brought to the ED 2 hours after an unknown ingestion. Gastric lavage would be most appropriate if he took:

   a. Scopolamine
   b. Ibuprofen
   c. Paroxetine
   d. Acetaminophen
   e. Cisapride

7. Your ED is called regarding an ingestion in a 15-month-old girl. You would recommend induced emesis with syrup of ipecac if the child had taken which of the following:

   a. Phenylpropanolamine
   b. Turpentine
   c. Lorazepam
   d. Sodium hydroxide
   e. *Dieffenbachia* plant leaf

8. Activated charcoal can be used for GI decontamination after ingestion of which of the following agents?

   a. Lithium
   b. Gasoline
   c. Aspirin
   d. Caustic cleaning agent
   e. Iron

9. Whole bowel irrigation may be useful in all of the following ingestions EXCEPT:

    a. Iron
    b. Cocaine packets
    c. Theophylline
    d. Lead
    e. Ibuprofen

10. An adolescent male patient flies back from Guam after visiting his father. He comes to the ED with complaints of tingling sensations and normally cold objects feeling extremely hot. A pharmacologic treatment to consider administering is:

    a. Trivalent botulism toxin
    b. Antihistamine
    c. Mannitol
    d. Cimetidine
    e. Ondansetron

11. A 4-year-old boy is found playing under the sink near several unmarked containers. Physical exam reveals several burns of the oropharynx. The next best step is:

    a. Administer steroids
    b. Simple dilution
    c. Consult social services
    d. Administer antibiotics
    e. Consult an endoscopist

12. A 6-year-old boy drinks furniture polish at home and coughs for approximately 5 minutes. He is asymptomatic when arrives at the ED, with a pulse oximetry reading of 100% O_2 saturation on room air. The next best step is to:

    a. Obtain a CXR immediately
    b. Obtain a CXR in 4 hours
    c. Discharge home without further interventions
    d. Administer antibiotics
    e. Administer steroids

13. An 18-month-old boy is brought to the ED vomiting blood. He was playing earlier in the day unsupervised in the kitchen. His vital signs are: T 37.5°C, HR 180, RR 24, and BP 80/palpable. Initial lab findings include Na 140 mEq/l, K 3.5 mEq/l, Cl 110 mEq/l, HCO_3 6 mEq/l, BUN 9 mg/dl, Cr 0.2 mg/dl, and glucose 180 mg/dl. Serum osmolarity is 290 mOsm/l. The best treatment is to administer:

    a. Activated charcoal
    b. Pyridoxine
    c. Dialysis
    d. Deferoxamine
    e. Fomepizole (4-MP)

14. An 11-year-old girl comes to the ED stating that she took an entire bottle of "pain pills" 12 hours ago. She is vomiting. Her vital signs are normal and her physical exam is normal except for some generalized, diffuse abdominal pain. Labs and ECG are normal. The best approach to this patient is to send an:

    a. Acetaminophen level upon arrival to the ED
    b. Acetaminophen level 4 hours after arrival to the ED
    c. Acetaminophen level and start N-acetylcysteine (Mucomyst) empirically
    d. Acetaminophen level upon arrival to the ED and 4 hours later
    e. Acetaminophen level and start urine alkalinization empirically

15. An 18-year-old girl is being evaluated for an overdose. She appears inebriated, but otherwise her exam is unremarkable. Lab findings include Na of 136 mEq/l, K 3.7 mEq/l, Cl 106 mEq/l, HCO_3 20 mEq/l, BUN 12 mg/dl, Cr 0.2 mg/dl, glucose 80 mg/dl, and a measured serum osmolarity of 320 mOsm/L. The most likely ingestion is:

    a. Ethanol
    b. Isopropyl alcohol
    c. Ethylene glycol
    d. Methanol
    e. Polyethylene glycol

16. A 15-year-old male patient is in the ED with an ECG that shows a PR interval of 0.12 seconds, a QRS interval of 0.08 seconds, a QT interval of 0.4 seconds, and an R-R interval of 0.64 seconds. Ingestion of which medication is most likely?

    a. Diphenhydramine
    b. Astemizole
    c. Cetirizine
    d. Loratadine
    e. Fexophenadine

17. A 17-year-old male has been camping in the woods with his high school friends. He developed nausea and vomiting with severe abdominal pain 8 hours ago, and now seems "confused." His friends deny having any medications or alcohols with them on the camping trip. The patient's vital signs are: T 37°C, HR 90, RR 16, and BP 110/65; O_2 saturation 100% on room air. His exam is notable for icteric skin and abdominal tenderness in the right upper quadrant. Lab workup is significant for elevated liver transaminases. After GI decontamination with charcoal, a treatment to consider is:

    a. Digoxin-specific antibody
    b. Physostigmine
    c. Anticonvulsants
    d. Penicillin
    e. Amyl nitrite

18. A teenager comes to the ED by ambulance after having been "found down." The patient was intubated in the field. Vital signs are: T 37°C, HR 50, RR 16 (bagged), BP 80/palpable despite atropine and IV fluids. On exam the pupils are 4mm and reactive; the patient's GCS score is 6 (Eye movement = 1, Verbal = 1, Motor = 4). Lab findings (blood chemistry profile) reveal serum levels of Na 140 mEq/l, K 3.8 mEq/l, Cl 110 mEq/l, HCO_3 14 mEq/l, BUN 8 mg/dl, Cr 0.8 mg/dl, and glucose 70 mg/dl. The patient's ECG is significant for sinus bradycardia of 48 bpm. GI decontamination and supportive measures are continued in the ED. The best antidote to use initially is:

    a. Naloxone
    b. Sodium bicarbonate
    c. Digoxin-specific antibody
    d. Nitroprusside
    e. Glucagon

19. A 21-month-old girl is sent by the primary care physician to the ED with a lead level of 55 mcg/dl found on routine screening. Physical exam is unremarkable. A KUB reveals small, multiple, scattered opacities in the small intestine. The next best step is to administer:

    a. Syrup of ipecac
    b. Activated charcoal
    c. Edathamil calcium disodium (Ca EDTA)
    d. 2,4-dimercaptopropanol (British Anti-Lewisite, or BAL)
    e. Polyethylene glycol

20. A 2-year-old girl is found near her grandmother's "diabetic pills." The child's bedside glucose level is 100 mg/dl. The agent most likely ingested is:

    a. Metformin
    b. Glipizide
    c. Glyburide
    d. Chlorpropamide
    e. Theophylline

21. An 18-year-old boy is working at his afterschool job cutting lawns when he develops eye tearing, nausea, and respiratory distress. On arrival to the ED, his vital signs are: T 37°C, HR 50, RR 20, and BP 110/70. His exam is significant for pupils that are 2mm reactive, moist eyes and mucous membranes, and wheezing on lung auscultation with pulses that are 2+. His abdominal exam is normal. His ECG shows sinus bradycardia at 50 beats per minute (bpm). The next best step is to:

    a. Administer atropine
    b. Administer atropine and pyridoxine
    c. Send a plasma cholinesterase level
    d. Administer atropine and pralidoxime
    e. Send a red blood cell (RBC) cholinesterase level

22. A 3-year-old boy is referred to the ED by the primary care physician for evaluation of a stiff neck. His mother states that the child has been well except for the "stomach flu" yesterday. There is no history of trauma. In the ED he is afebrile and has a completely normal exam except that his head is tilted to the left. The next step is to:

    a. Order neck films
    b. Perform a lumbar puncture
    c. Order a throat culture
    d. Administer activated charcoal
    e. Administer diphenhydramine

23. A 14-year-old female patient with known asthma is brought to the ED with a chief complaint of nausea and "the shakes." She is currently suffering from a URI. Her current medication regimen for asthma consists of albuterol, cromolyn sodium, and theophylline. All of the following medications are likely to worsen her symptoms EXCEPT:

    a. Cimetidine
    b. Phenobarbital
    c. Erythromycin
    d. Ciprofloxacin
    e. Clarithromycin

24. Lab results return for the patient in Question 23 and the theophylline level is noted to be 50 mcg/ml. The best treatment plan is:

    a. A single dose of activated charcoal
    b. Discharge patient without treatment
    c. Multiple doses of activated charcoal
    d. Multiple doses of activated charcoal plus dialysis
    e. Gastric lavage with normal saline

25. An 18-year-old female patient is brought to the ED for mental status changes. Vital signs are as follows: T 38.8°C, HR 120, RR 16, and BP 100/70. Her pupils are dilated, and she is delirious. Her ECG reveals a PR interval of 0.10 seconds, QRS interval of 0.12 seconds, and a corrected QT interval of 0.40 seconds. The best treatment is:

    a. Physostigmine
    b. Serum alkalinization
    c. Cardioversion
    d. Pralidoxime
    e. Defibrillation

26. All of the following medications are dangerous to toddlers in small doses (one or two doses) EXCEPT:

    a. Benzocaine
    b. Methyl salicylates
    c. Quinine
    d. Lindane
    e. *Philodendron* leaves

27. A 13-year-old boy is brought in to the ED by ambulance after he was found "acting strangely" at school. He developed ventricular fibrillation in route, and was unable to be resuscitated. The urine toxicologic screen that was sent to the inhospital lab is negative. The patient most likely ingested:

    a. Methylenedioxymethamphetamine
    b. Cocaine
    c. Halogenated hydrocarbon
    d. Gamma hydroxybutrolactone
    e. Phencyclidine

ANSWERS

1. c Pediatric poisonings are common medical emergencies. A multifactorial model has been proposed that considers the concordance of child, agent, and environmental factors that may lead to the possibility of a toddler ingestion. Children more likely to be poisoned include children that are 1–4 years old, male gender, hyperactive, and those with increased finger-mouth activity and pica. Likely agents to be ingested include those that are easy to obtain (e.g., in containers without a childproof cap) and ones that are attractive and/or palatable. Acute environmental stressors that could potentially put a child at risk would include a recent move, the holidays, or a new baby at home that could distract the parents. Children of caretakers with chronic disabilities also are predisposed to a higher likelihood of an ingestion. Overall, pediatric ingestions are more likely to occur in male children, are unintentional, usually consist of only one substance, and the most likely agents include household or personal care products as well as plants. The typical adult profile is an intentional ingestion that is due to many different drugs ("polypharmacy"), female gender, and is secondary to psychopharmacologic drugs (sedatives, tranquilizers, and antidepressants). Note that "nontoxic" ingestions in the pediatric population may not necessarily require any medical interventions, but will still require teaching about safety issues in order to provide the most optimal environment for the child.

2. b Drugs causing hypoglycemia can be remembered by the acronym "**HOBBIES**": H = hypoglycemia, O = oral hypoglycemics, BB = beta-blockers, I = insulin, E = ethanol, S = salicylates. Following this mnemonic, overdose with ethanol, propranol (beta-blocker), Pepto Bismol (bismuth and salicylates) and glipizide (oral hypoglycemic) can produce low blood sugars. The importance of checking a rapid blood glucose level early cannot be overemphasized. Hypoglycemia is corrected by giving 0.25–1.0 g/kg dextrose. Stimulants (caffeine, theophylline, beta agonists, epinephrine), calcium channel blockers, thiazides, and vacor cause hyperglycemia.

3. d The clinical scenario presented is typical of the opioid toxidrome (see Table 88.5 in *Textbook of Pediatric Emergency Medicine*, fourth edition), and therefore an empiric trial of naloxone should be given. Outside the neonatal period, it is safe to use a standard dose of 1–2 mg for acute overdose patients. Nalmefene and naltrexone are longer-acting opioid antagonists that may be useful in some clinical situations. Flumazenil, a benzodiazepine antagonist, should be administered in cases of a suspected benzodiazepine ingestions, but should NOT be used in cases of unknown overdoses such as possible tricyclic antidepressant (TCA) overdoses (this patient has a history of depression and may have access to such medications). The reason is that life-threatening seizures may be unmasked. Pyridoxine (Vitamin B6) is given for isoniazid overdoses (triad of metabolic acidosis, seizures, and coma). Glucose would not be indicated in a patient with a normal rapid bedside glucose test.

    The differential for miotic pupils is "**COPS**": C = cholinergics, clonidine, O = opiates, organophosphates, P = phenothiazines, pilocarpine, and S = sedative hypnotics. For mydriasis, the mnemonic is "**AAAS**": A = antihistamines, A = antidepressants, A = anticholinergics, atropine, and S = sympathomimetics. (APLS, third edition, 1999; American College of Emergency Physicians and the American Academy of Pediatrics, p 115)

4. b Opioids are contained in many medications. Paregoric is a camphorated tincture of opium that can be used in the treatment of diarrhea (to reduce GI motility and digestive secretions) or for neonatal opiate withdrawal. Cough and cold medications often contain dextromethorphan, which is an opioid derivative with potent antitussive but no analgesic or addictive properties. Propoxyphene (Darvon) is usually combined with acetaminophen (Darvocet) for use as an analgesic. Clonidine, an alpha-2 agonist, appears to interact with CNS opiate receptors, thus explaining the clinical symptoms of coma and miosis in overdose. Theophylline toxicity presents with nausea, vomiting, muscle tremors, seizures, and arrhythmias, not with lethargy and pinpoint pupils.

5. d It is important to be able to calculate both anion and osmolar gaps when evaluating toxicology patients. The anion gap = [Na] − [Cl] − [HCO$_3$] = 8–12 mEq/l. An elevated anion gap in the setting of metabolic acidosis can be caused by many different medications; "**MUDPILES**" is the mnemonic: M = methanol, metformin; U = uremia; D = diabetic ketoacidosis; P = paraldehyde, phenformin; I = isoniazid, iron, ibuprofen, inborn errors of metabolism; L = lactic acidosis; E = ethanol, ethylene glycol; and S = salicylates. The osmolar gap is calculated by subtracting the calculated osmolarity from the measured one. The formula for the calculated osmolarity is 2 [Na] + [glucose] ÷ 18 + [BUN] ÷ 2.8 = 290 mOsm/l. Rounding the denominator for glucose to 20 and the denominator for BUN to 3 can facilitate calculations. Overdoses of ethanol and other alcohols will elevate the osmolar gap. In this scenario, the calculated osmolarity is approximately 287 mOsm/l, and thus the osmolar gap is 3. Therefore, ingestion of an alcohol is unlikely; treatment with folic acid, fomepizole, Vitamin B1 (thiamine), and dialysis would not be indicated. Isoniazid presents with the triad of metabolic acidosis (one of the "I" medications in the MUDPILES mnemonic), seizures, and coma. Vitamin B6 (pyridoxine) will cause seizures and the metabolic acidosis to resolve.

6. a Gastrointestinal decontamination is the mainstay of management when the toxicology patient comes to the ED. While activated charcoal is preferred in most cases (see Question 8), gastric lavage can be useful in select instances. Gastric emptying is most effective if performed within the first hour ("golden hour") after ingestion, as the goal is to prevent the toxin from moving past the pylorus, where it can be systemically absorbed. Drugs with anticholinergic properties, however, may benefit from having lavage performed up to several hours after the ingestion, because gut motility has been slowed. Scopolamine is thus the most appropriate answer of the choices given in the question. The procedure does carry the risk of aspiration, mechanical trauma, and bradycardia (especially in elderly patients), and physical restraint may be needed. Therefore, gastric lavage is usually reserved for those patients who have ingested large amounts of potentially life-threatening medications, in cases where the procedure can safely be done within approximately 60 minutes of ingestion, and when activated charcoal alone may not be adequate.

7. e Gastric emptying can be accomplished either by induced emesis or gastric lavage (see Question 6). Syrup of ipecac is the only emetic agent approved for this use, and is derived from the roots of the *Cephaelis ipecacuanha* or *C. acuminata* plant. It is typically used in the home setting, often after plant ingestions (i.e. *Dieffenbachia*), and can be particularly beneficial for persons who live in rural communities that may be hours from a health care facility. Ipecac is used less frequently in urban areas, because it may interfere with the administration of activated charcoal once the patient reaches the health care facility. Induced emesis is contraindicated when patients have ingested caustics (e.g., sodium hydroxide) or hydrocarbons (e.g., turpentine), if they have uncontrolled hypertension (i.e., after ingestion of phenylpropanolamine) or increased intracranial pressure, and when there are issues of whether the airway is intact (for example, when lorazepam has been ingested).

8. c Activated charcoal is the primary method for gastrointestinal decontamination because it minimizes drug absorption into the body by adsorbing toxins onto its surface. The dose is 1 gram/kg in the pediatric population, up to a dose of 50–100 grams/kg in adolescents and adults. The majority of overdoses can be managed by administering charcoal; see Table 88.8 (in *Textbook of Pediatric Emergency Medicine*, fourth edition) for the small list of agents that are poorly adsorbed onto its surface. Quite simply, the major categories for which charcoal is not useful include the alcohols, hydrocarbons (e.g., gasoline), heavy metals (e.g., lithium/iron), caustics, and electrolytes and/or mineral acids and bases. Great care must be taken to ensure that the airway is protected, so that the charcoal is not aspirated.

9. e Whole bowel irrigation (WBI) is achieved by using large volumes and flow rates of a polyethylene glycol solution. It is not significantly absorbed nor does it exert an osmotic effect, making it safer than

the osmotic cathartics. This technique is particularly helpful in massive overdoses where charcoal does not bind the substance and when the patient presents late after ingestion, making gastric emptying less than optimal. Examples of cases where WBI may be useful would include ingestions of cocaine packets/crack vials, sustained-release medications (e.g., theophylline, lithium), and with heavy metal ingestions that either present late or when the efficacy of lavage is limited because of tube size.

10. c   Food-borne intoxications from consumption of contaminated marine life are second to the entero-toxins (*Salmonella*; *Shigella*; *Clostridium*, including botulinum; *Yersinia*; *E. coli*; and *Vibrio*) when working up a patient with presumed food poisoning. Guam, located in the South Pacific, is an endemic area for ciguatera poisoning. The toxin produced by the dinoflagellate *Gambierdiscus toxicus* is concentrated as it ascends the food chain. Humans become exposed when eating large fishes such as the barracuda, grouper, red snapper, and parrotfish. Patients may initially develop nausea and vomiting, followed by paresthesias. The classic symptom, though, is reversal of temperature sensation (paradoxical dysthesia). In severe cases, coma may be present. Treatment is primarily supportive; mannitol has been used to reverse neurologic manifestations. Trivalent antitoxin is recommended for all symptomatic patients exposed to botulism (as opposed to infant botulism). While diplopia, dysphagia, and dysarthria can be present in these cases, reversal of temperature is not. Antihistamines and/or cimetidine are helpful when a scombroid ingestion is suspected. The history would include eating tuna, bonita, skipjack, bluefish, or mahi-mahi. Because histamine is released, symptoms can include the acute onset of flushing, vomiting, pruritis, and wheezing. A peppery taste in the mouth is suggestive of scombroid poisoning. Although ondansetron could be considered in cases of prolonged GI symptoms, the nausea and vomiting associated with ciguatera poisoning is brief.

11. e   Caustic agents, also referred to as corrosives, can be either acidic, alkaline, or have a neutral pH. Many items stored under sinks are caustic, including oven cleaners, drain pipe cleaners, and toilet bowl cleaners. It can be difficult to identify the offending agent when unmarked containers are used to store them. Disc batteries lodged in the esophagus can be corrosive as well. A**C**idic products cause a superficial **C**oagulative necrosis; a**L**kaline ones penetrate deeply by means of **L**iquefactive necrosis, with possible subsequent perforation. Endoscopy is necessary to ascertain how much damage has taken place. Activated charcoal is not given, as this would obscure the mucosal surfaces. Simple dilution is not indicated for three reasons: 1) the child must be NPO for endoscopy, 2) fluids can extravasate into the mediastinum if perforation has occurred, and 3) an exothermic reaction could occur if the administered fluids are acidic or alkaline. Use of steroids is controversial. Most experts agree that first-degree burns will heal without complication, and that third-degree burns scar despite treatment. Second-degree burns, however, may benefit from steroids and empiric antibiotics. Neither steroids nor antibiotics would precede endoscopy. Social services would need to be consulted to ensure a safe environment for the child; again, this would not take precedence over endoscopy.

12. b   Furniture polish, lamp oils, and lighter fluids are aliphatic hydrocarbons that are commonly ingested in the pediatric population. The major concern is that these chemicals may be aspirated, resulting in a chemical pneumonitis. (See Figure 88.5 of *Textbook of Pediatric Emergency Medicine*, fourth edition.) If a child has no symptoms at home, then he or she can be observed there with close contact with a poison control center or ED for 12 hours. If symptoms develop and the child has symptoms upon presentation to the ED, a chest X-ray is obtained immediately and the child is admitted at that point if the film is abnormal. If it is normal, then the X-ray is repeated in 2–4 hours, because there may be a gradual evolution of abnormal radiographs. If the child is without symptoms at the time of arrival in the ED, then the X-ray may be obtained at 2–4 hours post ingestion. Children can be discharged home at 4–6 hours if they are asymptomatic; detailed instructions should be given to return if the patient develops fever or tachypnea, because evidence of pneumonitis may present at 12–24 hours post ingestion. Antibiotics are not recommended for prophylaxis but, instead, for a specific infection if it occurs. Steroids are not recommended because they have been shown to increase morbidity. Epinephrine is contraindicated because the hydrocarbons are known to cause ventricular irritability that can progress to fibrillation.

13. d   It is important to be able to calculate both anion and osmolar gaps when evaluating toxicology patients. The anion gap = $[Na] - [Cl] - [HCO_3] = 8–12$ mEq/L. An elevated anion gap in the setting of metabolic acidosis can be caused by many different medications/conditions; **"MUDPILES"** is the mnemonic: M = methanol, metformin; U = uremia; D = diabetic ketoacidosis; P = paraldehyde, phen-

formin; I = isoniazid, iron, ibuprofen, inborn errors of metabolism; L = lactic acidosis; E = ethanol, ethylene glycol; and S = salicylates. The osmolar gap is calculated by subtracting the calculated osmolarity from the measured one. The formula for the calculated osmolarity is 2 [Na] + [glucose] ÷ 18 + [BUN] ÷ 2.8 = 290 mOsm/l. Rounding the denominator for glucose to 20 and the denominator for BUN to 3 can facilitate calculations. In this particular scenario, the anion gap is 24 and the osmolar gap is 2. This patient most likely ingested iron, given that it is such a common ingestion and he is vomiting blood, is tachycardic, and hypotensive (symptoms of Phase I of iron intoxication). Deferoxamine is the chelator of choice and could be started empirically without waiting for an iron level given the history, exam findings, and laboratory information. Activated charcoal does not adsorb iron well (see Table 88.8 of *Textbook of Pediatric Emergency Medicine*, fourth edition). Any of the alcohols would give an elevation in the osmolar gap; thus dialysis and fomepizole would not be indicated. Finally, isoniazid is part of the MUD-PILES mnemonic, but the classic triad of symptoms is metabolic acidosis in conjunction with coma and seizures.

14. c   "Pain pills" is a term used by lay persons. The term can be used interchangeably to mean acetaminophen (APAP: N-acetyl-p-aminophenol), ibuprofen, aspirin (ASA), or a combination of these products. This patient presents with a history of an ingestion, is vomiting, and has diffuse general abdominal pain. It is highly probable that she did ingest APAP. She does not present with tinnitus, hyperpnea, or lethargy, which would be more suggestive of an aspirin overdose; also, her lab findings are normal (one would expect to see hypokalemia with a mixed respiratory alkalosis/metabolic acidosis on the arterial blood gas in a typical case of aspirin overdose). Therefore, it would be reasonable to wait for the aspirin level and start urinary alkalinization if the level is elevated. Although both an APAP and aspirin level should be sent upon arrival to the ED, this patient presents 12 hours out from the ingestion. The antidote N-acetylcysteine (NAC) is most protective against hepatotoxicity if given within 8 hours post ingestion. Given that 12 hours has passed, the loading dose of 140 mg/kg should be given immediately, and then once the APAP level is back, it can be used to determine possible hepatoxicity by plotting the level on the nomogram. If a patient presents less than 4 hours post ingestion, it is appropriate to wait until 4 hours post ingestion (not 4 hours after arrival to the ED) to draw the level. Patients who have ingested extended-release products should have a second APAP level drawn 4 hours after the first level to ensure that neither level is near the possible hepatotoxicity line on the nomogram. Liver function tests may not start to rise until 12–24 hours post ingestion.

15. b   Calculation of the anion and osmolar gaps once again can aid in making the correct diagnosis (see the answers to questions 5 and 13 for the calculations of these gaps). This patient's anion gap is 10 mEq/l and the osmolar gap is 40 mOsm/l. Although all of the alcohols (ethanol, isopropyl, ethylene glycol, and methanol) cause an elevated osmolar gap, isopropyl is the one alcohol that does not cause a high anion gap. This is because the metabolite is acetone. Isopropyl is approximately twice as intoxicating as ethanol and can cause myocardial depression at very high levels. Methanol is metabolized to formic acid, whereas ethylene glycol is broken down to both glycolic and oxalic acid.

16. b   The QTc (corrected QT interval) is calculated by dividing the QT interval (0.4 seconds) by the square root of the RR-interval (0.64 seconds) to give a QTc of 0.50 seconds. Antihistamines can cause cardiac toxicity in acute overdoses. Specifically, the nonsedating antihistamines terfenadine (i.e., Seldane, which is no longer available in the U.S.) and astemizole (Hismanol) cause QT interval prolongation and torsades-type atypical ventricular tachycardia. The other nonsedating antihistamines [e.g., cetirizine (Zyrtec), loratadine (Claritin), and fexophenadine (Allegra)] have not produced this change in the electrocardiogram. Diphenhydramine in massive overdoses can cause QRS prolongation and myocardial depression similar to the effects of a tricyclic antidepressant or class IA antiarrhythmic.

17. d   Plant ingestions are common in children at home as well as in older individuals who spend significant amounts of time outdoors. Adolescents and young adults may enjoy foraging for specific mushrooms (particularly *Psilocybe*) in order to experience hallucinogenic responses. Those mushrooms that produce symptoms within 6 hours (e.g., psylocybin and fungi with muscarinic, anticholinergic, and "Antabuse" effects) are usually benign in nature. However, when symptoms appear after 6 hours, *Amanita phalloides* must be considered. Symptoms include nausea/vomiting and abdominal pain that can progress to encephalopathy if fulminant hepatic failure ensues. Activated charcoal, especially multiple doses, is recommended to interrupt enterohepatic recirculation of amatoxin. Experimental therapies, such as high-dose penicillin (thought to inhibit liver uptake of amatoxin) and cimetidine (used for

cytochrome P450 system hepatoprotective effect), can be used after consultation with a toxicologist/regional poison control. If symptoms progress, liver transplantation may be required. Digoxin-specific antibodies are indicated in plant overdoses that have digitalis effects (i.e., lily-of-the-valley, foxglove, oleander). Atropine should be administered for ingestion of plants with atropinic effects (jimsonweed) and anticonvulsants should be given for ingestion of plants with nicotinic effects (e.g., tobacco) or those known to cause seizures (e.g., water hemlock). The Lily cyanide kit (amyl nitrite, sodium nitrite, and sodium thiosulfate) should be used to counteract toxic effects of plants that contain cyanogenic glycosides. Most plants (including *Dieffenbachia, Philodendron,* pokeweed, *Wisteria,* buttercup, and daffodils) merely cause gastrointestinal irritation. (See Table 88.16 of *Textbook for Pediatric Emergency Medicine,* fourth edition, for a complete listing of common plant toxidromes).

18. e   The patient presents with altered mental status, bradycardia and hypotension, which is a typical presentation for both beta-blocker and calcium channel blocker overdoses. The ECG can show sinus bradycardia, abnormal AV node conduction, or an accelerated junctional rhythm. Digoxin overdoses may present in a similar fashion; however, digoxin inhibits the sodium-potassium ATPase, and thus patients present with hyperkalemia after severe overdoses. Also, the ECG typically shows evidence of atrioventricular dissociation that appears as first- to third-degree heart block. Glucagon would be the best next step in management after decontamination and supportive measures. Glucagon is thought to increase intracellular cyclic AMP and thus improve both heart rate and blood pressure in both beta-blocker and calcium channel blocker overdoses; the mechanism of action is thought to be independent of both beta receptors and calcium antagonist action. Clonidine is a centrally acting alpha-2 agonist, causing a decrease in secretion of catecholamines into the synaptic cleft. Thus, patients present with decreased pulse and blood pressure, but these patients should also have pinpoint pupils (see Answer 3 for the differential of miotic pupils). Because clonidine seems to react at opiate receptors, naloxone can be used empirically. Early in the course of a clonidine overdose, alpha adrenergic effects at peripheral vascular receptors may result in hypertension; if an antihypertensive is needed, then a short-acting one such as nitroprusside can be utilized. Use of nitroprusside in this patient with a BP of 80/palpable would be absolutely contraindicated.

19. e   Lead poisoning in the pediatric population is usually secondary to lead paint exposure. The patient in this clinical scenario has lead paint chips throughout her small intestine. The mnemonic for radiodense substances is "**CHIPS**": C = chloral hydrate, H = heavy metals, I = iron, P = phenothiazines, S = sustained-release (enteric-coated) preparations (Schwartz, DT. In Goldfrank's *Toxicologic Emergencies,* sixth edition, Stamford, CT: Appleton & Lange, 1998, p 78). Gastric emptying, either by syrup of ipecac or gastric lavage, would not be indicated since the chips are past the pylorus. Activated charcoal does not bind lead. Whole bowel irrigation with polyethylene glycol (Go LYTELY) is the next best step in treating this child; chelation is *never* started until GI decontamination is completed. Asymptomatic children with lead levels in the 45–69 mcg/dl range are treated with edathamil calcium disodium (Ca EDTA). 2,4-dimercaptopropanol (British Anti-Lewisite, or BAL) is used in addition to Ca EDTA in symptomatic children or those with lead levels greater than 70 mcg/dl.

20. a   The oral hypoglycemics are used to treat adult-onset, or non–insulin-dependent, diabetes. Two major classes of these agents exist: the sulfonylureas (chlorpropamide, glipizide, glyburide) and the biguanides (metformin). The sulfonylureas lower blood glucose by stimulating endogenous pancreatic insulin secretion; thus, overdose with these agents will cause hypoglycemia. The biguanides, on the other hand, decrease hepatic glucose production and intestinal absorption of glucose but they do not stimulate insulin release. Therefore, overdose with metformin does not cause hypoglycemia, although lactic acidosis does occur. The elderly and those individuals with renal insufficiency are much more likely to have difficulties excreting metformin. Theophylline causes hyperglycemia. (Olsen, K. *Poisoning & Drug Overdose,* third edition, Stamford, CT: Appleton & Lange, 1999, pp 81–84).

21. a   This patient presents with a probable organophosphate ingestion from the chemicals he is using at work. Strict attention must be paid to protecting health care workers as they decontaminate these patients. Topical exposures, as in this case, should be approached by aggressive dermal decontamination as well as removing all contaminated clothing into plastic bags. The symptoms of an organophosphate exposure include the muscarinic, nicotinic, and central nervous system (CNS) effects. This patient presents with evidence of muscarinic involvement, which can be remembered by the mnemonics "**SLUDGE**" (S = Salivation, L = Lacrimation, U = Urination, D = Defecation, G = Gastrointestinal

cramping, E = Emesis) or "**DUMBELS**" (D = Diarrhea, U = Urination, M = Miosis, B = Bradycardia/Bronchorrhea, E = Emesis, L = Lacrimation, S = Salivation). Antidotal therapy begins with atropine to reverse these cholinergic effects. Severe poisonings that have evidence of nicotinic involvement (e.g., profound weakness, muscle twitching) would require the addition of pralidoxime (2-PAM). End point of therapy is when the patient no longer manifests cholinergic and neurologic signs. Because organophosphates inhibit cholinesterase, laboratory evidence may be obtained by measuring either red blood cell or plasma cholinesterase (the former is more specific). Levels are not available on a stat basis and would never preempt caring for the patient. Pyridoxine (Vitamin B6) is used as an antidote in isoniazid ingestions, with the clinical presentation being the triad of metabolic acidosis, seizures, and coma.

22.   e   Phenothiazines are not utilized as frequently in the pediatric population as they are in adults. Phenergan (promethazine) is commonly used as an antiemetic for children. Phenothiazine toxicity can present as a dose-dependent or dose-independent (idiosyncratic) phenomenon. For example, dose-dependent reactions would include CNS intoxication, cardiac conduction disturbances, and extrapyramidal effects. The dose-independent effect is the dystonic reaction, which is the presentation of this patient. These reactions are unrelated to the amount of ingested phenothiazine and may not have an onset of symptoms until 8–40 hours post ingestion. Given that this mother had not treated her child's "stomach flu" symptoms for at least a day, and these dystonic reactions can occur without an overdose, activated charcoal is not the best choice. Diphenhydramine, given either IM or IV, should reverse the problem. Torticollis can be secondary to many other entities (such as trauma or infection); in an afebrile, well-appearing child without a history of trauma, a medication reaction is the more likely etiology.

23.   b   Theophylline is not prescribed as often as it used to be for the treatment of asthma, due in part to its narrow therapeutic index. Theophylline's metabolism is by the hepatic mixed function oxidases (cytochrome P-450), and therefore numerous drug–drug interactions can occur. For example, a limited list of chemicals cause induction of cytochrome P-450 enzymes, thus lowering the theophylline level: phenobarbital, phenytoin, carbamazepine, and cigarette smoke (Shannon, MW. Theophylline and Caffeine. In Haddad, Shannon, & Winchester (eds.). *Clinical Management of Poisoning and Drug Overdose*, third edition. Philadelphia: WB Saunders, 1998; p 1095). The differential of drugs that reduce the metabolism of theophylline is broad; three frequently prescribed medications would be the H$_2$ antagonist cimetidine, the macrolide antibiotics (e.g., erythromycin and clarithromycin), and quinolones (i.e., ciprofloxacin).

24.   d   The therapeutic theophylline level is 10–20 mcg/ml. Clinical manifestations after acute ingestions can be predicted based on the level. For example, patients with a level in the range of 20–50 mcg/ml usually complain of nausea, vomiting, and muscle tremors. At levels above 60–70 mcg/ml, seizures and arrhythmias can occur. However, this correlation between serum level and symptoms is only true for acute overdoses and not for those persons with chronic intoxication. Activated charcoal is the mainstay of treatment. Multiple-dose activated charcoal (MDAC) is recommended, as theophylline elimination can be enhanced via gastrointestinal dialysis. Both hemoperfusion and hemodialysis also enhance elimination; however, hemoperfusion is not available in many medical centers. Both procedures are effective if done before seizures or arrhythmias develop; they do not change outcome if performed after these toxicities are seen. Hemoperfusion or hemodialysis is recommended if: 1) serum theophylline is greater than 80–100 mcg/ml in an acute ingestion, 2) serum theophylline is greater than 40 mcg/ml in a chronic ingestion, or 3) severe toxicity is present that is not responding to standard measures. Because this is a drug–drug interaction and not an acute overdose, there is no role for gastric lavage. It would not be appropriate to discharge a symptomatic patient home without treatment.

25.   b   This adolescent has ingested a tricyclic antidepressant. The clinical presentation of such patients can be remembered by the mnemonic "**TCA**": T = "tremors" (seizures), C = cardiovascular changes, and A = anticholinergic symptoms. Neurological symptoms can range from disorientation to seizures to coma. Cardiovascular changes include quinidine-like depression of the myocardium with subsequent arrhythmias and also hypotension from alpha adrenergic blockade. Anticholinergic effects are fever, delirium, urinary retention, pupil dilation, sinus tachycardia, and decreased GI mobility. A QRS interval of greater than 0.10 seconds increases morbidity and mortality significantly. Another ECG finding commonly seen in tricyclic overdoses is an R wave of less than 3 mm amplitude in lead aVR, suggesting that the distal conduction system of the right side of the heart may be more susceptible to the drug's toxic ef-

fects. (Liebelt, et al. ECG lead aVR versus QRS interval in predicting seizures and arrhythmias in acute tricyclic antidepressant toxicity. Annals Emergency Medicine 1995;26(2):195–201.) Serum alkalinization to maintain a pH of 7.45–7.55 will decrease drug binding to the myocardium and overcome sodium channel blockade in the conduction pathway. If the QRS does widen out and a ventricular arrhythmia develops, cardioversion (ventricular tachycardia with palpable pulses) or defibrillation (pulseless ventricular tachycardia or ventricular fibrillation) is mandated. Physostigmine is no longer recommended for treatment of the anticholinergic effects as the seizure threshold can be lowered and conduction defects may worsen. Urine alkalinization is used in overdoses such as aspirin, where the goal is to increase tubular secretion and inhibit tubular reabsorption (ion trapping). Pralidoxime is an antidote used in the treatment of organophosphate poisoning.

26. **e** A modest list of chemicals to be familiar with that may cause serious toxicity in the toddler in small doses is presented in Table 88.17 of *Textbook of Pediatric Emergency Medicine,* fourth edition. Although it is impossible to remember all of them, cardiac medications (beta-blockers, calcium channel blockers, clonidine, and the antiarrhythmics) lead the list. In addition, camphor, hypoglycemics, phenothiazines, theophylline, and tricyclic antidepressants are dangerous. Less obvious medications that are harmful in small doses to the young patient include both chloroquine and quinine, which exhibit quinidinelike cardiotoxicity. Also included in the list is benzocaine (which can cause methemoglobinemia and seizures), diphenoxylate (Lomotil, which can cause CNS/respiratory depression), lindane (which can cause seizures) and methyl salicylates (oil of wintergreen). *Philodendron* leaves may cause some mild GI irritation but are not usually dangerous in small doses.

27. **c** Inhalant abuse is very common among adolescents; of the 42 adolescent deaths in 1998 reported to the American Association of Poison Control Centers, 25% died from inhalant abuse. (Litovitz et al. American Journal of Emergency Medicine 1999;17(5):435–487.) These agents (e.g., glue, adhesives) are easy to use in school because the individual cannot be caught for possessing any type of illegal contraband. Though many of these agents merely produce inebriation when inhaled, the halogenated hydrocarbons can cause myocardial irritability/arrhythmias. The "sudden sniffing death" syndrome has been described. Toxicological screens may vary between institutions, but most are designed to detect common street drugs. Both methylenedioxymethamphetamine ("Ecstasy") and cocaine can also produce ventricular arrhythmias, but they should be picked up on the in-house urine toxicological screen. Phencyclidine (PCP) would rarely present with a dysrhythmia; it, too, is easily detected in the urine. Gamma hydroxybutyrolactone (GBL) is metabolized to gamma hydroxybutyrate (GHB) and is often used as a "date rape" drug. Individuals present with hypothermia, bradycardia, and coma; this coma usually lasts 1–2 hours. Most people can be managed with supportive care. GBL and GHB are not part of routine in-house toxicological screens at this point.

CHAPTER 89

Environmental Emergencies

VINCENT J. WANG, M.D.

QUESTIONS

1. A 3-year-old girl is brought to the ED after a near-drowning event. The mother was bathing her and had briefly left the room to obtain a towel. When she returned, she found her daughter under the water. The mother immediately pulled her out of the water. The patient coughed and choked, but was breathing spontaneously. In the ED, her vital signs are T 36.5°C, HR 100, RR 20, and BP 100/60. She is alert and interactive, in no acute distress. Her lung examination is normal, as is the rest of her examination. Your management includes:

   a. Obtaining a CXR
   b. Obtaining a CBC
   c. Administration of sodium bicarbonate
   d. Administration of cefuroxime IV
   e. Reassurance and discharge to home

The following case applies to Questions 2 and 3: A 5-year-old boy is brought to the ED after being found at the bottom of a pool. He had apparently hit his head after diving into the shallow end of the pool. His brothers pulled him out. When the paramedics arrived, the boy was noted to have shallow respirations and was minimally responsive. He is brought to the ED in C-spine precautions and on oxygen by facemask. In the ED, his vital signs are T 36.3°C, HR 120, RR 28, and BP 100/65, and an O_2 saturation of 99%. He is lethargic, but responds in full sentences when spoken to. You assign him a GCS score of 13 (Eye = 3, Verbal = 4, Motor = 6). He has a 3 cm hematoma over his forehead. His pupils are reactive bilaterally. His breath sounds are coarse, but symmetric. He is well perfused. The rest of his examination is normal.

2. Your initial management includes:

   a. Clearing his C-spine clinically
   b. Ordering a head CT scan only if his GCS changes
   c. Discontinuing the oxygen
   d. Restricting his fluids to ½ maintenance rate
   e. IV administration of methylprednisolone 30 mg/kg

3. The same boy's arterial blood gas analysis (ABG) reveals a pH of 7.0, Po_2 of 45 mmHg, Pco_2 of 70, and HCO_3 of 10 meq/l on 14 liters of oxygen by facemask. His CXR reveals diffuse pulmonary edema. He is not as responsive as before. Your management at this point should include all of the following, EXCEPT:

   a. Intubation
   b. Arterial cannulation
   c. Institution of hypothermia
   d. Administration of furosemide
   e. Administration of sodium bicarbonate

4. A 14-year-old boy is brought to the ED after being found face down in a lake. He was diving from a rock, but was not supervised by his parents. He was last seen 30 minutes prior to being found. He is brought to the ED apneic and pulseless, receiving bag-valve-mask ventilation and chest compressions. His core body temperature is 36°C. His physical examination is notable for no evidence of head trauma and for the smell of alcohol on his breath. His extremities are cool and mottled. Your management includes:

   a. Immediate intubation
   b. Institution of warming measures
   c. Obtaining an alcohol level
   d. Administration of epinephrine
   e. Discontinuing therapy

5. An 18-month-old girl is brought to the ED after being rescued from a house fire. She was found in the closet of her parents' bedroom. The fire appeared to start when an iron burned through the ironing board. On examination, she is alert and looking around. Her vital signs are: T 37°C, HR 110, RR 40, and BP 90/50. Her face is without soot and her lungs are clear, but she has mild retractions. You detect mild upper airway sounds. The rest of her examination is normal, and she does not have evidence of any cutaneous injuries. Your initial management should be:

   a. Immediate intubation
   b. Direct laryngoscopy
   c. Administration of a NS bolus 20 ml/kg IV
   d. Placement in a C-spine collar
   e. Observation for 2 hours and discharge to home

6. A 15-year-old boy is brought to the ED after being rescued from a school fire. He was found on the floor of the woodshop. His face is charred and his lips are swollen. He has extensive second- and third-degree burns over his face, legs, and trunk. Your management may include all of the following, EXCEPT:

   a. Immediate intubation
   b. Tracheostomy
   c. Administration of a NS bolus 20 ml/kg IV
   d. Placement in a C-spine collar
   e. Administration of steroids

7. A 9-year-old girl is brought to the ED because she has been lethargic. The mother returned home to find her in bed, minimally responsive. There are no medications at home and she has no other medical problems. It is the middle of winter and the home is being heated by an old coal furnace. On examination, she is minimally responsive. Her vital signs are: T 36.8°C, HR 110, RR 16, and BP 110/55; O_2 saturation is 99% on room air. Her skin is normal in color. Her lungs are clear and the rest of her examination is normal. You confirm your diagnosis by:

   a. Obtaining a CXR
   b. Obtaining a methemoglobin level
   c. Obtaining a carboxyhemoglobin level
   d. Obtaining a urine toxicologic screen
   e. Performing a lumbar puncture

8. A 7-year-old boy is rescued from a house fire. He is brought to you by the paramedics. His vital signs are: T 37.4°C, HR 120, RR 26, and BP 100/60; O_2 saturation is 99% on room air. He has no evidence of cutaneous injury, and his physical examination is normal. His GCS is 10 (Eye movement = 3, Verbal = 3, Motor = 4). You obtain a carboxyhemoglobin level, which reveals a level of 50%. Your management must include:

   a. Immediate intubation
   b. Administration of humidified oxygen via mist tent
   c. Placement in a hyperbaric oxygen chamber
   d. Administration of 100% oxygen
   e. Administration of 95% oxygen and 5% carbon dioxide

9. A 14-year-old girl is brought to the ED because of abdominal pain. She is a cross-country runner and had run a 10-kilometer race earlier in the day. While showering afterwards, she complained of severe abdominal pain. She felt as if her abdomen had "knots," as the pain lasted for several minutes. She denies fever, nausea, anorexia, or vomiting. The pain is now resolved. Her vital signs are: T 37°C, HR 120, RR 18, and BP 120/60. Her examination is normal and her abdomen is nontender. Which of the following tests would you obtain to confirm your diagnosis?

   a. CBC
   b. Serum electrolytes
   c. Abdominal x-ray
   d. Abdominal CT scan
   e. Urine pregnancy test

10. An 8-year-old boy is brought to the ED because of feeling faint at school. He had been rehearsing for the graduation ceremony that is to take place on the soccer field. He complains of how hot it was and that he felt extremely thirsty. Others described him as tired appearing and agitated. On examination, his vital signs are: T 38°C, HR 130, RR 24, and BP 100/60. His mucous membranes are dry, but the rest of his examination is normal. Your management includes:

    a. Obtaining an ECG
    b. Oral rehydration
    c. Rapid cooling measures
    d. Scheduling an EEG
    e. Urine toxicological screening

11. Another 8-year-old boy was with the boy from question 11. He had been complaining of similar symptoms, but in the commotion of the other child, he was overlooked. His classmates noted that he complained of headache and dizziness, and seemed to be confused. After the other ambulance had left, this child collapsed on the field. He is brought to you with the following vital signs: T 41°C, HR 150, RR 24, and BP 80/45. He has hot, dry skin that appears ashen. You send all of the following tests EXCEPT:

    a. Urinalysis
    b. Serum electrolytes
    c. CBC
    d. BUN and creatinine
    e. Calcium

12. A 15-year-old boy is brought to the ED because of lethargy. He had attended a friend's party that night, and was found on the front yard of the house lying on a snowbank, hours after the party was over. He is lethargic and has the smell of alcohol on his breath. His vital signs are: T 31°C, HR 60, RR 16, and BP 100/60. His skin is pale and cool to touch. He has no signs of trauma, and his physical examination is otherwise normal. His initial laboratory tests reveal an alcohol level of 240 mg/dl and a serum glucose of 80 mg/dl. Your best choice of rewarming techniques is:

    a. Use of blankets
    b. Immersion into a warm water bath
    c. Placement of electric blankets
    d. Inhalation of warm humidified air
    e. Peritoneal lavage

13. A 12-year-old girl is brought to you after being struck by lightning. She was playing golf in the rain when a bolt of lightning apparently struck her club. She is brought to you by the paramedics. Her vital signs are: T 37°C, HR 100, RR 18, and BP 110/60. Her physical examination is normal and she has no evidence of burns. Considerations in the treatment of this patient include:

    a. Wearing electrically insulated gloves when touching the patient
    b. Electrical defibrillation will be ineffective
    c. IV antibiotics should be given
    d. The patient should be admitted for observation
    e. No laboratory or ancillary studies need to be done

14. A 6-year-old boy is brought to the ED because he "shocked" himself when he placed a wire in an electrical socket. He sustained burns to his right hand, but is otherwise without complaint. On examination, he is alert and in NAD. He has minimal charring of the finger tips of his right hand, but no evidence of further burns. His neurovascular examination is normal in his hand. His physical examination is otherwise normal. Your management includes:

    a. X-ray of his right hand
    b. ECG
    c. CPK
    d. Urinalysis
    e. No further testing

ANSWERS

1. a   In this scenario, the patient appears to have had a minimal amount of time under the water. However, the patient could have aspirated water. Patients with significant hypoxemia may look well initially. Initial management includes obtaining a CXR and an O_2 saturation level on room air, with or without an ABG. If these are normal, the patient may be observed for further deterioration. In more severe events, a CBC, electrolytes, and a urinalysis should be obtained. Administration of sodium bicarbonate may be required to correct metabolic acidosis from resultant tissue hypoxia. However, this usually occurs with more severe episodes. Routine administration of antibiotics is not recommended.

2. d   Given his history of trauma and an abnormal neurological examination, a head CT scan is necessary and the C-spine should not be cleared unless the head CT scan is normal, and his GCS returns to normal. Administration of oxygen is important and should not be discontinued until it is determined that the patient is not hypoxemic and has not suffered a significant event. There is no proven benefit of steroid administration in near-drowners, and his neurological examination does not suggest a spinal cord injury. Since the patient's hemodynamic status is stable, fluids should be restricted to prevent potentially worsening pulmonary edema, thereby improving gas exchange.

3. c   This patient has severe respiratory distress, accompanied by hypoxemia and tissue hypoxia. The patient should be intubated and his acid-base status should be monitored with frequent ABG determinations, via arterial cannulation. Administration of furosemide is indicated to improve gas exchange. Sodium bicarbonate should also be given to correct the metabolic component of his acidosis. Even though studies are limited, mild hypothermia is neuroprotective. Patients who are hypothermic from a cold-

water near-drowning event may do well. However, there are no recommendations to institute hypothermia once in the care of physicians.

4. e Recent studies of drowning patients with asystole, but without hypothermia, have uniformly poor neurologic outcomes. In these cases the physician may reasonably discontinue resuscitative efforts. Determination of blood alcohol levels will not aid in the prognosis.

5. b Despite this child's well appearance, she is moderately tachypneic and shows signs of possible upper airway obstruction. Closed-space fires may cause inhalational injuries; this type of house fire may produce toxic gases from the combustion of various household goods. Direct laryngoscopy should be attempted to visualize the child's upper airway. If there is glottic, supraglottic, or pharyngeal edema, intubation should be considered. IV fluids are not necessary in the absence of shock. Likewise, cervical spine (C-spine) immobilization is not necessary since there is no history of trauma. If laryngoscopy is normal, the patient should be observed overnight.

6. e Management of a patient with severe burns over the face may include immediate intubation. Although some clinicians may choose to observe the patient closely, worsening edema over the next few hours may compromise the airway further, making the airway more difficult to secure. Tracheostomy may be necessary, as well, in this case. Given the significant burns, aggressive fluid resuscitation is warranted according to formulas discussed in Chapter 114 of the *Textbook of Pediatric Emergency Medicine*, fourth edition. Also, because a traumatic injury cannot be excluded, placement of a C-spine collar is recommended until the cervical spine can be appropriately evaluated. There is no role for steroids.

7. c Carbon monoxide poisoning should be suspected when children are exposed to potential sources, such as fires, automobile exhaust, or coal or wood-burning stoves and furnaces. The absence or presence of a "cherry red" color is of no diagnostic value; rather, the diagnosis should be made on the history and presentation. Pneumonia would likely cause more distress in a patient. Opiate or benzodiazepine ingestions and meningitis are potential causes of lethargy, but the other factors in the history and examination make these less likely.

8. d This patient has a severe intoxication from carbon monoxide poisoning. Treatment should include immediate removal from the fire environment and administration of 100% oxygen. Intubation may be required, but is not mandatory in this case. Humidified oxygen is recommended for smoke inhalations, but oxygen via mist tent is not recommended. The use of a hyperbaric oxygen chamber is somewhat controversial. If readily available, the chamber is helpful, but the transfer to a chamber should not jeopardize other conventional care. Inspired gas mixtures have not been shown to be of benefit.

9. b Heat cramps occur after significant muscle stress, as severe, brief, intermittent cramping of muscles. Cramps occur after the workload is done, typically while the individual is relaxing or taking a shower. Spasms last minutes and may be palpated as a mass in the affected muscle. Cramps may also occur in clusters. Laboratory investigation reveals hypochloremia and hyponatremia, and a decreased to absent urine sodium. Treatment involves repletion of these electrolytes. Occasionally, abdominal muscle cramps may resemble an acute abdomen, but given her history, this is less likely. Pregnancy (ectopic) should be considered in any appropriately aged female, but with an absence of other symptoms, this is very unlikely.

10. b Heat exhaustion may be manifest by either water depletion or salt depletion. In both cases, with a classic history of heat exhaustion, oral or IV rehydration is the predominant therapy. This patient does not have heat stroke, which would mandate rapid cooling measures as well. Other causes of syncope, such as prolonged QT syndrome or third-degree block, are unlikely given this history, and therefore an ECG is not indicated. Likewise, seizures or drug ingestion are unlikely.

11. c Complications of heat stroke include electrolyte abnormalities, rhabdomyolysis, hypocalcemia, shock, and neurologic dysfunction. Therefore each of the tests would be helpful, with the exception of a CBC.

12. e A number of strategies exist for rewarming a patient. Passive rewarming, such as the use of blankets, is inadequate for hypothermic patients with a body temperature below 32°C. Active rewarming may be divided into external and core rewarming techniques. External rewarming techniques include electric

blankets, hot water bottles, overhead warmers, and immersion into warm water baths. However, each of these may cause an "after-drop" of core temperature, as the warming of the skin and extremities leads to peripheral vasodilation and shunting of cold, acidemic blood to the vital organs. Core rewarming techniques are more rapid and less likely to cause after-drop. Peritoneal lavage, hemodialysis, extracorporeal blood rewarming, and mediastinal irrigation are all helpful, but require varying degrees of technical skill.

13. **d**   High-voltage injuries produced by lightning may cause significant injury. Contrary to popular belief, victims do not remain "electrified" and do not require insulating precautions. Also, defibrillation should be effective, and may be needed if arrhythmias develop. Risk of infection is increased, but routine use of prophylactic antibiotics is not indicated. Tetanus toxoid should be given if the patient is not up to date. Given the potential for injury, screening labs should be sent and the patient should be admitted for observation.

14. **e**   Minor household electrical injuries that are essentially asymptomatic do not require further testing. A thorough physical examination should exclude significant injuries. Fractures may be associated with significant electrocutions, but there are usually accompanying soft tissue signs of injury. An ECG would be recommended if the cardiovascular examination is abnormal, or in a high-voltage injury. Likewise, high-voltage injuries may cause renal and muscle damage, thereby warranting screening for these injuries. Treatment for this patient should be discharge to home and safety counseling for the child and the parents.

CHAPTER 90

Radiation Accidents

THOMAS H. CHUN, M.D.

QUESTIONS

1. A group of school children who were touring a nuclear power plant are brought to the ED for evaluation. While at the plant, the children were exposed to radioactive steam and radiation from the reactor, similar to the exposures experienced at "Three Mile Island." Appropriate radiation exposure precautions for ED personnel would be:

    a. Wearing radiation shielding (e.g., lead-lined equipment)
    b. Screening all patients for radioactivity with a Geiger counter
    c. Wearing radiation dosimeters, to keep track of total radiation exposure
    d. Undressing and showering all patients before they are seen by ED personnel
    e. No specific precautions needed

2. An explosion occurs at a nuclear weapons manufacturing plant. Two boys who were playing in their yards at the time of the explosion are brought to the ED for evaluation. The first child lives a quarter of a mile away from the plant and was in his yard for 15 minutes before his parents learned of the explosion. The second boy lives a mile away from the plant, but was in his yard for an hour before his parents brought him to the ED. There is an unobstructed field between the weapons plant and both homes. If any radiation was released from the explosion, the child who was exposed to more radiation is:

    a. The first child, by an insignificant amount
    b. The second child, by an insignificant amount
    c. The first child, by a large amount
    d. The second child, by a large amount
    e. There was equal exposure

The following case relates to Questions 3 and 4: Bart, Lisa, and Maggie, three siblings, are brought to an ED with an unusual assortment of linear lesions on their hands, buttocks, and thighs. The lesions vary widely and include areas of mild erythema, blisters, and frank necrosis. The children and their parents deny any history of thermal or burn injuries. They are unaware of how the lesions arose. The father, Homer, who works at the local pipe welding plant, does admit to occasionally bringing home objects from work, to be used as toys for the children.

3. Historical features of radiation injuries in children most often include:

    a. Accidental or covert exposure to radiation
    b. Employment of the child in an industry utilizing radiation
    c. Exposure to a known source of radiation
    d. Exposure to medical radionuclides
    e. Inadvertent ingestion of radium

4. Bart, Lisa, and Maggie's physical examinations are otherwise unremarkable. The children are afebrile, with normal vital signs, no signs of shock, and no other physical complaints. The course of their illness will most likely include:

    a. Bone marrow suppression
    b. Sepsis/death
    c. CNS and cardiovascular collapse
    d. Evolving tissue necrosis
    e. Gastrointestinal (GI) dysfunction

5. A 16-year-old girl comes to the ED for evaluation of possible radiation illness. Earlier in the day, she drove her father to a hospital for an appointment. Her father has a CNS tumor, for which he is receiving radiation therapy. After accompanying her father on the visit, she develops nausea and vomiting and believes that her symptoms are caused by radiation exposure she inadvertently received while sitting in the radiation oncology waiting area. The likely sequelae for this patient is:

    a. Psychiatric findings
    b. Decreased lymphocyte count
    c. GI tract sloughing
    d. Sepsis
    e. Bone marrow suppression

The following case relates to Questions 6–12: A nuclear weapon accidentally explodes in central Asia. It is estimated that the population of a nearby village was exposed to 300 rads of radiation. A disaster relief medical team is dispatched to the area to assist in the care of the victims.

6. A 9-year-old boy is seen approximately 48 hours after the accident. He presents with nausea, vomiting, fatigue, headache, and dizziness. Findings on his complete blood count (CBC) at this point in time would include:

   a. Anemia
   b. Lymphocytopenia
   c. Thrombocytopenia
   d. Neutropenia
   e. Leukemic infiltrates

7. Physical examination of the patient in Question 6 reveals an ill-appearing but nontoxic child. His vital signs are: T 37.2°C, HR 92, RR 18, and BP 104/78. His mucous membranes are moist and without evidence of sloughing or necrosis. His chest is clear to auscultation and he has a normal cardiovascular exam. Abdominal exam is unremarkable. His extremities are warm and well perfused. There are no focal neurologic deficits. He is eating and drinking without difficulty and has normal urine output. Appropriate management at this point would include:

   a. Bowel rest and parenteral hydration
   b. Sepsis workup and broad-spectrum antibiotics
   c. Transfusion of blood products
   d. Antioxidants, to decrease chromosomal damage
   e. Close observation, no specific interventions needed

8. A 17-year-old girl from the village was in a field next to the weapons facility at the time of the accident. Because of her proximity to the explosion, it is estimated that she received a dose of 5000 rads. Her initial clinical presentation and course is likely to be:

   a. The same as the first patient
   b. Similar to the first patient, with a longer prodromal stage
   c. Primarily severe nausea and vomiting
   d. Cardiovascular and CNS collapse
   e. Sepsis

9. A volunteer who has been assisting in rescue operations at the site of the accident is brought to you for evaluation. He denies any physical complaints. His clothing is covered with dirt from the accident site. For this patient and other health-care workers at the site, the risk of radiation injuries from the contaminated soil is:

   a. Patient—low risk; health-care workers—low risk
   b. Patient—high risk; health-care workers—low risk
   c. Patient—low risk; health-care workers—high risk
   d. Patient—high risk; health-care workers—high risk
   e. Risk cannot be determined without more information

10. In the initial care of the patient in Question 9, health-care workers should observe which of the following decontamination precautions?

    a. Decontamination by non–health-care workers
    b. Decontamination behind lead shielding
    c. Use of "universal precautions"
    d. Use of gloves only
    e. No precautions are necessary

11. In the decontamination of the patient in Questions 9 and 10, the single most effective procedure in eliminating external contamination is:

    a. Thorough irrigation of the skin
    b. Removal of his clothing
    c. Shaving of hair
    d. Scrubbing of the skin
    e. Use of soap and shampoo

12. The patient described in Questions 9–11 is not sure if he might have inhaled or accidentally ingested radioactive materials. He acknowledges that while he was at the accident site, he didn't always wash his hands before eating. An appropriate method for detecting internal contamination would be:

    a. Obtaining a CBC
    b. Scanning the patient with a Geiger counter
    c. Ophthalmic examination for cataracts
    d. Checking excretions for radioactivity
    e. Checking a sperm count

ANSWERS

1. e   There are no measurable acute biologic effects of radiation doses less than 10–20 rems. Radiation exposure to off-site medical personnel from "Three Mile Island" was 14 millirems (the radiation equivalent of 1 or 2 chest x-rays). Following the Chernobyl accident, which released much more significant levels of radiation, the highest radiation dose to off-site personnel was a few rems. It is thus extremely unlikely that caring for victims of a radiation accident such as these will injure ED personnel.

   The term *radiation* strictly refers to the transfer of energy from a source. *Ionizing radiation* includes x-rays, gamma, alpha, and beta rays, which are energetic forms of radiation that can strip electrons (ions) off atoms. Acute exposure to *non-ionizing radiation,* in the form of radio and microwaves as well as infrared, ultraviolet, and visible light, can cause thermal injuries. More severe cellular injury may result from chronic exposure to non-ionizing radiation. The term *radioactive* refers to an unstable atom, which spontaneously gives off radiation. A person who has been exposed to radiation is NOT radioactive, unless he or she has radioactive particles within the body or on its surface.

All Emergency Departments are required by the Joint Commission on Accreditation of Hospitals (JCAHO) to have a radiation emergency plan. ED physicians should familiarize themselves with their hospital's radiation emergency plan. Because these patients are not contaminated with radioactive particles, no specific decontamination or radiation screening measures are indicated. Radiation shielding equipment is cumbersome, impractical, and not warranted in the ED management of radiation-exposed patients.

2. c   The three factors that determine the amount of radiation exposure are *distance, time,* and *shielding.* The amount of radiation exposure follows the law of inverse squares: doubling the distance from the radiation source reduces the radiation dose by a factor of 4, tripling the distance reduces the dose by a factor of 9, and so on (see Figure 90.3 in the *Textbook of Pediatric Emergency Medicine,* fourth edition). The amount of exposure is directly proportional to the time exposed to the radiation. Shielding from the source of radiation in this instance was nonexistent. In most radiation accidents, shielding rarely provides meaningful protection, because high-energy radiation is involved.

Thus if radiation was involved in the explosion, the first child was exposed to four times the amount of radiation (16 times the intensity of radiation for one-fourth the amount of time) as the second child.

3. a   In the majority of reported pediatric radiation injuries, the child was either unknowingly or covertly and intentionally exposed (in a form of child abuse) to the source of radiation. Industrial exposure to radiation is the most common cause of radiation injury overall. Radiation is employed in many industries (e.g., sterilization of medical equipment or food industry equipment, checking pipe welds, etc.). Most victims exposed to these sources of radiation are adults, however. Medical radionuclides rarely cause radiation injury. They are engineered with short half-lives, which minimizes their potential to cause accidental injury. Children are not typically involved in radium painting, and are unlikely to have access to it.

Sources of radiation are often quite innocuous appearing, without safety or warning labels. Figure 90.4 in the *Textbook of Pediatric Emergency Medicine* (fourth edition) depicts the type of device that could have caused the injuries described in Question 3. Hands, thighs, and buttocks are common areas of accidental radiation injuries, incurred when victims picked up a radioactive object or placed it in their pockets. Fortunately, radiation injuries are uncommon in children, but should be considered in cases of unexplained burnlike injuries or focal tissue necrosis. Thermal burns are usually easily distinguished from local radiation injuries. The effects of a thermal burn are immediate and the patient almost always knows when and how the injury occurred.

4. d   Local radiation injuries rarely cause systemic symptoms (e.g., bone marrow suppression, GI, CNS, or cardiovascular effects) unless they are accompanied by significant whole body irradiation. Local radiation injuries are rarely life threatening. They are difficult to manage however, because they tend to evolve slowly over months or even years. The injuries evolve slowly because radiation causes progressive fibrosis of blood vessels, which in turns leads to tissue necrosis and poor healing. Lesions often have a waxing and waning course (appearing, disappearing, and reappearing over time), which can be confusing diagnostically. Local infections, gangrene, and amputation of structures are common complications. Systemic infections such as sepsis can occur but are not common. Skin grafting, especially musculo-cutaneous flaps, may be necessary.

5. a   This is a very low-risk situation for radiation exposure or illness. Perceived radiation exposure is by far the most common radiation-related complaint. Because of common misconceptions about radiation, any symptoms of illness are often attributed to radiation exposure. These perceptions can result in significant psychological stress and may be inadvertently reinforced by medical personnel who are unfamiliar with radiation biology. Sequelae of Acute Radiation Syndrome (e.g., gastrointestinal changes, bone marrow suppression, and/or sepsis) are unlikely in this scenario.

6. b   Acute Radiation Syndrome (ARS) occurs at radiation doses above 100 rems (see Table 90.5 in *Textbook of Pediatric Emergency Medicine,* fourth edition). ARS follows a predictable clinical course. The prodomal stage lasts for approximately 2 days after the radiation exposure. The latent stage ensues and

varies from 2 to 20 days in length. The next stage is that of "manifest illness," which may last up to 6 weeks (see Figure 90.6 in the textbook). This patient has the classic symptom complex of the prodromal stage. Lymphocyte counts decrease rapidly in the first 24 hours following radiation exposure. Thrombocytopenia, anemia, neutropenia, and leukemia (if it occurs) do not arise until at least 2 weeks into the course of ARS.

7. e   Estimating the amount of radiation exposure can very difficult, as the signs and symptoms of the prodromal stage of ARS are nonspecific. Nausea and vomiting are common but not specific for the severity of ARS. The lack of these symptoms however, would strongly suggest that the patient was not exposed to enough radiation to cause ARS. Treatment during the prodromal stage is entirely supportive. No survivable radiation injury requires immediate life-saving treatment. There are no acute treatments that prevent the development of ARS injuries.

This patient clearly does not need parenteral hydration, however. His greatest risk for sepsis will not arise for another 2 to 3 weeks. As discussed in the previous question, this patient is not at immediate risk of anemia or thrombocytopenia.

8. d   Although it is true that with increasing radiation exposure, the duration of the prodromal stage increases and the length of the latent stage decreases, doses above 700 rads cause different radiation syndromes. The "GI syndrome" occurs at doses greater than 700 rads. There is prompt onset of severe nausea, vomiting, and diarrhea. The latent stage is approximately 1 week, followed by recurrence of GI symptoms, sepsis, electrolyte imbalance, and (in most patients) death. These patients are at particular risk of sepsis secondary to bone marrow suppression and translocation of GI pathogens across radiation-damaged GI mucosa.

At doses over 5000 rads, CNS and cardiovascular symptoms predominate. Patients experience almost immediate nausea, vomiting, hypotension and increased vascular permeability. Patients develop CNS depression, ataxia, and seizures caused by cerebral edema and shock. Death usually occurs within 1 to 4 days.

9. a   External or internal radiation contamination is the only type of radiation injury that requires medical personnel to observe any radiation precautions. Even so, such contamination is rarely a significant medical problem. The majority of contaminated patients will not be highly radioactive; notable exceptions are patients covered with metallic particles or microscopic "hot particles," which can be intensely radioactive. The likelihood of contamination can usually be determined by an accurate description of the accident and/or radiation source. Use of a radiation detector (such as a Geiger counter) will quickly and easily identify which patients are radiation risks. Soil is not highly radioactive. This patient should be considered at low risk for radiation injury and for causing illness in his caregivers.

10. c   The easiest way to conceptualize appropriate decontamination precautions is to imagine that the patient is covered in a readily detectable noxious agent, such as sewage. The goals of decontamination are to prevent caregivers from becoming internally or externally contaminated and to contain the spread of the contaminated particles. Caregivers should at a minimum employ "universal precautions," wearing gown, gloves, and eye protection, as well as face masks with high filtering abilities to prevent respiratory uptake of contaminated particles. Ideally, aprons, shoe covers, and head coverings should also be used. If external contamination is widespread, covering the floor will help decrease the spread of contaminants. At the completion of the decontamination process, all equipment used should be placed in plastic bags and disposed of appropriately. Lead shielding is not necessary and would only make the task more cumbersome.

11. b   Removal of the patient's clothing will likely eliminate 70–90% of the external contamination. Patients should be washed repeatedly with a damp cloth and soap/shampoo, with particular attention paid to hair and the area under the nails, areas that may trap radioactive particles. Bathing with running water is an alternative; however, containing water runoff may be an added complication. Shaving and excessive rubbing of the skin (vigorous scrubbing with washcloths) should be discouraged, as this may increase absorption of radioactive particles through the skin.

A Geiger counter should be used to monitor decontamination efforts. Repeated washing may be necessary to remove all or most of the contamination. If radioactivity persists after cleaning, the contaminants may be internal or fixed to the skin.

12. **d**   A patient must undergo thorough external decontamination before being assessed for internal contamination. Checking moistened nasal swabs and excreta (including urine, stools, emesis, etc.) for radioactivity is the recommended method for screening for internal contamination. Unless the internal contamination is massive, CBC, ophthalmic, or sperm count abnormalities are more likely to be the result of whole body radiation exposure. A normal external scan with a Geiger counter does not rule out internal contamination.

If internal contamination is suspected, nonspecific interventions such as activated charcoal or alginate-containing antacids can be safely used. In cases of known radioactive iodine uptake, administration of stable iodine effectively blocks thyroid uptake of the radioactive isotope. Use of invasive procedures (such as pulmonary lavage) or other treatments should be undertaken only after consultation with radiation experts.

CHAPTER 91

Bites and Stings

VINCENT J. WANG, M.D.

QUESTIONS

1. A 6-year-old girl is brought to the ED shortly after brushing against a jellyfish in the water. The jellyfish is described as 15–30 centimeters in diameter and purple in color. When you examine the patient, the jellyfish tentacles are still embedded in the girl's leg. The first step in treatment is to:

   a. Apply baking soda to the site
   b. Soak the affected extremity in 40°C water
   c. Wash the area with lactated Ringer's solution
   d. Call the Marine Poison Control Center for jellyfish antivenin
   e. Administer phenytoin prophylactically

2. A 5-year-old boy was wading in shallow water off the coast of North Carolina and told his father that he had stepped on a "fish." He complains of intense pain in his leg. He also complains of weakness, nausea, and sweating. When the child is brought to you, you note a laceration of the thigh, but no other injuries. Management includes:

   a. Treatment with calcium carbonate
   b. Treatment with cephalexin
   c. Topical application of baking soda to the site
   d. Allowing the wound to bleed, since this will facilitate removal of the venom
   e. Submerging the wound in 40°C water

3. A 12-year-old boy was surfing when he was bitten by a shark. The patient sustained significant lacerations of the right thigh. He complains of weakness and appears pale. Management includes:

   a. Administration shark antivenin
   b. Administration of midazolam
   c. Pressor support for hypotension
   d. Careful inspection of the entire body for other bite sites
   e. Administration of ceftriaxone

4. A 5-year-old boy was camping in Arizona when he began screaming in pain just after he crawled into his sleeping bag. He is brought to your ED complaining of pain in his right leg. He is restless and has roving eye movements. On examination, there is no significant erythema or swelling at the site of his pain. Immediate management includes:

   a. Prophylactic intubation
   b. Sending a serum sample to the lab to determine the type of envenomation
   c. Applying a constriction band, followed by incision and suction to remove the venom
   d. Administering antivenin
   e. Providing supportive care only

5. An 8-year-old girl was playing in her grandmother's closet in New England earlier in the day. Approximately 3 hours later, she complained of generalized pain in her abdomen, flanks, thighs, and chest, which was described as cramping. She has also vomited twice. She has not had a fever. You suspect that:

   a. The patient has an appendicitis
   b. The patient has been bitten by a scorpion
   c. The patient has been bitten by a black widow spider
   d. The patient has been bitten by a brown recluse spider
   e. The patient has been bitten by a wolf spider

6. The most lethal spider bite is that of the:

   a. Tarantula (*Lycosa* species)
   b. Wolf spider (*Lycosa tarantula*)
   c. Black widow spider (*Latrodectus* species)
   d. Jumping spider (*Phidippus* species)
   e. Brown recluse spider (*Loxosceles reclusa*)

7. The mother of a 7-year-old girl reports that her daughter has been stung by a bee. The girl appears well, with no respiratory distress or rash at the time of presentation. The stinging apparatus is embedded in the girl's forearm. Initial treatment includes:

   a. Scraping, rather than pulling the stinger out
   b. Immediate subcutaneous (SC) injection of epinephrine at the site of the sting
   c. Immediate SC injection of epinephrine at any site
   d. Local wound care and oral diphenhydramine as needed
   e. Immediate incision and suction of the envenomation site

8. A 12-year-old boy was stung by a bee. He developed wheezing, difficulty breathing, and a muffled voice 10 minutes after the sting. Management includes:

   a. Local wound care and outpatient follow-up
   b. Oral diphenhydramine and outpatient follow-up
   c. Subcutaneous epinephrine and outpatient follow-up
   d. Subcutaneous epinephrine and admission to the hospital
   e. Immediate intubation and admission to the intensive care unit (ICU)

9. A 16-year-old girl was bitten by a snake in her family's garage. The girl's father is able to kill the snake and brings it to the ED. Which of the following characteristics makes you believe that she was NOT bitten by a member of the family Crotalidae (pit vipers)?

   a. Pits on the snake's head
   b. Round pupils
   c. Long, curved fangs
   d. Triangular-shaped head
   e. A single row of ventral scales

10. An 8-year-old boy was bitten by a rattlesnake approximately 30 minutes ago. In your assessment, you consider each of the following factors about the envenomation, EXCEPT:

    a. Venom toxicity
    b. Size and general health of the victim
    c. Site of the envenomation
    d. Size of the snake
    e. Victim's last meal

11. A 10-year-old boy sustained a snakebite in a desert in Arizona. He complains of immediate and intense burning pain after the bite. He presents in the ED approximately 20 minutes after the snakebite. On exam, you note two fang marks, 12 mm apart, with surrounding edema. You suspect that the patient was bitten by a:

    a. Coral snake (*Micruras euryxanthus*)
    b. Mojave rattlesnake (*Crotalus* species)
    c. Diamondback rattlesnake (*Crotalus atrox*)
    d. King snake
    e. Water moccasin (*Agkistrodon piscivorus*)

12. A 5-year-old girl was bitten by a snake. Which of the following characteristics would lead you to suspect this was a coral snake?

    a. Fang marks greater than 12 mm apart
    b. Intense local pain and swelling
    c. Paresthesias, fasciculations, and weakness
    d. Blood pressure of 70/30
    e. Respiratory rate (RR) of 20 breaths per minute, without retractions

13. You are hiking in the Southwest and your friend has just been bitten right above the ankle by a rattlesnake. The nearest medical facility is 30 minutes away. Immediate management of a rattlesnake envenomation includes:

    a. Stabilization and treatment in the field
    b. Elevating the affected extremity
    c. Applying a tourniquet distal to the wound on the extremity
    d. Applying a tourniquet proximal to the wound on the extremity
    e. Incision and suction of the wound

14. A 17-year-old boy is transported to your medical center after a rattlesnake envenomation. Three hours have elapsed since the bite. The site has surrounding erythema, edema, and ecchymoses. The patient is hypotensive, requiring high doses of pressor support. Appropriate therapy over the next hour would be:

    a. Supportive care alone
    b. Antivenin therapy, if the patient deteriorates
    c. Immediate administration of antivenin therapy
    d. Skin testing with antivenin, followed by antivenin therapy if the test is negative
    e. Incision and suction of the wound

15. A 2-year-old boy is brought to your ED in Florida after being bitten by an eastern coral snake (*Micrurus fulvius*). The bite occurred just minutes ago, and he is crying but well appearing on your examination. Appropriate management would be:

    a. Immediate application of a proximal constriction band
    b. Incision and suction of the wound
    c. Administration of antivenin
    d. Supportive care alone
    e. Administration of methylprednisolone and diphenhydramine

16. A 14-month-old boy is bitten on the arm by the family's German Shepherd. The dog is healthy and its immunizations are up to date. You evaluate the patient in the ED within an hour of the bite. He has small lacerations, but no puncture wounds, of his arm. He appears to have significant tenderness of the site. The boy's immunizations are also up to date. Management includes:

    a. Administration of tetanus toxoid
    b. Administration of rabies immune globulin and human diploid cell vaccine
    c. Obtaining radiographs of the limb to assess for fractures
    d. Arranging for delivery of the dog's head to the state lab
    e. Antibiotic prophylaxis

17. Antibiotic prophylaxis is NOT indicated in which of the following cases?

    a. Cat bite resulting in a superficial laceration of the lower leg
    b. Human bite resulting in a laceration of the forearm
    c. Dog bite producing superficial lacerations on the arm of an immunosuppressed patient
    d. Dog bite resulting in a superficial laceration of the face
    e. Dog bite resulting in a puncture wound in the hand

18. A 5-year-old girl is bitten on the arm by her pet cat. Appropriate prophylactic antibiotic therapy would include:

    a. Amoxicillin orally
    b. Trimethoprim-sulfamethoxazole orally
    c. Amoxicillin-clavulanic acid orally
    d. Neomycin cream topically
    e. Silvadene cream topically

19. An 18-year-old adolescent boy was involved in a fight. He sustained a laceration to his knuckles when he punched another youth in the mouth. The patient presents to you 2 days after the injury with moderate swelling and with pain on passive finger motion. Appropriate management would include all of the following, EXCEPT:

    a. Radiographs of the hand
    b. CBC and ESR
    c. Parenteral antibiotic therapy
    d. Oral antibiotic therapy
    e. Hepatitis B and HIV testing

20. In which of the following scenarios is rabies immune globulin and human diploid cell vaccine NOT indicated?

    a. A wild raccoon bites a child
    b. A bat is found hanging from the ceiling of the child's bedroom
    c. A stray cat scratches a child and then runs away
    d. A wild fox bites a child
    e. A rat bites a child

ANSWERS

1. **a** The nematocysts on a jellyfish's tentacles are the primary means for the organism to subdue, penetrate, anchor, and poison its prey. Venom is injected via nematocysts, but the mechanism of firing is not fully understood. Envenomation may occur even if the jellyfish is dead, and in fact, many injuries occur when these organisms wash ashore. Inactivation of the nematocysts may be achieved with topical application of baking soda, vinegar, or meat tenderizer (papain). The area should also be cleansed, preferably with sea water. Submerging the wound in hot water may be used for heat-labile toxins such as those of the stingrays, but this is not indicated for jellyfish envenomations. Removal of the tentacles is essential, since the nematocysts may continue to discharge venom while in contact with skin. Therefore the tentacles should be removed carefully with a gloved hand or with instruments. Routinely, antivenin therapy is not used, but in the case of the *Chironex fleckeri*, an antivenin is available. (The *Chironex fleckeri* is the most deadly of the jellyfish, but it is primarily found off of the coast of Australia.) There is no role for prophylactic phenytoin in this case.

2. **e** Most stingray injuries occur when the victim is wading in water and accidentally steps on the stingray. The envenomation is a defensive reflex as the stingray whips its tail toward the victim. The wound is a combination of a puncture and a laceration. Pain is noted immediately, followed by general-

ized symptoms such as weakness, nausea, vomiting, sweating, muscle fasciculations, and cramps. Paresthesias, hypotension, arrhythmias, and death may also occur. Treatment includes irrigating the wound with cold salt water, which will remove much of the venom. Bleeding should be controlled with direct pressure; there is no indication for allowing a wound to bleed. The affected area should be placed in hot water (40–45°C) for 30 to 90 minutes to inactivate the heat-labile toxin. Sea urchin spines are composed of calcium carbonate, and these spines may lodge deep in the flesh of the wound. These injuries are characterized by wounds on the feet, when the victim steps on the urchin. It would be unusual to have an injury from a sea urchin located on the thigh. In addition, systemic symptoms would be unlikely in a sea urchin injury. Divers will occasionally step on a stonefish, a fish with venomous spines protruding from its body. Typically the wound is on the patient's foot, rather than the leg, so the scenario is not consistent with this type of wound. Regardless, the stonefish's venom is heat labile, and a wound from that source would also benefit from submersion in hot water. Application of baking soda is effective for jellyfish envenomations, but it is not indicated in this scenario. Antibiotics should be considered if the wound becomes secondarily infected.

3. e Surfers are occasionally attacked by sharks, because surfboard shapes in the water may be mistaken for profiles of elephant seals, which are the natural prey of sharks. Sharks are not venomous and inflict their injuries via mechanical injury only. Hypovolemic shock is the immediate threat to life in shark attacks, and therefore bleeding must be controlled and fluids must be administered as needed, as with other cases of trauma. There is no role for pressor support. Although a thorough primary and secondary survey is indicated in any trauma patient, sharks usually bite once, and rarely inflict other injuries. Midazolam may exacerbate hypovolemic shock. Antibiotics, as well as tetanus toxoid and tetanus immune globulin if indicated, are recommended.

4. e Scorpion envenomation includes a neurotoxin, which produces symptoms such as pain, restlessness, hyperactivity, roving eye movements, and respiratory distress. Treatment options include cryotherapy, antivenin, and sedative-anticonvulsants; however, general supportive care is indicated first. Respiratory failure may occur, but this is not indicated now. There is no serological test to confirm scorpion envenomation. Applying a constriction band and beginning incision and suction is indicated in envenomations involving Crotalidae, but given the history and examination of this patient, scorpion envenomation appears more likely. In addition, incision and suction are helpful only if initiated immediately. Antivenin is helpful, but should be given after general supportive care and only if symptoms persist.

5. c The bite of the black widow spider is the leading cause of death from spider bites. The mortality rate is 4–5%, with death resulting from cardiovascular failure. Reaction to the bite consists of generalized pain and rigidity of muscles 1 to 8 hours after the bite. There are no local symptoms of the bite itself. *Latrodectus* antivenin is available and should be instituted as soon as a bite is confirmed. Brown recluse spider bites are characterized by a local reaction to a bite and by pain 2 to 8 hours after the bite. The bite is often unnoticed. Erythema then develops, with a central blister or pustule. This is followed by subcutaneous discoloration, and then by an ulcerated "crater." The bite of a wolf spider causes local reactions only. Appendicitis should be considered in a child with abdominal pain, vomiting, and fever. Even though a scorpion bite may be characterized by diffuse pain and vomiting, it would be exceedingly rare for a patient to have been bitten in New England.

6. c The black widow spider bite is the most significant with regard to mortality. The bites of the tarantula, the wolf spider, and the jumping spider inject mild venoms that cause local symptoms only. The brown recluse spider bite may cause significant erythema and ulceration, but does not usually cause death.

7. d The order Hymenoptera includes bees, wasps, hornets, and yellow jackets. Hymenoptera are responsible for 50% of human deaths from venomous bites and stings. The most common reaction to a sting is an allergic reaction, but other toxic reactions may be seen. The venoms of each species contain protein antigens that can elicit an IgE antibody response in victims. The venoms are similar and therefore cross-reactivity may occur. Treatment depends on the degree of allergic reactivity. If the stinger is still embedded in the patient, it should be removed immediately. Previously, scraping the stinger out was recommended; however, current recommendations are that the stinger should be removed immediately, and the mechanism of removal is irrelevant. For mild reactions (i.e., Group I or II—see next answer), local wound care and oral diphenhydramine as needed are the treatments of choice. Immediate subcuta-

neous injection of epinephrine at the site of the sting is not indicated for all stings. Subcutaneous epinephrine (injected at any subcutaneous site) is indicated for moderate to severe reactions. Incision and suction is indicated in Crotalidae envenomations only.

8. d   Group I reactions consist of local reactions at the site of the bite or sting and may be treated locally with cold compresses. Group II reactions consist of mild systemic reactions and may be treated with oral diphenhydramine. Group III reactions consist of severe systemic reactions such as wheezing, angioneurotic edema, nausea, and vomiting. These may be treated with subcutaneous epinephrine, oral diphenydramine, and an H_2 blocker. These patients should be observed for a period of time, and often require admission. Group IV reactions consist of life-threatening systemic reactions, such as laryngoedema, hypotension, and shock. In addition to epinephrine and supportive therapy, these patients should be observed in an ICU. They may require intubation, but only for signs of impending respiratory failure. In this scenario, the patient developed either a Group III or IV reaction with wheezing and possible laryngoedema. The patient should be admitted for observation.

9. b   The victim of a snakebite should bring the snake to authorities for identification, as long as this does not significantly delay transporting the patient, or endanger others. Snakes may bite reflexively even after being killed, so this feat must be undertaken with caution. The pit vipers in family Crotalidae (e.g., rattlesnakes, copperheads, and water moccasins) have each of the physical characteristics listed in Question 9 except "b"—their pupils are elliptical instead of round. Thus, this characteristic would make you suspect the patient was not bitten by a member of the family Crotalidae. However, coral snakes have round pupils. Therefore, a better identification of the snake in this scenario is needed; the bite may still be venomous.

10. e   The degree of effects of envenomation are multifactorial. Venoms are a mixture of necrotizing, hemotoxic, neurotoxic, nephrotoxic, and/or cardiotoxic substances. In addition to the venom itself, characteristics of the victim and the snake help to determine the overall toxicity. The victim's size and general health are important variables. The site of envenomation determines the speed of systemic spread. The snake's size and species will determine the amount of venom and the potency of the venom, respectively. In addition, an angry or hungry snake may inject more venom. A snake that has fed recently may have less venom, since it may have discharged much of it into its most recent prey. The victim's last meal would be important for airway management issues, but has no direct consequence regarding the envenomation.

11. c   Crotalidae envenomation is characterized by intense local pain, with the sensation of burning within several minutes. The pain can become worse; edema may follow. Victims of bites often complain of perioral, scalp, and peripheral paresthesias. The paresthesia may be accompanied by a metallic taste in the victim's mouth. Symptoms of systemic absorption include nausea, vomiting, chills, sweating, syncope, and other, more ominous signs. Different species may produce varying degrees of symptomatology. A coral snake bite usually leaves unimpressive local signs, with punctures at most 7–8 mm apart; nonetheless, the bite may be very serious. The Mojave rattlesnake envenomation may be as serious as that of other pit vipers, but the bite of this *Crotalus* species usually involves a relative lack of pain and swelling. King snakes are innocuous and are frequently mistaken for coral snakes. Water moccasin bites may produce similar symptoms to bites of other pit vipers, but this species is found in the Southeast.

12. c   Coral snakes leave 1 to 2 punctures, at most 7–8 mm apart. There is usually mild pain and little if any localized swelling, unlike Crotalidae envenomations, which cause intense pain, hemorrhagic blebs, and edema. Neurologic symptoms occur and include paresthesias, weakness, malaise, nausea, fasciculations, diplopia, and difficulty swallowing or talking. Respiratory failure may occur with coral snake envenomations. Coral snakes account for less than 1% of all envenomations annually.

13. e   Incision and suction is indicated if this can be started within 5–10 minutes of the envenomation, and if it does not delay transport of the victim. As with all medical emergencies, the ABC's (airway, breathing, and circulation) must be addressed when treating a victim of a snakebite. However, rapid transport to the nearest medical facility is critical. Therefore, the "scoop and run" technique of transport is especially pertinent, because the nearest medical facility is just 30 minutes away. The wound should be kept below the level of the heart and the affected extremity should be immobilized to decrease systemic absorption of the venom. Tourniquets are not recommended, but a constriction band placed proximal to the wound may be used to obstruct lymph and venous flow.

14. d Antivenin is available and effective for rattlesnake, water moccasin, and copperhead envenomations. Administration of antivenin should be considered for any patient with systemic signs of these envenomations. For maximal venom binding, antivenin is optimally given within 4 hours of the envenomation. Benefits of antivenin are questionable after 4 hours and up to 12 hours; and not indicated after 24 hours. Because antivenin is made from highly antigenic horse serum, skin testing is mandatory before institution of antivenin. Incision and suction of the wound is indicated immediately after the envenomation, but not 4 hours later.

15. c Application of constriction bands and incision and suction are not helpful to delay systemic absorption in coral snake envenomations. Antivenin is available for bites of eastern coral snakes, but not for those of the Arizona coral snake. As with rattlesnake antivenin, skin testing is mandatory. There is no role for methylprednisolone and diphenhydramine in this scenario.

16. c Dogs account for the majority of mammalian bites. Forces of 200–400 pounds per square inch have been documented in dogs. Therefore, a 14-month-old child sustaining a bite from a German Shepherd should have radiographs if the wound is severe or the patient has bony tenderness. Since the dog is the family dog and appears healthy, with its immunizations up to date, rabies immune globulin and human diploid cell vaccine is not indicated. However, the dog should be quarantined. If the animal is behaving suspiciously, definitive testing for rabies is available by sending the dog's head to the state lab. Antibiotic prophylaxis is indicated for high-risk wounds, which is not the case in this scenario.

17. d High-risk wounds include cat or human bites, wounds in immunosuppressed patients, puncture wounds, hand or foot wounds, and wounds given initial care after a delay of 12 hours or more. As a general rule, these wounds should not be sutured and prophylactic antibiotics are indicated. Dog bites resulting in a laceration of the face are wounds in which prophylactic antibiotics are not indicated. Some physicians would prescribe antibiotics if the wound requires suturing, however.

18. c The most common bacteria isolated from cat and dog bite wounds are *Staphylococcus aureus* and *Pasteurella multocida*. No single antibiotic is ideal, but amoxicillin-clavulanic acid comes close to ideal, providing coverage for *P. multocida* and *S. aureus*. Trimethoprim-sulfamethoxazole and amoxicillin do not provide adequate coverage. Topical antibiotics are insufficient. Silvadene cream is not indicated.

19. d The wound described above is a high-risk wound with what appears to be a deep-seated infection. Moderate swelling would suggest infection or fracture, and therefore radiographs would be indicated. Pain on passive finger motion suggests a more serious deep compartmental infection or tendonitis. Serum evaluation of CBC and ESR are helpful, and the patient will require parenteral antibiotic therapy. Given the case scenario, Hepatitis B and HIV screening would be reasonable. Oral antibiotics would be inadequate.

20. e Even though the incidence of rabies is low, rabies is uniformly fatal once contracted. Wild carnivores such as raccoons and foxes should be considered rabid. Currently, recommendations are that any exposure to a bat, even without a bite or scratch mark, warrants rabies treatment. Bites by strays and other domesticated mammals should be considered on a case-by-case basis and with consultation of the local health department. Bites of rodents and lagomorphs (e.g., rabbits) are considered no-risk bites.

CHAPTER 92

Allergic Emergencies

CYNTHIA JOHNSON MOLLEN, M.D.

QUESTIONS

1. A 3-year-old boy with a history of asthma is brought to the ED by his mother. She reports he has been ill for several days with cough, fever, and wheezing. In assessing the severity of his asthma exacerbation, you consider all of the following EXCEPT:

   a. Respiratory rate
   b. Temperature
   c. Level of alertness
   d. O_2 saturation
   e. Color

2. A 15-month-old girl is brought to the ED for wheezing. She has had episodes of wheezing associated with bronchiolitis in the past. The mother reports she was well until this afternoon, when she began coughing. At that time her mother noted a temperature of 37.0°C. The patient then began to wheeze. Her 3-year-old brother has asthma. On physical examination, the patient is in mild respiratory distress, with a RR of 44 and an O_2 saturation of 95% on room air. Her lung examination is significant for bilateral, high-pitched wheezes, which are more pronounced on the right. She has a small response to an initial bronchodilator treatment. Your next step is to:

   a. Administer oxygen therapy
   b. Obtain an ABG
   c. Obtain a CXR
   d. Continue bronchodilator therapy
   e. Administer corticosteroids

3. A 4-month-old girl is brought to the ED in February for her second episode of wheezing. She was born at 31 weeks gestation, and required mechanical ventilation for 4 days after her birth. This illness began 2 days ago with cough, rhinorrhea and fevers to 38.7°C. The mother reports that the infant has had poor feeding over the last 24 hours. The girl's wheezing has progressed over the last 24 hours. On examination, she is alert, in moderate respiratory distress, with a RR of 56 and an O_2 saturation of 94% on room air. She has diffuse wheezes bilaterally, with scattered crackles. Her most likely diagnosis is:

   a. Cystic fibrosis
   b. Asthma
   c. Diaphragmatic hernia
   d. Bacterial pneumonia
   e. Bronchiolitis

4. A 15-year-old boy with asthma has severe respiratory distress. His RR is 50, his O_2 saturation is 88% on room air, and his lung exam reveals few wheezes. He is complaining of chest pain. After oxygen therapy, multiple doses of bronchodilators, and a loading dose of steroids, he complains that his chest pain has worsened. Reassessment of his physical examination reveals an RR of 48, an O_2 saturation of 89% on room air, and few wheezes. The most likely cause of his symptoms is:

   a. Pneumonia
   b. Pneumopericardium
   c. Cardiac dysrhythmia
   d. Pneumothorax
   e. Anaphylaxis

The following case applies to Questions 5 and 6: A 3-year-old girl is brought to the ED with a 2-day history of worsening cough and wheezing. Her mother has been giving her nebulized albuterol treatments every 4 hours for the last 24 hours without much improvement. In the ED, her temperature is 38.5°C, her RR is 50, and her O_2 saturation on room air is 94%. Her lung examination reveals moderate work of breathing, decreased aeration throughout, and diffuse wheezes.

5. Your initial step in management is administration of:

   a. Subcutaneous (SC) epinephrine
   b. Repetitive inhaled beta$_2$-agonists
   c. Systemic corticosteroids
   d. Inhaled corticosteroids
   e. Inhaled ipratropium bromide

6. After appropriate treatment, the patient in Question 5 is much improved, with an RR of 30, and an O_2 saturation of 98% on room air. She continues to have a small amount of wheezing. Her instructions for discharge should be to:

a. Continue nebulized albuterol every 4 hours at home for 3 to 5 days

b. Stop all therapy, since she is better

c. Continue nebulized albuterol every 4 hours at home for 3 to 5 days, and to add oral prednisone for 5 days

d. Continue nebulized albuterol 3 times a day for 3 to 5 days, with 5 days of oral prednisone

e. Continue nebulized albuterol 3 times a day for 3 to 5 days

7. A 5-year-old boy is being treated in the ED for an acute asthma exacerbation. Systemic corticosteroids should NOT be used if:

a. He has a concomitant pneumonia

b. He is receiving antibiotics

c. His symptoms are much improved after frequent treatments with nebulized albuterol

d. He receives inhaled corticosteroids at baseline

e. He has had a recent exposure to varicella (chickenpox) and is unimmunized

The following case applies to Questions 8–10: A 6-year-old girl comes to the ED with respiratory distress. She has a history of asthma, and her mother reports that she has been wheezing for 4 days. She has not responded to nebulized albuterol given as often as every 1 to 2 hours in the last 24 hours. She is diaphoretic, with an RR of 60 and an O_2 saturation of 88% on room air. She is only able to speak in short phrases in between breaths. You immediately provide supplemental oxygen and continuous nebulized albuterol at 0.5 mg/kg/hr, as well as oral corticosteroids. After 30 minutes in the ED she has not improved.

8. Your next step is:

a. IV beta$_2$-agonist therapy

b. IV corticosteroids

c. Intubation and mechanical ventilation

d. IV theophylline

e. Antibiotics

9. The patient in Question 8 continues to deteriorate despite maximal medical therapy (continuous nebulized albuterol, IV terbutaline, IV methylprednisolone, and IV magnesium). She is obtunded, and her RR is 68. You decide she needs endotracheal intubation. Which agent is best included in the induction?

a. Morphine

b. Meperidine

c. Ketamine

d. D-tubocurare

e. Atracurium

10. The ideal mode of ventilation for the patient in Questions 8 and 9 is:

a. Volume-controlled ventilation with average tidal volumes

b. Volume-controlled ventilation with larger than usual tidal volumes

c. Volume-controlled ventilation with smaller than usual tidal volumes

d. Pressure-controlled ventilation with high pressures

e. Pressure controlled ventilation with low pressures

The following case applies to Questions 11 and 12: A 4-year-old boy is brought to the ED with cough and wheezing. He initially developed cough and wheezing several hours ago. Later, he complained of itchiness. The mother noted that he was breathing harder and that she could see his ribs when he breathed. He also appeared flushed.

11. You suspect:

a. Foreign body aspiration

b. Pneumonia

c. Asthma exacerbation

d. Bronchiolitis

e. Anaphylaxis

12. Upon further questioning of the boy's mother you determine that the symptoms described in Question 11 developed acutely while the boy was at the beach. He had been swimming earlier in the day. His mother remembered that he ate peanuts about 6 hours prior to the onset of symptoms, and shrimp about 1 hour before the symptoms began; she says he has had both of these foods in the past. He is currently taking amoxicillin for an otitis media infection; his last dose was about 8 hours ago. The most likely inciting factor for his symptoms is (are):

a. Peanuts

b. Amoxicillin

c. Shrimp

d. Cold

e. Sun

13. A 7-year-old girl is brought to the ED after being stung by a bee. She complains of dizziness, nausea, and itching. On physical examination, you note a RR of 40 and stridor. Her blood pressure is 104/65, and her HR is 110. She has diffuse urticaria and angioedema of her lips and tongue. Your first step in management is to:

a. Secure IV access

b. Prepare for endotracheal intubation

c. Administer nebulized epinephrine

d. Administer nebulized albuterol

e. Administer SC epinephrine

14. A 12-year-old boy develops a pruritic rash and mild swelling of the lips after taking trimethoprim-sulfamethoxazole. His vital signs are: T 37.2°C, RR 24, HR 86, and BP 123/78. He states he is not having difficulty swallowing or breathing, and his symptoms have not changed in 2 hours. Your treatment for him includes:

    a. Corticosteroids
    b. SC epinephrine
    c. Nebulized albuterol
    d. IV fluids
    e. Nebulized racemic epinephrine

15. A 3-year-old boy is brought to the ED for a fever. His mother states that he has had a fever to 38.8°C for 2 days, has been less active, and has developed a rash over the last 24 hours. On physical examination the boy appears tired but not toxic. His vital signs are: T 38.4°C, RR 30, HR 120, and BP 102/58. You note a maculopapular rash over his trunk and mild swelling and warmth of his knees and elbows, bilaterally. There are no other abnormal physical examination findings. Your first diagnostic test should be:

    a. CXR
    b. ECG
    c. CBC with differential
    d. Urinalysis
    e. Hepatic enzymes

16. A 4-year-old boy has a 3-day history of an urticarial rash, low-grade fevers, and hematuria. He completed an oral course of cefprozil (Cefzil) 14 days ago for otitis media. His treatment should include:

    a. Corticosteroids
    b. Trimethoprim-sulfamethoxazole
    c. Acetaminophen
    d. Amoxicillin-clavulanic acid
    e. Renal ultrasound (U/S)

17. A 9-year-old girl is brought to the ED because of rhinorrhea, pruritus of the nose, and red eyes. She reports that she has similar symptoms every fall. On physical examination, you note a dark discoloration below both eyes and pale nasal mucosa. Treatment in the ED may include all of the following EXCEPT:

    a. Oral antihistamines
    b. Oral decongestants
    c. Counseling to avoid environmental allergens
    d. Nasal corticosteroids
    e. Topical decongestants

ANSWERS

1. b   According to the Expert Panel Report of the National Heart, Lung, and Blood Institute (1991, 1997), several parameters can be used to estimate the severity of an asthma exacerbation. These include respiratory rate, alertness, dyspnea, accessory muscle use, color, wheezing, oxygen saturation, PEFR (peak expiratory flow rate), and $Paco_2$ (partial pressure of carbon dioxide). Even though temperature is an important factor for the general physical examination, it does not give any information about the severity of an asthma exacerbation.

2. c   This patient has several features in her history and physical examination that are suggestive of a foreign body aspiration. Most foreign body aspirations occur in children ages 6 months to 5 years; often a toddler-aged sibling with small toys is in the home. She had an acute onset of symptoms, and her lung examination is asymmetric. She respond only minimally to initial bronchodilator therapy, despite the mild nature of her symptoms. A chest x-ray should be obtained to look for clues to foreign body aspiration.

3. e   Bronchiolitis is an acute infection of the small airways caused by a virus (most commonly respiratory syncytial virus (RSV), but also parainfluenza, adenovirus, and influenza). The peak months for outbreaks are January through March. Patients are usually less than 1 year old, and have an upper respiratory infection that progresses to wheezing, feeding difficulty and respiratory distress. Even though most healthy infants are only affected by bronchiolitis once in a season, some infants have more than one episode. Bacterial pneumonia is possible, but is not usually associated with wheezing, and the clinical presentation is more consistent with bronchiolitis. Cystic fibrosis is unlikely to cause respiratory symptoms at this age, and foreign body aspiration is unlikely to occur in a 4-month-old child. Since this patient was intubated for several days after birth, diaphragmatic hernia would most likely have been

diagnosed earlier. Although this patient has risk factors for developing asthma, she has not yet manifested symptoms consistent with the chronic nature of asthma.

4. d Pneumothorax is a serious complication of asthma that should be suspected in any patient with severe chest pain, asymmetric breath sounds, or tracheal shift. It should also be suspected in patients with significant asthma exacerbations that do not respond to therapy as expected. Atelectasis is a common complication of asthma, but it does not cause symptoms as severe as those this patient is experiencing. Cardiac dysrhythmias are associated with adrenergic agents, but they do not cause asymmetric breath sounds and respiratory distress. Pneumonia can also occur in patients with asthma, but usually fevers, as well as localized findings on examination, are accompanying symptoms. Finally, even though anaphylaxis can cause wheezing and respiratory distress, this patient does not have any other finding to support this diagnosis.

5. b The mainstay of initial asthma therapy in children is repetitive, inhaled beta$_2$-agonist treatments with albuterol, a highly beta$_2$-selective agent and the agent of choice in the United States. Subcutaneous injection of either epinephrine or terbutaline should be reserved for the very ill patient, or the young patient whose condition is resistant to nebulized therapy. Systemic corticosteroids are indicated in most asthma exacerbations, and should be administered early in treatment, but are not the initial treatment. Inhaled steroids can be used instead of systemic steroids for patients who are chronically managed on this therapy and who are experiencing a mild exacerbation. Ipratropium bromide should be used in conjunction with albuterol for moderate to severe exacerbations, but not alone.

6. c Children who are discharged after an acute asthma exacerbation should receive intensified therapy over what they had been receiving at home. This usually includes frequent albuterol treatments and a short course of systemic steroids. Only regimen "c" provides this child with more therapy than she was receiving prior to her treatment in the ED.

7. e Exposure to varicella in the unprotected host is one of the few situations in which steroids may be avoided acutely—consideration must be given to the severity of the patient's symptoms, and the relative risks and benefits of avoiding steroids. Community-acquired pneumonia is not a contraindication to steroid therapy. Any patient whose exacerbation is severe enough to require more than one nebulized treatment should receive systemic steroids. Even patients who receive inhaled corticosteroids at baseline benefit from systemic corticosteroids during acute exacerbations.

8. a Intravenous beta$_2$-agonist therapy, such as IV terbutaline, is an option for children who fail continuous nebulized therapy. The dose should be titrated to effect, monitoring for unacceptable tachycardia. IV therapy should be tried prior to mechanical ventilation, because it may allow one to avoid intubation. There is no proven benefit of IV steroids over oral steroids; if the patient did not vomit her steroids, there is no need to repeat the dose IV. There is no role for theophylline in the acute management of an asthma exacerbation, and it is no longer recommended for hospitalized patients. There is no indication from this patient's clinical history and presentation that she will benefit from antibiotics.

9. c Ketamine is the preferred induction agent for asthmatic patients because it is a bronchodilator. The other agents listed may increase bronchospasm through histamine release and should be avoided.

10. b In order to ensure long expiratory times, volume-controlled ventilation with larger than average tidal volumes (10–20 cc/kg), normal respiratory rates, and high flow rates are preferred. Inspiratory pressures may be very high in this situation, but pressure-controlled ventilation with high pressures is not the preferred mode of ventilation. Controlled hypoventilation, with a Pa$_{CO_2}$ of less than 50 torr, can also help minimize barotrauma.

11. e Although all of the conditions listed can cause wheezing, increased work of breathing and retractions, only anaphylaxis will also cause diffuse flushing and pruritus.

12. c All of the agents listed can cause an anaphylactic reaction. Usually the patient has been exposed to the trigger within the preceding 1 to 2 hours, which makes the shrimp a more likely cause than amoxicillin or peanuts. The pathophysiology of the IgE-mediated reaction requires previous exposure to the agent for sensitization; therefore, the fact that he had eaten shrimp and peanuts in the past does not necessarily exclude them from the possibilities. Cold urticaria is an acute reaction to cold temperatures

with hives at the site of exposure; immersion in cold water can precipitate anaphylaxis, but the reaction is not delayed. Cold urticaria can be acquired, and often follows a viral infection. Solar urticaria is a reaction to light, with development of pruritis, erythema, and edema. Although this could have been the cause of this patient's symptoms, foods are more common triggers, and therefore shrimp is the best answer.

13. e   The first-line drug for anaphylaxis is epinephrine, and it should be administered as soon as possible. If the initial subcutaneous dose is ineffective, or if the patient is hypoperfused, the epinephrine can be given IV. Intravenous access is important, especially for the hypotensive patient, but this intervention should not delay the administration of epinephrine. This patient has some evidence of airway edema, but endotracheal intubation is not necessary at this point. Nebulized albuterol is useful in the treatment of anaphylaxis-induced bronchospasm, and there is some evidence that nebulized epinephrine can be useful, but these are not first-line treatments.

14. a   For patients with moderate reactions that are not evolving and do not involve the airway, treatment with antihistamines (H_1- and H_2-receptor antagonists) and corticosteroids are adequate. There is no need to administer SC epinephrine to this patient, and because he has a normal blood pressure, IV fluids are not indicated.

15. d   This patient's clinical picture suggests the diagnosis of serum sickness. Renal involvement is the most common complication, so all patients should have a urinalysis. Many other organ systems can be involved, and the physical examination and the level of uncertainty about the diagnosis should guide other diagnostic tests. A chest x-ray and ECG would be indicated if a friction rub or wheezing were present; a CBC could be sent to check for anemia, and hepatic enzymes should be checked if there is evidence of hepatomegaly, but these are not indicated for this patient.

16. a   This patient has serum sickness, most likely precipitated by his recent antibiotic use. He should be treated with antihistamines as well as corticosteroids because of the evidence of renal involvement. Antibiotics are not indicated at this point, because there is no current infection. NSAIDs such as ibuprofen would be preferable to acetaminophen because of the anti-inflammatory effects. A renal U/S should be performed at a later time if the hematuria does not resolve.

17. d   All of the agents listed are useful in treating allergic rhinitis. In fact, topical corticosteroids are first-line therapy for chronic allergic rhinitis. However, they are the least useful modality in the ED setting because patients may require treatment for as long as 2 weeks to achieve maximal relief. Therefore, antihistamines in conjunction with decongestants should be prescribed for more immediate relief, with follow-up by the primary care provider or an allergist. Topical (nasal) decongestants should only be prescribed for a maximum of 5 days, to avoid tachyphylaxis.

CHAPTER **93**

Gastrointestinal Emergencies

VINCENT J. WANG, M.D.

QUESTIONS

1. A 2-year-old boy has hematemesis. Which of the following suggests the need for nasogastric (NG) lavage?

   a. Associated epistaxis
   b. Protracted vomiting with hematemesis on the last emesis
   c. Associated diarrhea for several days
   d. Resting pulse (HR) 160
   e. Resting BP 85/50

2. A 6-month-old boy with a history of colic comes to the ED after a few episodes of hematemesis. He has had episodes of "spit-ups" for his entire life. He had one episode of blood-streaked emesis. He is otherwise well appearing. He is well perfused and his abdominal examination is benign. You suspect the etiology of his hematemesis is:

   a. Gastroesophageal reflux (GER)
   b. Mallory-Weiss tear
   c. Esophageal varices
   d. Swallowed foreign body
   e. Neonatal hepatitis

3. A 10-year-old girl has had an episode of hematemesis. She complains of lower abdominal pain and dysuria. She has had 5–6 episodes of emesis, with the last two associated with flecks of blood. Her examination is normal, with minimal vague abdominal pain. Diagnostic evaluation should include:

   a. NG lavage
   b. Abdominal CT scan
   c. Abdominal radiographs
   d. Urinalysis
   e. Pelvic ultrasound (U/S)

4. A 14-year-old boy complains of epigastric abdominal pain and one episode of coffee-ground emesis. He has a history of a dislocated shoulder and has been taking naproxen sodium for his pain. He complains of epigastric pain persisting for several days, but has not had fever or anorexia. His examination is normal, without abdominal tenderness. Treatment includes:

   a. Clarithromycin
   b. Ceftriaxone
   c. Sclerotherapy
   d. Ranitidine
   e. Ibuprofen

5. A 2-year-old girl has had several episodes of hematemesis. She is a former premature infant (born at 28 weeks gestation) who had a prolonged and complicated course of treatment in the neonatal intensive care unit (NICU). On examination in the ED, she is somewhat ill-appearing, with mild jaundice and ascites. After appropriate stabilization, treatment includes:

   a. Sclerotherapy
   b. Clarithromycin
   c. Sulfasalazine
   d. Hemodialysis
   e. Vasopressin

6. A 14-year-old boy with esophageal varices has had severe hematemesis. NG lavage at the transferring medical center confirms active bleeding despite vasopressin therapy. He arrives in your ED after 8 hours of vasopressin therapy. His hematocrit (hct) is 27% and he continues to have bloody NG output. Emergent treatment at this time includes:

   a. Further NG lavage
   b. Gastroesophageal balloon tamponade
   c. Vitamin K continuous IV infusion
   d. Epinephrine IV infusion
   e. Continued vasopressin IV infusion

7. A 3-day-old girl is brought to the ED by her parents after having one episode of hematemesis. Her perinatal history is unremarkable and she received vitamin K at the time of delivery. She has been nursing well and is otherwise without complaint. NG lavage produces pink aspirate. The test most likely to reveal the diagnosis is:

    a. Apt-Downey test of the emesis
    b. Heme testing of the emesis
    c. Upper GI series
    d. Esophageal pH probe
    e. Upper GI endoscopy

8. A 7-month-old girl has had mild diarrhea and blood-streaked stools. She began having diarrhea 2 days ago. She is taking adequate oral intake and is well hydrated. On examination you note a fissure of her anal sphincter. Treatment includes:

    a. Stool culture
    b. Loperamide
    c. Hydrocortisone topically
    d. Sitz baths
    e. Nystatin cream topically

9. A 3-year-old boy has rectal bleeding. He was previously diagnosed with an anal fissure and treated appropriately for this. On examination, he has perianal excoriations and mild erythema. Perianal culture is likely to reveal:

    a. *Staphylococcus epidermidis*
    b. *Neisseria meningitidis*
    c. *Streptococcus pyogenes*
    d. *Haemophilus influenzae* type b
    e. *Moraxella catarrhalis*

10. A 5-year-old girl complains of painless rectal bleeding, which has stopped. She is well appearing and in no distress, but has a palpable polyp on rectal examination. Her hematocrit is 33%. Immediate evaluation should include:

    a. Abdominal radiographs
    b. Barium enema
    c. Colonoscopy
    d. Abdominal ultrasound (U/S)
    e. Scheduled outpatient follow-up

11. A 3-week-old boy has blood-streaked loose stools. He is otherwise well appearing and feeds vigorously. He has not been crying. His rectal examination is normal. His stools are loose and mucoid. Heme testing of the stool demonstrates blood and a CBC demonstrates eosinophilia. The most appropriate treatment is likely to be:

    a. A new formula
    b. Surgery
    c. Air contrast enema
    d. Sulfasalicylic acid
    e. Steroid enema

12. A 7-year-old boy complains of fever, vomiting, abdominal pain, and diarrhea for 2 days. He has had poor oral intake and decreased urine output. On examination, he appears mildly dehydrated, but his abdomen is soft. His labs are significant for: WBC 6900, hgb 9, hct 27, platelets 63,000, Na 134, K 4.1, Cl 107, HCO_3 18, BUN 30, Cr 2.7. His symptoms are most consistent with:

    a. Henoch-Schönlein purpura (HSP)
    b. Crohn's disease
    c. Vascular (arteriovenous) malformation (AVM)
    d. Hemolytic uremic syndrome (HUS)
    e. *Salmonella* enteritis

13. A 16-year-old girl complains of abdominal pain. She has had abdominal pain for 3–4 months, associated with loose stools and a 4 kg weight loss. She has also had joint pain and blurry vision. Which of the following serum tests is likely to be elevated?

    a. Sodium (Na)
    b. Hematocrit (hct)
    c. Creatinine (Cr)
    d. Erythrocyte sedimentation rate (ESR)
    e. Serum IgE

14. A 17-year-old boy with ulcerative colitis complains of malaise, abdominal distension, diarrhea, and pain. He has had increasing symptoms over the day. On examination, his temperature is 38.6°C and his abdomen is diffusely tender, with mild distension. His WBC is 17,000 and his abdominal radiograph shows marked distension of his transverse colon. Treatment involves:

    a. Clear liquid diet
    b. Tylenol with codeine
    c. Loperamide
    d. Placement of an NG tube
    e. Penicillin alone

15. A 6-year-old girl complains of abdominal pain. She says her abdomen has hurt "all over" for the past week, and her mother reports occasional episodes of hematemesis. The abdominal pain awakens her from sleep. She has been afebrile. Her examination is normal, without focal abdominal tenderness, and her urinalysis is negative. Her urea breath test is positive. You make the diagnosis of:

    a. Functional abdominal pain
    b. Peptic ulcer disease (PUD)
    c. UTI
    d. Malrotation
    e. Mallory-Weiss tear

16. A 4-year-old boy is brought to the ED by his parents because of irritability. He initially developed chickenpox (varicella) 1 week ago. He was given oil of wintergreen. Today he began having vomiting and has been fussy. On examination, he is crying and is not consolable. He has hepatomegaly, but is without jaundice. The likely cause of these symptoms is:

a. Reye's syndrome
b. Meningitis
c. Varicella encephalitis
d. Pyelonephritis
e. Infectious mononucleosis

17. A 16-year-old girl with sickle-cell disease complains of a sudden onset of right upper quadrant (RUQ) tenderness. She says the pain is not her typical sickle crisis pain. She reports that it began after lunch today. She has not had fever. On examination her abdomen is tender in the RUQ. The most appropriate diagnostic test is:

a. Abdominal radiograph
b. Abdominal ultrasound (U/S)
c. Abdominal CT scan
d. Laparoscopy
e. Exploratory laparotomy

18. A 12-year-old boy has RUQ abdominal pain. He had a choledochal cyst removed as an infant. He has had abdominal pain for several days, as well as shaking chills, and a temperature of 39°C. You suspect he most likely has:

a. Acute cholecystitis
b. Acute cholangitis
c. Appendicitis
d. Hepatitis
e. Sepsis

19. A 9-year-old boy is brought to the ED after he fell onto his bicycle handlebars. He hit his abdomen and complains of sharp epigastric tenderness, with radiation to the back. He has severe epigastric tenderness and a bluish discoloration around the umbilicus. Which of the following serum tests should be elevated?

a. Creatinine
b. Hematocrit
c. LDH
d. Lipase
e. AST (aspartate aminotransferase)

20. An 11-year-old boy complains of anorexia and abdominal pain. He has a 2-month history of fatigue and malaise. He also complains of nausea and vomiting. He has been doing poorly in school recently. On examination he has minimal jaundice, mild hepatomegaly, and a brownish discoloration in the posterior part of the corneas bilaterally. Which diagnostic test is likely to make the diagnosis?

a. Coagulation profile
b. Hepatitis panel
c. Urine amino acids
d. Serum ceruloplasmin
e. Abdominal ultrasound

21. A 7-year-old girl complains of fatigue, nausea, and vomiting. She had a URI last week. On examination she has RUQ tenderness and jaundice. At times she is confused and/or combative. Laboratory findings consistent with the diagnosis include:

a. Decreased PT
b. Decreased total bilirubin
c. Increased sodium
d. Decreased glucose
e. Increased albumin

ANSWERS

1. d   Not every child with hematemesis requires NG lavage. NG lavage should be performed in patients who are suspected of having significant upper GI bleeding. NG lavage does not have any therapeutic role, but rather only a diagnostic role. Patients with epistaxis have a readily identifiable source of bleeding and do not require further diagnosis. Patients who have protracted vomiting may have a Mallory-Weiss tear, and unless unstable, do not need further investigation. Hematemesis associated with diarrhea is likely secondary to a gastroenteritis, and should not have significant upper GI bleeding. A BP of 85/50 is normal for a 2-year-old. However, a HR of 160 is tachycardic, and if this is a resting, non-agitated HR, further investigation is warranted.

2. a   Esophagitis due to GER is a common cause of hematemesis. If the patient had a history of protracted vomiting, a Mallory-Weiss tear would be possible. Esophageal varices are usually associated with extrahepatic obstruction or hepatic parenchymal disorders. A swallowed foreign body is more typical in an older child. Neonatal hepatitis would be rare in an otherwise healthy boy.

3. **d** Vomiting is commonly associated with urinary tract infections (UTI). Given the scant amount of blood associated with her emesis, further testing, other than a urinalysis and urine culture, is not indicated.

4. **d** Gastric mucosal lesions caused by NSAID use are a common cause of UGI bleeding. Therapy should consist of discontinuation of the NSAID and administration of ranitidine or another H_2 blocker. Omeprazole/clarithromycin/amoxicillin is a combination therapy used to treat peptic ulcer disease associated with *Helicobacter pylori* infections. Ceftriaxone is not indicated. Sclerotherapy would be necessary for active upper GI bleeding, but is not necessary in this vignette. Ibuprofen will not improve symptoms.

5. **e** Esophageal varices may be the result of portal hypertension, which is commonly associated with hepatic disease or obstruction. In this scenario, given her complicated NICU course, she is likely to have had an umbilical catheter, which may have predisposed her to having hepatic disease. Treatment for esophageal varices includes correction of any coagulation abnormalities with vitamin K, fresh frozen plasma (FFP), and platelets as needed. Antacids and H_2-blockers are administered, as well. Vasopressin will decrease blood flow through the portal circulation, and should stop the bleeding in most cases. Sclerotherapy may be necessary, but treatment with vasopressin should be attempted first.

6. **b** Indications for gastroesophageal balloon tamponade are massive, life-threatening hemorrhage or continued bleeding even after receiving vasopressin for 2 to 6 hours. Although balloon tamponade is effective in 50–80% of cases, the risk of complications and death is significant, and the procedure should only be performed by skilled physicians. In this case, vasopressin therapy has failed and therefore gastroesophageal balloon tamponade is indicated.

7. **a** Swallowed maternal blood may be a cause of melena or hematemesis in a newborn baby who is otherwise well. The Apt-Downey test involves distinguishing adult hemoglobin (Hgb A) from fetal hemoglobin, and will help to determine if the hematemesis is swallowed blood from breast feeding. The mother's breast milk may also be tested for blood. Heme testing of the emesis will only confirm the presence of blood, but will not determine the source. An upper GI series is indicated to evaluate for malrotation or obstruction. However, patients with these problems would appear toxic and should have protracted symptoms. A pH probe would help to diagnose GER, but this would be atypical with only one episode of emesis in a 3-day-old infant. Endoscopy could evaluate other lesions, such as esophageal varices or gastric ulcers, both of which are unlikely.

8. **d** Anal fissures may cause blood-streaked stools in patients of all ages. Treatment is supportive and includes stool softeners and local skin care. Sitz baths should be performed and a perianal lotion or protective ointment should be used. There is no indication for a stool culture or treatment with loperamide. Hydrocortisone cream and nystatin cream are also unnecessary.

9. **c** Peri-anal dermatitis occurs more frequently in boys, usually between the ages of 6 months and 10 years. (Darmstadt GL and Lane A. "Cutaneous Bacterial Infections: Perianal Dermatitis." In RE Behrman et al. (eds.). *Nelson Textbook of Pediatrics,* fifteenth edition. Philadelphia: W.B. Saunders, 1996; pp 1892–1893.) Associated complaints include erythema, anal fissures and excoriations, blood-streaked stools, and painful defecation. *Streptococcus pyogenes* is commonly cultured from this site, but *Staphylococcus aureus* may be cultured as well. Treatment involves antibiotics appropriate for the organisms cultured.

10. **e** Hamartomatous and adenomatous polyps are the major types of polyps diagnosed in childhood. Hamartomatous polyps are generally benign, whereas adenomatous polyps are potentially premalignant. The ED management of this patient should focus on hemodynamic stability, while arranging appropriate follow-up for the patient for further evaluation. The outpatient study of choice is a flexible colonoscopy.

11. **a** Dietary protein allergic syndromes, or allergic colitis, cause mucosal intestinal injury and enterocolitis as a result of various dietary proteins. Immunologic responses vary from mast cell activation to immune complex formation. Removal of the protein results in resolution of the symptoms. Typically a well-appearing infant less than 6 months of age develops blood-streaked, mucoid, diarrheal stools. Affected infants typically are otherwise feeding well, with appropriate weight gain. A CBC may demon-

strate eosinophilia, consistent with an allergic syndrome. Malrotation should present with vomiting in an ill-appearing child. The typical presentation of intussusception involves episodic crying, in addition to heme-positive stool. Crohn's disease and ulcerative colitis would be extremely unusual in this age group.

12. d HUS is characterized by a triad of oliguric renal failure, microangiopathic hemolytic anemia, and thrombocytopenia. The etiology of this condition is thought to be gastroenteritis or colitis secondary to infection with *Escherichia coli* 0157:H7. HSP is a systemic vasculitis, characterized by purpuric lesions often occurring on the lower extremities and buttock. Abdominal pain and rectal bleeding are common in HSP, but fever, diarrhea, and vomiting are not part of the clinical picture. Crohn's disease and AVMs do not have renal involvement, and should not present with such acute symptoms. *Salmonella* enteritis may present with similar symptoms, but should not have anemia and renal insufficiency.

13. d Inflammatory bowel disease (IBD) may present in children 10 years and older. Symptoms include abdominal pain, diarrhea, GI blood and protein loss, anemia, weight loss, and growth failure. In addition, extra-intestinal manifestations such as arthritis, erythema nodosum, chronic hepatitis, sclerosing cholangitis, and uveitis may be seen, although these are more common with Crohn's disease. Associated laboratory findings include: anemia, hypoalbuminemia, and leukocytosis. The sodium, creatinine, and IgE levels should be unaffected by IBD. ESR is typically elevated.

14. d Toxic megacolon is a complication of ulcerative colitis, a life-threatening emergency that requires immediate attention. Treatment includes fluid resuscitation, gastrointestinal decompression with an NG tube or a Miller-Abbott tube, broad-spectrum antibiotics, and ICU observation. Opiates and anticholinergic medications may precipitate toxic megacolon, and should be discontinued.

15. b PUD is characterized by ulcers within the stomach or duodenum, which is manifested by abdominal pain, vomiting, hematemesis, melena, and feeding difficulties (in infants). Pain may awaken patients at night, a characteristic that distinguishes PUD from functional abdominal pain. There is a strong association between PUD and *Helicobacter pylori* infection. The urea breath test confirms the presence of *H. pylori*. Malrotation generally presents acutely, and a Mallory-Weiss tear should not cause abdominal pain.

16. a Reye's syndrome is a reversible syndrome characterized by fatty degeneration of the viscera and severe noninflammatory encephalopathy. It is far less common now than previously, with the decreased use of aspirin. Typically, children develop an acute febrile illness, usually a URI or varicella. This is followed by protracted vomiting, and then encephalopathy. Physical examination may reveal tachycardia, tachypnea, encephalopathy, and hepatomegaly without jaundice. Meningitis and encephalitis do not cause hepatomegaly. Pyelonephritis should not cause encephalopathy and hepatomegaly. Infectious mononucleosis is unlikely to cause encephalopathy, and is unlikely to be the cause of this patient's symptoms, especially given the other risk factors.

17. b Acute cholecystitis is a complication of cholelithiasis, which may be associated with patients who have hemolytic anemias. Inflammation develops as a reaction to chemical injury caused by obstruction of the cystic duct by a pigment stone. Abdominal U/S is the test of choice for diagnosis. Other, non-emergent tests include a cholecystography or radionuclide testing.

18. b Acute cholangitis should be suspected in patients who have Charcot's triad: RUQ abdominal pain, shaking chills, and fever. Usually there is a history of previous abdominal surgery. Early diagnosis of acute cholangitis is critical because sepsis can develop rapidly. Hepatitis and acute cholecystitis should not have fever and chills. RUQ abdominal tenderness would be an atypical presentation of appendicitis, but this diagnosis should still be considered.

19. d Pancreatitis may follow upper abdominal trauma and is characterized by epigastric tenderness, with or without radiation to the back. A bluish discoloration of the flanks (Grey Turner's sign) or around the umbilicus (Cullen's sign) are indicators of a hemorrhagic pancreatitis. Serum amylase and/or lipase levels will be elevated in acute pancreatitis. The creatinine level should be unaffected. The hematocrit may be decreased or normal in an acute hemorrhage. Unless the patient sustained hepatic trauma, the LDH and AST levels should be normal.

20. d   Wilson's disease is a disorder of copper metabolism. (Balistreri WF. "Metabolic diseases of the Liver: Wilson Disease." In RE Behrman et al. (eds.). *Nelson Textbook of Pediatrics,* fifteenth edition. Philadelphia: W.B. Saunders, 1996; pp 1139–1140.) When diagnosed in childhood, hepatic symptoms predominate, but in adult patients, neurologic symptoms predominate. Hepatic manifestations include asymptomatic hepatomegaly, hepatitis, or fulminant hepatic failure. Ascites and portal hypertension may also be present. Neurologic symptoms may develop insidiously: poor performance in school, behavioral changes, an intention tremor, or dysarthria. Kayser-Fleischer rings are found as a brownish discoloration of the eyes. A serum ceruloplasmin level is the best screening test.

21. d   The PT level is the most commonly used marker to determine the severity of liver disease, but the PT level should be prolonged in liver failure. In addition, other laboratory findings are an increased total bilirubin, increased transaminase levels, hypoglycemia, and hypoalbuminemia. The sodium level should not be affected.

CHAPTER 94

Pediatric and Adolescent Gynecology

JACQUELINE BRYNGIL, M.D.

QUESTIONS

1. You are evaluating a 6-year-old girl for complaint of a foul-smelling discharge on her panties. Questions directed to the mother about her caretakers reassure you that abuse is unlikely. The child denies abdominal pain, fever, urinary frequency, hesitancy, and dysuria. Your most appropriate course of action at this time is:

   a. Perform a speculum examination for cultures
   b. Bimanual examination with culture of the discharge
   c. Examination of child in frog-leg position for cultures
   d. Referral to gynecology for speculum examination under anesthesia
   e. Discharge without cultures on regimen of sitz baths

2. A 13-year-old girl who experienced menarche at age 11 years complains of abdominal pain. She denies vaginal discharge and urinary frequency, urgency, and dysuria. She has had several episodes of vomiting over the past week, is afebrile, and has not had diarrhea. Her mother is present during your evaluation. She denies sexual experience and her periods have been irregular by history, her last menstrual period being 2 months prior to the visit. The most likely cause of her symptoms is:

   a. Gastroenteritis
   b. Appendicitis
   c. Constipation
   d. Pregnancy
   e. Strep pharyngitis

3. You are examining a 2-year-old girl brought in by the parents because of vaginal odor. On her examination she is well appearing. She is Tanner stage I. You do not note vaginal discharge, but are aware of the presence of a foul smell at the introitus. Rectal examination of the patient is without finding. The patient is afebrile. The most likely reason for her symptoms is:

   a. Bacterial vaginitis
   b. Poor hygiene
   c. Vaginal candidiasis
   d. Premature adrenarche
   e. Vaginal foreign body

4. A 6-month-old girl is brought to the ED for evaluation of a lower abdominal mass. The parents also report that the infant has a history of constipation and urinary straining. They also comment that the child's genitalia do not appear "normal." There is no history of fever. Your most likely finding on physical examination, aside from a lower abdominal mass, is:

   a. Absence of deep tendon reflexes in the lower extremities
   b. A protruding hymen
   c. Respiratory distress
   d. Atrophy of the muscles in the lower extremities
   e. Poor rectal tone

5. You are evaluating a 15-year-old girl for primary amenorrhea. She has a history of tetrology of Fallot and polydactyly syndrome. On her physical examination, she is Tanner stage 3–4. She has a fullness in the suprapubic region. Urine pregnancy test is negative. You attempt a digital examination of her vagina but cannot fully insert your gloved finger. Recto-abdominal examination reveals a palpable, full uterus and cervix. In this child's family there is most likely a history of:

   a. Consanguinity
   b. Cervical cancer
   c. Maternal DES exposure
   d. Delayed puberty
   e. Uterine fibroids

6. A 17-year-old female patient complains of abdominal pain. When obtaining a gynecological history, you find that she is premenarchal and virginal. She denies fever, vomiting, or diarrhea. Her physical examination reveals the presence of Tanner 4 breast development with Tanner 1 pubic hair development. Rectal examination is negative for masses. Urine HCG is negative. On a workup for this patient's primary amenorrhea you will most likely find:

   a. Hematometrocolpos
   b. Karyotype XY
   c. Decreased levels of FSH (follicle-stimulating hormone)
   d. Karyotype 45XO
   e. Decreased levels of LH (luteinizing hormone)

7. You are seeing a 2-week-old girl for her second hepatitis vaccination. The mother is alarmed because she feels her daughter's vagina is closed. On inspection, you note a thin membrane with a median raphe below the labia majora. Initial treatment of this condition may include:

   a. Referral to a urologist
   b. Application of estrogen cream
   c. Manual separation at the raphe
   d. Surgical separation at the raphe
   e. Referral to a geneticist

8. A 4-year-old African-American girl is brought to the ED with a chief complaint of vaginal bleeding. Your examination reveals the presence of a purple, doughnut-shaped mass protruding from the labia majora. The most appropriate management of this patient would be:

   a. Refer immediately to surgery
   b. Order sitz baths and estrogen cream
   c. Refer to oncology
   d. Apply hyrdocortisone cream
   e. Obtain a biopsy

9. You are examining a 14-year-old girl whose chief complaint is severe cramping with her periods. She experienced menarche 8 months ago and has had regular, monthly bleeding. She describes the pain as generalized to the lower abdomen and associated with nausea and diarrhea. She has never been sexually active. Her condition is most likely due to:

   a. Increased serum levels of FSH
   b. Increased serum levels of prostaglandins
   c. Increased serum levels of LH
   d. Decreased serum levels of FSH
   e. Decreased serum levels of prostaglandins

10. A 17-year-old female patient complains of painful periods for the past 6 months. She is sexually active and uses condoms occasionally as her only form of contraception. She states the pain is often associated with headaches and back pain and lasts approximately 1–2 days. It is not associated with increased bleeding. This patient would benefit most by treatment with:

   a. Starting norgestril/ethinyl estradiol (Lo/Ovral)
   b. Drinking more caffeine
   c. Using naproxen
   d. Using aspirin
   e. Using acetaminophen

11. You are called in to see a 15-year-old girl with a HR of 130, BP 110/60, and pallor. She states that her period has lasted for 10 days and she has gone through at least 5 pads per day since its onset. The bleeding is painless. Her symptoms are most likely the result of:

   a. Thrombocytopenia
   b. Pregnancy
   c. Anovulation
   d. Polycystic ovary syndrome
   e. Pelvic inflammatory disease

12. A hematocrit obtained on the patient in Question 11 is 22 mg/dl. Your most appropriate next step in her management would be:

   a. Transfuse with 2 units of type-specific packed RBCs
   b. Administer conjugated estrogens IV
   c. Administer cefixime and azithromycin PO
   d. Transfuse with 6 units of platelets
   e. Administer a combined estrogen-progestin tablet PO

13. You are assessing a 9-year-old girl brought in by her mother for suspicion of sexual abuse. In questioning the patient, she divulges an encounter with a male relative 1 week ago. Your next most appropriate step in managing this case is:

    a. Full examination, including rape kit, speculum examination, and full STD screening
    b. Speculum examination and full STD screening only
    c. STD prophylaxis only
    d. Rape kit only
    e. Limited examination of external genitalia and selective STD screening

14. During examination of a 2-month-old girl for rash, you note a thin, yellowish vaginal discharge. The infant is afebrile and has no external signs of vaginal trauma or irritation. Your most appropriate management of this patient is:

    a. Culture of discharge and metronidazole
    b. Counseling of parent on perineal hygiene
    c. Culture of discharge and IM ceftriaxone
    d. Social services consultation
    e. Gynecologic examination with cultures under sedation

15. A 19-year-old female patient complains of severe abdominal pain, flushing, headache, and vomiting. While taking her history, you detect the smell of alcohol on her breath. She states she is on "some medication" for a vaginal infection. Characteristics of her vaginal infection are most likely to be:

    a. A purulent discharge with pruritis
    b. Inguinal adenopathy and a palmar rash
    c. A curdlike, whitish discharge with dysuria
    d. A frothy, yellow-green, pruritic discharge
    e. Lower abdominal pain without discharge

16. A 17-year-old female patient complains of a vaginal discharge. She states it is foul smelling, white, and nonpruritic. She has had similar symptoms in the past and her history includes the birth of a 32-week, 2-pound infant. Microscopic examination of her discharge is most likely to reveal:

    a. Hyphae
    b. Clue cells
    c. Motile flagellates
    d. Polymorphonuclear leukocytes with diplococci
    e. None of the above

17. An 18-year-old female patient complains of vaginal pain. On examination, you note an erythematous, fluctuant bulge at the vestibule. There is no discharge present. The most appropriate treatment of this patient would be:

    a. Incision and drainage (I&D) only
    b. Sitz baths
    c. Ceftriaxone IM
    d. I&D, Word catheter placement, and ceftriaxone IM
    e. I&D, Word catheter placement, and culture of pus

18. You are examining a 14-year-old girl with abdominal pain. Her axillary temperature (T) is 38.2°C, HR 94, RR 16 and BP 110/75. On pelvic examination you note copious discharge. The patient has both cervical motion and bilateral adnexal tenderness on bimanual examination. On rectovaginal examination you feel a fullness on the right. The most appropriate management for this patient would be:

    a. Outpatient management only, with ceftriaxone IM single dose and doxycycline PO to complete 14 days
    b. Admit for cefoxitin IV and doxycycline IV for a full 14 days
    c. Outpatient management with ceftriaxone IM, single dose only
    d. Admit for IV cefoxitin and IV doxycycline until clinically improved, then outpatient management with doxycycline PO to complete 14 days
    e. Outpatient management with ofloxacin PO and metronidazole PO for 14 days

19. You are counseling a 16-year-old sexually active female patient about birth control. She states that she had engaged in her first intercourse at age 12 years and has had at least 7 sexual partners. She has already been treated for two cases of chlamydia-positive cervicitis. Which of the following statements is true?

    a. The use of barrier contraception will not change her risk for subsequent cervicitis
    b. Her risk of infertility is greater than 15%
    c. Oral contraceptives can prevent a lower-tract gonorrheal infection from ascending
    d. She is at low risk for developing pelvic inflammatory disease (PID)
    e. She is a good candidate for an intrauterine device (IUD)

20. During a routine pelvic examination, you note the presence of several flat, velvety lesions ranging from 0.5–1 cm in diameter around the patient's perineum. On further examination you are most likely to find:

    a. Flat, palmar macules
    b. Cultures positive for human papilloma virus (HPV) type 2
    c. Positive serum RPR
    d. Koilocytes on Pap smear
    e. Presence of cheesy vaginal discharge

ANSWERS

1. c   In a premenarchal child, a standard pelvic examination is usually unnecessary except for cases of vaginal bleeding secondary to trauma or abuse. In these cases, the examination should be performed under sedation. Most children can be examined and cultured lying on their backs in a frog-leg position. Bimanual examination in the absence of abdominal pain, referral to gynecology for speculum examination and discharging the patient without cultures would all be inappropriate in this case.

2. d   It may be extremely difficult to elicit an accurate sexual history from an adolescent patient, particularly when a parent is present. It would be most important to check a serum or urine HCG in this patient, because there is a high likelihood that pregnancy is the cause of her symptoms. Gastroenteritis without diarrhea would be a diagnosis of exclusion, as would appendicitis in the absence of fever. Constipation rarely causes vomiting. Streptococcal pharyngitis without other complaints indicating this condition would be unlikely.

3. e   In many instances, the presence of a vaginal foreign body cannot be detected on rectal examination because most are composed of toilet tissue. Symptoms include a foul odor and sometimes a discharge from the vagina. Vaginitis and candidiasis cause discharge. Premature adrenarche is characterized by vaginal bleeding. There is nothing in the history to suggest that poor hygiene is the cause of this patient's symptoms, and this must be a diagnosis of exclusion.

4. b   Presence of an abdominal mass, constipation, and urinary symptoms are all found with hydrocolpos, or imperforate hymen. Fluid and discharge from the vagina build up and cause obstruction of the urethra, leading to bladder distension. This can result in constipation and sometimes urinary tract findings of hydronephrosis. It is also associated with hypoventilation, as opposed to respiratory distress. Absence of deep tendon reflexes, muscle atrophy, and poor rectal tone are all symptoms of neurologic disease, none of which are seen with hydrocolpos.

5. a   McKusick-Kaufman syndrome is found in consanguineous families and includes the presence of transverse vaginal septum, polydactyly, and congenital heart disease. The presence of a transverse vaginal septum is the cause of this child's primary amenorrhea. Cervical cancer at this age is rare, and would not present in this manner. Vaginal cancers from maternal DES exposure are no longer seen in this age group, and uterine fibroids are very rarely found in this age group. Since this patient is Tanner stage 3–4, there is no evidence to support familial late puberty as a reason for her primary amenorrhea.

6. b   Testicular feminization syndrome or gonadal dysgenesis syndrome is the result of end-organ insensitivity to androgens. Patients with this syndrome are phenotypic females but genetic males. They lack a uterus, have a blind vaginal pouch and experience breast development. Hematometocolpos, the result of imperforate hymen, would be noted on the examination. Serum measurements of FSH and LH may be elevated in this syndrome. Patients with karyotype 45XO have Turner's syndrome, and do not fit the description of the patient above.

7. b   Labial adhesions are common in children and generally do not require treatment. If necessary, application of estrogen cream over a period of weeks will break down the adhesions. This condition should never be treated with manual or surgical separation, as these procedures will lead to scarring and further adhesion. Neither a urologic nor a genetics consultation is warranted for workup of this condition.

8. b   Sitz baths along with topical estrogen cream is the preferred initial management of urethral prolapse. Urethral prolapse is characterized by the presence of a red/purple doughnut-shaped mass, which is often accompanied by symptoms of bleeding and urinary retention. It occurs most frequently in African-Americans. If the prolapse fails to recede after conservative measures have been tried, surgical excision with reanastomosis may be necessary. This is not a tumor and biopsy and/or oncologic consultation is unnecessary. Hydrocortisone cream is ineffective in treating this condition.

9. b   Prostaglandins F_2 and E_2, which are synthesized by endometrial tissue, are responsible for increasing uterine resting tone, and the amplitude and frequency of myometrial contractions. This, in turn, can produce tissue ischemia and lead to menstrual pain, or dysmenorrhea. This patient suffers from primary dysmenorrhea, a condition affecting many women with ovulatory menstrual cycles in the absence

of pelvic pathology. Although FSH and LH are responsible for the hormone surges that lead to ovulation and, eventually, to myometrial sloughing, it is the increased levels of prostaglandins that produce the painful contractions characteristic of dysmenorrhea.

10. a The patient described in this question is sexually active and is not using birth control. Birth control pills provide both contraception and pain relief, and would therefore provide treatment for both of her needs. Nonsteroidal anti-inflammatory drugs (such as naproxen) are first-line treatment for most cases of dysmenorrhea, but would not provide this patient with protection against unwanted pregnancy. Acetaminophen, aspirin, and caffeine do not have action against prostaglandins and would not produce adequate relief of symptoms of dysmenorrhea.

11. c Dysfunctional uterine bleeding (DUB) is irregular, prolonged or excessive menstrual bleeding associated with anovulation and unrelated to pregnancy. In this patient, with her history of irregular menses prior to this event, it is likely that her cycles are still anovulatory. Although DUB is the most likely cause of her symptoms, other etiologies of prolonged bleeding must be considered, however. Bleeding disorders such as thrombocytopenia and von Willebrand's disease, endocrine disorders like polycystic ovary syndrome, and pelvic diseases caused by *Chlamydia* or gonorrhea should be considered if associated signs are noted. However, in this setting, DUB is the most likely cause.

12. e Management of DUB consists of stopping the bleeding, changing the state of the endometrium from proliferative to secretory, and controlling the sloughing. This is best accomplished with a combination of estrogen, which supports the endometrium and acutely stops the bleeding, and progestin, which induces the secretory state. Antibiotics should also be administered if PID is diagnosed, however, in this case there is no evidence to support infection in the patient. Transfusion may be necessary if the patient is hemodynamically unstable or thrombocytopenic. Intravenous estrogen is rarely indicated; however, it may be necessary in cases of severe or prolonged bleeding.

13. e In the case of a prepubertal girl in which a sexual encounter occurred more than 72 hours from presentation, the most appropriate management is a physical examination limited to the external genitalia with appropriate, selective STD cultures. If the child has any evidence of vaginal trauma (such as bleeding not readily visualized from an external source), a speculum examination under anesthesia would be indicated. Full STD screening (vaginal, rectal, oropharynx) is not recommended universally in prepubertal females, as the yield is low. Rape kits have little usefulness when the event occurred more than 72 hours before the ED visit, and STD prophylaxis should be restricted to high-risk children (children whose assailant has an STD or in cases where multiple assailants are involved).

14. a Trichomonal vaginitis may be seen in infants who have acquired the infection perinatally through an infected mother. These patients are generally asymptomatic except for the discharge. Culture of the discharge reveals flagellated trichomonads. The treatment of choice is metronidazole for 7 days. Discharge associated with gonococcal infections is usually thick or purulent. Although poor perineal hygiene often presents with vaginal secretions, it usually is associated with irritation of the perineum and, in older patients, pruritis. Unless *Neisseria gonorrhea* is cultured or the patient has obvious signs of perineal trauma, social services does not need to be contacted in this case. A full gynecologic examination should be reserved for cases in which evidence of perineal trauma exists.

15. d Postpubertal females with trichomonal vaginitis present with a characteristic frothy, yellow-green pruritic vaginal discharge. Treatment of trichomoniasis is metronidazole in a single dose in these patients. When ingested with alcohol, this medication can produce a disulfiram-like ("Antabuse") reaction characterized by flushing, abdominal pain, headache, and vomiting. This reaction is not seen with medications used to treat the other infections described [gonorrhea (a), syphillis (b), *candida* vulvovaginitis (c), chlamydia (e)].

16. b This patient has symptoms consistent with bacterial vaginosis. Most cases of bacterial vaginosis are secondary to infection with *Gardnerella vaginallis*. Clue cells, epithelial cells studded with bacteria, are commonly seen on microscopic examination. Bacterial vaginosis has also been shown to be associated with endometritis, chorioamnionitis, and low-birth weight, premature births. Hyphae are characteristic of infection with *Candida albicans*. Candidal vulvovaginitis is characterized by the presence of cheesy or curdlike, whitish vaginal discharge and pruritis. Motile flagellates, or trichomonads, are seen in vaginal trichomoniasis, which typically presents with pruritis and frothy yellow discharge. The presence of

diplococci in polymorphonuclear leukocytes is diagnostic of infection with *N. gonorrhea*. Typical discharge from this infection is thick and whitish or greenish, and is usually associated with pruritis.

17. d   All patients with a Bartholin's gland abscess should be treated for presumed infection with *N. gonorrhea*. Incision and drainage of these abscesses should be accompanied by either placement of a Word catheter or marsupialization to prevent recurrence. Culture of pus should be obtained as well, but since 10–50% of all abscesses are infected with gonococcus, treatment with antibiotics is recommended for all patients with abscess formation. Sitz baths, I&D alone, or treatment of the infection with antibiotics alone are ineffective.

18. d   The patient in Question 18 with PID meets criteria for admission secondary to fever and possible presence of a tubo-ovarian abscess (TOA). Correct management would include admission until clinical improvement is obtained, and then outpatient treatment for the remainder of a 14-day course of doxycycline. Outpatient management of a patient with a suspected TOA, or whose clinical disease is significant or associated with fever, would be inappropriate. Admission for a full 14 days is likely to be unnecessary.

19. c   The patient in the above scenario is a high-risk candidate for PID, and already has had two proven lower-tract infections. Oral contraceptive pills have been shown to decrease the likelihood that a lower-tract infection with gonorrhea will develop into ascending disease. There is no history given that this patient has had an ascending infection, so her risk of infertility is not known. After one episode of salpingitis, however, the infertility risk is estimated at 15% and becomes higher with each subsequent episode. Using barrier contraceptive methods (condoms, sponges, diaphragms, spermicides) decreases the overall risk of contracting gonorrheal and chlamydial cervicitis, whereas using an IUD increases a patient's risk of developing ascending infection in the presence of lower-tract disease.

20. d   The patient above has condyloma accuminata, genital warts most often caused by HPV types 6 and 11. The presence of koilocytes on a Pap smear is diagnostic of cervical HPV infection. Although HPV type 2 may be found in these lesions, it is uncommon. Flat palmar macules and a positive serum RPR are symptoms of syphilis. Syphilis may also be associated with the presence of a type of flat wart called condyloma lata. It is a highly contagious form of secondary syphilis. Cheesy vaginal discharge is commonly seen with candidal vulvovaginitis, and is not an associated finding with genital warts.

CHAPTER 95

Pulmonary Emergencies

JOHN J. REEVES, M.D.

QUESTIONS

1. With regard to causes of death due to pulmonary disease, which of the following is true?

   a. Primarily because of improvements in neonatal care, mortality rates from respiratory illness related to HIV disease in newborn infants is slowly decreasing

   b. In children less than 4 years of age, more children die of sudden infant death syndrome (SIDS) than from all other respiratory diseases combined

   c. Because of the high rate of teen suicide, most deaths from suffocation occur in this age group

   d. Although pneumonia is still the leading cause of death in children older than 10 years of age, asthma deaths continue to increase in this age group

   e. If current trends continue, respiratory deaths due to problems from prematurity will continue to increase

2. A 10-year-old boy with multiple congenital anomalies, including severe scoliosis, is being treated in the ED for severe respiratory distress and hypoxia secondary to pneumonia. After intubation, the child is being ventilated with 100% FIO_2 at the following parameters: RR 15, peak inspiratory pressure (PIP) 20 cm of H_2O, positive end-expiratory pressure (PEEP) 4 cm of H_2O and an inspiratory/expiratory (I:E) ratio of 1:2. The patient continues to be hypoxic (O_2 saturation of 82%). Assuming correct tube placement and patency, what is the next appropriate measure to improve his oxygenation?

   a. Decrease the I:E ratio
   b. Increase the respiratory rate
   c. Decrease the PEEP
   d. Increase the PIP
   e. Obtain an arterial blood gas (ABG)

3. A 6-year-old with pneumonia confirmed radiographically at another hospital is brought to the ED by the hospital transport team. On arrival, the patient is being ventilated via an endotracheal tube on 50% FIO_2. The current parameters are: RR 30, PIP of 38 cm of H_2O, PEEP 4 cm H_2O, and an I:E of 1:2. An ABG on arrival shows an arterial pH of 7.37, $Paco_2$ 52, Pao_2 91, and O_2 saturation of 96%. What should be done next?

   a. Increase the PIP to 45 and maintain current FIO_2
   b. Increase PIP to 45 and increase FIO_2
   c. Decrease PIP to 32 and maintain the current FIO_2
   d. Decrease the PIP to 32 and increase the FIO_2
   e. None of these maneuvers is needed at this time

4. A 12-year-old girl with a history of asthma comes to your ED in severe respiratory distress. She fails to improve after nebulizer treatments with a beta-agonist and is intubated successfully and placed on a ventilator. With regard to mechanical ventilation of this patient, which of the following is true?

   a. Higher than normal peak inflating pressures (PIP) may be required to ensure adequate ventilation and oxygenation

   b. A higher than normal respiratory rate (RR) may be required to prevent CO_2 retention

   c. An increased I:E ratio may be needed

   d. The RR and PIP should be slowly increased until a CO_2 of 35–40 is achieved

   e. PEEP should be higher than normal to prevent airway collapse

5. An emergency physician working at a rural community hospital calls your ED to arrange for transfer of a premature infant who was born 2 hours ago at 32 weeks gestational age. He states that the child is in severe respiratory distress and that an ABG shows acidosis, hypoxia, and hypercapnia. The physician is planning on intubating the patient and he asks for your recommendations regarding ventilator settings. What do you recommend?

   a. PEEP should be used to prevent airway collapse

   b. A volume-cycled ventilator mode would be preferable to prevent overexpansion of the lungs

   c. Lower than usual pressures should be used to prevent acute worsening of the hyaline membrane disease

   d. A slow respiratory rate and a prolonged expiratory phase may be beneficial to prevent hypercarbia

   e. Hypoxia is usually better tolerated than hypercarbia in a newborn infant, so correction of the CO_2 to a range of 35–40 should be the primary goal

6. An 8-year-old boy has been intubated in the ED because of severe asthma. The patient has been stabilized and is being adequately ventilated using the following settings: RR 22, PIP 42, I:E 1:3, and PEEP 3. The patient is otherwise hemodynamically stable. Which statement about IV fluids for this patient is true?

   a. Increased fluid may be required to compensate for expiratory moisture lost in the ventilation circuit

   b. Increased fluids may be required to help to increase the production of surfactant and to mobilize secretions

   c. Decreased fluids may be required to prevent pulmonary edema

   d. Determination of ongoing fluid requirements will require placement of a central venous catheter

   e. The patient may require increased fluids to improve his cardiac output

7. A 3-month-old, ex–35-week premature infant is brought in to the ED in January for evaluation. The mother reports that her regular physician diagnosed the child with a respiratory virus 4 days ago. She states that the child has been eating well and has not seemed to have much breathing difficulty. She is concerned because earlier today she thinks that the child stopped breathing while he was taking a nap. She states that she was holding the child on her lap and she noticed that the child did not take a breath for about 30 seconds. She gently shook the child and he began breathing again on his own. Since then the child has been acting fine. On your examination the child is quiet but nontoxic appearing. He is well hydrated and is in no respiratory distress. His RR is 45 and his O_2 saturation by pulse oximetry is 97%; the rest of his vital signs are unremarkable. Other than a small amount of nasal secretions, the rest of the physical examination is normal. What would be your next step in management of this child?

a. The child should be admitted for observation

b. The child may be safely discharged to home after parental instruction

c. The child may be discharged home with close observation

d. The child should be admitted and treated with disease-specific IV immunoglobulin

e. Before a treatment plan can be initiated, an ABG should be obtained

8. With regard to interstitial pneumonitis, which of the following are true?

   a. The more common form of this disorder (usual interstitial pneumonitis) is typified mainly by cellular infiltrates, whereas the more acute form of the disease (desquamative interstitial pneumonitis, or DIP) is characterized by sloughing of respiratory epithelium and progressive fibrosis

   b. Although interstitial pneumonitis is normally seen in older children and adults, where the etiology is often unknown, neonatal interstitial pneumonitis is associated with HIV infection in the majority of cases

   c. Although lung transplantation is required in many cases of interstitial pneumonitis, even this is only palliative, because the disease will often relapse and redevelop in the transplanted organs

   d. Treatment with steroids is most useful in the desquamative form of the disease, because dramatic improvement is often seen

   e. Although decreased macrophage activity is common late in the course of the disease, anemia is a common early finding

The following case relates to Questions 9–11:   While performing procedural sedation for an orthopedic procedure on an otherwise healthy 6-year-old child, the patient vomits, coughs, and has an acute episode of desaturation, which resolves after 45 seconds.

9. Which of the following is true?

   a. Although aspiration of food or organic material is generally more severe than aspiration of clear, acidic stomach fluid, the pathologic response is similar

   b. Aspiration of acidic fluids is more dangerous than aspiration of nonacidic fluids, partly because acidic aspirates are more likely to result in bacterial infection

   c. In contrast to this patient, patients with bowel obstruction are more likely to have a more severe course, primarily because they tend to have gastric contents of lower pH

   d. The type of bacterial infection seen following an aspiration event is primarily dependent on the patient's oral flora and is less influenced by other factors

   e. Children with some types of aspiration events, specifically hydrocarbon aspirations, often have severe symptoms despite normal CXRs

10. What can be said regarding the expected clinical findings in aspiration pneumonia?

    a. Immediate hypoxia is due to reflex airway closure, because pulmonary edema and surfactant destruction occur only after a latent period of several hours

    b. Although bacterial infection is uncommon initially, this child will likely develop a delayed bacterial infection

    c. The presence of fever would be unusual in this child

    d. A thorough medical workup should be sought to determine the cause of the aspiration

    e. Because of the brief duration of the aspiration event and the quick resolution of symptoms, this child is unlikely to suffer any further complications

11. In addition to treatment for his orthopedic injury, what else should be done for this patient?

    a. It is important to place an NG tube in order to check the pH of the stomach contents

    b. He should receive a course of antibiotics

    c. Brief observation (1–2 hours) is probably all that is necessary

    d. A normal CXR would be very helpful in this situation

    e. A course of oral corticosteroids should be started

12. Upon reviewing a chest radiograph on a previously healthy, acutely distressed infant, you note that the child has significant pulmonary edema. Which of the following cardiac lesions is LEAST likely to be associated with this finding?

    a. Ventricular septal defect (VSD)

    b. Hypoplastic left heart syndrome

    c. Tetralogy of Fallot

    d. Patent ductus arteriosus (PDA)

    e. Aortic stenosis

13. You are called from the ED to assist with a patient in the nursery. The child is a 2-month-old boy, who was recently extubated after repair of severe tracheal stenosis. The child initially did well following extubation, but over the last several hours the child has gradually developed hypoxia (O_2 saturation 89%) and respiratory distress. On exam, the child has no stridor, but tachypnea and grunting are noted. Chest examination reveals bilateral rales. Which of the following is LEAST likely to help this patient?

    a. Reintubation

    b. Steroids

    c. Continuous positive airway pressure (CPAP)

    d. Beta-blockers

    e. Furosemide

14. An 11-year-old boy is brought to the ED with severe bleeding from the mouth and nose. His mother reports that the child has been complaining of increased cough, shortness of breath, and abdominal pain for the past 2 days. Yesterday his stool was noted to be black. She found him this morning with "lots of blood all over his pillow." The child is noted to be pale, with shallow, labored respirations. He is minimally responsive but responds to sternal rubs. He is actively coughing or vomiting up large amounts of blood; his breathing is labored and he is being assisted with bag-valve-mask (BVM) ventilation at an RR of 30. HR is 160, BP is 72/41 mmHg, and O_2 saturation is 88%. IV access has been established and a normal saline (NS) bolus is being given. Which of the following should be done FIRST?

    a. Place an NG tube to check for bloody stomach fluid

    b. Order a blood transfusion

    c. Endotracheal intubation

    d. Arrange for an urgent endoscopy

    e. Arrange for urgent pulmonary arterial embolization

The following case relates to Questions 15–17: A 19-year-old, previously healthy girl has been ill with high fever and cough for 5 days. A CXR reveals a pulmonary infiltrate with pleural effusion. While reviewing the radiograph, you note that a fluid meniscus is seen on both the AP and the lateral view; however, the diaphragms are obscured only at the angles.

15. How large is the effusion?

    a. Less than 100 ml

    b. 100–200 ml

    c. 200–500 ml

    d. More than 500 ml

    e. More information is required

16. A diagnostic thoracentesis is performed. Which of the following combinations of test results would you expect to see in this patient? Assume a normal range for serum LDH (lactate dehydrogenase) of 150 units per liter (U/l).

	Pleural Fluid LDH	Pleural Fluid Protein	Serum Total Protein
a.	95 U/l	2.5 g/dl	6.0 g/dl
b.	120 U/l	3.0 g/dl	7.2 g/dl
c.	110 U/l	2.9 g/dl	6.5 g/dl
d.	110 U/l	3.5 g/dl	6.0 g/dl
e.	120 U/l	3.2 g/dl	7.0 g/dl

17. A chest tube should be placed:

    a. Immediately in the ED

    b. If the pH of the pleural fluid is less than 7.2

    c. Within 24 hours in the OR

    d. If the WBC count of the pleural fluid is greater than 10,000/mm²

    e. If the pleural fluid to serum fluid glucose is low (less than 0.5)

18. A previously health 8-year-old boy is sent to the ED for psychiatric evaluation. His mother reports that his performance in school has deteriorated and that he has been fighting with his peers. You perform a medical clearance examination prior to contacting psychiatry. Which of the following symptoms is most concerning for the presence of an underlying medical problem?

    a. Violent behavior
    b. Obesity
    c. Hyperactivity
    d. Snoring
    e. Withdrawn behavior

19. A 10-year-old boy comes to the ED with a history of daytime sleepiness, a restless sleep pattern, and poor school performance. Which of the following is true?

    a. Snoring is present in most if not all patients with this disorder
    b. This disorder rarely leads to serious medical complications
    c. Most children with this disorder can be managed with medical therapy alone
    d. Night sweats are an uncommon symptom in this disorder
    e. This child is most likely severely obese

ANSWERS

1. b   More children die from SIDS than from all other causes in the first few years of life. Although neonatal care is improving, HIV-related respiratory disease is on the increase in the neonate. Strangulation is a common method of teen suicide, especially in males; however, many more infants die in this manner. Pneumonia is the second most common pulmonary cause of teen deaths; asthma continues to lead in this area. Overall respiratory deaths from causes related to prematurity are currently on the decrease.

2. d   In a child with restrictive lung disease (scoliosis and pneumonia) increased inflating pressures may be required to improve oxygenation. Increasing (not decreasing) the I:E ratio would help to recruit collapsed alveoli. Increasing the RR may help to control an elevated CO_2 level, but it would not impact much on oxygenation. Decreasing the PEEP would likely worsen airway collapse and have a detrimental effect on oxygenation. Although obtaining an ABG may help in further assessing this patient's ventilatory status, hypoxia is the initial primary concern and should be addressed first.

3. e   This child has satisfactory ABG values at this time. This level of hypercarbia is acceptable in a child on these ventilatory parameters. Increasing the RR and decreasing the I:E ratio are acceptable maneuvers; however, of the options given, watchful waiting is most reasonable. Increasing the PIP from 38 (already high) to 45 would likely run the risk of increasing barotrauma and is probably unnecessary. An O_2 saturation of 96% is tolerable in a child with pneumonia.

4. a   The goals of ventilation in an intubated asthmatic child are to provide adequate oxygenation and to obtain a normal or slightly acidic pH. Complete correction of hypercarbia is usually difficult to obtain and should not be the main focus. Increased peak airway pressures, which will improve oxygenation, should be anticipated. Hyperventilation to decrease CO_2 should be of lesser concern. Increasing the PEEP in a child with reactive airway disease (RAD) will increase the risk of barotrauma and will worsen air trapping. A decreased I:E ratio is more likely to help an asthmatic patient.

5. a   In a child with decreased lung volumes such as in hyaline membrane disease (not to be confused with older children with bronchopulmonary dysplasia—BPD), PEEP should be used in order to recruit collapsed alveoli. In addition, higher airway pressures and an increased I:E ratio may be required. Use of a volume-cycled ventilator (which delivers a set volume within preselected pressure limits) in an unstable patient, especially a newborn, provides no benefit over conventional pressure-limited ventilation. Hypoxia is rarely tolerated well.

6. e   Several changes occur in the intubated patient, which may affect their fluid requirements. They have decreased fluid losses through the respiratory tree as a result of the humidification equipment present on nearly all ventilators. As a result of increased intrathoracic pressure from positive-pressure ventilation, the risk of pulmonary edema is actually relatively decreased. The increased intrathoracic pressure

can impinge on cardiac filling and may need to be overcome with increased fluid requirements (this is often achieved with IV fluid boluses based on the cardiovascular status of the patient). Increased fluids may have a theoretical benefit in clearing of secretions, but this is rarely the philosophy behind increasing fluid administration in an intubated patient. Central venous line placement may be useful for fluid monitoring, but it is rarely essential.

7. a   This child has a history consistent with respiratory syncytial virus (RSV) and a story for apnea at home. Despite a very unremarkable examination in the ED, a credible story for apnea requires hospital admission at the minimum. Apnea can be the sole presentation of an RSV infection and should be taken seriously. Further treatment with RSV immunoglobulin is not currently recommended for an otherwise healthy child with RSV infection. An ABG would presumably add little information.

8. d   Cellular infiltrates predominate in DIP, whereas fibrosis is more common in usual interstitial pneumonia (UIP). Although there is an increased relationship between lymphocytic interstitial pneumonitis and HIV infection in neonates, the vast majority of cases are idiopathic. Steroids are very effective in the desquamative form of the disease, but they are ineffective in the other forms of the disease. Lung transplant is curative; the disease does not reoccur in the transplanted organs. The presence of macrophages and anemia both present later in the disease.

9.–11. b, e, c   This child had a brief, self-limited event and is previously healthy. He is likely to recover fully and requires nothing other than observation. Steroids and prophylactic antibiotics are not indicted. A CXR should be obtained to assess the lungs after an aspiration insult; however, a normal radiograph does not rule out lung injury. Placement of an NG tube would increase the risk of further vomiting and aspiration and would not drastically alter management. The initial hypoxia is probably due primarily to reflex airway closure, but direct lung injury, destruction of surfactant, and pulmonary edema can contribute to the initial hypoxia. The risk of developing complications such as hypoxia and bacterial infection are related most to the child's underlying risk factors and the amount and composition of the aspirate. As the acidity increases, so does the risk of serious complications. Acidic aspirates cause more severe direct lung injury and result in a neutrophilic infiltrate. The composition of a bacterial infection, once it develops, is most related to underlying factors (e.g., the presence or absence of chronic medical problems, bowel obstruction, and chronic hospitalization). Hydrocarbon aspirations often present with minimal symptoms but a very impressive chest radiograph. Fever is a nonspecific finding and is often present in children after an aspiration event (or any other traumatic event, for that matter) and does not necessarily indicate an infection.

12. c   Pulmonary edema can be caused from many causes; one of these is exposure of the pulmonary circulation to systemic blood pressure. Of the preceding choices, all except tetralogy of Fallot (uncorrected) are associated with increased arterial pressures in the pulmonary circulation.

13. b   This child is suffering from postintubation pulmonary edema, not upper airway edema. True "grunting" respirations indicate a parenchymal/alveolar process (i.e., pulmonary edema). The patient is pushing air against a closed glottis in an attempt to maintain patency of the alveoli. Initiation of positive airway pressure via CPAP or intubation, furosemide, and beta-blockers will all help this condition. Steroids, which are useful in upper airway edema, have no role in the treatment of pulmonary edema in this patient.

14. c   ABCs. This child has severe cardiovascular collapse from bleeding of unclear etiology. He requires protection of his airway as an initial step, followed by treatment of his hypoxia and hypotension. Intubation should be performed with a low dose of a cardioprotective medication (e.g., etomidate or ketamine). Placement of a nasogastric (NG) tube for diagnosis is unnecessary because it will be positive no matter what the source of the bleeding. An NG tube may required for cold saline lavage as a treatment modality, but certainly not as a first step. Transfusion should be ordered, but it will take some time. Endoscopy or arterial embolization will have to await stabilization of the patient.

15.–17. c, d, b   In an adult it is possible to estimate the size of a simple pleural effusion. A fluid collection visible on the lateral radiograph only is approximately 50 ml. If the fluid is visible on the AP radiograph as well, but the diaphragms are not obscured, then the fluid collection is approximately 200 ml. At 500 ml the hemidiaphragm is obscured. An exudate, as would be expected in this child with pneumonia, is distinguished from a transudate by several features. If any one of the following is found, then the fluid can be considered an exudate:

- A pleural fluid to serum protein ratio greater than 0.5
- A pleural fluid to serum LDH ratio greater than 0.6
- A pleural LDH concentration that is more than two-thirds of the upper limit of normal for serum

    The need for chest tube placement is controversial. Of the answers given, only "b" is entirely correct. Immediate placement of a chest tube in the ED or deferred placement in the operating room may be practiced at many institutions depending on multiple factors. It should be recognized that guidelines are unclear in this area. A diagnostic thoracentesis clearly does not need to be followed by chest tube placement in all cases. Most children can safely undergo successful chest tube placement in the ED with either local anesthetic alone or with carefully performed procedural sedation. In adult patients, a pleural effusion pH of less than 7.2 correlates with failure of effusion resolution and need for chest tube placement. A pH less than 7.0 can be associated with empyema, collagen-vascular disease, or esophageal rupture. Other fluid parameters (e.g., glucose concentration and surprisingly high WBC count) do not reliably translate into useful clinical guidelines.

18.   d   Obstructive sleep apnea (OSA) is an organic disorder that is often misdiagnosed as hyperactive attention deficit disorder (HADD). Although hyperactivity, violent behavior, and behavior changes can be seen in a variety of medical and psychological disorders, the presence of snoring, disordered sleep, or daytime sleepiness should cause a further investigation into the possibility of OSA. Obesity is present in a large number of children and even though it is of general concern from a medical standpoint, it does not normally imply a specific medical diagnosis.

19.   a   Obstructive sleep apnea is a complex and poorly understood disorder. Most children snore due to nighttime upper airway obstruction. Although obese children are at increased risk of OSA, not all children with this disorder are overweight. Night sweats are a common complaint in children with OSA, which is likely due to their increased catecholamine release, stimulated by hypoxia and respiratory distress. Although weight reduction is important in obese children, medical management alone of OSA is rarely successful, because most patients need either surgical excision of redundant tissue or nighttime respiratory support with either a special appliance or positive airway pressure. Pursuit of resolution of OSA is essential, because most children are at risk for serious psychological and medical complications.

CHAPTER 96

Cystic Fibrosis

ANDREA STRACCIOLINI, M.D.

QUESTIONS

1. You are called to the nursery to evaluate a neonate who is now 14 hours old. The infant has had four feedings of formula. After the last feeding, the infant's abdomen became distended. The child has had no meconium stools. On examination, you note a distended abdomen with visible peristaltic waves. An abdominal plain film (KUB) shows dilated loops of bowel and a bubbly granular density in the lower abdomen. There is no free air. The best next step in caring for this infant is:

    a. Laparotomy
    b. Abdominal CT
    c. Contrast enema
    d. Ultrasound (U/S)
    e. Sweat test

2. A 2½-year-old girl with cystic fibrosis (CF) is brought to the ED because the mother has just noticed that the girl has pink mucosal tissue protruding from her rectum. The only pertinent history is that the child has been non-compliant with taking her pancreatic enzymes. As the ED physician, you:

    a. Attempt manual reduction
    b. Obtain a surgical consult
    c. Order a Fleet's enema
    d. Admit the child
    e. Obtain a contrast enema

3. A 15-year-old boy with CF is brought to the ED because of abdominal pain. He has been vomiting for the past 8 hours. On physical examination, there is abdominal distension, the bowel sounds are decreased, and there is tenderness in the right lower and middle quadrants. The KUB shows dilated loops of bowel and multiple air fluid levels. There is a paucity of bowel gas distally. The next step in the evaluation and treatment of this patient is:

    a. Contrast enema
    b. Mineral oil orally
    c. N-acetylcysteine (NAC)
    d. External abdominal pressure
    e. Abdominal CT

4. A 6-month-old girl with CF is brought to the ED by her parents. She is lethargic and pale. The family has been vacationing at the beach. The infant has had a URI for the past few days. Her oral intake abruptly decreased, and she then became lethargic. She has had no urine output for 8 hours. The best initial treatment for this infant is:

    a. IV 3% NaCl solution 20 ml/kg bolus
    b. IV 20 ml/kg NS with KCl 20mEq/l bolus
    c. IV D5 ½ NS with 20mEq KCl/l maintenance
    d. IV 30 ml/kg ½ NS bolus
    e. IV 20 ml/kg NS bolus

5. An 18-year-old male patient with CF comes to the ED complaining of a sudden onset of chest pain referred to the shoulder. He complains of pain with deep breaths. He denies trauma, palpitations, or drug use. The likely treatment for this patient will include:

    a. IV antibiotics
    b. Sublingual (SL) nitroglycerine
    c. Tube thoracostomy
    d. Bronchoscopy
    e. Intubation

6. A 15-year-old girl with CF comes to the ED because she has been having hemoptysis for the past 2 days. She initially had intermittent blood streaking of the sputum. Today she reports approximately 50 ml of bright red blood. Your immediate care of this patient may include all of the following, EXCEPT:

    a. Vitamin K
    b. IV antibiotics
    c. Hospital admission
    d. PT and PTT
    e. Bronchoscopy

7. A 20-year-old man with CF is brought to the ED with respiratory distress. He wears oxygen at home and has had an increase in sputum production, dyspnea, and fever for the past few days. Over the last few hours he has required more oxygen and has had significantly increased work of breathing. On physical examination, he is tachycardic and tachypneic. He has pronounced clubbing, diffuse crackles, and an enlarged tender liver. The most effective treatment in the acute care of this patient is:

a. Albuterol
b. Atenolol
c. Digoxin
d. Furosemide
e. Antibiotics

ANSWERS

1. c   Neonatal manifestations of cystic fibrosis (CF) may be intestinal obstruction from meconium ileus. This child has a typical history of abdominal distension after a few feedings and passage of no or little meconium stool. An abdominal mass may be palpable and peristaltic waves may be visible. A three-view radiographic examination should be obtained promptly. If there are no signs of perforation, a radiographic examination following contrast enema is indicated and will typically show a microcolon of disuse and impacted meconium in the terminal ileum. Other abnormalities or complications include volvulus, which can be seen easily on barium enema. Immediate laparotomy is not warranted without evidence of perforation. Ultrasound is not as useful as contrast enema in outlining the anatomy and cause for obstruction. A sweat test is indicated, but not in the acute management of this patient.

2. a   Rectal prolapse occurs most commonly in children less than 3 years old. The association with CF is frequent and a sweat test is indicated for an undiagnosed child who has had rectal prolapse. In a child who is known to have CF, rectal prolapse usually results when pancreatic enzyme therapy has been inadequate, as in this case scenario. The prolapse can often be easily reduced by placing the infant in a comfortable position and using a lubricated glove for manual reduction. Fleet's enema and admission to the hospital are not necessary. Surgical consult and contrast enema should be obtained if you suspect intussusception or other complications.

3. a   Acute abdominal pain is common in CF patients, and an associated fecal mass in the right lower quadrant is often present. Intestinal obstruction occurring in CF patients beyond the neonatal period is referred to as *meconium ileus equivalent*. These patients often have signs and symptoms of intestinal obstruction. The fecal mass may serve as a leading edge for either an intussusceptum or a volvulus. When the roentgenogram of the abdomen shows signs of obstruction, such as dilated loops of bowel or air fluid levels, a barium or diatrizoate methylglucamine enema must be performed. If only a fecal mass is present—without an associated volvulus or intussusception—medical management may be tried. External pressure to the abdomen is contraindicated. In cases of fecal impaction without complete obstruction, and after intussusception and volvulus have been ruled out, enemas, oral mineral oil, and NAC have been reported to be effective.

4. e   During periods of hot weather, the increased loss of sodium and chloride in the sweat of patients with CF may lead to severe and symptomatic electrolyte depletion. In patients who present with lethargy and decreased urine output, prompt fluid replacement with isotonic saline (NS) is critical; 20–30 ml/kg should be given within 15 minutes if there are signs of shock, or within 1 hour in less severely ill patients. Potassium chloride (KCl) should be administered as soon as urine output is established. Hypotonic fluids should not be given in the acute management of this patient.

5. c   Sudden onset of chest pain often referred to the shoulder and associated with the acute onset of increasing dyspnea and cyanosis is most likely the result of a pneumothorax in the CF patient. Rupture of a subpleural bleb introduces air into the pleural space. Recurrences are common and tension pneumothorax has been reported in as many as 30% of these cases. CF patients with a pneumothorax of larger than 10% of the area of the hemithorax should be treated with tube thoracostomy.

6. e   A small amount of hemoptysis is a fairly common occurrence in CF patients. There is no need for a major change in the patient's usual home care regimen other than considering antibiotic therapy to treat potential infection. Significant hemoptysis is defined as the expectoration of at least 30–60 ml of fresh blood. Hospitalization for observation is indicated. Blood should be sent for a type and cross-match as well as a hematocrit and PT/PTT. IV antibiotics against *Staphylococcus* and *Pseudomonas* should be started. Large-bore IV access should be obtained in case rapid transfusion becomes necessary. Vitamin K should be given if the PT is prolonged. Bronchoscopy is not performed in the acute setting without massive (300–2500 ml) hemoptysis, in which case ligation of a bleeding vessel is often required.

7. d   Patients with CF who have moderately severe pulmonary insufficiency and hypoxia will eventually develop right ventricular hypertrophy resulting from pulmonary hypertension. Increased hypoxia during an exacerbation of pulmonary symptoms in such patients may precipitate an acute episode of congestive heart failure (CHF), as in this case scenario. The patients often present with cyanosis, tachypnea, tachycardia, and an enlarged liver, and may have a gallop rhythm, peripheral edema, and ascites. Most patients will have digital clubbing. Oxygen and diuretics (furosemide 1 mg/kg IV) are most effective. Digitalis and pulmonary vasodilators have not been shown to be of proven benefit. Some CF centers, however, will use digitalis during an acute episode of heart failure and/or significant biventricular dysfunction on echocardiography.

CHAPTER 97

Endocrine Emergencies

KAREN DULL, M.D.

QUESTIONS

1. A 6-year-old girl is brought to the ED with vomiting, abdominal pain, and a 10-pound (or 5 kg) weight loss. Despite the vomiting, she has been urinating every hour and waking in the night to urinate. She has also had excessive thirst for 2 weeks. On exam she is tachypneic and appears moderately dehydrated. Her electrolytes show Na 145 mEq/l, K 4.8mEq/l, Cl 100mEq/l, HCO_3 10mEq/l, BUN 23 mg/dl, Cr 0.9 mg/dl, and glucose 445 mg/dl. Initial treatment should include:

   a. Administration of 20 ml/kg of isotonic saline (NS) given over 1 hour, followed by ½ NS + 80 mEq/l KCl/l
   b. Administration of 20 ml/kg of isotonic saline (NS) given over 1 hour, followed by ¼ NS + 40 mEq/l KCl/l + 50 mEq $NaHCO_3$/l
   c. Administration of 20 ml/kg of isotonic saline (NS) given over 1 hour, followed by ½ NS + 40 mEqKCl/l
   d. Administration of 20 ml/kg of isotonic saline given over 1 hour, followed by ½ NS
   e. Administration of 20 ml/kg of D5NS given over 1 hour, followed by D5 ½ NS + 40 mEqKCl/l

2. A true statement about the insulin therapy for the patient in Question 1 is:

   a. Insulin should be started when the child is able to tolerate liquids and solids
   b. The rate of insulin infusion should be adjusted to sustain a fall in the blood glucose of about 100 mg/dl/hour
   c. If the glucose falls too rapidly, the dose of the insulin should be discontinued
   d. The insulin may be given intravenously (IV), intramuscularly (IM), or subcutaneously (SC)
   e. The starting dose of insulin is 1 U/kg/hr

3. A 3-year-old boy is brought to the ED with restlessness and anxiety for several hours. He has had vomiting and diarrhea for the last 24 hours and has refused to eat or drink. On examination he is alert but has a sluggish capillary refill time and dry mucous membranes. A reagent strip for glucose registers 20–40 mg/dl and you order a serum glucose. What is the treatment of choice for his condition?

   a. 1 ampule of D50
   b. 1.0 ml/kg of 25% dextrose
   c. 2.0 ml/kg of 50% of dextrose/kg
   d. 10 ml/kg of 10% glucose
   e. None, pending the serum glucose level

4. A 10-year-old girl is brought in to the ED in December by a friend's mother, with whom she had been staying for a week. She has had intermittent vomiting, diarrhea, and progressive lethargy for 5 days. Her friend's mother reports that she thinks the patient has a problem with her kidneys, but she is not sure of a specific diagnosis. On exam the girl is afebrile, with HR 140, BP 80/30, and RR 10. She is minimally responsive to pain. She has bluish extremities, which are cold. You notice a tanned appearance of her skin, despite being the middle of winter. You immediately give her 60 ml/kg of NS IV, with no change in her vital signs or clinical picture. The next step in her management is to administer:

   a. Hydrocortisone
   b. 3% NS
   c. 9-alpha-fluorocortisol
   d. Glucose, followed by insulin
   e. Dobutamine

5. A 4-week-old boy is brought to the ED with poor feeding, vomiting, lethargy, and irritability for the last 2 weeks, which has rapidly progressed over the last 24 hours. On exam he is cachectic appearing, with HR 150, BP 78/48, and RR 28. His electrolyte levels are: Na 129 mEq/l, K 6.9 mEq/l, Cl 100 mEq/l, HCO$_3$ 10 mEq/l, BUN 30 g/dl, Cr 0.8, and glucose 120 mg/dl. His ECG is unremarkable. The next step in correcting the metabolic abnormalities includes:

   a. 0.1 U/kg of insulin, followed by 1 gm/kg glucose
   b. 20 ml/kg of NS
   c. 100 mg/kg of 10% calcium gluconate
   d. 2 mEq/kg of sodium bicarbonate
   e. 3 ml/kg of 3% NS

6. A 6-year-old boy is brought to the ED with headache and vomiting for 2 weeks. On physical exam he is tired appearing and his mucous membranes are very dry, despite drinking more than 2 liters of fluids earlier in the day. You also note papilledema in both eyes and decreased vision in his lateral visual fields. His HR is 140, RR 20, and BP 60/40. Serum electrolytes show Na 170, K 4.0, Cl 120, and HCO$_3$ 15. The initial management of his condition would be:

   a. 20 ml/kg of ¼ NS IV bolus
   b. 20 ml/kg of ½ NS IV bolus
   c. 20 ml/kg of D5W IV
   d. 20 ml/kg of NS IV bolus
   e. D5W at 120 ml/hour IV

7. A 3-year-old girl arrives from an outside hospital for the management of suspected meningitis. She received ceftriaxone and two IV boluses of normal saline (NS) for hypotension. On the way to your hospital she begins to have a generalized seizure that is unresponsive to two doses of 0.1 mg/kg of lorazepam and 15 mg/kg of phosphenytoin. Upon arrival in the ED her vital signs are: T 38.5°C (rectally), HR 110, BP 120/80, RR 20, and an O$_2$ saturation of 100% on face mask O$_2$. Her pupils are equal, round, and reactive to light symmetrically. She continues to have generalized tonic-clonic seizure activity. Her electrolytes show Na 124 mEq/l, K 4.0 mEq/l, Cl 102 mEq/l, and HCO$_3$ 19 mEq/l. The next step in the management should be:

   a. Emergent head CT
   b. 10 mg/kg of phenobarbital
   c. 20 mg/kg of phenobarbital
   d. 0.1 mg/kg of midazolam
   e. 3 ml/kg of 3% NS

8. A 1-year-old girl who was born at 24 weeks gestation presents with right wrist swelling and pain for the last week. There is no known trauma. Radiographs reveal widening and irregularity of the distal radial epiphyseal plate and cupping of the metaphysis. Which of the following would support her diagnosis?

   a. Elevated alkaline phosphatase
   b. Hypercalcemia
   c. Hyperphosphatemia
   d. Periosteal elevation of the tibia
   e. Bucket-handle fractures of the humerus

9. An 18-year-old adolescent with hyperthyroidism presents with fever to 41°C, associated with restlessness and sweating. On examination she is tremulous, with a temperature of 40.0°C and BP 180/90. Which of the following should be given acutely?

   a. Propylthiouracil
   b. Methimazole
   c. Propranalol
   d. Aspirin
   e. Nitroprusside

ANSWERS

1.   c Fluid replacement should begin with 20 ml/kg of NS IV to replenish intravascular volume. This may need to be repeated if indicated by the physical exam. One-half normal saline (½ NS) should be started after the initial bolus of NS. All children with DKA are total body potassium depleted; therefore, the maintenance fluid should have potassium added. The use of sodium bicarbonate should be reserved for severe cases in which the pH is less than 7.1 and for patients who cannot hyperventilate to control the CO$_2$.

2.   b Insulin is necessary to stop ketone body production. The insulin should be started early in the rehydration process. Insulin may be given intravenously or intramuscularly, but subcutaneous routes should be avoided if the child is acidotic because of the unpredictability of its absorption via this route. The starting dose of insulin is 0.1 U/kg/hour. The rate of insulin infusion should be adjusted to attain the goal of decreasing the glucose by 100 mg/dl/hour. If the glucose falls too rapidly, glucose should be added to the IV fluids, or the rate of insulin infusion may be decreased, but the insulin should not be stopped as long as the child remains acidotic.

3. b   The initial symptoms of hypoglycemia are nonspecific. They include palpitations, anxiety, tremulousness, hunger, and sweating. They can progress to fatigue, confusion, seizure, and unconsciousness. Therapy should be instituted if the screen is suggestive of hypoglycemia. The treatment of choice is 0.25 g of dextrose per kilogram. This is 2.5 ml/kg of 10% dextrose, or 1.0 ml/kg of 25% dextrose. The serum glucose should then be maintained with an infusion providing dextrose at a rate of 6–8 mg/kg/minute.

4. a   This patient has adrenal insufficiency. Acute adrenal insufficiency is commonly precipitated by stressors such as infection, trauma, or surgery. It is manifested as an inappropriate decompensation to one of these stressors. Biochemical changes include hyponatremia, hyperkalemia, and hypoglycemia. Treatment consists of rapid volume reexpansion and administration of hydrocortisone (IV 50–100 mg/m^2). Clinical improvement in the peripheral circulation should occur within the first hour. Mineralocorticoid therapy with 9-alpha-fluorocortisol is important for long-term management, but it is rarely important in the acute phase.

5. b   This infant has the salt-losing form of congenital adrenal hyperplasia (CAH). The most common form of CAH presenting in infancy is 21-hydroxylase deficiency. 21-hydroxylase is involved in the production of cortisol and aldosterone. The lack of production of cortisol stimulates an increase in ACTH (adrenocorticotropic hormone) production, which stimulates the adrenal glands to increase steroid hormone production. Because cortisol synthesis is impaired, there is accumulation of the cortisol precursors. Females are often virilized in utero and, therefore, the diagnosis is usually made in the newborn period. Males have normal genital development and usually present with salt-wasting crisis. The sodium is characteristically low and the potassium is elevated. Hydrocortisone (50 mg/m^2 or 50–100 mg) IV bolus, followed by 50–100 mg/m^2/24 hours as a continuous infusion should be given as soon as the diagnosis is suspected. Only hydrocortisone and cortisone have some of the necessary mineralocorticoid effects. Volume repletion with NS bolus is usually the only measure needed to correct the potassium level. If an arrhythmia develops, IV 10% calcium gluconate should be used. Therapy with glucose and insulin is contraindicated because of the possibility of inducing hypoglycemia.

6. d   The child described has diabetes insipidus (DI), which is due to an inability of the kidneys to concentrate urine secondary to a lack of antidiuretic hormone (central DI) or the inability of the kidneys to respond to the ADH (nephrogenic DI). In this case, the DI is secondary to a craniopharyngioma that is affecting the patient's vision and causing increased intracranial pressure (ICP). Other common causes of central DI include brain radiation, trauma, meningitis, and neurosurgery. There will characteristically be an elevated serum osmolality (greater than 290 mOsm/l) and an elevated serum sodium (greater than 145 mmol/l) with a dilute urine (less than 150 mOsm/l). The treatment of DI is similar to that for hypernatremic dehydration. If the child is hypotensive, initial volume expansion is necessary using 20 ml/kg of normal saline. After the child has been intravascularly repleted, fluid replacement should be started to slowly lower the serum sodium by 0.5 to 1 mEq/hour. Rapid fluid shifts can cause water to move into brain cells, producing cerebral edema. If the diagnosis is strongly suspected, DDAVP in doses of 5–20 µg intranasally or 0.2 to 0.4 µg/kg subcutaneously may be used. DDAVP (desmopressin acetate) acts to promote tubular resorption of free water.

7. e   This child has the syndrome of inappropriate antidiuretic hormone (SIADH). There is excessive secretion of ADH, with normal or low plasma osmolality and a low serum sodium. The urine osmolality and sodium will be elevated. More than 50% of children with bacterial meningitis develop SIADH. Hypertonic saline is the treatment of choice for children with seizures or who are comatose secondary to hyponatremia. It should be given in doses of 3 ml/kg, which can be repeated. Phenytoin inhibits ADH release and may also be of help in the patient with seizures attributed to central nervous system causes of SIADH. Asymptomatic children may be treated with fluid restriction as long as the child is not hemodynamically compromised.

8. a   Children with rickets usually present with limb pain and swelling, bowed legs, seizures, failure to thrive, hypocalcemia, or as an incidental finding on radiographs. It is commonly seen in premature infants, children with malabsorption problems or renal disease (Fanconi's syndrome), or children who are not exposed to light. The characteristic radiographic findings include broadened, frayed metaphysis; fractures; and bowing of the weight-bearing legs. The characteristic laboratory findings include low or normal calcium, low phosphate, elevated alkaline phosphatase, and elevated parathyroid hormone. Because rickets may also be associated with Fanconi's syndrome, renal disease should also be investigated.

The treatment for rickets is vitamin D. Calcium supplementation may also be needed if serum calcium levels are low. Bucket-handle fractures are seen in abuse cases, and periosteal elevation is seen in syphilis.

9. c   Thyroid storm is very rare in children. It usually presents in a patient with a history of hyperthyroidism, with fever greater than 41°C with symptoms of acute hyperthyroidism. The initial treatment involves adrenergic blockade with propranolol. Iodide decreases thyroid hormone release, but it is only effective for 3–5 days. Propylthiouracil prevents release of thyroid hormone and inhibits the peripheral conversion of thyroxine (T_4) to tri-iodothyroine (T_3). In the acute situation the effects of propylthiouracil are minimal. Glucocorticoids are used in the acute situation. They may inhibit the release of thyroid hormone and decrease conversion of T_4 to T_3. Although lowering the body temperature is very important during a thyroid storm, the use of aspirin is contraindicated because it is a potential uncoupler of oxidative phosphorylation, which may increase the metabolic state.

CHAPTER 98

Metabolic Emergencies
(Inborn Errors of Metabolism)

RON L. KAPLAN, M.D.

QUESTIONS

The following case relates to Questions 1–4: A 1-year-old boy with a history of developmental delay and failure to thrive is brought to the ED because of progressive lethargy and decreased responsiveness. He has had episodic vomiting and decreased intake for several days, with no fevers or diarrhea. He has been hospitalized twice in the past for vomiting and dehydration. Both times he responded quickly to IV fluids.

1. Which of the following tests is most likely to determine the need for an immediate potentially life-saving treatment?

   a. Plasma ammonia
   b. Bedside glucose determination
   c. ABG analysis
   d. Serum sodium (Na)
   e. Serum potassium (K)

2. The following laboratory data are obtained: ammonia 496 µg/dl, blood glucose 64, pH 7.37, Na 143, K 5.1, BUN 3, Cr 0.3; urine dipstick is positive for ketones. What is the most likely diagnosis?

   a. Galactosemia
   b. Isovaleric acidemia
   c. Medium-chain acyl-CoA dehydrogenase (MCAD) deficiency
   d. Phenylketonuria (PKU)
   e. Ornithine transcarbamylase deficiency

3. Which of the following acute treatments is NOT indicated in this patient?

   a. IV arginine
   b. D10W ¼ NS at twice maintenance
   c. IV sodium bicarbonate
   d. IV sodium benzoate
   e. Enteral sodium phenylbutyrate

4. Results of which test are most likely to suggest the specific diagnosis?

   a. Liver biopsy
   b. State newborn screening tests
   c. Serum amino acids
   d. Urine organic acids
   e. Acylcarnitine profile

5. A 2-week-old infant presents with vomiting, diarrhea, poor feeding, and jaundice. Cataracts are noted on exam. Which of the following findings is likely?

   a. Increased anion gap metabolic acidosis
   b. Pronounced indirect hyperbilirubinemia
   c. Glucosuria
   d. Hemolysis on peripheral blood smear
   e. Negative test for urine reducing substances

The following case relates to questions 6 and 7: A 2-week-old infant is brought to the ED with a history of irritability for several hours, followed by rapid progression to unresponsiveness. He is hypotonic and obtunded. Temperature is 35.2°C rectally. Initial laboratory findings include neutropenia, hypoglycemia, and metabolic acidosis. A faint smell of sweaty socks is noted.

6. Which of the following treatments is most important to institute during the initial resuscitation?

   a. IV antibiotics
   b. Hemodialysis
   c. Enteral L-carnitine
   d. IV glycine
   e. IV arginine

7. Long-term management of this patient would include:

   a. Decreased dietary carbohydrate intake
   b. Oral thiamine supplementation
   c. Oral glycine
   d. A high protein diet
   e. Oral folic acid

ANSWERS

1. **b** This child has a history suggestive of an inborn error of metabolism. These patients may have failure to thrive and developmental delay. Symptoms are more likely to appear during times of stress or catabolism. Failure of a metabolic pathway results in the accumulation of toxic metabolites and depletion of cellular energy stores. Nonspecific symptoms (e.g., vomiting) may progress rapidly to obtundation and coma. Metabolic disorders may present with profound hypoglycemia, which may be fatal if not rapidly identified and treated.

2. **e** The combination of severe hyperammonemia with a low BUN suggests a defect in the urea cycle, which is responsible for the conversion of ammonia to urea. Patients with organic acidemias (e.g., isovaleric acidemia) may have a milder degree of hyperammonemia and would be expected to have significant acidosis. MCAD deficiency is a defect in fatty acid oxidation, which results in hypoketotic hypoglycemia; some degree of hyperammonemia may be seen as well. Hyperammonemia is not a feature of galactosemia, which is a disorder of carbohydrate metabolism, or PKU, which is a disorder of amino acid metabolism.

3. **c** Treatment involves delivering glucose to provide an energy source and turn off the catabolic state, and enhancing the elimination of toxic metabolites. Arginine, sodium benzoate, and sodium phenylbutyrate treat hyperammonemia by favoring the production of metabolites that are excreted in the urine. Sodium bicarbonate treatment is indicated only for severe metabolic acidosis.

4. **c** Urea cycle defects may be identified by the serum amino acid profile. Liver biopsy will identify glycogen storage diseases. Newborn tests screen for galactosemia. Urine organic acids are abnormal in the organic acidurias, and carnitine profiles may be abnormal in errors of fat metabolism.

5. **d** Gastrointestinal symptoms, failure to thrive, jaundice, and cataracts are findings associated with galactosemia. Galactosemia results in failure of conversion of dietary galactose to glucose and hypoglycemia. This results in the presence of reducing substances in the urine in the absence of glucosuria. A hyperchloremic acidosis may be seen secondary to renal tubular dysfunction. The hyperbilirubinemia may initially be indirect, but a significant direct hyperbilirubinemia is characteristic after a week or two. Hemolysis may be a prominent finding, particularly in newborns.

6. **a** Although this infant may have a metabolic disorder, this presentation is consistent with sepsis and must be treated as such until proven otherwise. Hemodialysis may be indicated in some inborn errors of metabolism to remove toxic metabolites. Carnitine supplementation is often included in the long-term treatment of some metabolic diseases. Glycine is an adjunctive therapy for isovaleric acidemia that favors the excretion of toxic metabolites. Arginine facilitates the treatment of hyperammonemia associated with some urea cycle defects.

7. **c** The smell of sweaty socks is associated with isovaleric acidemia. Glycine therapy may significantly reduce the level of isovaleric acid in these patients. Because this is a disorder of protein metabolism, a low protein diet is indicated and modification of dietary carbohydrate would not be expected to have an effect. Thiamine is used in the treatment of maple syrup urine disease and folic acid in the treatment of methylmalonic aciduria.

CHAPTER 99

Dermatology

MICHELE M. BURNS, M.D.

QUESTIONS

The following case relates to questions 1 and 2:

1. A mother brings her 10-month-old girl in to the ED for a "bad rash." She had been told in the past that her child has atopic dermatitis. Physical exam findings consistent with this disorder include all of the following, EXCEPT:

   a. Scaling scalp
   b. Pityriasis alba
   c. Coin-shaped, scaling plaques
   d. Follicular accentuation
   e. Hyperlinear palms and soles

2. Your diagnosis for the patient in the preceding question is supported by:

   a. Increased IgE levels
   b. Cell-mediated reactions to antigenic material
   c. Cultures positive for *Candida albicans*
   d. Alterations in the ratio of surface fat levels
   e. A positive Tzanck test

The following case relates to questions 3 and 4:

3. An 8-year-old male comes to the ED with scaling lesions on the scalp. Irregular, scattered areas of alopecia are present. This patient's problem is most likely due to:

   a. Seborrheic dermatitis
   b. *Microsporum audouini*
   c. Pediculosis capitis
   d. *Rhus* dermatitis
   e. *Trichophyton tonsurans*

4. Your diagnosis is supported by:

   a. History of contact with shrubs and vines
   b. Culture of the lesions
   c. Fluorescence under Wood's lamp
   d. Visualization under a magnifying lens
   e. A positive family history

5. A 10-year-old boy comes to the ED with a coin-shaped lesion of the right wrist. Diagnoses to be considered include all of the following, EXCEPT:

   a. Tinea corporis
   b. Nummular eczema
   c. Xerosis
   d. Pityriasis rosea
   e. Contact dermatitis

6. You are sending a 2-year-old child home with amoxicillin to treat his first ear infection. The father asks you what drug reactions could occur. Which of the following is most likely?

   a. Urticaria
   b. Maculopapular eruptions
   c. Target lesions
   d. Erythema with satellite lesions
   e. Tender, erythematous nodules

The following case relates to Questions 7 and 8:

7. A mother brings in her 6-month-old infant with a confluent, erythematous diaper rash. She states that the rash has been present for 2 months, despite putting over-the-counter diaper creams on it and changing the diapers frequently. The older sibling had a similar diaper rash when he was an infant. Your diagnosis is:

   a. Seborrheic dermatitis
   b. Moniliasis
   c. Atopic dermatitis
   d. Occlusion dermatitis
   e. Secondary infection with *S. aureus*

8. Treatment for this child's diaper rash would include:

   a. Oral cephalexin
   b. Topical mupirocin
   c. Topical nystatin
   d. Avoidance of tightly fitting diapers
   e. Low-potency topical steroids

The following case relates to Questions 9 and 10:

9. A 4-year-old child is brought in to the ED by her mother with concerns of a severe sunburn. The child is febrile and irritable. On exam, there is generalized, tender erythema, with areas of sloughing when pressure is applied. Your diagnosis is:

    a. First-degree burn
    b. Stevens-Johnson syndrome
    c. Toxic epidermal necrolysis (TEN)
    d. Staphylococcal scalded skin syndrome (SSSS)
    e. Fixed drug eruption

10. Treatment for this patient includes all of the following, EXCEPT:

    a. Steroid therapy
    b. Antibiotic therapy
    c. IV fluids to maintain hydration
    d. Electrolyte monitoring
    e. Burn management of extensive denuded skin

11. A 12-year-old boy returns from camp and comes to the ED with linear lesions on his lower extremities. The lesions consist of papulovesicles and are pruritic. All of the following statements about this condition are true, EXCEPT:

    a. The child should be bathed as soon as possible
    b. All contaminated clothing should be laundered
    c. Lesions will continue to spread from vesicular fluid
    d. Calamine lotion and antihistamines are useful for pruritus
    e. Topical steroids are minimally effective

12. A 15-year-old girl comes to the ED with brown, scaling macular lesions on her upper trunk. She thinks she may have had a reaction in sunlight when she applied perfume there. Your diagnosis is:

    a. Tinea corporis
    b. Tinea pedis
    c. Tinea capitis
    d. Tinea cruris
    e. Tinea versicolor

13. All of the following statements regarding bites and infestations in childhood are true, EXCEPT:

    a. Mosquitoes are the most common cause of insect bites in childhood
    b. The major type of louse infection in children is the body louse
    c. Systemic illness after a tick bite can include Rocky Mountain spotted fever (RMSF), tick paralysis, and Lyme disease
    d. The brown recluse spider produces most skin reactions caused by the bite of a spider
    e. Once a scabies infestation occurs, it takes approximately 1 month for sensitization and pruritus to develop

14. A 5-year-old boy comes to the ED with urticaria. You tell his father that the lesions can be caused by all of the following factors, EXCEPT:

    a. Cholinergic stimulation
    b. Solar exposure
    c. Dermographism
    d. Xerosis
    e. Parasite infection

The following case relates to Questions 15 and 16:

15. A 5-year-old girl is brought to the ED with a lesion on her right hand. This lesion is a round papule with a white center that is umbilicated. Your diagnosis is:

    a. Cold panniculitis
    b. Verruca plana
    c. Molluscum contagiosum
    d. Pyogenic granuloma
    e. Verruca vulgaris

16. The etiology of the lesion described in Question 15 is:

    a. Human papilloma virus (HPV)
    b. Previous trauma at site of lesion
    c. Cold injury to fat
    d. Poxvirus
    e. Drug exposure

17. Physical exam findings in a patient with congenital herpes simplex virus (HSV) infection could include all of the following, EXCEPT:

    a. Hypothermia
    b. Fever
    c. Poor feeding
    d. Congenital heart disease
    e. Vesicular lesions

18. The differential diagnosis for congenital HSV infection includes all of the following, EXCEPT:

    a. Bullous impetigo
    b. Toxic epidermal necrolysis (TEN)
    c. Congenital syphilis
    d. Neonatal pustulomelanosis
    e. Cytomegalovirus (CMV) infection

19. A 2-week-old infant is brought to the ED because of "dark spots" in the facial area. All are possible diagnoses, EXCEPT:

    a. Addison's disease
    b. Nevus of Ota
    c. Peutz-Jeghers syndrome
    d. Benign juvenile melanoma
    e. Tuberous sclerosis

ANSWERS

1. c   Atopic dermatitis affects about 3% of children, with lesions typically beginning at 1–2 months of age. In infancy, the erythematous, exudative lesions appear on the cheeks and extensor surfaces, with the characteristic flexural involvement becoming prominent by age 2 years. Other symptoms include areas of hypopigmentation of the cheeks (pityriasis alba), a scaling scalp with or without hair loss, patchy or diffuse, fine papules (follicular accentuation), and hyperlinear palms and soles that may desquamate. Coin-shaped, scaling plaques are characteristic of the lesions seen in nummular eczema.

2. a   Patients with atopic dermatitis have immune system dysregulation that includes increased production of IgE by B cells. In addition, elevated prostaglandin E_2, abnormal lymphokine secretion profiles, and abnormalities of Langerhans cells are noted. Cell-mediated reaction to antigenic material would support the diagnosis of allergic contact dermatitis, which is a type IV delayed type of hypersensitivity. Lesions occur after 6–18 hours. Alterations in the ratio of surface fat levels are found in individuals with seborrheic dermatitis. Differentiation of atopic and seborrheic dermatitis may be difficult in infancy; seborrheic dermatitis usually will also have lesions in the intertriginous areas, the scaling lesions are often a greasy and yellow, and there often is a lack of pruritus. Both atopic and seborrheic dermatitis lesions can become secondarily infected, but a culture positive for *Candida albicans* or a positive Tzanck test for HSV would not help to differentiate various scaling lesions.

3. e   Tinea capitis is a common infection in school-aged children. *Microsporum* species caused the majority of infections in the past; *Trichophyton* species are more common today. The two different species have different clinical presentations. *Microsporum* species cause round patches of scaling alopecia that will fluoresce a blue-green color under a Wood's lamp. *Trichophyton* species, on the other hand, cause a scattered alopecia with indistinct margins. The lesions do not produce fluorescence. Seborrheic dermatitis presents with salmon-colored patches with yellow, greasy scales. These lesions are seen in infancy and then again in adolescence. In fact, scaling lesions seen in this age group are usually atopic dermatitis or tinea capitis. True seborrheic dandruff does not appear until puberty, secondary to excess sebum production. *Rhus* dermatitis is secondary to exposure to the most common allergen (i.e., poison ivy, oak, sumac) that is attributed to contact dermatitis. Lesions are typically present on exposed areas of the extremities, not just confined to the scalp. Pediculosis capitis would present with visualization of nits along the hair shaft. Alopecia is not seen.

4. b   The diagnosis of tinea capitis can be made with a positive KOH prep, but this will not distinguish the *Microsporum* species from the *Trichophyton* group. As noted above, only the *Microsporum* species will cause a blue-green fluorescence under a Wood's lamp. A positive family is seen in both atopic and seborrhea dermatitis. A hand-held magnifying lens can aid in the visualization of nits in those patients with pediculosis capitis. Nits present 15 cm from the scalp indicate an infestation that is 9 months old. A history of exposure to shrubs and vines would lead the physician to consider the diagnosis of *Rhus* dermatitis.

5. c   The differential diagnosis for a coin-shaped lesion includes tinea corporis, nummular eczema, pityriasis rosea, contact dermatitis, and granuloma annulare. Xerosis, or dry skin, appears as rough, red, scaling skin and looks similar to "chapped hands and cheeks." This condition is seen commonly in patients who bathe frequently, use harsh soaps, and live in climates with low humidity and temperatures. Tinea corporis lesions appear as scaly patches with areas of central clearing. These lesions are often confused with nummular eczema, which also presents with coin-shaped plaques. A KOH prep is important to obtain if the diagnosis is not certain. Pityriasis rosea is an exanthematous, red-scaling eruption with oval, slightly raised scales that follow the lines of cleavage in a "Christmas tree" distribution. In 80% of children, a Herald's patch precedes the eruption; this large, oval solitary lesion is usually on the trunk. The etiology is unknown, although drug eruptions and viral infections have been implicated. When pityriasis rosea appears in adolescence, serologies should be obtained to rule out secondary syphilis. Granuloma annulare appears as papules or nodules that are grouped in a ringlike distribution. These patients may be at risk for developing diabetes mellitus. A wristwatch on the back of the wrist could produce a coin-shaped area of erythema. Nickel-containing jewelry is often responsible for such lesions.

6. a   Drug reactions are any reactions in the skin when a child is taking a medication. Hospitalized patients are 30% more likely to have a reaction because of multiple exposures. Penicillins, sulfonamides,

and blood products are responsible for the majority of these reactions. Urticaria, or hives, is the most common expression of drug sensitivity, with lesions being seen within 1 week of drug exposure. Maculopapular eruptions are the second most common rash and present with symmetrical erythematous macules and papules with areas of confluence. Ampicillin often produces this type of reaction, particularly in patients with mononucleosis. Erythema multiforme is secondary to exposure to drugs (i.e., penicillins, sulfonamides, hydantoins, barbiturates) or infections. The classic target or iris lesion is seen. Last, erythema nodosum lesions appear as deep, tender, erythematous nodules of the extensor surfaces of the extremities. Although hypersensitivity to infections (i.e., streptococcal pharyngitis, TB, coccidioidomycosis, histoplasmosis), inflammatory bowel disease, sarcoidosis, and malignancies are common etiologies for erythema nodosum, drugs can cause this phenomenon. Erythema with satellite lesions is suggestive of a diaper dermatitis secondary to *Candida albicans.*

7. c   Diaper dermatitis is a common complaint seen by pediatricians. The different types include occlusion dermatitis, atopic dermatitis, seborrheic dermatitis, moniliasis, and a mixed, not diagnosable rash with possible secondary infection. Occlusion dermatitis presents with erythema, especially in areas where contact/friction with the diaper is greatest (inner thighs, lower abdomen, prominent surfaces of the genitalia, and buttocks). The rash often has a shiny, glazed appearance. Atopic dermatitis can be challenging to differentiate from occlusion dermatitis, but the chronicity and difficulty in treating the lesions can be clues to the correct diagnosis. There is often a family history of atopy, and physical exam may disclose lesions on the extensor surfaces in children less than 2 years of age and on the flexor surfaces in children more than 2 years of age. Seborrheic dermatitis will usually have salmon-colored patches with yellow, greasy scales. Moniliasis causes the most characteristic diaper rash—an area of confluent erythema that has a sharp border is seen, with satellite lesions extending beyond the demarcation edge. If the problem is chronic, seeding from the GI tract or from a mother with monilial vaginitis should be considered. There is often a mixture of the various categories that complicates making an accurate diagnosis. Secondary infection can occur. If blistering develops, secondary infection with *S. aureus* should be considered.

8. e   Treatment is dictated by the etiology of the diaper rash. Proper skin care, with decreased frequency of washing, use of mild soaps, and leaving the diaper off as much as possible will help, despite the etiology. Occlusion dermatitis can be avoided if tight-fitting diapers and, especially, plastic-covered paper diapers are avoided. Chronic exposure to moisture is known to be one of the major instigating factors in the development of diaper dermatitis. When atopic dermatitis is the diagnosis, topical steroids are necessary. High-potency or fluorinated steroids, however, cannot be used in the diaper area because the occlusion by the diaper enhances the steroid effect and is more likely to cause skin atrophy and striae. A low-potency topical steroid (e.g., 1% hydrocortisone) is therefore recommended. These low-potency topical steroids are useful in patients with seborrheic dermatitis as well. Topical nystatin is helpful for patients with monoliasis, and can be obtained in many over-the-counter remedies. Oral cephalexin would be indicated if blistering lesions suggestive of infection with *S. aureus* were visualized.

9. d   Generalized erythema can be due to numerous causes. Concerning diagnoses to consider would include toxic epidermal necrolysis (TEN), staphylococcal scaled skin syndrome (SSSS), and Stevens-Johnson syndrome. Although a sunburn or first-degree burn could also produce erythema, the child should not be febrile (fever is possible if secondary infection of blisters occurs later). Illness in SSSS is caused by circulating staphylococcal exotoxin. The children present with malaise, fever, and irritability. The "sunburn" (erythema) is very tender to touch. The skin will rub off with pressure (Nikolsky's sign). Skin biopsy reveals epidermal cleavage in the epidermal layer. SSSS is often confused with TEN, which also presents with tender erythema; however, TEN is much more common in the adult population. A history of medication use (i.e., antibiotics, barbiturates, hydantoins, sulfonamides) can often be obtained, although infections have also been implicated and many cases are thought to be idiopathic. Skin biopsy in TEN shows dermal-epidermal separation. Stevens-Johnson syndrome, or erythema multiforme major, will typically present with target lesions and extensive mucosal involvement; however, vesicular-bullous lesions can be seen in Stevens-Johnson syndrome. A fixed drug eruption produces a localized round dermatitis at the same location each time there is exposure to an offending drug. The lesions are erythematous but are not generalized over the body surface.

10. a   SSSS is usually a self-limiting disorder. Antibiotics may shorten the course of the disease. Neonates and children less than 1 year of age should be admitted to the hospital for IV antibiotics (e.g., cefazolin,

oxacillin) after blood cultures are obtained. If an older child appears toxic or has severe skin involvement, they, too, should be admitted. Older children can potentially be managed at home with oral antibiotics (e.g., cephalexin, dicloxacillin, erythromycin) if they are not toxic and have limited desquamation. Particularly when large areas of skin are involved, these patients are treated like burn patients; they are closely monitored for their hydration status, electrolyte imbalance, and they may need coverage of their skin with sterile dressings. Steroids clearly have no benefit in SSSS, and they may actually exacerbate the dermatitis by increasing the ability of the organism to proliferate and produce greater amounts of epidermolytic toxin. Steroids are probably not helpful in TEN or Stevens-Johnson syndrome, either. If used, they must be started within 2 days of the eruption to be effective, and should not be used after 5 days if the reaction is continuing to progress. In addition, if skin denudation is greater than 20% of the child's body surface area, steroid therapy should be avoided. Consultation with a pediatric dermatologist can be quite helpful.

11. c   The active ingredient in the urushiol oil is pentadecylcatechol. The average time to the appearance of the rash is 48 hours. Patients present with pruritus, inflammation, and grouped or linear papulovesicles or bullae. The eruption can last from 1 to 3 weeks. Avoidance of exposure is the best prophylaxis in treatment. Once exposure has occurred, the body should be bathed as soon as possible and all contaminated clothing removed and laundered. Once the oil has been removed, spread does not occur, even from vesicular fluid. Lesions that erupt later in time indicate exposure to a lesser dose of the offending oil initially. Calamine lotion and antihistamines can reduce pruritus. Topical steroids are minimally effective; with generalized reactions, systemic steroid therapy may be indicated.

12. e   Superficial fungal infections of the skin occur commonly, and are named based on the location of the principal site of infection. Tinea capitis occurs on the head, whereas tinea corporis can be found in multiple places on the body. Sites of predilection include the forearm and neck. Lesions of tinea corporis consist of sharply circumscribed scaly patches with areas of central clearing; there is no fluorescence under Wood's lamp. Tinea versicolor occurs primarily on the trunk and differs from tinea corporis in that lesions consist of brownish scales with areas of either hypopigmentation or hyperpigmentation. Wood's light examination shows yellowish-brown fluorescence, and KOH prep shows hyphae in the "spaghetti and meatballs" pattern. Treatment is with selenium sulfide shampoo over the entire body and topical antifungal agents for local areas of involvement. Tinea cruris, or "jock itch," occurs in males in the genitourinary region, whereas tinea pedis, or "athlete's foot," occurs on the feet. Tinea versicolor, tinea cruris, and tinea pedis are more common in warm, humid environments.

13. b   Mosquitoes are the most common cause of insect bites in childhood, followed closely by fleas. Although mosquito bites typically occur in warm months, flea bites happen year round because of pets living indoors. There is no specific treatment for insect bites, although antihistamines, calamine lotion, or topical steroids may have a limited effect. Prevention by using prophylactic insect repellant is the best way to avoid these lesions. There are three forms of lice that infest humans: the head louse (pediculosis capitis), the body louse (pediculosis corporis), and the pubic louse (pediculosis pubis). The major louse infestation in children involves the scalp. Treatment of both head and pubic louse consists of 1% permethrin (Nix), with nits being removed with a fine-toothed comb. Because the body louse resides in clothing, treatment is aimed at disinfecting clothing with steam under pressure. Ticks typically only produce local reactions. They should be removed with a pair of forceps, tweezers, or fingers protected with gloves, pulling upward with a steady even force. Systemic illness (e.g., Rocky Mountain spotted fever, tick paralysis, or Lyme disease) is possible after a tick bite. The spider responsible for most skin reactions is the brown recluse spider, or *Loxosceles reclusus*. This spider is known for its violin-shaped lesion on the dorsal cephalothorax. Its venom contains necrotizing, hemolytic, and spreading factors that are responsible for the hemorrhagic blisters that can progress into a gangrenous eschar. Treatment consists of oral steroids within 6–12 hours of the bite, antibiotics to prevent secondary infection, and possible surgical removal of the necrotic area. Finally, scabies infestations present with intense pruritus, with lesions typically concentrated on the hands, feet, and body folds (e.g., the finger webs). It usually takes 1 month from infestation until sensitization and pruritus develop. Treatment is with 5% permethrin (Elimite). Lindane is no longer recommended for the treatment of lice or scabies because it causes seizures (see Chapter 88: Toxicologic Emergencies, in *Textbook of Pediatric Emergency Medicine*, fourth edition).

14. d   Urticaria is frequently encountered in pediatrics, occurring in approximately 2–3% of children. No etiology is found in 90% of these children. Possible etiologies of urticaria include ingestion of drugs or foods (e.g., strawberries, nuts, eggs, shellfish) and infections (e.g., viral, bacterial, and parasites). There have also been physical factors (e.g., dermographism, cholinergic stimulation [heat, exercise, emotional tension], cold [acquired and familial], and solar exposure). Last, substances that cause degranulation of mast cells (e.g., radiocontrast material) can cause urticaria. Xerosis, or dry skin, is not a known cause. Lesions typically resolve after 24–48 hours. Acute urticaria is the term applied when the lesions last less than 6 weeks; chronic urticaria is defined as those that last more than 6 weeks.

15. c   Molluscum contagiosum presents as a papule with a white center that is often umbilicated. They can occur at any age, and are frequently seen in swimmers, wrestlers, and persons with atopic eczema. Lesions favor intertriginous areas. Removal of the white core will cure the lesion. Molluscum can be confused with verruca plana, or flat warts. These lesions are commonly seen on the face, arms, and knees but do not have a white, umbilicated center. Verruca vulgaris, or the common wart, resembles a tiny cauliflower. Cold panniculitis lesions appear as red, indurated nodules, and are often seen on the cheek after the infant holds an ice popsicle in their mouth. Pyogenic granulomas are bright red to brownish vascular nodules that are often pedunculated.

16. d   Molluscum contagiosum is caused by the common poxvirus, whereas warts are produced secondary to infection with human papilloma virus (HPV). Cold panniculitis is secondary to cold injury to fat. Pyogenic granulomas are vascular nodules that occur at the site of an injury (e.g., a cut, scratch, insect bite, or burn). Histology reveals proliferating capillaries in a loose stroma, and the lesions are seen often in children on the fingers, face, hands, and forearms. Drug exposure can lead to a fixed drug eruption, but the localized, round area of dermatitis is initially erythematous, and then resolves with a violet hue postinflammatory hyperpigmentation.

17. d   The risk of acquiring congenital herpes simplex virus (HSV) during pregnancy is small. If a primary infection occurs shortly before labor, however, neonatal HSV can occur in up to 50% of newborns. The incubation period is 2–30 days following exposure. Clinical manifestations are diverse, but more than 50% have cutaneous involvement consisting of grouped vesicles on erythematous bases. Constitutional symptoms include fever, irritability, poor feeding, hypothermia, and lethargy that can usually be attributed to encephalitis. Disseminated disease involving the liver and adrenal glands can be present as well. Treatment consist of intravenous acyclovir. Congenital heart disease is seen typically in congenital rubella.

18. b   The differential diagnosis of vesiculopustular lesions in the newborn include bullous impetigo, congenital cutaneous candiasis, congenital syphilis, neonatal pustulomelanosis, and cytomegalovirus (CMV) infection. Differentiation relies on Gram stains, KOH preps, serologic studies for syphilis, and cultures. Children with disease limited to the integument are often mistakenly treated for impetigo. TEN can be caused by infections but typically occurs in older patients and the lesions would not appear as vesicles with erythematous bases.

19. e   Hyperpigmented lesions can occur in several disease states. For example, Addison's disease can present with pigmentation lesions near the oral mucosa, gingivae, tongue, palate, and buccal mucosa. More commonly, the hyperpigmentation lesions are seen in the sites of intense flexures. The nevus of Ota affects the dermal pigment in the distribution of the ophthalmic branch of the fifth cranial nerve; the palate and sclera may be hyperpigmented as well. Peutz-Jeghers syndrome is an autosomal dominant familial polyposis characterized by frecklelike lesions of the lips, buccal mucosa, nose, finger, and subungual areas. Multiple hamartomatous polyps in the small intestine, large intestine, and stomach may lead to abdominal pain, melena, and intussusception. Single or multiple papules/nodules on the face or extremities of pediatric patients can be confused with malignant melanoma; hence, the name *benign juvenile melanoma*. Ninety percent of patients with tuberous sclerosis have a hypopigmented lesion known as the "ash-leaf" macule.

CHAPTER 100

Oncologic Emergencies

BEN WILLWERTH, M.D.

QUESTIONS

1. A 3-year-old boy with Down syndrome is brought to your ED because of fatigue, irritability, pallor, and a petechial rash. He has not had any fever, URI symptoms, vomiting, or diarrhea. On your exam, you find a pale, lethargic boy with diffuse lymphadenopathy and hepatosplenomegaly. The test most likely to yield a definitive diagnosis is:

   a. Echocardiogram
   b. Liver biopsy
   c. Blood culture
   d. Lymph node biopsy
   e. Bone marrow biopsy

2. A child who is diagnosed with acute lymphoblastic leukemia (ALL) currently has an approximate 75% long-term survival rate. Of the complications of ALL noted, the highest mortality is associated with:

   a. Infection
   b. Tumor lysis syndrome
   c. Hemorrhage
   d. Thrombosis
   e. Heart failure

3. A 4-year-old girl with neurofibromatosis comes to your ED with fever, lethargy, and bone pain. You note splenomegaly on physical exam. Her laboratory studies are: WBC count of 150,000/mm³, with 65% blasts; Na 137 mEq/l; K 6.0 mEq/l; Cl_3 110 mEq/l; bicarbonate 18 mEq/l; BUN 12 mg/dl; Cr 0.6 mg/dl; Ca 7.5 mEq/l; Mg 2.1 mEq/l; Ph 7.1 mEq/l; and uric acid 8.0 mg/dl. Your plan includes:

   a. Furosemide
   b. Immediate chemotherapy
   c. Alkalinization and allopurinol
   d. Plasmapheresis
   e. Exchange transfusion

4. A 10-year-old boy with Wiskott-Aldrich syndrome comes to the ED because of swelling in his neck. The swelling began 1 week ago and seems to be enlarging. He denies fever, fatigue, or night sweats. He denies exposure to cats. He is well appearing with a 3 × 4 cm unilateral firm, nontender cervical mass. You find no neck, axillary, or inguinal lymphadenopathy. A CBC and CXR are normal. You recommend:

   a. Outpatient monitoring
   b. Oral antibiotics
   c. IV antibiotics
   d. Lymph node biopsy
   e. Incision and drainage

5. An 8-year-old boy comes to the ED with a large neck mass and respiratory distress. The swelling began approximately 2 weeks ago, and has now worsened, despite taking cephalexin as prescribed. The boy's RR is 50, O_2 saturation is 90% after supplementation with 100% oxygen, HR is 100, and BP is 100/50. On exam, you note an ill-appearing boy in severe respiratory distress. You find a 4 × 5 cm firm, fixed, nontender, unilateral neck mass. An emergent CXR reveals an anterior mediastinal mass. You plan to:

   a. Intubate without medication
   b. Arrange for intubation in the operating room
   c. Intubate with a small dose of midazolam only
   d. Intubate using midazolam and fentanyl
   e. Intubate using midazolam, fentanyl, and succinylcholine

6. A 2-year-old girl comes to the ED because of status asthmaticus. On your routine physical exam, you note a large abdominal mass in an otherwise well-appearing girl with mild bilateral wheezing. You obtain a CBC, which demonstrates a normal WBC and platelet count and a hematocrit (hct) of 30. A urinalysis demonstrates a small amount of blood. A KUB is suggestive of a right-sided mass, but is otherwise normal. The most likely oncologic cause of this mass is a:

   a. Rhabdomyosarcoma
   b. Neuroblastoma
   c. Hepatoblastoma
   d. Burkitt's lymphoma
   e. Wilm's tumor

7. A 12-year-old boy comes to the ED because of unilateral leg pain, which is waking him at night. He remembers striking his leg against a table 2 weeks ago, but has not noticed any bruising of his leg. He denies constitutional symptoms. On exam, you find the middle of his tibia to be mildly swollen and tender. A radiograph of this region demonstrates periosteal elevation and lytic lesions, but no fracture. Your treatment plan is:

   a. Rest and pain control with ibuprofen
   b. Splint and follow up with orthopedics in 3–5 days
   c. Oncology consultation and bone culture/biopsy
   d. Short leg cast and repeat radiographs in 1 week
   e. Blood culture and oral antibiotics for 6 weeks

8. A 4-year-old girl is brought to your ED by ambulance. According to the paramedics, the girl has been complaining of headaches, vomiting, and gait problems over the past week, and today became lethargic. There is no history of trauma. On your exam, she is obtunded, has fair respiratory effort with normal breath sounds, and normal perfusion. She is afebrile. Her other vital signs are HR 60, RR 15, and BP 140/90. Her pupils are sluggishly reactive and equal. Her deep tendon reflexes are increased. She has an IV catheter placed. Your next action would be:

   a. Lumbar puncture
   b. Head CT scan
   c. Head MRI
   d. Endotracheal intubation
   e. Lower head of the bed

9. A 14-year-old boy is sent to the ED by his oncologist because of a fever. The boy's mother tells you that he has had a T of 38.7°C, rhinorrhea, and cough for 1 day. He has been active and taking fluids well. He is on maintenance chemotherapy for osteosarcoma, with his last administration of chemotherapy 2 weeks ago. His vital signs are currently T 38.6°C, HR 95, RR 20, and BP 120/70. He is well appearing. There are no localizing physical findings. The WBC is 4000, with 8% neutrophils on the differential. A urinalysis is normal. Blood and urine cultures are sent. A CXR shows normal aeration of the lungs. Your plan at this time includes:

   a. Cefuroxime PO
   b. IV cefuroxime
   c. IV ceftriaxone
   d. IV vancomycin and IV cefotaxime
   e. IV ceftazidime and IV gentamicin

10. A 7-year-old boy with acute myelogenous leukemia (AML) who is undergoing maintenance chemotherapy comes to the ED because of right-sided abdominal pain. The patient complains of several hours of waxing and waning right lower quadrant abdominal pain. He has vomited a few times, but had no bowel movements. He is unsure if he has been febrile. He denies dysuria or perirectal pain, and has been having normal bowel movements prior to today. He is currently afebrile. He is pale and quiet. His abdomen is firm with particular tenderness in the right lower quadrant. A CBC reveals a WBC of 2000, with 10% neutrophils. A urinalysis is normal. A KUB suggests an ileus, and an abdominal CT reveals a thickened cecal wall. The most appropriate management of this patient at this time is:

    a. Air contrast enema
    b. Fleet's enema
    c. Inpatient observation
    d. Broad-spectrum antibiotics
    e. Emergency laparotomy

11. A 6-year-old girl with a history of neuroblastoma comes to your ED complaining of low back pain and a right leg weakness and numbness. She has no other pain. She has developed urinary retention and bowel incontinence today. On exam, she has tenderness over her lower lumbar spine that is exacerbated with flexion of her back. Her rectal tone is diminished. She has weakness and numbness of her right lower extremity. Your next step is:

    a. Discharge with ibuprofen (Motrin)
    b. Plain radiographs of the back
    c. CT of the back and spine
    d. Steroid administration
    e. Radiation therapy

12. You are treating a 5-year-old boy who is undergoing maintenance chemotherapy for acute lymphoblastic leukemia (ALL). He is complaining of malaise, coryza, and a vesicular rash. He is well appearing and afebrile, with 10 vesicles scattered over his trunk. His CBC, liver function tests, and creatinine level are normal. Your management includes:

   a. Discharge and follow-up with his oncologist the following day
   b. Administration of varicella-zoster immune globulin (VZIG) and follow-up with his oncologist the following day
   c. Oral acyclovir and follow-up with his oncologist the following day
   d. Single dose IV acyclovir, with subsequent oral acyclovir and follow-up
   e. Admission and IV acyclovir each 8 hours (q8h)

ANSWERS

1. e   A bone marrow aspirate or biopsy demonstrating a hypercellular marrow with a monotonous population of blasts makes the diagnosis of leukemia. Detailed diagnosis and treatment is based on karyotyping, immunophenotyping of surface markers, and histochemical stains. Other than fatigue and hepatosplenomegaly, this child's presentation is inconsistent with heart failure; thus, echocardiography is not indicated in this scenario. Performing a blood culture in this child with fatigue, irritability, and a petechial rash is reasonable, but the lack of a fever and presence of lymphadenopathy suggest a different process. Lymph node biopsy may be appropriate for diagnosis of other malignancies (e.g., lymphoma), but it is not diagnostic of leukemia.

2. a   Infection remains the leading cause of death in children with acute leukemia because these patients nearly always have quantitative and qualitative cellular immune dysfunction at the time of diagnosis. Blood and urine cultures, as well as a CXR, should be obtained and broad-spectrum IV antibiotics should be started in a patient presenting with a fever and a new diagnosis of leukemia. Hemorrhage is the second most common cause of death in children with leukemia, because severe thrombocytopenia, infection with disseminated intravascular coagulation, or consumptive coagulopathy in some forms of leukemia can all compromise the clotting system. Tumor lysis syndrome leading to hyperkalemia, thrombosis from initial leukocytosis or L-aspariginase treatment, or heart failure from long-term use of adriamycin all have significantly lower levels of mortality.

3. c   Tumor lysis syndrome refers to the release of potassium, phosphates, and nucleic acids into the circulation as a result of the lysis of massive numbers of tumor cells. Leukemia or, less commonly, lymphoma patients may present with this syndrome, although it usually occurs after the initiation of antineoplastic therapy. IV hydration, alkalinization, and initiation of allopurinol therapy helps prevent tumor lysis syndrome from developing, although it may still occur despite this appropriate therapy. Furosemide may temporarily lower the serum potassium, but it would not address the underlying problem in this scenario. Immediate initiation of chemotherapy without initiation of IV hydration, alkalinization, and allopurinol increases the risk of tumor lysis syndrome. Although this patient has a marked leukocytosis, it is not significant enough to warrant plasmapheresis or exchange transfusion.

4. d   Children with inherited immunodeficiency states (e.g., Wiskott-Aldrich syndrome, severe combined immunodeficiency, and X-linked hypogammaglobulinemia) have a markedly increased risk of non-Hodgkin's lymphoma (NHL). Thus, a high degree of suspicion must be maintained in these patients, and early biopsy of an enlarging cervical mass is indicated in this child. NHL presents as localized disease (e.g., cervical or inguinal lymphadenopathy, nasopharyngeal masses, mediastinal masses, or bone pain) in 25% of childhood patients.

5. b Children with respiratory distress from an anterior mediastinal mass must be treated with extreme caution. Sedation of these children can lead to hemodynamic compromise secondary to compression of great vessels by the mass. Thus, a child with an anterior mediastinal mass who requires intubation should have this done in the most controlled setting possible (i.e., the operating room).

6. e This child is most likely to have a Wilm's tumor. Wilm's tumor is the fourth most common malignancy in children less than 5 years old. Seventy percent of patients with Wilm's tumor have an abdominal mass discovered incidentally. The mass is usually deep in the flank. Twenty-five percent of patients with Wilm's tumor have hematuria. Neuroblastoma, which can also present with an abdominal mass, is the most common solid tumor in childhood. Children with neuroblastoma usually have other symptoms at presentation, including irritability, anorexia, weight loss, pallor, and/or bone pain. Neuroblastoma does not cause hematuria, and often causes calcifications that can be seen on plain radiographs (both not present in this vignette). Rhabdomyosarcoma, Burkitt's lymphoma, and hepatoblastoma are much less common malignancies in childhood.

7. c This child's clinical presentation is consistent with a bone tumor (e.g., osteogenic sarcoma or Ewing's sarcoma) or osteomyelitis. Children with malignant bone tumors usually complain of pain or a painful lump, but they are usually otherwise asymptomatic. As in this case, a recent traumatic event is often identified and the pain is often worse at night. Because of this patient's symptoms, physical findings, and radiographs, further investigation for oncologic disease (oncologic consultation and subsequent bone biopsy) and osteomyelitis (bone culture) is warranted. More conservative treatments are not appropriate in this scenario.

8. d This child is demonstrating signs of increased intracranial pressure (ICP), including obtundation, bradycardia, and hypertension secondary to a brain tumor, and should be treated aggressively to reduce her ICP. Intubation with mild hyperventilation (aiming for a P_{CO_2} of 30–35) is indicated in this scenario. Dexamethasone should be given, and mannitol may be used in some cases of increased ICP. Lumbar puncture should not be performed in a patient in whom increased ICP is suspected, because brain herniation could result. Brain CT or MRI would help to identify this child's tumor, but they would be performed after stabilization of the child. Raising, not lowering, the child's head may help reduce ICP. Although children with brain tumors will usually present with more subtle signs (e.g., personality changes, headache, lethargy, vomiting, or ataxia), obtundation and increased ICP may be the presenting signs of a brain tumor.

9. e Infection remains a leading cause of morbidity and mortality in cancer patients; thus, febrile illnesses in these children must be taken very seriously. Initial workup should include sampling of the blood and urine, and a CXR should be obtained if respiratory symptoms exist. Treatment is dependent on the presence or absence of neutropenia, which is defined as an absolute neutrophil count (ANC) of less than 500. The ANC can be determine be multiplying the total WBC by the percentage of neutrophils, in this case $4000 \times 0.08 = 320$. Because the ANC is less than 500 in this case, this patient should be admitted for empiric broad-spectrum IV antibiotics. Gram-positive and gram-negative organisms (including *Pseudomonas*) must be treated; thus, piperacillin/tazobactam or ceftazadime must be among the antibiotics chosen.

10. d This child's presentation is consistent with typhlitis, which is a necrotizing colitis of the cecum seen most commonly in patients with AML who are neutropenic. Treatment consists of broad-spectrum antibiotics, serial abdominal exams (watching for perforation), and no oral intake (NPO). The clinical presentation of typhlitis is similar to that of appendicitis, with fever, right lower quadrant abdominal pain, and tenderness of the abdomen with palpation. This symptomatology, in combination with radiographic studies that show a thickened cecal wall or air in the cecal wall, makes the diagnosis. Despite appropriate treatment with broad-spectrum antibiotics, there is a high mortality rate with this disease. Air contrast or Fleet's enemas would be appropriate if concern of intussusception or constipation were present, but the clinical and radiographic findings are inconsistent with these illnesses. Exploratory laparotomy is unnecessary in this scenario because the diagnosis has been established.

11. d This scenario is highly suggestive of spinal cord compression secondary to metastatic oncologic disease. Thus, high-dose steroid administration, MRI of the spine, and neurologic and/or neurosurgical consultation should be done emergently. Immediate infusion of steroids may be critical in preserving

neurologic function and should be one's initial therapy. Surgery, radiation therapy, or chemotherapy may be indicated depending on the clinical scenario.

12. e   Varicella-zoster virus is currently the most common cause of death for patients with ALL in remission. These patients are high risk for serious disseminated infection because of their altered cell-mediated immunity. Thus, oral therapy is inadequate for this patient, and he should be admitted for admitted for IV acyclovir therapy. Immunoglobulin for varicella-zoster virus (VZIG) should be given to immunocompromised patients without a history of previous varicella or documented titers to varicella as soon as possible after an exposure to varicella. VZIG is not helpful, however, once active disease is present.

CHAPTER 101

Rheumatologic Emergencies

BARBARA WALSH, M.D.

QUESTIONS

1. A 4-year-old girl comes to the ED with high spiking fevers for a few weeks now. She has been seen by other doctors in the past 2 weeks and has had blood work and a bone marrow study reported as unremarkable. On exam the patient has a temperature (T) of 39.4°C. You note an erythematous macular rash on her trunk, as well as joint inflammation in the knees, ankles, and wrists. She has diffuse lymphadenopathy. Which of the following additional findings is most likely in this patient?

   a. Leukopenia
   b. Hepatosplenomegaly
   c. Positive antinuclear antibody (ANA)
   d. Positive rheumatoid factor
   e. Nonpurulent conjunctivitis

2. A 5-year-old boy comes to the ED with swollen ankles for several months. He has no history of tick bites, fever, or trauma. He has been stiff and limping. His mother tried giving him ibuprofen for a short while, with transient improvement. Which diagnostic test is most likely to make the diagnosis?

   a. ANA
   b. Erythrocyte sedimentation rate (ESR)
   c. C-reactive protein (CRP)
   d. Rheumatoid factor
   e. None of the above

3. A patient has been taking hydroxychloroquine for the treatment of refractory juvenile rheumatoid arthritis (JRA). The patient accidentally took too many pills over the past 2 weeks and comes to the ED for concern of toxicity. The organ system to be most at risk for toxicity is the:

   a. Eye
   b. Liver
   c. Kidney
   d. Bone marrow
   e. Lungs

4. A 5-year-old female with JRA comes to the ED with fever for 3 days. She has a cough and rhinorrhea as well as a sore throat. On physical examination she has an exudative pharyngitis. Her knees are tender, with limited range of motion (ROM). There is no overlying erythema and both joints may be moved about 5–10 degrees with some discomfort. Swelling of the joint is prominent. Her only medication is naproxen. Her WBC is 6800 with a normal differential. Rapid group A strep test is positive. What is the most appropriate management at this time?

   a. Arthrocentesis for cell count and culture
   b. Amoxicillin and prednisone PO
   c. Ceftriaxone and sulfasalazine
   d. Pulse dose steroids and IV cefotaxime
   e. Amoxicillin PO alone

5. A 15-year-old girl with JRA comes to the ED with fever and chest pain. She has been sick for 1 week. Her temperature is 39°C, HR 120, BP 110/65, and RR 24, with an O_2 saturation of 100%. You note a friction rub on cardiac auscultation. An ECG reveals diffuse ST segment elevations. A CXR shows a normal heart size. The best management of this patient would be:

   a. IV pulse Solu-Medrol
   b. Prednisone PO
   c. Naproxen PO
   d. Pericardiocentesis
   e. No further treatment

6. A 12-year-old girl with known JRA comes to the ED with cough and dyspnea. She also complains of joint swelling in both of her knees and right ankle. All the symptoms occurred simultaneously. She is febrile to 38.7°C, HR 92, RR 28, and BP 112/72. O₂ saturation is 94% on room air. She has decreased breath sounds at her lung bases but no crackles. CXR shows small bilateral pleural effusions. The best management option for this patient would be which of the following?

   a. Prednisone and amoxicillin PO
   b. IV solumedrol
   c. Ibuprofen and amoxicillin PO
   d. Ibuprofen PO alone
   e. Methotrexate and sulfasalazine

7. A 14-year-old boy with JRA comes to the ED with sudden onset of bilateral eye pain, photophobia, tearing, and redness. Which of the following tests is most likely to be abnormal?

   a. Fundoscopic exam
   b. Visual field testing
   c. Slit lamp exam
   d. Fluoroscein exam
   e. Ocular tenometry

8. A 19-year-old girl with arthritis comes to the ED with fever and dysuria. She takes naproxen and methotrexate for her arthritis. Her urine shows 20–50 WBCs/hpf. Which medication would be contraindicated in treating this patient?

   a. Cefixime
   b. Amoxicillin
   c. Cephalexin
   d. Trimethoprim-sulfamethoxazole
   e. Ciprofloxacin

9. A 4-year-old boy with chronic arthritis on multiple medications comes to the ED with a diffuse erythematous rash. He is febrile to 38.9°C with RR 24 and BP 110/70. The rash is papular, with central clearing and surrounding erythema. He has been scratching at the lesions. He is miserable and refusing to drink. The drug most likely to cause this reaction is:

   a. Methotrexate
   b. Gold injections
   c. Sulfasalazine
   d. Penicillamine
   e. Plaquenil

10. A 16-year-old girl with SLE on prednisone 60 mg PO every day (qd) and naproxen for arthritis and lupus nephritis comes to the ED with cough, fever, and tachypnea. She appears dehydrated. Vital signs are: T 39°C, HR 116, RR 32, and BP 105/64. O₂ saturation is 95% on room air. She has rales in her left lower chest posteriorly. A blood culture is sent. The best treatment for this patient is:

    a. Oral prednisone 60 mg b.i.d. and oral clindamycin
    b. Oral prednisone 60 mg b.i.d. and oral augmentin
    c. Oral prednisone 60 mg b.i.d. and IV penicillin
    d. Oral prednisone 60 mg t.i.d. and IV cefotaxime
    e. Oral prednisone 60 mg t.i.d. and IV vancomycin

11. A 13-year-old girl with known SLE comes to the ED with pallor. She has a T of 37.1°C, RR 32, HR 140, BP 108/72, and O₂ saturation is 100% on room air. She was well until two days ago. She has no other complaints. Her physical exam shows scleral icterus. Hematocrit (hct) is 18%. Reticulocyte count is 8.4%. Treatment should be started with:

    a. Transfusion of packed RBCs
    b. Ferrous sulfate
    c. Prednisone
    d. Exchange transfusion
    e. Erythropoietin

12. A 14-year-old girl comes to the ED with rash for 1 week. On exam she had diffuse petechiae and purpura. She has been taking methotrexate long term for SLE. She has otherwise been well. CBC shows WBC 1200, hct 22.8%, and platelet count of 24,000. Her smear is normal. Reticulocyte count is 0.5%. Her platelets appear small on peripheral smear. The most likely explanation for her rash is:

    a. Systemic vasculitis
    b. Idiopathic thrombocytopenic purpura (ITP)
    c. Bone marrow suppression
    d. Acute lymphoblastic leukemia (ALL)
    e. Coagulopathy

The following case applies to Questions 13 and 14.

13. A 22-month-old toddler comes to the ED with fever to 103°F (39°C) for 6 days. On exam he is febrile to 39.7°C and very irritable. You note conjunctival erythema without any purulent discharge. He also had red/cracked lips and a red tongue. He has a diffuse erythematous maculopapular rash on his trunk and extremities, and enlarged cervical adenopathy on the right. All of the following tests should be done, EXCEPT:

   a. ESR
   b. Throat culture
   c. Echocardiogram
   d. Blood culture
   e. ANA

14. The best treatment course for the patient in Question 13 would be:

   a. Penicillin
   b. Cephalexin
   c. IV immunoglobulin
   d. No treatment
   e. Prednisone

15. A mother brings her 2-year-old son to the ED for evaluation of fever and rash for 3 days. She is concerned that her child might have Kawasaki disease. Which of the following types of rash would be most inconsistent with this diagnosis?

   a. Papular
   b. Erythrodermal
   c. Macular
   d. Vesicular
   e. Urticarial

The following case applies to Questions 16 and 17.

16. A 10-year-old boy comes to the ED with acute onset of bilateral knee pain and swelling as well as fatigue. He denies any trauma. He is afebrile and has slightly swollen and tender knees on physical examination. The mother reports a large rash several weeks ago that was red and oval on his left leg. It went away on its own and was not bothersome to the patient. Which of the following tests would be most helpful?

   a. Blood culture
   b. ANA
   c. ESR
   d. Serology for *Borrelia burgdorferi*
   e. Rheumatoid factor

17. What would be the best management option for the patient in Question 16?

   a. Arthrocentesis
   b. Prednisone
   c. Ibuprophen
   d. Doxycycline
   e. Clindamycin

ANSWERS

1. **b**   In systemic-onset JRA a patient may present with a constellation of symptoms that resemble an infectious disease or malignancy. Thus, these two categories of illness must be explored. Hepatosplenomegaly is commonly seen in systemic-onset JRA, along with lymphadenopathy, rash, high fevers, and leukocytosis. It most often occurs in children less than 5 years of age. ANA and rheumatoid factor are negative in systemic-onset JRA.

2. **e**   Because there are no laboratory abnormalities specifically characteristic of JRA, the diagnosis is based on clinical grounds. Patients under 16 years of age should have chronic arthritis in one or more joints lasting over 6 weeks as well as exclusion of other diseases associated with chronic synovitis. ESR and CRP may be helpful, but in many patients with JRA they may be normal or only mildly elevated. The ESR is usually increased with the number of inflamed joints. The hematocrit is usually low from anemia of chronic disease, iron deficiency, or both, but certainly will not make the diagnosis. ANA is helpful only if it is a criteria used for looking at risk factors or in a patient where you are considering the diagnosis of SLE. Rheumatoid factor is unique to a subgroup of polyarticular JRA; however, this subgroup accounts for only 15% of cases overall and is usually associated with severe arthritis in older girls.

3. **a**   The eye is the organ system that is affected the most when doses of hydroxychloroquine exceed 7 mg/kg/day. The usual manifestations are macular degeneration and corneal deposition.

4. b This patient is presenting to the ED with strep throat and otitis media. The bacterial infection has likely triggered a mild flare of her arthritis, which is very common. Thus, treating the underlying infection and the flare simultaneously with antibiotics and steroids is the best treatment. This can be done as an outpatient. Sulfasalazine is a longer-acting medication that will not help in the acute setting. This patient has a normal WBC and her differential is unremarkable, which is reassuring. Arthrocentesis should be performed only when there is concern for a septic joint. In a patient with a septic joint there is pronounced limitation of the ROM, with severe muscle spasm and pain with the slightest movement; however, in JRA the joint can usually be moved 5–10 degrees even if the inflammation is severe. In addition, in a septic joint there is usually overlying erythema. This is rare in a joint flare.

5. c This patient has pericarditis. Her case appears to be mild in that her vital signs are stable and she has no evidence of pericardial effusion. Even in mild cases, however, it is still recommended that patients be admitted for close observation, NSAID/salicylate therapy, and bed rest. In more severe cases where there is evidence of massive pericardial fluid accumulation or a smaller effusion that does not respond to salicylates/NSAIDs, corticosteroids should be started. Other than the tests mentioned, an echocardiogram should also be done to assess ventricular function and pericardial fluid accumulation.

6. b This patient is most likely experiencing a flare of her systemic disease with both arthritis and pleural effusion, both of which are very common. The treatment of choice would be admission and IV steroids to control the systemic inflammation and monitor the pleural effusion. Antiobiotics would be necessary only if there were concern for infection. The patient described in this scenario has had ongoing inflammation and is unlikely to have an infection as well. Methotrexate and sulfasalazine would not be the best treatment option in the acute care setting.

7. c This patient is presenting with acute iridocyclitis. The appropriate way to diagnose this disease process is to identify cells in the anterior chamber using the slit lamp. Consultation with an ophthalmologist is essential when making this diagnosis. Treatment usually includes topical steroids and mydriatics.

8. d This patient has a urinary tract infection (UTI). Most of the medications listed would be acceptable in treating the UTI except Bactrim (trimethoprim-sulfamethoxazole) because of the concurrent use of methotrexate. Bactrim and methotrexate use together will increase the risk of bone marrow suppresion with pancytopenia and thus should be avoided.

9. c Sulfasalazine is associated with a variety of rashes, with Stevens-Johnson syndrome being potentially the most aggressive kind. Other rashes associated with this medication are photosensitivity eruptions and less severe types of hypersensitivity reactions.

10. d This patient is presenting with a focal pneumonia. Her underlying disease as well as the prednisone she takes makes her prone to opportunistic infections. Not all patients with SLE presenting with fever need be admitted to the hospital; however, patients who are acutely ill, those with absolute neutrophil counts below 1000, suspicion of meningitis, or pneumonia should be admitted and treated with broad-spectrum antibiotics. Because she has been on chronic steroids she also needs to be covered during the acute illness with stress-dose steroids which should be at least three times her physiologic dose.

11. c This patient is presenting with an acute autoimmune hemolytic anemia, which is a known complication of SLE. Prednisone is the initial treatment of choice. Transfusion should be reserved for cases of rapidly dropping hemoglobin concentrations or in those cases complicated by congestive heart failure. Erythropoietin would have no role in treatment.

12. c This patient has been on long-term methotrexate, which can cause significant bone marrow suppression. Her smear is normal; thus, she is unlikely to have acute leukemia, although a definitive test to rule out leukemia would be a bone marrow aspirate. ITP and systemic vasculitis would not give the low WBC. GI bleeding would give her symptoms of anemia but is unlikely to cause purpura and petechiae as her presenting symptoms.

13. e This patient is presenting with many features of Kawasaki disease. There is no gold standard test to make the diagnosis. The clinical criteria used to diagnose Kawasaki disease are: cervical lymphadenopathy, bilateral, nonexudative conjunctivitis with limbal sparing, cracked, red lips and a strawberry tongue, rash, which is polymorphous and never vesicular or bullous, and edema of the extremities or desquamation of the toes or fingertips. Laboratory studies can be helpful and support a diagnosis; how-

ever, an echocardiogram, if it shows coronary abnormalities, is the closest tool to support the diagnosis. A normal echocardiogram on the other hand, does not exclude the diagnosis of Kawasaki disease. All of the other tests except for the ANA would be done to exclude other etiologies. The ANA would not be helpful in this patient.

14. c   The treatment of choice is IV immunoglobulin. It has been shown to prevent and reduce the morbidity associated with coronary artery aneurysms.

15. d   The rash of Kawasaki disease is polymorphous and can appear in many different forms. A vesicular or bullous rash, however, is not typical and should prompt a search for another diagnosis.

16. d   This patient's presentation is very suspicious for Lyme disease. The study of choice would be serology for *Borrelia burgdorferi*. Many laboratories are becoming more experienced at running this test, especially in endemic areas.

17. d   In patients greater than 8 years of age, doxycycline is the treatment of choice. Amoxicillin is the second-line choice and should be used in patients less than 8 years of age. In cases of recurrent/persistent arthritis, or where there is evidence of carditis or meningitis/encephalitis, ceftriaxone would be the drug of choice.

CHAPTER **102**

Problems of the Very Early Neonate

JACQUELINE BRYNGIL, M.D.

QUESTIONS

1. You are called to the newborn nursery to assess tachypnea in a full-term infant 4 hours after a cesarean section birth. The child is vigorous. Vital signs at this time include T 37.2°C, HR 122, RR 72, BP 70/40, and room air O_2 saturation 97%. There is no cyanosis, and physical examination reveals clear lungs, regular heart rate with no murmur, and a normal abdominal examination. Your most appropriate next step in management would be:

    a. Full sepsis workup, including blood, urine, and CSF
    b. Stat cardiology consult
    c. Intubation
    d. CXR, continuous pulse oximetry, and re-evaluation
    e. None of the above

The following case applies to Questions 2 and 3: In evaluating a 7-day-old infant who comes to you for evaluation of "fussiness," you note a vesicular and pustular rash over the trunk.

2. Your initial step in confirming your diagnosis would be:

    a. Skin biopsy
    b. Referral to dermatology
    c. Culture of the lesion
    d. Application of potassium hydroxide (KOH) to a slide specimen
    e. Peripheral smear for eosinophilia

3. Your next step in the management of this patient would be:

    a. IV ceftriaxone
    b. IV acyclovir
    c. Topical corticosteroids
    d. Cephalexin PO
    e. Reassurance

4. You are evaluating a newborn during a well-child visit when you notice a bluish-black discoloration over the lumbosacral region. He has been feeding well and has no other symptoms. His physical examination is otherwise normal. Your most appropriate next step in the management of this patient is:

    a. CBC, including platelet count and PT/PTT
    b. Skeletal survey
    c. MRI of the spine
    d. Dermatology evaluation
    e. Reassurance

5. You evaluate a 3-day-old boy brought to the ED for a lump on his head. He is otherwise well appearing. He was born at home and was delivered by a midwife without any complications. He has done well at home and has been feeding well. The parents cannot recall any trauma. The swelling is unilateral, somewhat boggy, and approximately 4 × 4 cm in dimension. The suture lines are intact. Workup of this child should include:

    a. CT of the head
    b. Skeletal survey
    c. Bilirubin level
    d. Lumbar puncture
    e. Ophthalmology consult

6. A 7-day-old boy is referred to your ED for evaluation of weight loss. His birth weight was 6 pounds 7 ounces. On Day 2 of life, when he left the hospital, his weight was 6 pounds 6 ounces. He is taking 3–4 ounces of formula every 3 hours and is having normal stools and urine. His weight at this visit is 6 pounds 2 ounces. At this time, your management of this patient should be:

    a. Serum antigliaden antibody test
    b. Switch to 24 calorie-per-ounce formula
    c. Referral for sweat testing
    d. Stool test for eosinophils
    e. Reassurance and weight check in 1 week

7. You are called to evaluate a 4-hour-old infant in the newborn nursery. He is vigorous with a loud cry. His vital signs are T 37.6°C, HR 188, RR 32, and BP 74/palpable. You note that his hands and feet have a bluish discoloration. His pulse oximetry reading is 97% O_2 saturation on room air. The most likely finding on his physical examination would be:

   a. Bilateral rales
   b. Absent femoral pulses
   c. Hepatomegaly
   d. No change with supplemental oxygen
   e. A harsh pansystolic murmur

8. A 6-day-old girl is brought to your ED for evaluation of a "neck strain." She was born without difficulty and has been feeding well at home. On examination, you palpate a mass within the sternocleidomastoid muscle on the left. Her physical examination is otherwise normal. The most appropriate management of this infant would be:

   a. Cervical spine x-ray
   b. Ultrasound of the neck
   c. Karyotyping
   d. Passive stretching exercises
   e. CT of the neck

9. You evaluate a 1-month-old boy for a cough. The mother reports that he was treated for watery conjunctivitis at 10 days of age. Vital signs at the time of his visit reveal a T 37.8°C, HR 160, RR 64, and BP 80/palpable. You obtain a CBC, which shows WBC 14,800 with 55% granulocytes, 30% lymphocytes, 12% eosinophils, and 3% band forms. A CXR shows patchy interstitial infiltrates. Your most appropriate treatment of this patient consists of:

   a. IM ceftriaxone
   b. Discharge home on amoxicillin PO for 10 days
   c. Admission for IV ampicillin and gentamicin
   d. Discharge home on azithromycin PO for 5 days
   e. Admission for IV erythromycin

The following case applies to Questions 10 and 11: You are examining an infant in the ED who has had decreased feeding. On his skin you note several raised, red and blue lesions over his trunk and extremities. He is slightly tachycardic and tachypneic. He appears slightly pale. Stool for guaiac is hemoccult negative.

10. Your next step in the workup of this patient should be:

    a. Obtain a dermatology consult
    b. Perform a lumbar puncture
    c. Obtain a GI consult
    d. Obtain a CBC with platelet count
    e. Obtain a CXR

11. Another common finding on the physical examination of this patient would be:

    a. Cyanosis
    b. Weight below third percentile
    c. Hepatomegaly
    d. Hemiparesis
    e. Bulging fontanelle

12. A 6-day-old girl is referred to you for evaluation of an absent red reflex. The patient had a normal delivery and has been feeding well. Her physical examination is normal, except for an absent red reflex in the left eye. Your next appropriate course of management is:

    a. Referral to an ophthalmologist
    b. Admission for IV ampicillin and gentamicin
    c. Reassure the parents that this is normal
    d. CT of the head
    e. Prescribe erythromycin ophthalmic ointment

13. You are evaluating a 5-day-old girl in the ED who has been crying for the past 12 hours. She is afebrile and has been taking formula well. Evaluation of this patient should include all of the following EXCEPT:

    a. Fluorescein staining of the eyes
    b. Stool guaiac
    c. Skeletal survey
    d. Examination of fingers and toes
    e. Urinalysis

14. You are examining a 2-week-old boy and notice a cystic structure along the maxillary mucosa. The infant is otherwise well and the rest of his examination is normal. The cystic lesion is 1–2 mm in diameter, located towards the left of the maxillary mucosa. There are no other lesions. Your most likely diagnosis is:

    a. Epstein's pearl
    b. Dental lamina cyst
    c. Bohn's nodule
    d. Natal tooth
    e. Rhabdomyosarcoma

15. You are examining a 2-week-old girl brought in to the ED for breast enlargement. Upon examination, you notice that the left breast is erythematous and slightly indurated. Manipulation of her breast causes the expression of fluid from the nipple. She is afebrile. Your most appropriate next step is:

    a. Culture of the fluid
    b. Warm compresses and recheck in 1 day
    c. Cephalexin PO
    d. Admission for IV ampicillin
    e. Reassurance

16. A newborn is brought to you for evaluation of a rash. On examination, you notice a sacral hair tuft and dimple. On probing, there is an unclear terminus. The most appropriate next step in the evaluation of this newborn would be:

    a. CT scan
    b. Plain lumbosacral (LS) spine films
    c. MRI of the spine
    d. Lumbar puncture
    e. Reassurance

17. You are examining an infant in the ED with a complaint that he has not been moving his left arm. You notice that he has a "clawed" left hand, with fixed flexion of the left elbow. History of this patient is most likely to reveal:

    a. Child abuse
    b. Large-for-gestational-age infant
    c. Seizure disorder
    d. Abnormal bilateral upper extremity radiographs
    e. Cesarean birth

18. You are called to assess an infant at 12 hours of life who was noted to have a brief episode of "shaking." The infant is currently awake and alert. You order electrolytes, a CBC, and urinalysis. The most likely etiology of this child's activity is:

    a. Glucose of 80 mg/dl
    b. Calcium of 8 mg/dl
    c. Potassium of 6 mEq/l
    d. Sodium of 120 mEq/l
    e. Magnesium of 2 mEq/l

19. You are examining a lethargic infant in the ED and notice that he has a weak cry. When you lift him in a prone position you note that he cannot hold his head against gravity and his arms and legs hang down. Birth history reveals a full-term infant with no perinatal complications. Likely findings on further evaluation may include all of the following EXCEPT:

    a. Seizures
    b. Absence of deep tendon reflexes (DTRs)
    c. Poor suck
    d. Shallow respirations
    e. Sweet-smelling urine

20. You are evaluating a 3-day-old boy in the ED for diarrhea. He is being cared for by his new foster parents, who are unaware of his perinatal medical history. You observe that he appears irritable, jittery, and sweaty. You ask the foster mother to feed him, and you note that he feeds poorly. You feel that he also meets admission criteria for dehydration and decide to admit for IV fluid hydration. In addition to the management of dehydration you suggest all of the following, EXCEPT:

    a. Urine drug screen
    b. Social services consultation
    c. Swaddling of the infant
    d. Phenobarbital
    e. Sepsis evaluation

ANSWERS

1. d   Transient tachypnea of the newborn (TTN) is seen in term infants at 2–6 hours of life after Cesarean section and is generally believed to be secondary to a delay in the absorption of normal fetal lung fluid. Evaluation for this condition should include a chest x-ray, re-evaluation, and pulse oximetry. The condition usually resolves in 72 hours. Congestive heart failure in the newborn is accompanied by hepatomegaly. Sepsis should be considered if the child becomes ill appearing or develops temperature instability.

2. c   Neonatal herpes simplex virus (HSV) infections are associated with significant morbidity and mortality. Most are caused by HSV Type 2, acquired during delivery secondary to maternal genitourinary infection. A primary maternal infection at the time of delivery is associated with a 40–50% risk of transmission. Infants become symptomatic at 4–7 days of life and a vesicular or pustular rash may erupt at this time. Culture of the lesion for HSV is the gold standard for diagnosis. If the culture of the lesion is inconclusive, a dermatology consult should be obtained. Peripheral smear for eosinophilia and KOH preparations will be negative in a viral infection. Skin biopsy is not indicated in this patient.

3. b   Prompt management with IV acyclovir can improve the morbidity and mortality of this condition. Neonates suspected to have HSV infections should be admitted for IV acyclovir. Because this infection is viral, antibiotics and corticosteroid treatment are not indicated.

4. e   Mongolian spots are generally located in the lumbosacral region as well as on the buttocks and lower extremities in 80–90% of African-American children and some Caucasian and Asian-American chil-

dren. The spots typically fade after several years. Although child abuse must always be considered, a skeletal survey would not be indicated in an otherwise asymptomatic child, with no other evidence of nonaccidental trauma. Evaluation for coagulopathies, spina bifida occulta, or other dermatologic lesions are not necessary.

5. c Cephalohematomas occur because of normal vaginal birth trauma. They are primarily unilateral, and do not cross suture lines. Large cephalohematomas can be related to neonatal jaundice and anemia, and screening for these is recommended. Given a history of trauma, a CT scan and/or skeletal survey would be indicated. Ophthalmology should be consulted if there is suspicion of child abuse or if the child is ill appearing. A lumbar puncture would not be indicated in this child without other symptoms of sepsis.

6. e The normal newborn will lose about 5–10% of his birth weight during the first several days of life and regain this weight by 10–14 days of life. At this time, repeat weight checks are indicated. If weight loss is persistent, attempts should first be made to assure adequate caloric intake with a feeding diary and formula manipulation. If this is unsuccessful, then testing for milk allergy, malabsorption syndromes, and cystic fibrosis should be considered.

7. d Acrocyanosis, or cyanosis confined to the hands, feet, and sometimes the circumoral region, is a normal finding in otherwise healthy newborns. It does not improve with supplemental oxygen, and room air O_2 saturation is normal. Acrocyanosis is often caused by cool ambient temperature. The presence of bilateral rales, a pathologic murmur, hepatomegaly, and absent pulses all represent significant cardiac abnormalities, which are more likely to be associated with generalized cyanosis, hypoxia, and an otherwise ill-appearing child.

8. d Congenital muscular torticollis is a common birth-related finding. Treatment for this is passive stretching. In the presence of a low hairline, Klippel-Feil syndrome must be ruled out. X-rays of the cervical spine showing bony fusion would support this diagnosis. Karyotyping for conditions such as Turner's syndrome may be indicated if the neck is webbed. Ultrasound and CT of the neck are indicated if the condition fails to resolve with stretching exercises, or the mass lesion changes in size.

9. e *Chlamydia trachomatis* is the most frequently recovered pathogen in children with afebrile pneumonias between 4 and 12 weeks of age. In symptomatic patients, treatment consists of admission and administration of erythromycin at 40 mg/kg/day. Chlamydia is preceded by conjunctivitis in 50% of cases and is characterized by eosinophilia and interstitial infiltrates. The use of other antimicrobials is insufficient to treat *C. trachomatis*, and the patient's respiratory rate indicates he has mild respiratory distress; therefore, outpatient therapy would not be indicated.

10. d Kasabach-Merritt syndrome involves multiple rapidly enlarging hemangiomas with associated thrombocytopenia and a consumptive coagulopathy. Evaluation of a patient with multiple hemangiomas, pallor, tachycardia, and tachypnea should include a CBC and platelets. GI bleeds may cause symptoms of decreased volume; however, the stool was guaiac negative. Although CHF may also cause these symptoms, the presence of hemangiomas leads one away from that diagnosis. Sepsis should be considered if the patient looks ill and has temperature instability.

11. c In Kasabach-Merritt syndrome, intraparenchymal hemangiomas are not uncommon, and hepatomegaly is a common finding. Hemiparesis may be found with other vascular lesions (e.g., Sturge-Weber syndrome). In isolated feeding issues, failure to thrive (weight below third percentile) may be a finding as well. Cyanosis sometimes accompanies CHF; however, it is unlikely in Kasabach-Merritt syndrome.

12. a Failure to obtain a normal pupillary light reflex is never normal in a newborn and can represent several ophthalmologic conditions of varying severity (e.g., retinoblastoma, retinopathy of prematurity, cataracts, retinal detachment, and colobomas). Immediate referral to an ophthalmologist is indicated. A CT of the head is not indicated at this time and erythromycin ointment without the presence of infection would be an inappropriate choice. Likewise, IV antibiotics are not indicated.

13. c The crying infant poses many problems to the physician. The infant often shows no focal findings suggestive of a specific etiology. It is important to rule out common causes such as corneal abrasions, hair tourniquets, UTIs and GI issues, which may not be evident on a routine examination. An unlikely

cause in an otherwise asymptomatic infant would be child abuse, although a skeletal survey would be indicated if other signs suggestive of abuse were present.

14. b Dental lamina cysts are benign gingival cysts that most commonly occur along the maxillary and mandibular mucosa. Epstein's pearls are keratin-filled lesions found along the midline of the palate. Bohn's nodules are generally not solitary and form along the gums and palate. Natal teeth appear as teeth and are calcified. It is rare to find a rhabdomyosarcoma in a child of this age.

15. a Neonatal mastitis affects prepubertal children between 2 and 5 weeks of life, and culture of the fluid generally yields the pathogen. 90% of cases are due to *Staphylococcus aureus* and should be treated with IV oxacillin, or another appropriate parenteral antibiotic, after the culture is obtained. Outpatient management is not appropriate. Although gynecomastia is a common finding in neonates, the presence of redness and induration indicates infection.

16. c Presence of a sacral dimple with or without a hair tuft is suggestive of spina bifida occulta. If you cannot determine whether there is a sinus tract connecting to the intradural space, MRI and neurosurgical consultation are indicated. If the terminus of the dimple is visible, either no workup or plain LS spine films to look for vertebral anomalies would be appropriate. Lumbar puncture in the absence of suspected infection and CT scan of the area would be inappropriate choices.

17. b Congenital brachial plexus injuries mostly occur during birth trauma in vaginal deliveries of large-for-gestational-age infants. Injuries of the C8–T1 nerve roots result in damage to the muscles of the hand and a fixed flexion at the elbow (Klumpke's paralysis, or "claw-hand"). Injuries to C5–C6 result in shoulder adduction, elbow pronation, and wrist flexion (Erb's palsy, or "waiter's tip" posture). Abnormal bilateral radiographs may be indicative of TARR syndrome, with an absent radius. These findings are unlikely with cesarean births or strokes. Trauma postnatally is unlikely to give an isolated brachial plexus injury.

18. d With a serum sodium level of 120 mg/dl, hyponatremia is the most likely cause of seizures in this infant. The other laboratory values are normal. Possible etiologies of hyponatremia in an infant of this age include adrenal insufficiency, dehydration, congestive heart failure and renal abnormalities. Other likely causes would be hypoglycemia, hypocalcemia, and hypomagnesemia. Changes in potassium are more likely to be associated with cardiac abnormalities.

19. b This infant has symptoms of central hypotonia, with lethargy and a weak cry. Inborn errors of metabolism (e.g., maple syrup urine disease) may be a likely cause of central hypotonia in an infant who becomes progressively lethargic. In central hypotonia, DTRs are typically normal or increased. Infants with lower-motor neuron dysfunction generally have absent DTRs. Poor muscle tone may lead to shallow respirations and poor suck. Seizures are a common finding in disorders with features of central hypotonia.

20. e This infant has symptoms of withdrawal to narcotics. Aside from management of this infant for probable dehydration, consideration should be given to the child's welfare. A urine drug screen may be sensitive for up to 7 days for substances such as cocaine. Most children respond best to swaddling in a stimulus-free environment; however, some children require treatment with phenobarbital. Given the presentation, sepsis would be an unlikely source of this child's symptoms.

SECTION IV Trauma

CHAPTER 103

An Approach to the Injured Child

ATIMA CHUMPA, M.D.

QUESTIONS

1. A 15-year-old boy is brought to your ED after sustaining a head injury. He flipped and landed on his head while skateboarding. He had a helmet on, but had loss of consciousness (LOC) for 2–3 minutes. He is now sleepy and complains of a headache. His Glasgow Coma Scale (GCS) score is 12. You would do each of the following, EXCEPT:

   a. Obtain C-spine x-rays
   b. Immobilize his C-spine
   c. Obtain a head CT scan
   d. Perform serial GCS examinations
   e. Endotracheal intubation

2. A 10-year-old girl is brought to the ED by her parents after she was hit by a car while riding her bicycle. She was hit on her right side and then thrown in the air, landing approximately 5 feet away. She had a helmet on and had no LOC. On arrival, her vital signs are: T 36.8°C, HR 110, RR 18, BP 100/70. She is awake, alert, and crying. She complains of chest and abdominal pain. You immediately:

   a. Obtain a CXR
   b. Immobilize her C-spine
   c. Obtain IV access
   d. Obtain an ECG
   e. Perform needle thoracostomy

3. A 12-year-old boy is brought to your ED after sustaining a neck injury. He was at a cookout when he fell off a tree from a height of 8 feet. A barbecue fork became embedded into the right side of his neck, approximately 2 cm deep. There was no LOC. On arrival, his vital signs are: T 37.6°C, RR 24, HR 100, BP 112/78, and O_2 saturation 98% on room air. He is breathing spontaneously. You would do each of the following, EXCEPT:

   a. Remove the fork and repair the wound
   b. Leave the fork in place and explore the wound
   c. Immobilize his C-spine and examine the airway
   d. Obtain IV access
   e. Obtain a C-spine x-ray

4. A 15-year-old boy, who is a gang member, is brought to your ED after being stabbed in the abdomen with a knife. On arrival, his vital signs are: T 36°C, HR 110, BP 110/76, RR 24, and O_2 saturation 96%. His airway is intact and he has equal breath sounds bilaterally. He also has strong pulses with good perfusion. His wound is approximately 2 cm in length and located in the right lower abdomen. The knife remains in the wound. Your first step in management is:

   a. Explore the wound
   b. Obtain IV access
   c. Consult surgery for exploration
   d. Obtain abdominal CT
   e. Remove the knife

5. An 8-year-old girl is brought to the ED after falling while riding her bicycle. She says she fell forward onto her handlebar when she was coming down the hill. There was no LOC. She is brought in a C-spine collar. She complains of severe abdominal pain upon arrival. Her initial HR is 110 and her BP 120/80. Her airway is intact and her breath sounds are clear bilaterally. You are unable to assess her abdomen because of guarding and pain. Her neurological examination is normal. After obtaining IV access, you would immediately:

   a. Obtain an intravenous pyelogram (IVP)
   b. Perform a diagnostic peritoneal lavage
   c. Obtain a head CT scan
   d. Administer midazolam
   e. Obtain an abdominal CT scan

ANSWERS

1. e   Because the history suggests a severe injury, and he has a GCS score of 12, a head CT scan should be obtained. Serial evaluations of GCS are important and should be performed in this patient. The initial score serves as the baseline for the detection of subsequent deterioration. Given the mechanism of injury, the C-spine should be immobilized. At first, a cross-table lateral x-ray of the cervical spine should be obtained with the patient immobilized. If the first radiograph shows all C-spine vertebrae to be intact and properly aligned, a complete radiologic evaluation of the cervical spine can be performed. Intubation, which is required in severe head injuries, is not indicated at this time.

2. b   Based on her history and complaints, this patient might have sustained multiple injuries. An approach to the patient with multiple injuries should follow an order of primary assessment, resuscitation (initial treatment), secondary assessment, and definitive care. The primary assessment includes assessing Airway, Breathing, Circulation, Disability (neurologic status), and Exposure (completely undressing the patient, but preventing hypothermia). In trauma victims, while assessing and managing the patient's airway, great care should be taken to prevent excessive movement of the cervical spine. Appropriate C-spine immobilization should be obtained at this time. In this patient, therefore, airway assessment and C-spine immobilization should take priority, followed by assessment and management of breathing and circulation.

3. a   This patient sustained a penetrating neck wound and blunt trauma from falling. The initial approach should be directed at immobilizing the C-spine and at assessing the airway, followed by assessing breathing, assessing circulation, and establishing vascular access. Given that he fell from 8 feet, a C-spine x-ray should also be obtained. Protruding objects should be left in place by the physician in the ED. Wounds superficial to the platysma muscles are appropriate for repair in the ED. Wounds deep to the platysma require surgical evaluation.

4. b. Stab wounds produce variable degrees of internal injury. A patient with stable vital signs and a stab wound that is superficial to the peritoneum may be considered to have a mild injury. Stab wounds that violate the peritoneum should be considered moderately serious and surgical consultation should be obtained. Stab wounds that lead to unstable vital signs are considered severe. Assessing a patient who sustained a stab wound follows the ABC rules of priority. The first intervention in this patient following airway, breathing, and circulation assessment should be establishing IV access. The evaluation should be followed by local exploration, lavage, or laparotomy.

5. e   This patient sustained an isolated but forceful blow from the handlebars to the abdomen. After assessing her ABCs, at least one IV catheter should be inserted. Abdominal CT should be obtained in this patient because a handlebar injury to the abdomen is often associated with significant duodenal or splenic injury. An IVP is helpful in patients who are unstable and need an emergent evaluation of the renal system. If a patient is stable, an abdominal CT scan is preferred over a diagnostic peritoneal lavage because the CT scan will yield more information. Head CT is not indicated, because this appears to be an isolated injury and her neurological examination appears to be normal. Midazolam should not be administered because it may alter or mask a patient's mental status.

CHAPTER **104**

Major Trauma

ATIMA CHUMPA, M.D.

QUESTIONS

1. An 8-year-old boy was brought to your ED after he was hit by a car while in-line skating. On arrival, he is awake, anxious, and pale. His vital signs are: T 37°C, HR 120, RR 40, and BP 80/40, with an O_2 saturation of 90% on supplemental oxygen. On your examination, he is moving air well, with no evidence of airway obstruction. His breath sounds are decreased on the right with the trachea shifted to the left. A puncture wound was noted on the right side of his chest. His abdomen is tender and distended, with a large abrasion on the right side. You would immediately:

   a. Explore the puncture wound on the chest
   b. Obtain a CXR
   c. Place two large-bore IVs
   d. Perform needle thoracostomy
   e. Perform diagnostic peritoneal lavage (DPL)

2. A 4-year-old boy who was previously healthy was found unresponsive in a pool. Friends saw him jumping in the pool and noted that he did not resurface. His father rescued him immediately. After resurfacing, he was noted to be breathing spontaneously, but was unresponsive and seizing. His father brought him to your ED. On arrival, the boy has generalized tonic-clonic seizures, but his airway is intact. You would immediately:

   a. Obtain IV access
   b. Administer rectal diazepam (Valium)
   c. Immobilize his C-spine
   d. Warm him with a radiant warmer
   e. Obtain his O_2 saturation level

3. A 17-year-old boy was brought to your ED after a motor vehicle accident. He was a restrained driver of a truck when he hit his head traveling at a moderate to high speed. He was intubated at the scene and brought to your ED by air transport. He was given a normal saline fluid bolus of 40 cc/kg en route. On arrival, his vital signs are: T 37.2°C, HR 110, BP 96/88, RR 20, and O_2 saturation 92% on 100% oxygen. On examination, he had equal breath sounds bilaterally, distant heart sounds, thready pulses, and an open femur fracture. At this time, you would:

   a. Obtain a central venous access
   b. Perform pericardiocentesis
   c. Administer IV cefazolin
   d. Order a blood transfusion
   e. Obtain an EKG

4. A 9-year-old girl was brought to your ED after she was hit by a car while riding her bicycle. She was thrown in the air and landed approximately 6 feet away. She was wearing a helmet, and there was no loss of consciousness. IV access was established by the paramedics. On arrival, she is difficult to arouse, and she is pale. Her vital signs are: T 36.8°C, HR 136, RR 32, and BP 72/58. O_2 saturation is 94% on supplemental oxygen. Her airway is intact. Breath sounds are clear bilaterally. She has weak pulses and cool extremities. Her abdomen is distended and tender on palpation. You establish another peripheral IV, and then give 20 cc/kg NS bolus twice. After boluses, her BP is 80/54, and HR 140. You would immediately:

   a. Start a dopamine drip
   b. Consult surgery for emergency laparotomy
   c. Obtain hematocrit level
   d. Obtain abdominal CT scan
   e. Transfuse O-negative blood

5. A 16-year-old football player was brought to your ED after he was tackled while playing football. He was unable to move after he collided head on with another player. He had no loss of consciousness. He complains of numbness and a tingling sensation on his fingers. He is unable to move his arms or legs. On arrival, he is awake, alert and breathing spontaneously. He still has his helmet on, but there is no obvious facial or airway trauma. You would immediately:

   a. Obtain C-spine x-rays before removing the helmet
   b. Obtain IV access and administer high dose steroids
   c. Consult neurosurgery
   d. Break the helmet open and examine the C-spines
   e. Remove the helmet, then obtain C-spine x-ray

The following case applies to Questions 6 and 7: A 10-year-old girl was transferred to your ED from another ED after a motor vehicle accident. She was a restrained front seat passenger in a van that hit another car in oncoming traffic. She had loss of consciousness. She was brought to a local ED where her mental status deteriorated and she was subsequently intubated. Her head CT scan revealed a right parietal epidural hematoma; therefore, she was transferred for further neurosurgical care at your institution. She had stable vital signs prior to leaving the first ED, but during transport her BP started to drop. A normal saline 20 ml/kg IV bolus was given twice. On arrival, she is sedated and intubated. Her vital signs are: T 36.8°C, HR 120, BP 82/64, RR 24, and O_2 saturation 95% on 100% O_2. On exam, she has clear breath sounds bilaterally. She arrives with a peripheral IV. Her pulses were weak. Her abdomen was slightly distended with lap belt mark noted on the abdomen. She also has right thigh swelling and deformity. The surgeon immediately performs a DPL, which shows 50,000 RBCs/mm³ and 200 WBCs/mm³ in the aspirate after installing 10 ml/kg Ringer's lactate.

6. You interpret this result as:

   a. She most likely has a pelvic fracture as well
   b. She requires immediate laparotomy
   c. The result is uninterpretable because the DPL technique was wrong
   d. She most likely has laceration of spleen or liver
   e. Pancreas or duodenum injuries cannot be ruled out

7. After DPL, the child dropped her O_2 saturation to 88% on 100% oxygen. Her breath sounds are decreased on the right. You would immediately:

   a. Withdraw the endotracheal tube (ETT)
   b. Obtain a CXR
   c. Check the ETT position and suction
   d. Perform needle thoracotomy on the left side of the chest
   e. Obtain KUB

8. A 9-year-old boy sustained injuries from a fall when he climbed up a tree and fell down from approximately 10 feet. He landed on his right side, but did not hit his head. He denies neck pain, tingling sensations or numbness. On examination, he has an abrasion on the right hip and the right side of the abdominal wall. His abdomen is nondistended and nontender. There are a few drops of blood noted on the scrotum. You would perform all of the following, EXCEPT:

   a. Insert Foley catheter
   b. Urethrogram
   c. Pelvis x-ray
   d. Obtain liver function tests
   e. Abdominal CT scan

9. Abdominal CT scan is indicated in all of the following cases, EXCEPT:

   a. A 4-year-old girl who was an unrestrained backseat passenger who was ejected from the car in a motor vehicle collision. Her abdomen is nondistended and soft. She is lethargic and has a Glasgow Coma Scale score of 13.
   b. A 13-month-old girl who is a victim of nonaccidental trauma. She has a skull fracture and bruises on her chest and abdomen.
   c. An 8-year-old boy who was a restrained front seat passenger of a car that was rear-ended by another vehicle. There is a lap-belt mark present on the abdominal wall. His abdomen is soft and nontender, and he has a normal mental status with no evidence of head injury.
   d. A 6-year-old girl who fell from a swing and landed on her back. She has no CVA or spine tenderness. Her abdomen is soft and nontender, and the rest of her examination is normal. Her urinalysis showed 5–10 red blood cells per high-power field.
   e. A 5-year-old boy who fell off monkey bars and landed on his right side. His AST is 200 U/l and ALT is 180 U/l.

10. A 7-year-old boy was brought to the ED after a motor vehicle accident. He was a restrained front seat passenger in a car going at a high speed when it hit a tree. There was major damage to the front of the car. He did not have loss of consciousness, but he broke his leg. On arrival, he is awake and alert. His airway is intact. His spine is immobilized in a cervical collar and backboard. His breath sounds are equal bilaterally. His pulses are strong and symmetric. He has an open femur fracture with active bleeding from the wound. You would immediately:

   a. Establish vascular access
   b. Apply hemostats to the bleeding vessels
   c. Apply tourniquet above the bleeding site
   d. Apply a splint to that leg
   e. Apply direct pressure to the bleeding site

ANSWERS

1. d The presentation of respiratory distress, hypotension, and decreased breath sounds with a shifted trachea in this child is consistent with a tension pneumothorax. Once tension pneumothorax is recognized, immediate needle thoracostomy should be performed, followed by tube thoracostomy. The approach to a trauma patient should follow in order of priority: airway, breathing, and circulation during the primary survey. In this case, relief of the tension pneumothorax takes precedence over IV access or the other interventions listed.

2. c In addition to seizures, the child in this scenario might have sustained trauma to his head or neck while jumping into the pool. While the choices given above are all appropriate interventions, airway assessment and C-spine immobilization take priority.

3. b This patient has hypotension, a narrow pulse pressure and distant heart sounds, all of which are indicative of cardiac tamponade. In addition, cardiac tamponade may cause distended neck veins. The symptoms may be difficult to distinguish from tension pneumothorax, which might cause distended neck veins and a narrow pulse pressure, as well as diminished breath sounds and a shifted trachea. Because airway and breathing have already been assessed and stabilized, however, cardiac tamponade should be immediately relieved by pericardiocentesis.

4. e The symptoms of tachycardia, hypotension, and poor perfusion are consistent with shock. Shock after trauma is usually hypovolemic. The treatment should begin promptly with crystalloid infusion, followed by blood transfusion in severe hypovolemic shock. This child still has signs and symptoms of shock after being given 40 ml/kg of crystalloid solution. Blood transfusion should be initiated. Fully cross-matched or type-specific blood is preferred. Type O-negative blood may be given if fully cross-matched or type-specific blood is not available. The diagnosis and management of hypovolemic shock should not rely on the hematocrit value because a near-normal hematocrit does not exclude the possibility of a significant blood loss. Diagnostic testing and definitive treatment should follow stabilization. Vasopressors do not play a role in the initial management of hypovolemic shock.

5. a This patient has a stable airway and is breathing spontaneously. In this situation, a C-spine series x-ray can be obtained before helmet removal. When it is necessary to remove the helmet before the neck is cleared, a two-person technique ensuring neck immobilization should be used. C-spine stabilization and radiography should take priority over neurosurgical consultation or administration of steroids.

6. e The results of DPL are considered positive when the initial aspirate is grossly bloody or if the aspirate after instilling 10 ml/kg of Ringer's lactate reveals greater than 100,000 RBCs/mm^3, greater than 500 WBCs/mm^3, a spun effluent hematocrit greater than 2%, or the presence of bile, bacteria, or fecal material. The DPL in this child, therefore, is negative. The result may be falsely negative despite injuries to pancreas, duodenum, genitourinary tract, aorta, vena cava, and diaphragm. False-positive results may also be caused by a pelvic fracture.

7. c The approach to every child with major trauma should follow a rapid and reproducible schema of primary survey, resuscitation, secondary survey, and eventual triage. The order of priority is airway, breathing, and circulation (A, B, C). If there is deterioration at any point during the secondary survey or subsequent care, the primary survey should be repeated in the order of A, B, and C. Following this approach, the first response to the deterioration in this child is to evaluate the airway by checking the ETT position and suctioning. The ETT may be displaced or obstructed. Re-intubation may be necessary if the patient's condition does not improve with suctioning or ETT repositioning.

8. a When there is blood at the urethral meatus or on the scrotum, urinary catheterization should not be attempted before a retrograde urethrogram has ruled out a urethral injury. Pelvis x-ray, liver function tests, and abdominal CT scan are appropriate diagnostic studies in this patient, who may have a pelvic fracture and intra-abdominal injury.

9. d An abdominal CT scan is indicated in a hemodynamically stable victim of blunt trauma who has clinical signs of intra-abdominal injury, transaminase elevation of greater than 100 U/l, hematuria greater than 20 RBCs/hpf, or a worrisome mechanism of trauma in the presence of neurologic compromise.

10. **e**   Following the order of A, B, and C during the primary survey, this patient has a stable airway and breathing status. During circulation assessment, external hemorrhage should be controlled immediately by direct pressure or pneumatic splints. Application of extremity tourniquets or hemostats to bleeding vessels is less useful and potentially harmful. After the primary survey, vascular access should be established.

CHAPTER 105

Neurotrauma

DAVID GREENES, M.D.

QUESTIONS

1. An 8-year-old boy comes to the ED comatose after being thrown from an automobile. His left pupil is 6 mm and nonreactive, and his right pupil is 4 mm and reactive. Which of the following therapies would be contraindicated?

   a. Rapid-sequence intubation with ketamine and rocuronium
   b. Positive-pressure ventilation with mild hyperventilation
   c. IV mannitol administered at a dose of 1 g/kg
   d. Elevation of the head of the bed at an angle of 30 degrees
   e. Immobilization of the neck in a semi-rigid cervical collar

2. A 14-year-old boy is transported by EMTs after a diving accident. He is unresponsive with dilated pupils bilaterally, and he is intubated. An inline end-tidal CO_2 monitor is applied. What is the optimal end-tidal CO_2 for this boy while awaiting head CT?

   a. 15 mm Hg
   b. 20 mm Hg
   c. 30 mm Hg
   d. 40 mm Hg
   e. 50 mm Hg

3. An 8-month-old boy falls from a height of 5 feet onto a cement floor. He is seen 6 weeks after the fall with persistent boggy swelling of the scalp. What is the most likely diagnosis?

   a. Depressed skull fracture
   b. Subgaleal hematoma
   c. Leptomeningeal cyst
   d. Basilar skull fracture
   e. Epidural hematoma

4. A 16-year-old football player loses consciousness for several seconds after being tackled. He is confused for approximately 20 minutes and has headache, nausea, and dizziness for several hours. He asks you when he can resume playing football. Your reply is that:

   a. He may return as soon as he is feeling better
   b. He should sit out for the rest of the season
   c. He may return after being asymptomatic for 1 week
   d. He may return after being asymptomatic for 2 weeks
   e. A head CT must be performed before deciding

5. A 5-year-old boy is struck by an automobile traveling at high speed. On initial evaluation, he has diminished strength in both arms but good strength in both legs. What anatomic injury would be most consistent with these findings?

   a. Complete transection at the level of C-5
   b. Injury to the central portion of the cord at the level of C-5
   c. Hemisection of the cord at the level of C-7
   d. Complete transection at the level of T-1
   e. Conversion reaction, with no anatomic injury

6. Which of the following trauma patients is a candidate for IV glucocorticoid therapy?

   a. An 8-year-old boy with an epidural hematoma and a Glasgow Coma Scale (GCS) score of 15
   b. A 2-year-old girl with diffuse axonal injury and a GCS score of 7
   c. A 13-year-old boy, normal neurologic exam, fracture through posterior elements of C-2
   d. A 10-year-old boy, alert, diminished strength and tone in both lower extremities
   e. A 6-month-old boy with a subdural hematoma and a GCS score of 12

7. A 2-year-old child was thrown from an automobile. On arrival to the ED, there is obvious contusion to the scalp and deformity of the skull. Which of the following physiologic changes could not be explained by the head injury?

   a. Irregular respirations
   b. Bradycardia
   c. Hypotension
   d. Mydriasis
   e. Hemiparesis

8. A 14-year-old boy is struck by an automobile traveling at high speed. He is transferred to your ED after being seen at another hospital, where he was intubated for inadequate respiratory effort. On initial assessment, his HR is 40 and BP is 85/40. The most likely explanation for these findings is:

   a. Increased intracranial pressure (ICP)
   b. Intra-abdominal hemorrhage
   c. Spinal cord injury
   d. Overdose of sedative medications
   e. Tension pneumothorax

9. A 10-month-old boy presents with a parietal scalp hematoma. His neurologic examination is normal. The family reports that he rolled off a bed 3 days ago, but that he seemed fine at the time. They seem appropriately concerned and involved in his care. Head CT shows a linear parietal skull fracture with a 2-mm epidural hematoma. What is the most appropriate course of action?

   a. Contact the state's child protective services
   b. Immediate operative evacuation of the epidural hematoma
   c. Admit to intensive care unit (ICU) with follow-up head CT in 6 hours
   d. Semi-elective surgical repair of the skull fracture
   e. A brief period of clinical observation and discharge to home

10. A 15-year-old boy suffers a gunshot wound to the head. On arrival to the ED, he is somnolent and intermittently agitated. There is an entrance wound noted on the right temple. Which of the following steps is NOT an appropriate step of ED management?

    a. Place 2 large-bore IVs
    b. IV cefazolin 30 mg/kg
    c. Cervical spine (C-spine) immobilization
    d. Exploration and irrigation of the wound
    e. Immediate head CT

11. An 11-year-old gymnast complains of neck pain and tingling of her right leg, which began abruptly after she fell from the uneven bars and landed on her head, hyperflexing her neck. The injury occurred 10 hours ago. She has some mild diffuse tenderness over the posterior aspect of the spinal column, ranging from C-5 to C-7. Neurologic examination is normal, except for the complaint of right leg paresthesias. X-rays of the cervical spine show no fracture or subluxation. The most appropriate course of management at this time is:

    a. Transfer to another facility for immediate MRI of the cervical spine
    b. Discharge to home with a soft collar and ibuprofen
    c. Admit to the hospital for bedrest, with immobilization of the neck in a hard collar
    d. Initiation of high-dose methylprednisolone and admission to the ICU
    e. CT of the neck to look for occult fracture, and discharge if normal

12. A 10-year-old girl is referred to your hospital from an outside facility. The patient fell off of a unicycle several hours earlier, landing on the pavement on the side of her head. She was not wearing a helmet. Physical examination is notable for purple discoloration on the bony prominence behind the left ear. Her neurologic status is normal. Skull radiographs performed at the outside hospital showed no fracture. The additional finding that would be of greatest significance in changing your management of the patient would be which of the following?

    a. Discovery of a subtle fracture through the temporal bone on head CT
    b. Fluid in the mastoid air cells on head CT
    c. Intracranial air (pneumocephaly) on head CT
    d. Periorbital ecchymoses ("raccoon eyes") noted on physical examination
    e. Serosanguinous drainage from the left ear on physical examination

13. A 9-year-old boy is "horsing around" in the house and falls, hitting the side of his head on the corner of a fireplace mantel. He does not lose consciousness, but he is dazed for a few seconds. Thereafter, he goes outside to play for about 2 hours, but then comes in saying he does not feel well, and he begins to vomit. By the time his parents get him to the ED, he is very difficult to arouse. The most likely diagnosis is:

    a. Epidural hematoma
    b. Cerebral contusion
    c. Subdural hematoma
    d. Diffuse axonal injury
    e. Concussion

ANSWERS

1. a Rapid-sequence intubation is appropriate for a comatose, head-injured patient. Ketamine would be contraindicated, however, because it may elevate increased intracranial pressure. Other sedative agents, such as thiopental, midazolam, and fentanyl—which do not lead to elevations of intracranial pressure—would be preferred. The other therapies listed are all appropriate. Mild hyperventilation, administration of mannitol, and elevation of the head of the bed are all appropriate therapies for patients with clinical signs of increased ICP. Immobilization of the cervical spine is always appropriate in a traumatized patient who is unconscious and therefore cannot cooperate with a complete physical examination to evaluate for cervical spine injury.

2. c Therapeutic hyperventilation is recommended as initial therapy for patients who have clinical signs of increased ICP. Therapeutic hyperventilation leads to reflex vasoconstriction of the cerebral vasculature, thereby decreasing intracranial blood volume and, subsequently, intracranial pressure. Researchers have increasingly found that prolonged or severe hyperventilation of head-injured patients is deleterious, probably because it leads to too much cerebral vasoconstriction, resulting in compromised cerebral blood flow. Most authorities now recommend mild hyperventilation, to a Pco_2 of approximately 30 mm Hg, as initial therapy to prevent cerebral herniation while awaiting head CT and/or surgical intervention.

3. c Leptomeningeal cyst, or growing skull fracture, is a rare complication of skull fracture in infants, in which a portion of the meninges, sometimes accompanied by brain tissue, herniates through a fracture line. The herniated tissue prevents proper healing of the fracture, which persists, and sometimes appears to widen, over time. Growing skull fracture usually presents as a persistent boggy swelling of the scalp, often accompanied by seizures, developmental delay, or focal neurologic signs attributable to the herniated brain tissue. A depressed skull fracture may present with a palpable abnormality of the skull, but one would not expect persistent swelling so long after an injury. A subgaleal hematoma may have a similar appearance on physical examination, but it should resolve within approximately 2 weeks after an injury. Basilar skull fractures are usually diagnosed on the basis of clinical signs of vascular injury or cerebrospinal fluid (CSF) leak. Because of the location of the fracture in the basal skull, the actual fracture site is not accessible on physical examination. Epidural hematoma refers to bleeding beneath the skull, in the epidural space. Although epidural hematomas are usually associated with an overlying skull fracture, the epidural hematoma itself is not palpable on physical examination.

4. c According to guidelines published by the Centers for Disease Control (CDC), the patient's injury would be classified as a Grade 3 concussion (head injury associated with initial loss of consciousness). The guidelines recommend abstinence from contact sports for 1 week if the loss of consciousness is brief, and 2 weeks if it is prolonged. Although many clinicians would perform a head CT for a head-injured patient who suffered loss of consciousness, a head CT is not required in order to use the guidelines. If an intracranial lesion is noted on head CT, the guidelines recommend that the patient abstain from contact sports for the remainder of the season.

5. b The "central cord syndrome" may occur with hyperextension injuries to the neck. This unusual injury pattern injures the central gray matter of the cord without affecting the more peripheral white matter. This leads to a clinical pattern of neurologic deficits to more proximal structures with sparing of more distal functions. This pattern is in contrast to that of most other cord injuries, which lead to deficits below the level of the cord injury, with sparing of more proximal functions. This more typical pattern of distal deficits is what would be expected with a complete transection of the cord, or with a hemisection.

   Some patients do have conversion reactions manifesting as motor weakness; many such patients have an anatomic distribution of weakness that is not consistent with a true nervous system injury. Although it is conceivable that this patient is having a conversion reaction, it is imperative to recognize that the clinical presentation is consistent with a spinal cord injury, and the patient must be treated as such.

6. d The North American Spinal Cord Injury Study (NASCIS) found improved outcomes for patients with spinal cord injuries if they were treated with high-dose IV methylprednisolone within 8 hours of the time of the injury. Patients should be considered candidates for this therapy if they have neurologic

deficits that indicate spinal cord injury. Patients with injury to the spinal column, but without neurologic deficits, should not be treated. There is no indication for glucocorticoid therapy as treatment for intracranial injury.

7. c   Patients with increased intracranial pressure who are experiencing tentorial herniation may exhibit some or all of the characteristic vital sign changes known as *Cushing's triad:* bradycardia, hypertension, and irregular respirations. These changes are thought to represent compression of autonomic control centers in the brainstem. In addition, patients suffering from herniation develop a mydriatic or "blown" pupil because of compression of cranial nerve III by the herniating temporal lobe. Hypotension, however, cannot be explained by the head injury. With the possible exception of very young infants (especially premature infants), patients cannot lose enough blood volume into their heads to suffer hemodynamic instability. In the setting of head trauma, therefore, hypotension must be assumed to be a result of an extracranial injury. Most commonly, hypotension reflects blood loss, either external (e.g., from a bleeding laceration) or internal (e.g., into the abdomen or pelvis).

8. c   The combination of bradycardia, hypotension, and inadequate respiratory effort is most consistent with spinal "shock," an interruption of the autonomic impulses carried in the spinal cord. Most cases of hypotension in trauma are a result of hypovolemia or decreased venous return. In these cases, such as with intra-abdominal hemorrhage (B) or tension pneumothorax (E), tachycardia would be expected. Increased intracranial pressure, if it causes tentorial herniation, will cause bradycardia and hypertension. Although sedative medications might cause some bradycardia and hypotension, the degree of bradycardia seen in this case would be unusual. The patient should be treated as if there is a spinal cord injury until proven otherwise.

9. e   It is not unusual for an infant's parents to first discover an abnormality several days after a skull fracture occurs, when the subgaleal hematoma begins to liquefy and a "boggy" swelling is noted. Linear skull fractures require no specific therapy; they will generally heal well without any intervention. Epidural hematomas, if they accumulate quickly, may be life threatening. Larger epidural hematomas must be evacuated immediately to prevent progression to brain injury and/or tentorial herniation. Many small epidural hematomas may be managed nonoperatively, however. Because this patient has a small epidural hematoma that apparently has not progressed significantly in 3 days, he is at little risk for subsequent deterioration. Although some clinicians might favor admission for a brief period of in-house observation, it is probably not necessary to provide ICU-level monitoring, repeat brain imaging, or surgical evacuation of the hematoma. Although skull fractures certainly can be a result of child abuse, the vast majority result from household falls, many from heights of less than 3 or 4 feet. Epidural hematomas are less commonly seen in child abuse than are subdural hematomas. It is always appropriate to consider a diagnosis of child abuse when an infant is injured, but the scenario as presented does not raise any particular concerns for abuse.

10. d   Most patients with gunshot wounds to the head will be taken to the operating room for exploration, debridement of the superficial aspects of the wound, and repair of the dura. It is not necessary to attempt exploration or irrigation of the wound in the ED. Initial management in the ED focuses on stabilizing the patient and excluding other life-threatening injuries. As with all traumatized patients, it is appropriate to obtain IV access immediately. Cervical spine immobilization should also be maintained because some patients with gunshot wounds to the head will experience migration of the bullet to the neck, with possible injury to the spinal column or spinal cord. Immediate head CT is essential to exclude intracranial hematoma that may require emergent evacuation. Finally, it is appropriate to institute prophylactic antibiotic therapy. An antibiotic that covers skin flora, such as cefazolin, is recommended.

11. c   This patient has evidence of possible spinal cord injury, with sensory symptoms that would be consistent with a lower cervical spine injury. The absence of hard neurologic findings on physical examination suggests that the patient will likely have a good prognosis, but it does not exclude the possibility of a spinal cord contusion. The absence of abnormalities on x-ray does not exclude spinal cord injuries because many spinal cord injuries in pediatrics occur in the absence of evident bony abnormalities (a syndrome known as "spinal cord injury without radiographic abnormalities," or SCIWORA). The most appropriate management is to assume some instability of the spinal column and to admit the patient to monitor for any progression of symptoms and to ensure full immobilization. Because the patient has a

normal neurologic examination, and because the injury occurred 10 hours ago, high-dose IV glucocorticoids are not indicated. Neck CT might reveal an occult fracture missed by plain x-ray, but even a normal neck CT would not exclude the possibility of spinal cord injury. MRI might help delineate the exact nature of the cord injury, but it would be unlikely to change management. Emergent MRI of the spine is only indicated for patients with incomplete but progressing signs of cord compression, who might have a surgically reparable lesion.

12. e   The purple discoloration overlying the mastoid bone is known as Battle sign, which is one of the classic clinical signs of basilar skull fracture. Other clinical findings in basilar skull fracture include hemotympanum, periorbital ecchymoses ("raccoon eyes"), CSF rhinorrhea, and CSF otorrhea. Fractures of the basal skull are often not evident on skull radiographs. The fracture line may be difficult to detect on head CT as well. More commonly, associated signs indicating basilar skull fracture (e.g., pneumocephaly or fluid in the mastoid air cells or paranasal sinuses) are noted on head CT. There is some risk for meningitis to develop as a complication of basilar skull fracture. For most patients, this risk is low, and prophylactic antibiotics are not indicated. However, patients with ongoing CSF leak (CSF rhinorrhea or otorrhea) clearly have a persistent defect in the dura and are at high risk for the development of infectious complications. Patients with these signs are usually admitted to the hospital for observation and IV antibiotics. In some cases, if the CSF leak persists, surgical interventions are pursued.

13. a   Epidural hematoma is classically caused by an injury that causes deformation to the temporal or parietal skull, causing a laceration to the middle meningeal artery, which courses underneath. A fairly minimal force is often involved, and the brain tissue itself is not primarily injured. Patients become symptomatic only several hours later, when the epidural hematoma begins to exert a mass effect and symptoms of intracranial hypertension appear. In the interim, they may appear totally well (the so-called lucid interval). In contrast, cerebral contusion and diffuse axonal injury both indicate primary brain injury, and patients will most commonly have some symptoms from the moment of impact. A more severe mechanism of injury will often be reported. Subdural hematoma is also usually caused by fairly high-force acceleration/deceleration mechanisms, which are usually associated with primary brain injury as well.

CHAPTER 106

Neck Trauma

NEIL SCHAMBAN, M.D.

QUESTIONS

1. Which of the following statements regarding neck injury in children is true?

    a. Because of their larger head size and lower fulcrum, children are predisposed to lower cervical (C-spine) injuries

    b. Children with C-spine injuries always have bony abnormalities seen on plain film

    c. Although C-spine injuries are less common in children than adults, they are associated with a higher mortality

    d. Anatomy of the neck in children makes it more accessible to direct trauma

    e. Because of the anatomy of a child's neck and head, children are less prone to acceleration/deceleration injuries than adults

2. A 3-year-old boy is brought to the ED with a triangular piece of wood lodged in the left lateral aspect of the neck. Vital signs are as follows: T 37.4°C, HR 150, RR 28, and BP 100/60. O_2 saturation on room air is 98%. Appropriate management in the ED is:

    a. Immediate endotracheal intubation

    b. Removal of foreign object and local wound exploration

    c. Immediate surgical consultation

    d. Send patient for lateral neck and CXR

    e. Send patient for contrast CT scan

3. A 4-year-old girl involved in a moderate impact motor-vehicle collision is brought to the ED immobilized on a backboard, with a C-spine collar. She is alert and appropriate on arrival. No obvious evidence of head injury is noted. There is no reported loss of consciousness (LOC). The child does not complain of neck pain or tenderness and the neurological exam is normal. Lateral cervical spine films demonstrate 2 mm of anterior displacement of C-2 on C-3. The most appropriate next step in management would be:

    a. CT scan of the neck

    b. MRI of the neck

    c. Flexion/extension views of the neck

    d. Assess posterior cervical line on plain film

    e. Remove collar and discharge home

4. A 9-year-old boy is involved in a high-speed motor-vehicle collision. The patient is brought to the ED immobilized in a C-spine collar and on a backboard. The patient complains of neck pain. His examination reveals lower extremity weakness and paresthesias. His Glasgow Coma Scale (GCS) score is 15 and his vital signs are stable. C-spine films do not reveal any bony abnormalities. Which of the following is most appropriate?

    a. Obtain flexion/extension views of the neck

    b. Immediate endotracheal intubation

    c. Administer 0.5 g/kg of IV mannitol

    d. Administer 30 mg/kg of IV methylprednisolone

    e. Psychiatric consult

ANSWERS

1. c Cervical spine injuries in young children, although less frequent than they are in adults, are associated with a higher mortality. This is largely due to the fact that because of the larger size of the head, relatively weak musculature, poor protective reflexes, and a higher fulcrum, C-spine injuries tend to be in the upper cervical spine. The relatively larger head size also predisposes children to acceleration and deceleration injuries more commonly than in adults. Spinal injury is often present, but it is not apparent on plain films of the spine (spinal cord injury without radiographic abnormality, SCIWORA). Finally, the larger head and relatively shorter neck makes the anterior neck less susceptible to direct trauma.

2. c Penetrating injuries to the neck always warrant surgical consultation. Objects lodged in the neck should never be removed outside of the operating suite. They may be tamponading a vessel or may cause more damage upon removal. Patients should be observed in the ED. Films (e.g., a lateral neck x-ray and a CXR) may be very useful, but they should be obtained as portable radiographs. Immediate endotracheal intubation is not necessarily indicated if there is no respiratory compromise. Fiberoptic laryngoscopy is preferred so that the subglottic airway may be directly visualized prior to passing an endotracheal tube.

3. d The finding described in this case most likely represents pseudosubluxation of C-2 on C-3, which is common in cervical radiographs of children. It occurs in up to 25% of children less than 8 years of age and can occur up to age 16 years. It is due to ligamentous laxity, weak neck muscles, relatively horizontal facets, and cartilage artifact. Assessment of the posterior cervical line, as described in the chapter, can help to distinguish pseudosubluxation from actual subluxation due to an underlying injury. This should be done prior to any further testing. A finding consistent with pseudosubluxation in this case scenario would support sending the patient home without further testing.

4. d Neurological findings after a motor vehicle collision are worrisome for spinal cord injury. Treatment is directed at reducing swelling of the cord and improving neurological outcome. Currently, the recommended therapy is an IV loading dose of methylprednisolone, 30 mg/kg. Subsequent doses of 5.4 mg/kg/hour should be administered for the next 24 hours. Intubation is not necessary because the patient has no airway compromise and a GCS score of 15. Mannitol administration is used to decrease ICP. Flexion/extension views of the neck on plain film are contraindicated because any movement or manipulation could worsen an underlying injury. The patient should remain in appropriate C-spine immobilization with appropriate C-spine precautions.

CHAPTER **107**

Thoracic Trauma

ATIMA CHUMPA, M.D.

QUESTIONS

1. A 10-year-old boy is brought to the ED after he was hit by a car while riding his bicycle. He had a helmet on and there was no loss of consciousness (LOC). On arrival he is crying. His vital signs are: T 37.4°C, HR 140, RR 40, BP 90/60, and O_2 saturation 92% on room air. He has an intact airway and is placed in a cervical collar. His trachea is shifted to the right. His breath sounds are absent on the left. His extremities are cool and skin is poorly perfused. You would immediately:

   a. Administer 20 ml/kg NS bolus
   b. Perform intubation
   c. Perform pericardiocentesis
   d. Perform needle decompression
   e. Obtain an emergent portable CXR

2. An 8-year-old boy is brought into your facility after he fell off his tree house approximately 8 feet onto the ground. He landed on his right side and did not have LOC. On arrival in the ED, he is awake and alert. His vital signs are: T 36.8°C, HR 100, RR 24, BP 112/78, and O_2 saturation 98% on room air. He denies any pain. On exam, there is no C-spine tenderness and his breath sounds are equal bilaterally. There is an abrasion on his anterior chest. His CXR reveals a pneumothorax approximately 10% on the right. ECG is normal. Your next step is to:

   a. Discharge home, follow-up CXR tomorrow
   b. Perform tube thoracostomy
   c. Obtain an ABG
   d. Perform percutaneous catheter thoracostomy
   e. No intervention, but admit him for observation

3. A 14-year-old boy is brought into the ED after he was stabbed by a knife in the left side of his chest during an altercation. He complains of shortness of breath and chest pain. His vital signs are: T 37.9°C, HR 120, RR 28, BP 110/70, and O_2 saturation 94% on 100% O_2. On exam he is pale, his trachea is midline, and breath sounds are slightly decreased on the left side. There is a 2-cm laceration over the anterior chest wall, between the fifth and sixth intercostal space. You would do all of the following, EXCEPT:

   a. Obtain CXR
   b. Obtain IV access
   c. Insert a chest tube at the opening site
   d. Apply occlusive dressing
   e. Order cross-match for blood

4. A 16-year-old girl is brought into the ED after a motor vehicle accident. She was an unrestrained front-seat passenger in a car with no passenger airbag. The car hit a truck at high speed. On arrival her vital signs are: T 37°C, HR 100, RR 28, BP 130/88, and O_2 saturation 94% on room air. She is awake, alert, and complains of chest pain. Her airway is intact with midline trachea and she is in a cervical collar. Her breath sounds are equal bilaterally and her abdomen is soft and nontender. IV access is established. Her CXR reveals a pneumothorax approximately 30% on the left. You then perform tube thoracostomy, which relieves her chest pain. Twenty minutes later, however, she becomes diaphoretic, difficult to arouse, and her BP drops to 86/72. Breath sounds are equal bilaterally, and extremities are cool, with a capillary refill time greater than 3 seconds. You immediately perform endotracheal intubation. Which of the following interventions should be done next?

   a. Start vasopressor
   b. Transfuse 2 units of blood
   c. Replace the chest tube
   d. Perform pericardiocentesis
   e. Perform thoracostomy

5. A 6-year-old boy is brought to the ED after a lawn mower ran over his chest. His vital signs on arrival are: T 36.8°C, HR 140, RR 40, BP 110/70, and O_2 saturation 94% on 100% O_2. He is screaming and thrashing. On exam, his airway is intact, with a midline trachea and subcutaneous emphysema over the neck. His breath sounds are equal bilaterally. IV access is established. His CXR shows pneumomediastinum, but no pneumothorax. Which of the following interventions is indicated?

   a. Bronchoscopy
   b. Tube thoracostomy
   c. Endotracheal intubation
   d. Pericardiocentesis
   e. Admit for observation

6. A 16-year-old girl is brought into the ED after a motor vehicle accident. She was a restrained driver in a car hit by a high-speed pick-up truck on the driver's side. She had no LOC. Her vital signs are: T 37.4°C, HR 128, RR 28, BP 120/74, and O_2 saturation 99% on 100% O_2. On exam, she is awake, alert, crying, and complains of chest and abdominal pain. Her airway is intact. Trachea is midline. Breath sounds are slightly decreased on the left side. Suprasternal and subcostal retractions are present. Her abdomen is noted to be scaphoid, with generalized tenderness on palpation. CXR reveals no pneumothorax and an elevated left hemidiaphragm. Which of the following interventions is indicated?

   a. Bronchoscopy
   b. Esophagoscopy
   c. Exploratory laparotomy
   d. Echocardiogram
   e. Tube thoracostomy

7. A 15-year-old boy is brought to the ED after he was stabbed in the chest. His vital signs on arrival are: T 36.8°C, HR 128, RR 36, BP 110/70, and O_2 saturation 94% on 100% O_2. He complains of chest and abdominal pain. Breath sounds are equal bilaterally. There is a 2-cm stab wound on the anterior chest wall as well as subcutaneous emphysema. After IV access is established you obtain a CXR, which shows pneumomediastinum and an air-fluid level in the mediastinum. The following interventions are indicated, EXCEPT:

   a. Give 20 ml/kg NS bolus
   b. Place an NG tube
   c. Administer IV ampicillin, gentamicin, and clindamycin
   d. Perform tube thoracostomy
   e. Perform esophagoscopy

8. A 7-year-old boy is transferred to your ED after a boulder fell onto him while he was playing on a rocky coastline. He was trapped underneath for approximately 20 minutes before the fire department removed the boulder. Vital signs on arrival are: T 37°C, HR 120, RR 36, and BP 100/60. O_2 saturation is 95% on 100% O_2. The boy appears sleepy, but responds to verbal stimuli. Physical exam reveals an intact airway and midline trachea. Mild suprasternal retractions are noted. There is ecchymosis and an abrasion on his anterior right chest wall. Breath sounds are slightly decreased on the right. In addition, he has subconjunctival hemorrhages, periorbital edema, and petechiae noted on his head and neck examination. Which of the following statements is true regarding this condition?

   a. Intracranial hemorrhage is a common finding
   b. Aortography should be performed
   c. Pulmonary contusion and hepatic injuries are commonly seen
   d. Surgical repair of superior vena cava is the definitive treatment
   e. Abnormal bleeding diatheses cause these findings

9. A 13-year-old girl is brought to the ED after she was hit by a car while in-line skating. There was no loss of consciousness. Her vital signs on arrival are: T 36°C, HR 100, RR 24, and BP 116/78; O_2 saturation is 98% on 100% O_2. She is awake, alert, and complains of chest pain. Her airway is intact and the trachea is midline. Breath sounds are decreased on the left side. No retractions are noted. Her extremities are cool and clammy. Her abdomen is tender in the left upper quadrant. IV access is established. CXR shows fifth, sixth, and seventh rib fractures and a pulmonary contusion on the left. You would:

   a. Administer morphine sulfate
   b. Perform endotracheal intubation
   c. Apply pressure dressing at the fracture sites
   d. Avoid chest physiotherapy
   e. Transfuse 2 units of blood

10. A 17-year-old boy is brought to the ED after a motor vehicle accident. He was an unrestrained driver in a car without an airbag that ran into a pole. His vital signs on arrival are: T 36.6°C, HR 128, RR 24, and BP 100/60; O_2 saturation is 96% on 100% O_2. He is pale, diaphoretic, and responds to verbal stimuli. He complains of chest and back pain. His airway is intact with a midline trachea. There is a large area of redness over the anterior chest. His breath sounds are equal bilaterally. IV access is established. CXR shows a widened mediastinum, left-sided pleural cap, pulmonary contusion, and no pneumothorax. Which of the following interventions is indicated?

   a. Pericardiocentesis
   b. Aortography
   c. Tube thoracostomy
   d. Endotracheal intubation
   e. Bronchoscopy

11. A 12-year-old girl is brought into the ED after hitting her chest on a springboard. She was diving at a pool and hit her chest on the springboard on the way down after she made a flip in the air. Since then she has complained of chest pain. On arrival her vital signs are: T 37.8°C, HR 100, RR 24, and BP 120/80; O$_2$ saturation is 98% on room air. She is awake, alert, and anxious. Her airway is intact, with a midline trachea. There is erythema and tenderness on palpation of the anterior chest wall. Breath sounds are equal bilaterally. Her CXR shows no pneumothorax and normal heart size. ECG shows second-degree AV block. All of the following statement are true, EXCEPT:

a. CPK-MB is a specific diagnostic test
b. Transesophageal echocardiogram should be performed
c. This condition is self-limited
d. A new heart murmur or congestive heart failure may develop
e. ST changes may also be found with this condition

12. A 15-year-old boy is brought into the ED after he was shot in the midchest. On arrival he is awake, alert, pale, and anxious. Vital signs are: T 36°C, HR 120, RR 36, and BP 96/70; O$_2$ saturation is 90% on room air. His airway is intact, with a midline trachea. Breath sounds are decreased on the left side. There is a gunshot wound noted on the anterior midchest. He has weak pulses and cool extremities. You would immediately perform:

a. Needle decompression
b. Exploration of the wound
c. Endotracheal intubation
d. Thoracotomy
e. Tube thoracostomy

ANSWERS

1. d   The presentation of respiratory distress, shifted trachea, absent breath sounds on one side of the chest, hypotension, and poor perfusion is consistent with tension pneumothorax. Tension pneumothorax occurs when there is progressive accumulation of air within the pleural cavity, which collapses the ipsilateral lung and compresses the contralateral lung. Mediastinal structures can also be shifted to the contralateral side, resulting in reduced blood return to the heart and hypotensive shock. Although the patient needs volume resuscitation and other sources of blood loss need to be sought, tension pneumothorax needs to be released immediately with needle decompression. This is performed by inserting a needle in the midclavicular second intercostal space of the ipsilateral side. If there is a tension pneumothorax, an immediate release of air should be noted and tube thoracostomy should then be performed. Chest x-ray should not be used to diagnose tension pneumothorax in the symptomatic patient.

2. e   A pneumothorax less than 15% is considered to be small. If the pneumothorax is small and the patient is asymptomatic, observation in the hospital and administration of 100% oxygen is all that is necessary. Tube thoracostomy is indicated in symptomatic patients, patients undergoing positive pressure ventilation, and those requiring air transport. Even an asymptomatic patient with a small pneumothorax should be admitted to the hospital for observation because of possible progression to a tension pneumothorax.

3. c   The decreased breath sounds and open wound on the left side of the chest suggest an open pneumothorax. Chest thoracostomy should be done immediately to prevent development of a tension pneumothorax; however, the chest tube should be inserted at a different site than the open wound. An occlusive dressing should be applied at the wound site. CXR should be obtained to assess intrathoracic injury. IV access needs to be established, followed by fluid resuscitation. Blood should be readily available in any patient with penetrating thoracic trauma, because hemothorax can cause significant blood loss.

4. d   Pericardial tamponade should be suspected in a patient with thoracic trauma who presents with hypotension, narrow pulse pressure, and poor perfusion. Patients may also have distant heart sounds and pulsus paradoxus. CXR may show cardiomegaly. ECG may show low-voltage QRS waves. Pericardial tamponade occurs when there is injury to the myocardium and blood accumulates in the pericardial sac. Cardiac output decreases secondary to decreased venous return and stroke volume. This patient developed hypotensive shock. After the airway is controlled, pericardiocentesis should be performed,

along with volume resuscitation. Pericardiocentesis is performed by inserting a 20-gauge spinal needle below the xiphoid process at a 45-degree angle toward the left shoulder. The patient may show transient improvement after blood is removed from the pericardial sac. This should be followed by creation of a pericardial window performed in the operating room (OR) for continual drainage of blood.

5. **a** Subcutaneous emphysema, pneumomediastinum, and respiratory distress caused by crush injury to the chest suggest airway rupture. Symptoms may also include cyanosis and hemoptysis. In the absence of a pneumothorax, tracheal rupture should be suspected if a pneumomediastinum or cervical emphysema is present. If a pneumothorax is present with these findings, a bronchial rupture should be suspected. Bronchoscopy should be performed to identify and locate the lesion, followed by surgical repair. If the airway is stable, endotracheal intubation should be performed in the OR under bronchoscopic guidance because a partial tear may become complete after endotracheal intubation.

6. **c** This patient has the clinical presentation of a diaphragmatic injury. This includes chest pain, respiratory distress, scaphoid abdomen, and elevated hemidiaphragm. Diaphragmatic injuries are more common in blunt trauma, especially with a lateral torso impact in motor vehicle accident. Approximately 80% of diaphragmatic injuries occur on the left and 20% occur on the right. The left diaphragm is relatively unprotected, whereas the liver protects the right side. Other diagnostic studies (e.g., chest and abdominal CT with contrast or upper and lower GI series) can help confirm the diagnosis. In this case, abdominal CT should be performed to identify any intra-abdominal trauma. Exploratory laparotomy and surgical repair should be performed when a diaphragmatic hernia is strongly suspected; because of the motion of the diaphragm with respiration, diaphragmatic defects do not heal spontaneously.

7. **d** Esophageal injury should be highly suspected in a child with pneumomediastinum, air-fluid levels in the mediastinum, and subcutaneous emphysema in the setting of penetrating trauma. The most common cause for esophageal perforation in the pediatric population is iatrogenic, followed by penetrating trauma. Patients with an esophageal perforation in the cervical region may have neck pain, cervical subcutaneous emphysema, or odynophagia. Those with an esophageal perforation in the thoracic region may present with chest pain, dyspnea, abdominal pain, and guarding or subcutaneous emphysema. CXR may show a pneumothorax, pneumomediastinum, or an air-fluid level in the mediastinum. When esophageal perforation is suspected, patients should receive volume resuscitation and antibiotics covering Gram-positive, Gram-negative, and anaerobic bacteria. An NG tube should also be placed. The diagnosis of an esophageal perforation can be made by either esophagoscopy, esophagography, or both. Once the diagnosis is made, immediate surgical correction is mandatory. Complications of an esophageal perforation include mediastinal sepsis and death.

8. **c** The clinical presentation in this child is consistent with traumatic asphyxia. Traumatic asphyxia results from direct compression of the chest or abdomen. The most common mechanism is a child run over by a motor vehicle or pinned underneath a heavy object. Positive pressure is transmitted to the mediastinum and blood is forced out of the right atrium into the venous and capillary system. Areas drained by the superior vena cava are mostly affected. Clinical presentation includes subconjunctival hemorrhages, upper body petechiae, periorbital edema, cyanosis, respiratory distress, and altered mental status. The primary goal of treatment is to stabilize the patient and identify associated injuries. Pulmonary contusion and hepatic injuries are commonly seen with traumatic asphyxia. Neurological injury usually results from hypoxia, not intracranial hemorrhage.

9. **a** Fracturing two or more ribs on the same side may result in a flail chest. This occurs when that particular chest wall segment loses continuity with the thoracic cage, causing paradoxical movement of the chest wall. Crush injury to the chest is the most common mechanism for a flail chest. Flail chest is uncommon in children because of the marked compliance of the chest wall. When a flail chest occurs, it is usually associated with an intrathoracic injury. Any patient with respiratory distress should be intubated and placed on positive-pressure ventilation. In addition to protecting the airway, the positive pressure provides optimal expansion and splinting of the injured segment. In this case the patient does not need to be intubated. Aggressive pulmonary physiotherapy and pain control is the treatment of choice.

10. b   The evidence of a widened mediastinum and left-sided pleural cap on CXR in this patient is consistent with traumatic rupture of the thoracic aorta. Symptoms may include ecchymosis and tenderness over the chest, difference in pulses between the arms and legs, paraplegia, and anuria. CXR may show a widened mediastinum, loss of the aortic knob, left-sided pleural cap, tracheal deviation, and NG tube deviation. Early diagnosis of traumatic rupture of the thoracic aorta is imperative. The gold standard for diagnosis is aortography. In an unstable patient, a transesophageal echocardiogram can be performed while the patient's other life-threatening injuries are being treated.

11. a   Cardiac contusion should be suspected in this patient, given the mechanism of injury and the evidence of cardiac arrhythmia. Patients with blunt cardiac injury may also present with a new murmur or congestive heart failure. Transesophageal echocardiogram should be performed in patients who sustain thoracic trauma and present with an abnormal ECG, arrhythmia, or a new heart murmur. CPK-MB ratios have a high false-positive rate. Cardiac contusions are usually self-limited, unless ventricular fibrillation, which is rare, develops.

12. e   Hemothorax and pneumothorax are the most common complications of penetrating thoracic injuries, which almost always require tube thoracostomy. This child presents with respiratory distress, hypotension, and decreased breath sounds on the injured side of the chest. His airway is stable. Tube thoracostomy should be performed immediately. The patient should also receive IV fluid resuscitation. If type-specific blood is not available, O-negative blood should be at the patient's bedside as soon as possible. Pericardial tamponade should also be considered in this patient.

CHAPTER 108

Abdominal Trauma

BARBARA M. GARCIA PEÑA, M.D., M.P.H.

QUESTIONS

1. A 10-year-old unrestrained back-seat passenger is brought to the ED with unstable vital signs, bilateral femur fractures, multiple rib fractures, and an open head injury. His abdomen is soft and nondistended. His condition quickly deteriorates and he expires in the ED despite life-saving measures. What is the likelihood that he has sustained an abdominal injury?

   a. 20%
   b. 40%
   c. 60%
   d. 80%
   e. 100%

2. A 2-year-old restrained back-seat passenger comes to the ED after a low-speed motor vehicle collision. He had no loss of consciousness at the scene, but cried immediately after the impact. On examination, vital signs include HR 120, RR 20, BP 80/50, and O_2 saturation of 100% on room air. His examination is normal except for mild abdominal distension. The abdomen is otherwise soft and nontender. Rectal examination is negative for occult blood. The most likely cause for this child's abdominal distension is:

   a. Hemoperitoneum
   b. Peritonitis
   c. Bladder injury
   d. Pneumothorax
   e. Swallowed air

3. A 16-year-old boy was an unrestrained front-seat passenger and is brought to the ED after a high-speed motor vehicle accident. Vital signs are stable in the ED and examination is remarkable for blood at the urethral meatus. Rectal examination is negative. Which of the following is the most appropriate next step in management?

   a. Insertion of Foley catheter
   b. Pelvic ultrasonography
   c. Pelvic CT
   d. Retrograde urethrogram
   e. Intravenous pyelogram (IVP)

4. A 16-year-old girl restrained driver is brought to the ED after her car collided with a pole while traveling at a speed of 70 miles per hour. She is boarded and collared at presentation. Her vital signs are stable and she is conversant and alert. You secure IV access and send the appropriate laboratory studies. Which of the following is true?

   a. The absence of hyperamylasemia precludes pancreatic injury
   b. Screening for intra-abdominal injuries by evaluating transaminase levels is not universally accepted
   c. Patients with AST levels greater than 250 U/l and ALT levels greater than 150 U/l should always undergo abdominal CT
   d. Arterial blood gas (ABG) determinations should be sent on all patients with abdominal trauma
   e. A decreasing hematocrit on serial determinations usually suggests a need for aggressive IV crystalloid fluid resuscitation

5. A 13-year-old boy is brought to the ED with a penetrating stab wound to the abdomen. He is bleeding profusely. He is obtunded, HR 150, and BP 80/40. After securing the airway and establishing adequate respirations, you obtain IV access and begin infusion of:

   a. Normal saline (NS), starting at 10 ml/kg
   b. Lactated Ringer's (LR), starting at 20 ml/kg
   c. LR, starting at 30 ml/kg
   d. NS, starting at 30 ml/kg
   e. LR, starting at 40 ml/kg

6. A 6-year-old male restrained back-seat passenger is brought to the ED after a severe automobile collision. His vital signs are stable at presentation; however, his abdomen is becoming progressively distended. HEENT examination reveals significant distortion to the maxilla. Which of the following is required in this child?

   a. NG tube stomach decompression and urinary bladder catheterization
   b. Orogastric tube stomach decompression only
   c. NG tube stomach decompression only
   d. Urinary bladder catheterization only
   e. Orogastric tube stomach decompression and urinary bladder catheterization

7. A 4-year-old boy comes to the ED after being struck while on foot by an automobile moving at 20 mph. There was a questionable loss of consciousness at the scene. He arrives to the ED boarded and collared, crying, and fearful. His vital signs are: T 37.6°C, HR 130, RR 30, BP 94/64, and 0_2 saturation of 100% on 100% O_2. His examination is unremarkable except for diffuse abdominal tenderness to palpation and mild distension. After ensuring adequate airway, breathing, and circulation, which of the following is the most appropriate next step in management?

   a. Admit for inpatient observation
   b. Perform diagnostic peritoneal lavage (DPL)
   c. Perform urgent laparotomy
   d. Obtain abdominal CT
   e. Obtain abdominal ultrasound (U/S)

8. A 12-year-old bicyclist comes to the ED after being struck by a car. His vital signs are stable and his GCS score is 15. His examination is normal except for some bruising and mild tenderness of his upper abdomen. His CXR, pelvis films, and C-spine series are normal. You decide to further image this child's abdomen. Which of the following is the best radiographic study to perform and why?

   a. Abdominal CT with IV contrast, due to its high sensitivity for pancreatic injury
   b. Abdominal CT without IV contrast, due to its high sensitivity for pancreatic injury
   c. Abdominal CT with IV contrast, due to its high sensitivity for hepatic injury
   d. Abdominal CT without IV contrast, due to its high sensitivity for hepatic injury
   e. Abdominal U/S, due to its high sensitivity for the detection of intraperitoneal fluid in children

9. A 9-year-old female unrestrained passenger comes to the ED after a severe automobile collision. Upon presentation, her vital signs include a pulse of 150, RR 30 and shallow, and BP 70/40. Her right pupil is fixed and dilated, whereas her left pupil is reactive to 3 mm. She requires immediate craniotomy and there is not sufficient time to obtain an abdominal CT. You consider performing diagnostic peritoneal lavage (DPL). Which of the following is true?

   a. DPL should be performed through a supraumbilical incision
   b. DPL has a low sensitivity for the detection of small amounts of blood
   c. DPL should be performed before the placement of an NG tube and urinary bladder catheter
   d. DPL does not affect subsequent physical examination findings
   e. DPL should be performed with 20 ml/kg of lactated Ringer's, instilled into the peritoneal cavity over a 10-minute period

10. Which of the following clinical scenarios is NOT an indication for immediate laparotomy?

    a. A 17-year-old restrained passenger with evidence of pneumoperitoneum on plain film
    b. A 15-year-old unrestrained driver with persistent and significant hemodynamic instability and with evidence of abdominal injury
    c. A 12-year-old with a gunshot wound to the abdomen
    d. A 14-year-old with stab wound to the back
    e. A 5-year-old struck by car with abdominal distension associated with persistent hypotension

11. A 10-year-old boy pedestrian was struck by a motor vehicle traveling at high speed. His vital signs at presentation to the ED are: HR 140, RR 28, and BP 80/35. He is alert and is complaining of abdominal pain. His abdomen is distended and is covered with abrasions and ecchymoses. Which of the following injuries would be most likely associated with a fatal outcome for this patient?

    a. Splenic
    b. Gastric
    c. Intestinal
    d. Hepatic
    e. Pancreatic

12. An 8-year-old boy comes to the ED with epigastric abdominal pain 1 week after falling onto the handlebars of his bicycle. His vital signs are stable and his abdominal examination is remarkable for midepigastric tenderness and a palpable mass in this area. Which of the following is true regarding this injury in childhood abdominal trauma?

    a. It is usually not apparent on initial CT scan
    b. It almost always presents with epigastric pain, palpable abdominal mass, and laboratory abnormalities
    c. It is unlikely in the absence of laboratory abnormalities
    d. It usually has a spontaneous resolution of 50%
    e. It requires internal surgical drainage once it has persisted beyond 4 weeks

13. A 15-year-old restrained driver comes to the ED after a high-speed motor vehicle accident that occurred 1 day prior. He rapidly decelerated from a speed of 75 mph to avoid collision. He had no loss of consciousness (LOC) at the scene. His vital signs are stable in the ED, but he has a fever of 38.6°C and diffuse abdominal pain. The diagnosis is usually made with:

    a. Plain abdominal radiograph
    b. Abdominal U/S
    c. Abdominal CT
    d. DPL
    e. Laparotomy

14. A 4-year-old boy comes to the ED with epigastric abdominal pain and distension associated with bilious emesis. Further history informs you that the child was kicked in the abdomen by his older brother approximately 2 weeks ago. Which of the following is the most likely diagnosis?

    a. Pancreatic pseudocyst
    b. Hematobilia
    c. Duodenal hematoma
    d. Splenic laceration
    e. Bowel perforation

15. A 16-year-old girl comes to the ED with right-sided abdominal pain and hematemesis 2 days after a motor vehicle accident. She was an unrestrained back seat passenger in a high-speed motor vehicle accident. She states that she only had mild abdominal pain and did not seek medical attention at the time of the accident. Which of the following is the most likely diagnosis?

    a. Pancreatic pseudocyst
    b. Hematobilia
    c. Duodenal hematoma
    d. Splenic laceration
    e. Bowel perforation

16. A 15-year-old male is brought to the ED by the EMTs after being stabbed in the midabdomen. Which of the following organs is most likely to have sustained an injury?

    a. The bowel
    b. The stomach
    c. The liver
    d. The spleen
    e. The urinary bladder

17. A 10-year-old girl is brought to the ED immediately after being shot in the abdomen. She is alert with a GCS score of 15. Her vital signs are: T 37.9°C, HR 120, RR 25, and BP 90/65. Her examination is normal except for an entrance wound in the left lower quadrant of the abdomen. The bleeding is controlled. Which of the following is the next appropriate step in patient management?

    a. DPL
    b. Abdominal CT
    c. Local exploration
    d. Laparotomy
    e. Antibiotics and observation

18. A 17-year-old boy comes to the ED with a stab wound by a penknife to the abdomen. His vital signs are: HR 90, RR 20, and BP 100/70. His abdominal examination is remarkable for a 1-cm wound 2 cm to the left of the umbilicus. He does not have abdominal tenderness or distension. His rectal examination is heme negative. KUB is negative. Which of the following is the next appropriate step in patient management?

    a. Abdominal U/S
    b. Abdominal CT
    c. Local exploration
    d. Laparotomy
    e. Antibiotics and observation

19. A 4-year-old boy restrained back-seat passenger comes to the ED after a high-speed automobile accident. On examination, his vital signs are stable. His abdominal exam reveals ecchymosis in the pattern of a belt. Which of the following is true regarding this type of injury in children?

    a. He is at risk for a Chance fracture
    b. He has a 75% risk of an intra-abdominal injury
    c. A normal abdominal CT scan excludes ruptured viscus
    d. Lumbosacral (L-S) spine radiographs are not necessary if abdominal CT is normal
    e. Intra-abdominal injury is unlikely if urine analysis is normal

ANSWERS

1. a Trauma causes approximately 70% of deaths from age 5 to 19 years with head and thoracic injuries accounting for the majority. Abdominal injuries occur in 20% of children with fatal polytrauma and abdominal trauma is the most common unrecognized cause of fatal injuries.

2. e Although abdominal distension may be due to hemoperitoneum or peritonitis, the abdominal distension in this patient is most likely due to air swallowed by crying. The history of the injury is benign and he has no other concerning findings on abdominal or rectal examination.

3. d Blood at the urethral meatus, a boggy or high-riding prostate, or a distended bladder may be seen with urethral disruption and a retrograde urethrogram should be performed to rule this out. A Foley catheter should not be inserted if disruption of the urethra is suspected. Pelvic U/S, pelvic CT, or IVP are not helpful in the diagnosis of urethral disruption.

4. b Screening for intra-abominal injuries by evaluating transaminase levels (alanine aminotransferase [ALT] and aspartate aminotransferase [AST]) is not universally accepted because sensitivity and specificity of testing varies widely in the literature. Markedly elevated transaminase levels (AST greater than 450 U/l and ALT greater than 250 U/l) correlate well with hepatic injuries, however, and the evaluation of these patients should include abdominal CT. Hyperamylasemia is sometimes present with pancreatic injury, but its absence does not exclude injury. ABG determinations are helpful in the evaluation of pulmonary injuries and may indicate metabolic acidosis when volume resuscitation is not adequate. A decreasing hematocrit on serial determinations suggests ongoing blood loss.

5. b This patient is in hemorrhagic shock. This is treated with the infusion of isotonic crystalloid solution of either LR or NS, starting at 20 ml/kg, per ATLS protocol. More fluid may be needed, however, if the patient does not respond to the initial IV bolus. As the crystalloid solution is infusing, one should also consider obtaining O-negative blood for transfusion.

6. e The abdomen in this child is becoming distended and needs to be decompressed. Any patient with maxillofacial trauma should have an orogastric tube placed, not an NG tube. Catheterization of the urinary bladder helps monitor urine output and may provide evidence of genitourinary system injury. If urethral disruption is suspected, however, bladder catheterization is contraindicated.

7. d The child in this vignette has diffuse abdominal tenderness and mild distension. Abdominal imaging with CT scan is indicated when there is any suspicion for intraabdominal injuries. Abdominal U/S is used readily in the adult population as a screening modality in abdominal trauma. In children, however, the primary and more sensitive imaging modality is CT. The primary indication for DPL in children is on an urgent "need to know" basis (e.g., if the child is hemodynamically unstable or requires immediate craniotomy).

8. c The child with abdominal trauma who is stable yet warrants further imaging is best evaluated with CT using intravenous contrast. However, abdominal CT has its lowest sensitivity for pancreatic injury and small intestinal perforations. The sensitivity for liver and splenic lacerations is high, however.

9. a DPL is not frequently performed on children with abdominal trauma; however, there are some situations that warrant it (i.e., a child who is hemodynamically unstable or who requires immediate craniotomy). DPL is often too sensitive in children. The technique in children involves a small supraumbilical incision in order to avoid the bladder. A nasogastric tube and urinary bladder catheter should be in place prior to performing the DPL. Lactated Ringer's (10 ml/kg with a maximum volume of 1 l) is instilled into the peritoneal cavity over 10 minutes and is then removed for analysis. After DPL, physical examination findings are affected because the procedure causes peritoneal irritation.

10. d Indications for immediate laparotomy in children with abdominal trauma are: multisystem injuries, with indications for craniotomy in the presence of a positive DPL or free peritoneal fluid on ultrasound; persistent and significant hemodynamic instability in the presence of abdominal injury; penetrating wounds to the abdomen; pneumoperitoneum; or significant abdominal distension associated with hypotension. A stab wound to the back in a patient with stable vital signs is not an indication for immediate laparotomy, although the wound should be fully explored.

11. d Blunt liver trauma is the most common fatal abdominal injury in children. The other choices less readily result in mortality.

12. a Blunt abdominal injury, particularly from bicycle handlebars, is the most common cause of pancreatic pseudocyst formation in children. Abdominal U/S and CT are used to diagnose pseudocysts, although the original CT at the time of the injury usually does not detect the acute pancreatic injury. The classic triad of epigastric pain, a palpable abdominal mass, and hyperamylasemia is very rare in children and usually develops slowly. The absence of hyperamylasemia does not rule out pancreatic trauma because an elevated amylase is detected in 16–80% of cases of pancreatic injury. Nonoperative management is usually used for children with pancreatic pseudocyst caused by blunt trauma. Spontaneous resolution occurs in approximately 25% of children. Surgical internal drainage is performed once a pseudocyst has persisted beyond 6 weeks.

13. e Most bowel perforations and transections are found at laparotomy, which is usually performed due to advancing peritonitis or unexplained persistent fever. Plain abdominal radiographs, U/S, and CT are not particularly sensitive for diagnosing bowel perforation. Although DPL may demonstrate amylase in the peritoneal fluid, the diagnosis of the majority of perforations will be made at laparotomy.

14. c Duodenal hematomas are an uncommon injury that result from a direct blow to the epigastrum or from rapid deceleration and may cause either partial or complete bowel obstruction. Bleeding into the duodenal wall causes compression and symptoms of intestinal obstruction (e.g., pain, gastric distension, and bilious vomiting). Although pancreatic pseudocysts and hematobilia are also late presentations of abdominal trauma, they do not present in this fashion. Splenic lacerations and bowel perforations would have an earlier presentation.

15. b Hematobilia is a result of pressure necrosis from an intrahepatic hematoma or direct injury to the biliary tree. Children with hematobilia present several days after the abdominal trauma with abdominal pain and upper GI bleeding. Pancreatic pseudocysts and duodenal hematomas do not present with hematemesis. Splenic lacerations and bowel perforations would present with earlier symptoms. Hematemesis in these entities would also be unlikely.

16. a Intra-abdominal organs are at risk for penetrating trauma, depending on their size and location. The small bowel and colon are large in volume and are the most commonly injured structures, followed by the liver, spleen, and major vessels.

17. d Laparotomy is mandated in all gunshot wounds to the abdomen. Broad-spectrum antibiotics (e.g., ampicillin, gentamicin, and clindamycin) should be used prophylactically; however, the patient should not be solely observed without operative intervention. Imaging is not necessary because the patient requires laparotomy: Imaging will only delay treatment. Local exploration is not justified in gunshot wounds to the abdomen.

18. c Local exploration in minor stab wounds is necessary to determine if penetration of the peritoneum has occurred. Anterior stab wounds should be explored by laparotomy if there is hemodynamic instability or signs of peritonitis. This patient is hemodynamically stable with a benign abdominal examination. Abdominal U/S or CT will not show the extent of the injury. Inpatient observation is not necessary if the wound is explored in the ED and found not to penetrate the peritoneum.

19. a Children who are restrained only by lap belts in automobiles involved in rapid deceleration crashes are at risk to suffer Chance fractures, which are compression or flexion-distraction fractures of the lumbar spine, in association with intra-abdominal injuries (the lap-belt complex). As many as one-half of children with Chance fractures will have intra-abdominal injuries. The hallmark indicator of the lap-belt complex is abdominal or flank ecchymosis in the pattern of a belt or strap. A normal abdominal CT does not exclude ruptured viscus. L-S spine films are necessary to rule out Chance fractures even if the abdominal CT is normal.

CHAPTER **109**

Genitourinary Trauma

VINCENT J. WANG, M.D.

QUESTIONS

1. A 12-year-old girl is brought to the ED after being struck by an slowly moving car. She is alert and cooperative on presentation. Her vital signs and examination are normal except for mild abrasions over her back. She has no contusions or abrasions over her perineum. However, her urinalysis reveals microscopic hematuria of 30 RBCs per high-power field (hpf). Appropriate management/evaluation includes:

   a. Discharge and outpatient follow-up
   b. Repeat urinalysis (UA) in an hour
   c. Diagnostic peritoneal lavage (DPL)
   d. Abdominal CT scan
   e. Exploratory laparotomy

2. A 16-year-old boy is brought to your hospital as a passenger in a high-speed motor vehicle accident. He is initially alert and complains of chest pain. He is tachycardic and hypotensive. His CXR reveals a slightly widened mediastinum and a hemothorax. He has diminished femoral pulses. He has microscopic hematuria of 30 RBCs/hpf. A chest tube is placed, and the cardiothoracic surgeons wish to do a thoracotomy in the operating room as soon as possible. A DPL is negative. Which of the following is indicated before this patient is transferred to the OR?

   a. Abdominal CT scan
   b. Radionuclide imaging
   c. Intravenous pyelogram (IVP)
   d. Angiography
   e. No further studies are needed

3. A 6-year-old boy was a restrained passenger (wearing a seat belt) in a low-speed motor vehicle accident. There was minimal damage to the car. No one else was injured. The patient is brought to you immediately after the accident. On examination, he is tachycardic, but his blood pressure is normal. He has mild right flank tenderness, but no other tenderness. His urine is significant for gross hematuria. CT imaging is likely to reveal:

   a. Splenic rupture
   b. A vascular pedicle injury
   c. Renal vascular injury with contained hemorrhage
   d. Avulsion of the renal hilum
   e. Wilm's tumor

4. A 12-year-old boy is brought to your ED seizing after a four-story fall. He has been intubated and paralyzed. He has required multiple IV fluid boluses and remains hypotensive. Upon examination, you note a flank hematoma and a palpable flank mass on the right. His urine microscopy, however, shows an RBC count of 0 per high-power field (hpf). As an isolated injury, you suspect the following etiology:

   a. Vascular pedicle injury
   b. Parenchymal contusion of the kidney
   c. Ruptured bladder
   d. Transection of the right ureter
   e. Wilm's tumor

5. A 12-year-old boy was injured in a motor vehicular accident. He initially appears stable. Which of the following test results mandates further renal evaluation?

   a. Cervical spine (C-spine) films suggesting rotatory subluxation
   b. CXR demonstrating a pneumothorax
   c. Urine microscopy with 10 RBCs/hpf
   d. Pelvic films showing a pelvic fracture
   e. Femur films showing a femur fracture

6. In a patient originally suspected to have an isolated ureteral injury, which of the following CONTRADICTS that diagnosis?

   a. CT scan demonstrating no injury
   b. IVP demonstrating no injury
   c. Normal urinalysis
   d. An enlarging flank mass over the hospital course
   e. Hypotension over the hospital course

7. A 12-year-old boy is involved in a skiing accident. He had collided with a tree branch, injuring his pelvis. He complains of not being able to void. On examination he has a palpable fluid wave in his abdomen, but he is normotensive and minimally tachycardic. Laboratory findings consistent with this diagnosis include:

   a. Elevated serum BUN
   b. Elevated serum creatinine
   c. Hyperammonemia
   d. Elevated hepatic transaminases
   e. Anemia

8. A 5-year-old boy is brought to the ED after falling onto the supporting bar frame of his bike. He complains of pain over his genitalia. His examination is normal, except for a penile shaft contusion and blood at the urethral meatus. The most helpful diagnostic test/maneuver for the suspected injury is:

   a. The ability to pass a Foley catheter
   b. CT scan
   c. Ultrasonography
   d. Retrograde urethrography
   e. Urinalysis

9. A 14-year-old boy complains of scrotal pain after being kicked in the scrotum while playing soccer. On examination, he has swelling over the right hemiscrotum and exquisite tenderness over the right testicle. Which test is most helpful?

   a. IVP
   b. CT scan
   c. Ultrasonography
   d. Retrograde urethrography
   e. Microscopic urinalysis

10. A 17-year-old boy complains of a scrotal injury after wrestling with his friend. He has a small ecchymosis of his scrotal sac, but no apparent testicular injury. Appropriate management includes:

    a. Ice packs and scrotal support
    b. Ultrasonography
    c. Retrograde urethrogram
    d. Operative surgical exploration
    e. Drainage of the ecchymosis under local anesthesia

11. A 3-year-old boy is brought to your ED after sustaining penile trauma from a toilet seat falling onto his penis while voiding. Appropriate management includes:

    a. Operative surgical exploration of the wound
    b. Supportive care and warm soaks
    c. Urethral catheterization until healed
    d. Placement of a suprapubic tube
    e. Antibiotics

12. A 6-year-old girl is brought to your ED after a straddle injury. She complains of significant pain and bleeding from her vaginal area. The examination is difficult because of pain and anxiety. From your limited examination, she has a laceration of her perineum, extending to the vaginal wall. Appropriate management includes:

    a. Operative surgical exploration of the wound
    b. Supportive care and warm soaks
    c. Voiding into a tub of warm water and sitz baths
    d. Urethral catheterization until healed
    e. Laceration repair under local anesthesia

ANSWERS

1. d Hematuria of 20–30 RBCs/hpf warrants further diagnostic imaging. Hematuria may result from an injury anywhere along the urinary tract, from the kidneys to the urethral orifice. In the absence of genitalia injury, however, external urethral injuries are not likely. A DPL does not exclude a retroperitoneal injury. Although the IVP has been the traditional modality, CT scan is the current study of choice in a stable patient. Operative intervention is not indicated in a stable patient.

2. c In the unstable patient requiring operative intervention for other injuries, the IVP will rapidly assess the overall integrity and functioning of the renal system, and is the currently recommended imaging modality for these patients. Abdominal ultrasound (U/S) may have some utility if it is readily available; however, its sensitivity in diagnosing renal injury is only 70%. Angiography has been replaced by the CT scan, but obtaining a CT scan would not be indicated in an unstable patient. Radionuclide imaging has no role in an unstable patient.

3. e Signs of significant renal injury with only minimal trauma suggests the presence of a pre-existing anomaly such as a Wilm's tumor, horseshoe kidney, pelvic kidney, or ureteropelvic junction obstruction. Each of the other diagnoses suggest an injury associated with a more significant traumatic mechanism.

4. a   The absence of hematuria does not exclude renal injuries. Hematuria may be absent in 30% of ureteral transections and in up to 50% of pedicle injuries. Given the significance of the fall, the presenting symptoms and signs, and the absence of hematuria, suspicion for a vascular pedicle injury should arise. Parenchymal contusions are likely to produce hematuria, but are unlikely to cause shock. A ruptured bladder would present with abdominal pain and extravasation of urine into the intraperitoneal cavity or into the extraperitoneal space, depending on where the laceration is located. This injury would be unlikely to cause shock, however. In addition, bladder injuries usually present with hematuria. Transection of the ureter would also be unlikely to produce shock, but it is often associated with other significant injuries that might cause significant circulatory compromise. Congenital renal anomalies or tumors should be suspected when the hematuria is out of proportion to the degree of injury.

5. d   The initial screening tests for patients sustaining trauma are helpful for guiding further evaluation of the patient. The presence of any abnormality should lead to a higher index of suspicion for other injuries. Abnormalities on C-spine films and CXRs do not necessarily suggest renal injury, however. A rib fracture or lower spine fracture may suggest renal injury. Urine microscopy with greater than 20–30 RBCs/hpf has been used as a threshold for further evaluation. A pelvic fracture, but not a femur fracture, would suggest possible renal injury.

6. d   Ureteral injuries are difficult to diagnose, with less than 50% diagnosed within 24 hours of presentation. The physical examination may be normal. However, an enlarging flank mass over the hospital course may suggest urinary extravasation. CT and IVP are helpful, but they have low sensitivity, detecting only 33% of injuries. Hematuria may be absent in up to 30% of cases. Hypotension in this setting is indicative of ongoing blood loss, but it does not necessarily suggest ureteral injury.

7. a   Intraperitoneal bladder ruptures are associated with a palpable fluid wave in the peritoneal cavity and with elevated levels of blood urea nitrogen (BUN) because of rapid peritoneal reabsorption of urea. An elevated serum creatinine level suggests intrinsic renal pathology. Hyperammonemia would be expected with defects of the urea cycle. Elevated hepatic transaminases would be seen in hepatic injury. Anemia might be present with shock, but it may be absent early in the course.

8. d   Retrograde urethrography is the test of choice for diagnosing a urethral injury. Passing a Foley catheter is contraindicated in patients with suspected urethral trauma because of the possibility of converting a partial urethral tear into a complete transection. A CT scan and ultrasonography are not adequate. Hematuria is associated with an injury anywhere along the upper and lower urinary tract and would not adequately assess this patient's urethra.

9. c   Ultrasonography is the test of choice for diagnosing a testicular injury. If the sonogram is equivocal, radionuclide scanning may be helpful.

10. a   With minor isolated injuries of the scrotal sac, ice packs and scrotal support are sufficient. Ultrasonography is helpful for diagnosing testicular injuries, but this is not indicated here. Retrograde urethrogram will help with urethral injuries. Surgical exploration is indicated when there are large testicular hematomas or the possibility of testicular rupture. Drainage is not indicated.

11. b   Blunt penile trauma from this mechanism has been reported. If the history does not match the injury, however, sexual abuse should be considered. Supportive care and warm soaks are indicated for this injury. There is no role for the other interventions.

12. a   Given this scenario, the patient has a significant laceration. A laceration involving deeper structures may be revealed with an optimal examination. The patient should be examined under anesthesia and repaired in the operating room. Warm soaks and sitz baths are indicated for minor abrasions or lacerations. Voiding into a tub of warm water may help alleviate pain associated with minor injuries. Urethral catheterization is contraindicated now because an inadequate examination has been performed and the possibility of urethral injury has not been eliminated.

CHAPTER 110

Facial Trauma

RON L. KAPLAN, M.D.

QUESTIONS

The following case relates to Questions 1 and 2: A 10-year-old boy falls off his bike, striking his chin on a gravel driveway. He has a 1-cm-deep laceration with several centimeters of surrounding abrasion with particulate matter embedded in the skin. He has difficulty opening his mouth and decreased sensation of the lower lip.

1. You suspect:
   a. Fracture of the angle of the mandible
   b. Bilateral subcondylar fractures
   c. Parasymphyseal fracture and contralateral subcondylar fracture
   d. Parasymphyseal fracture and ipsilateral subcondylar fracture
   e. Injury to the marginal mandibular branch of the facial nerve

2. If mandibular fractures are not present, which statement regarding wound care is true?
   a. Removal of particulate matter with a scalpel blade may be necessary
   b. Lidocaine with epinephrine should not be used for anesthesia
   c. Topical antibiotics are indicated to prevent infection
   d. The laceration should be left open and repaired with delayed primary closure
   e. The patient should receive IV antibiotics, followed by oral antibiotics as an outpatient

3. A 16-year-old boy is hit in the eye by a line drive at a baseball game. He has limitation of upward gaze on the left. Which additional finding would be most likely?
   a. Enophthalmos
   b. Exophthalmos
   c. Orbital dystopia
   d. Decreased sensation of the ipsilateral forehead
   e. Decreased sensation of the ipsilateral cheek

4. Which finding would indicate the need for urgent surgical consultation for the patient in Question 3?
   a. Enophthalmos
   b. Exophthalmos
   c. Orbital dystopia
   d. Inability to gaze upward fully
   e. Hyphema

5. A 5-year-old girl is running through the house when she gets hit in the nose by a swinging door. She has moderate swelling and tenderness of the nose. Which statement is true?
   a. Nasal x-rays are unnecessary because fractures will be clinically evident
   b. Nasal x-rays should be obtained immediately
   c. Septal hematoma is an uncommon minor complication
   d. CT scan should be obtained
   e. She may be discharged with reevaluation in 2–3 days

The following case relates to Questions 6–8: A 17-year-old involved in a motor-vehicle accident hit his face on the dashboard.

6. Which finding would be consistent with a complete fracture of the zygoma?
   a. Orbital dystopia
   b. Exophthalmos
   c. Decreased sensation along the distribution of the buccal nerve
   d. Superior displacement of the zygoma
   e. Difficulty closing the mouth

7. The patient has loss of anterior projection of the nose on lateral view, rounding of the medial canthi, and increased intercanthal distance. Extraocular muscles are intact. There is no orbital dystopia, and he is able to open and close his mouth without difficulty. What is the most likely diagnosis?

   a. LeFort I fracture
   b. LeFort II fracture
   c. LeFort III fracture
   d. Orbital blowout fracture
   e. Naso-orbito-ethmoid fracture

8. Which diagnostic procedure is most likely to confirm a diagnosis?

   a. Sinus x-rays
   b. Panorex x-rays
   c. CT scan
   d. Lateral facial x-rays
   e. Water's view x-rays

9. A 6-year-old girl comes to the ED with a deep laceration of the cheek. Which finding might you expect that would indicate the need for further evaluation?

   a. Decreased sensation along the distribution of the frontal branch of the facial nerve
   b. Excessive tearing
   c. Upward pull of the corner of the mouth on the affected side
   d. Clear fluid from Stenson's duct with parotid massage
   e. Decreased smile on the affected side

ANSWERS

1. c A fall on the chin is likely to result in a fracture anteriorly near the mandibular symphysis, and there is often an associated fracture in the opposite subcondylar region. The mental nerve exits the mental foramen, which is an anterior opening in the mandible on a common vertical line with the second premolars. Injury to this nerve results in anesthesia to the lower lips and lower incisors. The marginal mandibular branch of the facial nerve courses 1–2 cm below the border of the mandible and is responsible for depression of the corners of the mouth.

2. a After local anesthesia, vigorous cleansing of the wound is the most important step in preventing wound infection. Lidocaine with epinephrine is indicated unless there is concern for tissue viability or in end-arterial systems such as the earlobe or tip of the nose. Debridement may require vigorous scrubbing and removal of particulate matter with a scalpel blade. The laceration may then be repaired. If an open mandibular fracture is not present, IV antibiotics are not necessary.

3. e The infraorbital nerve exits the maxilla just below the orbital rim and may be injured with fractures of the orbital floor. This leads to decreased sensation of the cheek, upper lip, and upper gums on the affected side. An acute increase in the orbital space occurs due to disruption of the orbital floor. This may lead to enophthalmos, or a sunken-in appearance to the globe, and orbital dystopia, or asymmetry in the horizontal level of the two eyes. Both of these findings may not be present acutely due to the presence of periorbital edema, but usually become apparent within 5–7 days.

4. d Inability to fully gaze upward indicates entrapment of the inferior rectus in the fracture gap in the floor of the orbit. This is an indication for immediate surgical consultation.

5. e Nasal x-rays contribute little to the acute management of nasal fractures. Fractures may be difficult to detect clinically because of marked swelling. If no other injuries are present, the patient can be discharged with ENT evaluation in 2–3 days when the swelling has subsided. If a septal hematoma is not identified and treated promptly, cartilage necrosis and septal perforation may occur.

6. a A complete fracture of the zygoma results from fractures at the zygomaticofrontal, zygomaticotemporal, and zygomaticomaxillary regions. Attachment of the masseter muscle to the zygoma results in its downward displacement. The increase in apparent orbital volume leads to enophthalmos and orbital dystopia. Impingement on the mandibular condyle may cause difficulty opening the mouth. Decreased sensation along the distribution of the infraorbital nerve may be seen.

7. e   Loss of anterior projection of the nose on lateral view and traumatic telecanthus are characteristic of naso-orbito-ethmoid fractures, which involve complete separation of the nasal bones and medial walls of the orbits from the frontal bone. Separation of the nasal and orbital bones allows the medial palpebral ligaments to drift laterally, producing rounding of the medial canthi and increased intercanthal distance. LeFort I fractures extend through the zygomaticomaxillary region separating the maxilla from its attachments. The LeFort II fracture extends more superiorly to the infraorbital rims and across the nasofrontal sutures. The LeFort III pattern, also known as *craniofacial dissociation,* extends across the zygomatic arch, zygomaticofrontal region, floor of the orbit, and nasofrontal sutures, separating the facial bones from the skull base. Fractures of the floor of the orbit, otherwise known as *orbital blowout fractures,* are associated with enophthalmos and orbital dystopia that may not be present acutely due to the presence of periorbital edema. Other findings may include decreased sensation in the distribution of the infraorbital nerve and limitation of extraocular movements if muscles become entrapped in the fracture gap.

8. c   CT scan is the procedure of choice for diagnosis of most bony facial fractures. Panorex views are useful in diagnosing mandibular fractures and also give information about tooth root anatomy and condylar position. Sinus films may show opacification of the maxillary sinuses when orbital floor fractures cause blood and fat to sink into the maxillary sinuses. Lateral facial views provide some information about the mandible on that side and the nasal bones. The Water's view is useful for viewing the orbital rims and maxillary sinuses.

9. e   Deep cheek lacerations must be examined carefully for evidence of injury to deeper vascular, neural, and glandular structures. Injury to the buccal nerve produces decreased ability to smile on the affected side. Injury to the parotid duct is evaluated by massaging the parotid gland and observing the expression of fluid from Stenson's duct. Clear fluid suggests an uninjured duct. Absence of fluid or bloody fluid suggests injury to the gland or duct. Injury to the frontal branch of the facial nerve may be seen with lacerations of the lateral periorbital region. Excessive tearing associated with lacerations of the medial periorbital region suggests lacrimal duct injury.

CHAPTER **111**

Eye Trauma

CYNTHIA JOHNSON MOLLEN, M.D.

QUESTIONS

1. A 5-year-old boy is brought to the ED after a softball struck him in the eye. He is holding his hand over his eye and is resistant to being examined. You can see ecchymoses over the superior ridge of the orbit. When he moves his hand there is significant swelling, and an almost 360-degree subconjunctival hemorrhage is visible. Your next step should be:

   a. Anesthetic eye drops to allow for a more comfortable, thorough examination
   b. Placement of a patch and ophthalmology consultation
   c. Placement of an IV for antibiotic therapy
   d. Placement of a shield and ophthalmology consultation
   e. Further examination using the direct ophthalmoscope

2. A 2-year-old boy was unintentionally hit in the eye by a baseball bat being carried by his 5-year-old brother. He has pulsating proptosis of his right eye, and is unable to look down. His most likely injury is a(n):

   a. Corneal abrasion
   b. Inferior wall orbital fracture
   c. Ruptured globe
   d. Traumatic iritis
   e. Superior wall orbital fracture

3. A 7-year-old boy was involved in a playground fight in which several children threw handfuls of gravel and sticks at each other. He is brought to the ED because of a 2-cm-deep laceration to his eyelid. Management of this injury involves:

   a. 2-octyl cyanoacrylate topical skin adhesive (Dermabond) closure
   b. Two-layer closure of the laceration
   c. No treatment because suturing is contraindicated
   d. Single-layer closure of the laceration
   e. Staple closure

4. Upon further examination of the patient in Question 3, it is noted that his left pupil has an irregular shape. This physical finding raises suspicion for which ocular injury?

   a. Hyphema
   b. Ruptured globe
   c. Corneal abrasion
   d. Traumatic iritis
   e. Blowout fracture

5. A 10-year-old girl complains of right eye pain. She was experimenting with her mother's eye makeup when she began complaining of pain in her right eye. Initial examination demonstrates a normal periorbital area, with redness of the conjunctiva. She is in too much pain to allow further examination. The next step in her evaluation should be:

   a. Instillation of a topical anesthetic
   b. Forced examination of the eye using a retractor
   c. Referral to ophthalmology
   d. Placement of IV for antibiotics
   e. Discharge home with warm compresses

6. Fluorescein staining of the patient in Question 5 reveals an abrasion near the center of the cornea. Treatment may include all of the following, EXCEPT:

   a. Gentamicin ointment
   b. Cycloplegic drops
   c. Steroid-containing drops
   d. Ophthalmologic exam in 24 hours
   e. Pressure patch over the eye

7. A 9-year-old boy was helping his mother in the grocery store. While reaching up for a can of corn, several other cans fell from the shelf. He is brought to the ED with periorbital swelling and ecchymosis. Further examination demonstrates a round, reactive pupil; a small subconjunctival hemorrhage; and a large amount of blood in the anterior chamber of the eye. Within the next week, the complication that poses the greatest risk to the patient is:

   a. Permanent loss of vision
   b. Rebleeding
   c. Glaucoma
   d. Secondary infection
   e. Persistent periorbital ecchymosis

8. A 6-year-old outfielder is brought to the ED the day after being hit in the left eye with a softball. She is complaining of severe pain. It is difficult for her to tolerate evaluation with the direct ophthalmoscope because of discomfort. You note that the pupil of the left eye is more constricted than the right. Her most likely diagnosis is:

   a. Ruptured globe
   b. Corneal abrasion
   c. Blowout fracture
   d. Hyphema
   e. Traumatic iritis

9. A 12-year-old boy is brought to the ED by his mother, who states that he has been unable to see since he was a passenger in a motor-vehicle accident earlier that day. He sustained a blow to his head during the accident. In the ED, he is unable to write his name when given a paper and pen. His red reflex and direct ophthalmoscope exams are unremarkable. He has a large contusion of his occiput. You suspect:

   a. Feigned visual loss
   b. Transient cortical blindness
   c. Retinal detachment
   d. Traumatic cataract
   e. Optic nerve injury

ANSWERS

1. **d** The patient is at high risk for a ruptured globe, given the mechanism of injury and the presence of a 360-degree subconjunctival hemorrhage, which is often associated with a ruptured globe. If a ruptured globe is suspected, eye drops should never be instilled, and a patch should never be applied. Both interventions could worsen the injury. Instead, a plastic shield should be placed over the eye, with the rim making contact only with the bony surfaces of the orbit. Even though broad-spectrum antibiotics are indicated, agitation from IV placement may worsen the injury; therefore, this procedure may be performed after the ophthalmologic examination. Finally, further examination is not necessary by the ED physician because enough evidence exists that this patient may have a ruptured globe.

2. **e** The mechanism and physical findings are most consistent with a blowout fracture of the superior ridge of the orbit. This injury often results in "pulsating proptosis" because of communication between the orbit and the intracranial cavity. The hallmark of blowout fractures is decreased extraocular movement because of entrapment of a nerve in the fracture. When this occurs, the patient cannot look away from the fracture. At times, hemorrhage may displace the eye away from the fracture and restrict the patient's ability to look toward the fracture, although this is less common. This patient is at risk for a ruptured globe, but the physical findings present are not consistent with this injury.

3. **d** Lacerations of the superficial eyelid can be managed by standard skin closure techniques: Single-layer closure is best in this case. Deep sutures are not recommended because they may result in a cicatrical eversion of the lid margin. Skin adhesive is not ideal given the risk of ocular exposure. Staples are not indicated in the face.

4. **b** Patients with eyelid lacerations may have several associated injuries. In this case, the irregular shape of the pupil, often in the shape of a teardrop, suggests a ruptured globe. Immediately after disruption of the globe a small amount of choroid plugs the wound. Because of this movement, the pupil becomes

disrupted, with the narrowest segment pointing toward the rupture. It is important to remember to examine the eye fully after trauma, even if the injury seems to be minor.

5. a   The history suggests the patient may have a corneal abrasion and/or a foreign body. If a superficial injury is suspected, use of a topical anesthetic can be diagnostic—the pain will be relieved if the injury is confined to the ocular surface. Her mechanism of injury is not concerning for more severe injuries, so immediate referral to ophthalmology is not required. There is no indication for antibiotics in this scenario. Further examination is necessary before discharge, but there is no need to examine the patient forcefully when anesthetic drops are safe and may make the exam easier.

6. c   An antibiotic ointment (not containing neomycin) can be used for 2–3 days for comfort and to prevent infection. Some studies suggest that patching does not accelerate healing, especially for small abrasions; however, many physicians still prefer to patch the affected eye for 24 hours. Use of cycloplegic drops should be limited to the ED. These may be used to relax of the ciliary muscle to relieve spasm, making the patient more comfortable. Ophthalmologic evaluation is recommended for patients with large abrasions, those with abrasions involving the visual axis, or those in whom pain persists after 24 hours. Steroid drops should never be used by the emergency physician.

7. b   This patient has a hyphema. Such patients have a vulnerable period 3–5 days after the injury when spontaneous rebleeding can occur. Patients with hemoglobinopathies are at particular risk, so all patients in high-risk ethnic groups should be tested. Glaucoma is a late complication, and is unlikely to manifest in the first week. Even though visual loss can be a complication of hyphema, the larger the hyphema the smaller the risk; therefore, this is not the primary concern for this patient. Finally, periorbital ecchymoses are likely to persist for several weeks; this is expected and requires no treatment.

8. e   Even though this patient is at risk for several different injuries because of the mechanism, the constellation of symptoms, as well as the time of presentation, suggests a traumatic iritis. Such patients often present 24–72 hours after the injury and have severe pain, photophobia, a red eye, and occasionally vision loss. Careful evaluation should be performed in the ED to exclude other injuries, but this patient requires slit-lamp examination by an ophthalmologist even if no other injuries are found.

9. a   Patients who are feigning visual loss will usually be unable to write their names; patients with true visual loss maintain this ability. Another test is to pass a checkered surface in front of the patient to check the optokinetic reflex; if the patient can see, they will reflexively follow the pattern as it passes over their field of vision. Transient cortical blindness is a consideration in this patient because it usually develops after occipital head trauma with an otherwise normal exam; however, this patient does not appear to have true blindness. The other selections will have associated abnormalities of the physical examination.

CHAPTER 112

Otolaryngologic Trauma

JEFFREY P. LOUIE, M.D.

QUESTIONS

1. A 3-year-old boy is brought to the ED with complaints of left ear pain. His mother thinks that he may have put a plastic bead into his ear recently. Otoscopic examination reveals a foreign body adjacent to the tympanic membrane and surrounded by cerumen. The most appropriate technique to remove this foreign body is:

   a. Attempt to scoop the bead out with a curette
   b. Dislodge the bead from the cerumen using an 18-gauge needle
   c. Use an alligator forceps to grab the bead
   d. Irrigate the ear to dislodge the foreign body
   e. Instill alcohol, then attempt removal with forceps

2. A 16-year-old girl comes to the ED after being assaulted by her father. She complains of right ear pain. On physical exam there is bruising of the pinna and tragus, a small amount of blood is noted in the external canal, and a perforated tympanic membrane is noted on otoscopic exam. All of the following are possible complications of this injury, EXCEPT:

   a. Vertigo
   b. Sensorineural hearing loss
   c. Facial nerve palsy
   d. Cholesteatoma
   e. Mastoiditis

3. A 7-year-old girl comes to the ED with significant nasal swelling after she was struck by a football thrown by her brother. Nasal bleeding was noted by the mother after the incident. Other than the obvious swelling, you note a small amount of lateral deviation as well as a palpable step-off. The remainder of the exam is normal. Which of the following should be done?

   a. Attempt manual reduction
   b. Immediate surgical consultation
   c. Discharge home with follow up in 4 days
   d. Obtain a full series of nasal radiographs
   e. Obtain a CT scan of the nose

4. A 16-year-old boy is brought to the ED by the police after an altercation in which he was struck in the nose. On examination, he has severe swelling externally. The left nostril is obstructed by bulging of the septum laterally. The right side shows some active bleeding posteriorly. You should do which of the following?

   a. Apply direct pressure
   b. Cauterize the area
   c. Drain immediately
   d. Place nasal packing
   e. Obtain nasal x-rays

5. A 3-year-old boy is brought to ED after falling with a popsicle stick in his mouth. He is crying and blood is noted in his mouth. The stick was recovered completely intact. On exam, a 1-cm horizontal laceration is noted along the posterior pharynx. What should be done next?

   a. Discharge the patient home on antibiotics
   b. Probe the wound for a foreign body
   c. Obtain a CT scan of the area
   d. Obtain soft tissue lateral x-ray of the neck
   e. Obtain an angiogram immediately

6. A 2-year-old girl comes to the ED after a choking spell. The patient admits to eating a carrot before the episode. The parents state the she has appeared well since the incident except for an occasional cough. She appears to be in no distress and her lung exam is normal. Formal chest radiographs (AP and lateral) appear normal. What should now be explained to the parents?

   a. Their daughter can be safely discharged home
   b. Their daughter will require antibiotics
   c. An invasive procedure will be required
   d. More x-rays will need to be done
   e. She will need to swallow contrast medium for an esophagogram

ANSWERS

1. d   Irrigation is the best option in this scenario. Other appropriate methods to remove an external canal foreign body are to use an ear curette, small alligator forceps, or even application of "Super glue" on the end of a wooden cotton swab. When a foreign object is adjacent to the tympanic membrane, however, irrigation is the preferred modality because there is less risk of traumatic injury to the eardrum. Alcohol should be instilled into the ear in cases where a live insect is present to kill the foreign invader prior to removal.

2. e   Mastoiditis is not associated with middle-ear trauma, but can be a complication of acute and chronic middle-ear infections. Vertigo, sensorineural hearing loss, and facial nerve palsy are possible complication of middle-ear trauma that require urgent otolaryngological evaluation. A cholesteatoma can arise secondary to traumatic perforation of the tympanic membrane when the edges of the membrane fold inward. If not removed, the cholesteatoma can invade the surrounding structures and spread into the intracranial cavity.

3. c   This patient has most likely sustained a nasal fracture. Immediate intervention is not needed and imaging studies will add little to the management. The most appropriate evaluation consists of ensuring that there is no septal hematoma or other injuries to facial structures. The patient should follow up with a surgeon within 7 days for possible reduction if there is still significant deformity after the swelling has subsided.

4. c   This patient has a septal hematoma. Septal hematomas are true emergencies that should be drained immediately. Complications can range from infection, necrosis of nasal cartilage, and the development of a saddle nose.

5. d   A soft-tissue injury of the neck should be assessed by lateral neck radiographs for the presence of air in the tissues of the posterior pharynx extending down the retropharyngeal space. Foreign bodies (e.g., a popsicle stick) may not show up on plain films; therefore, it should be determined if the object was removed intact, because surgical exploration may be required if there is suspicion that foreign material remains. Surgical consultation should be obtained in this case because the patient is at risk for serious vascular injury. An angiogram should be considered in this case; however, plain films should be done initially. A CT scan is not the study of choice (unless a foreign body is suspected). Probing the wound is contraindicated as this may precipitate bleeding.

6. d   The next radiographs that should be done (depending on the child's ability to cooperate) are left and right decubitus, or inspiratory and expiratory films to look for air trapping as a sign of foreign body aspiration. Given this patient's history, the threshold to consult an ear, nose, and throat (ENT) surgeon for bronchoscopy should be low irregardless of the radiographic results.

CHAPTER 113

Dental Trauma

VINCENT J. WANG, M.D.

QUESTIONS

1. A 2-year-old boy comes to the ED after injuring his mouth. He had tripped and fallen 2 hours ago. The mother said that he cried immediately, but she was alarmed when she saw blood in his mouth. On examination, you note a 4-mm superficial laceration of the left side of his tongue. His dentition is normal. He has no other injuries. Treatment involves:

   a. Copious irrigation with normal saline
   b. Closure with chromic gut sutures
   c. Closure with nylon sutures
   d. Panorex films of his mandible
   e. Observation without suture closure

2. An 11-year-old girl complains of tooth pain. She had tripped and hit her tooth on a chair yesterday. On examination, she has a fracture of the upper left incisor. The lower half of the visible tooth is fractured and avulsed, with bleeding from the central core of the tooth. There is no other dental trauma and the dentition is in normal position. Treatment includes:

   a. Analgesics and follow-up with the dentist tomorrow morning
   b. Analgesics, oral antibiotics, and follow-up with the dentist tomorrow morning
   c. Facial bone radiographs
   d. Emergency dental consultation that night
   e. Reassurance and follow-up with the dentist as needed

3. A 9-year-old boy fell and injured his upper incisors. On examination, he has tenderness to percussion of his left upper incisor. The incisor has minimal mobility, but no displacement. Treatment includes:

   a. Analgesics and follow-up with the dentist in the morning
   b. Saline rinses and oral antibiotics
   c. Emergency dental consultation that night
   d. Splinting of the upper teeth
   e. Tooth extraction

4. A 7-year-old girl with newly erupting upper incisors comes to the ED after sustaining oral trauma. She fell onto her mouth and complains of pain of her upper incisors. On examination, her incisors are minimally visible and you note swelling of the surrounding soft tissue. The mother thinks that the teeth are less visible than before. Immediate management includes:

   a. Obtaining Panorex films
   b. Obtaining a CT scan of her facial bones
   c. Extraction of the teeth
   d. Emergent pulpectomy
   e. Discharge and outpatient follow-up

5. A 3-year-old girl fell and injured her lower incisors. The mother reports that her tooth fell out approximately 15 minutes ago. On examination, you note minimal soft tissue injury, as well as an avulsed lower incisor with the tooth intact in the father's possession. Management at this point is:

   a. Placement of the tooth in milk until the dentist can reinsert the tooth
   b. Placement of the tooth in Frank's solution until the dentist can reinsert the tooth
   c. Emergency splinting
   d. Placement of the tooth in the socket in the ED
   e. Saline rinses and follow-up as needed

6. A 12-year-old boy has jaw pain and is unable to close his mouth. He had been undergoing a dental procedure, and has had to open his mouth for a prolonged period of time. After the procedure, he was unable to close his mouth. There is no history of trauma. Attempts by the dentist at reduction of what he thought was a mandibular dislocation failed. On your examination, he has no swelling or tenderness of the temporal mandibular joint. He is unable to close his mouth. Treatment includes:

a. Emergent consultation with the oral surgeon
b. Reduction by applying traction similar to the chin lift maneuver for airway compromise
c. Reduction by applying downward and backward pressure on the posterior teeth
d. Reduction by hyperextending the neck slowly over several minutes
e. Reduction by applying pressure behind the mandible in the anterior direction, one side at a time

7. A 2-year-old boy comes to the ED after biting on an electrical cord. He is alert and playful. On examination, you note erythema and minimal charring of the distal tip of his tongue. He has been able to drink without difficulty. Treatment includes:

a. Oral hygiene care and follow-up with a dentist in the morning
b. Serum coagulation studies
c. Antibiotics and an outpatient re-check in the morning
d. Debridement of the injured areas
e. Admission and IV hydration

ANSWERS

1. e   For minimal lacerations of the tongue, it is common practice not to suture these lacerations. These wounds heal well and provide no future cosmetic problems. Panorex films are indicated if there is dental trauma. Irrigation with normal saline or any other medium is difficult to perform in a 2-year-old child, who is likely to swallow the fluid. If the child were older, swishing and spitting with a saline solution would be an alternative to irrigation. Treatment in this child is likely to consist of drinking plenty of fluids and eating a soft diet until the wound heals.

2. d   Complicated tooth fractures involve the pulp of the tooth. This may be diagnosed by seeing bleeding from the central core of the fractured tooth. Dental pulpal treatment must be instituted within 24 hours of the injury to obtain optimal preservation of tooth viability. Because the injury occurred yesterday, emergency dental consultation would be indicated, rather than follow-up the following day. Facial bone radiographs are not necessary in the absence of other trauma.

3. a   Periodontal injuries may be divided into five categories: concussion, subluxation, intrusion, extrusion/lateral luxation, and avulsion. This patient sustained a concussion, with percussion tenderness, but no displacement or excessive mobility. Treatment is supportive; however, arrangements should be made for a dental follow-up visit to obtain baseline radiographs. There is no role for antibiotics.

4. a   Intrusion injuries are seen clinically as teeth that are displaced directly into the socket. The teeth are occasionally not visible, and they may give the false impression that the teeth are avulsed. A Panorex film of the dentition is necessary to evaluate this and to search for other injuries to the alveolar socket. Treatment of permanent teeth involves repositioning and splinting the teeth. Extraction is defined as removal of the teeth, and is not indicated. Pulpal treatment may be indicated at a later time if the pulp becomes nonvital, but this is not indicated emergently. A facial bone CT scan is not necessary because plain radiographs of the area are adequate.

5. e   Treatment for avulsed primary teeth is dental cleansing, analgesics, and outpatient follow-up. Timely replacement of secondary, or permanent teeth, is critical for viability. Replacement of the primary tooth in the socket, however, risks aspiration in this age group and may interfere with development of the secondary tooth. If it is uncertain if the tooth is primary or secondary, the tooth may be placed in Viaspan, Hanks' solution, or milk (best alternative solution) until the assessment can be made. Frank does not have a solution.

6. c   Mandibular dislocations may occur after prolonged, extreme mouth opening. Initial attempts with reassurance and gentle massage of the muscles of mastication should be made first. If this has failed, the

patient may be given a benzodiazepine for relaxation, and gentle downward and backward pressure should be applied to the occlusive surfaces of the posterior teeth. The clinician should be careful to wrap his/her thumbs with gauze or other padding to protect from accidental bite injuries during the procedure.

7. a Electrical burns of the mouth occur when children bite through an electrical cord, with the saliva acting as a conductor to complete the circuit. The initial assessment should be that of airway, breathing, and circulation. If stable and the symptoms are mild, as in this vignette, the patient requires meticulous oral hygiene and outpatient follow-up. A bland, soft diet is also recommended. If the patient is unable to take any food by mouth, admission for IV hydration is warranted. With severe burns of the lips or mouth, severe arterial bleeding may occasionally occur 5–8 days later. Admission may be warranted, or, if the patient is discharged, close follow-up should be guaranteed.

CHAPTER 114

Burns

ANDREA STRACCIOLINI, M.D.

QUESTIONS

1. A 2-year-old girl is brought to the ED with a burn covering the dorsum of her hand extending to the wrist. The mother explains that the child was sitting on her lap and spilled hot soup onto her hand and arm. On physical examination the burn is erythematous throughout with large ruptured bullae. The child cries when the burn is touched. She is able to move all of the fingers and the wrist. The neurovascular examination is normal. The correct classification for this burn is:

    a. First-degree/partial-thickness burn
    b. Second-degree/full-thickness burn
    c. Second-degree/partial-thickness burn
    d. Third-degree/partial-thickness burn
    e. Third-degree/full-thickness burn

2. Appropriate management of the burn described in Question 1 would include:

    a. Debridement of the ruptured bullae, sterile dressing, IV antibiotic therapy
    b. Sterile dressing without debridement, plastic surgery consult in the ED, systemic antibiotics
    c. Sterile dressing after debridement, follow up with PCP as needed, topical antibiotic ointment
    d. Sterile dressing after debridement, follow up in the ED the next day, topical antibiotic ointment
    e. Sterile dressing after debridement, follow up with plastic surgery in one week, file a child abuse report

3. An 18-month-old boy sustained a burn to the distal forearm after he brushed up against a hot iron about an hour ago. The burn is erythematous and tender. The parents of this child call you for advice regarding the initial care for this burn. You tell them to:

    a. Apply ice directly to the burn and then wrap the burn with clean gauze or cloth
    b. Apply petroleum jelly and wrap the burn with a clean cloth or gauze
    c. Run cool water over the injured area and then wrap the burn in a clean gauze
    d. Rupture all intact blisters and then wrap the burn in a clean gauze
    e. None of the above

4. A 4-year-old boy is brought to the ED after being involved in a house fire. He is awake and alert. From your initial assessment you note that he has burns over 20% of his body surface area (BSA), including his face. The initial care of this child should include:

    a. Primary assessment of ABCs, C-spine immobilization
    b. Care of the burns maintaining sterile technique
    c. Immediate intubation of the trachea
    d. IV access, systemic antibiotics
    e. IV morphine sulfate

5. A 2-year-old girl who was involved in a fire is brought to the ED by the EMTs. She has extensive burns over 30% of her body. She has no facial burns and her airway is patent. Her vital signs are: RR 28, HR 135, and BP 110/45. Her room air O_2 saturation is 99%. She is alert and moving all extremities. IV access is obtained. The correct initial fluid management for this patient is:

    a. NS bolus 40 ml/kg
    b. 20 ml/kg albumin bolus
    c. 20 ml/kg lactated Ringer's bolus
    d. ½ NS at maintenance
    e. Lactated Ringer's 4 ml/kg/%BSA burn

6. A 2-year-old is brought to the ED with a scald burn over his buttocks. The parents tell you that he went to sit in the bathtub and the hot water burned him. On physical examination you note second-degree burns over the buttocks. The child is well nourished and there are no other burns or signs of injury. The most important treatment for this child should include:

a. Tetanus immunoglobulin
b. IV antibiotics
c. 20 ml/kg NS bolus
d. Child abuse evaluation
e. Plastic surgery consult

7. An 18-month-old girl is brought to the ED by her parents. She was found chewing on an electrical cord from a lamp in the living room. She presents with burns to both corners of her mouth. She is most at risk for:

a. Severe arrhythmias including ventricular fibrillation and asystole
b. Infection of the wound
c. Bleeding from the labial artery in 1–2 weeks
d. Permanent damage to the facial nerve
e. None of the above

8. An 18-year-old boy spilled battery acid onto his right hand and forearm while fixing his car. On physical examination, you note scattered vesicles and bullae with surrounding erythema. He has full range of motion of the fingers and wrist and the pulses are strong. He has no other injuries. Correct treatment for this injury includes all of the following, EXCEPT:

a. Tetanus prophylaxis
b. Plastic surgery consultation
c. Copious irrigation
d. Morphine sulfate
e. Neutralization

ANSWERS

1. c Most burns treated in the ED are partial thickness or second-degree burns. A first-degree burn is characterized by redness and a mild inflammatory response confined to the epidermis, without significant edema or vesiculation. Superficial second-degree burns involve the epidermis and less than half of the dermis. Blistering is often present. These injuries are usually painful because intact sensory nerve receptors are exposed. Scarring is usually minimal. Third-degree/full-thickness burns involve destruction of the epidermis and all of the dermis. They are usually pale or charred in color. Destruction of the cutaneous nerves in the dermis make them nontender, although surrounding areas of partial thickness burns may cause pain. Most of these burns require skin grafting.

2. d Correct management of this partial-thickness/second-degree thermal burn includes debridement of the ruptured bullae to remove damaged tissue that would serve as a medium to nourish bacterial growth. Removal of this material by cleansing and debridement reduces substrate for bacterial proliferation. Aggressive topical antimicrobial therapy is indicated to prevent infection. There is no role for systemic antibiotics in the initial management of a burn. Daily follow-up to assess wound healing is necessary. Plastic surgery follow-up would be appropriate for this injury because it involves the hand and crosses a joint.

3. c Emergency physicians are often asked about immediate care of minor burns. The first step is to stop the burning and help dissipate the heat. Running cool water over the injured area accomplishes both of these goals. Applying ice directly to the wound is painful, and the extreme cold could worsen the injury. Parents should be reminded not to put grease, butter, or any ointment on the burn because they do not dissipate heat well, and they may contribute to contamination. Intact blisters should not be broken. The burn should be covered with a clean cloth or bandage.

4. a This child would be classified as having a major burn because it is greater than 15% BSA. Most life-threatening burns are the result of house fires. The inhalation of hot gases can injure the upper airway, leading to progressive edema and airway obstruction. Any child with burns to the face is at high risk. The initial assessment of the ABCs is indicated. A history of trauma may not be available at the time of

airway management; thus, C-spine immobilization and management of the airway with the neck in neutral position is indicated. Immediate intubation is not required if the child is alert and vital signs are stable, although it should be performed urgently after a primary assessment, oxygenation, stabilization of the C-spine, and IV access. Edema of the burned airway will worsen over the first 24–48 hours. Knowledge of the time course of airway swelling and any signs of airway compromise may warrant early intubation of the trachea to prevent later difficult airway management of this child. General surgical consultation is often required in the management of major burns, although this is not necessary for the initial care of this patient in the ED.

5. c   Prompt treatment of the hypovolemia is important in children with severe thermal burns. An initial bolus of 20 ml/kg lactated Ringer's solution is recommended while assessment of the extent of the burns takes place. Extravasation of water and sodium through abnormally damaged permeable capillaries continues for about 24 hours after the injury. Crystalloid is recommended during the first 24 hours because colloid may extravasate through leaky capillaries and worsen interstitial edema. Care must be taken not to overhydrate children with major burns because it can worsen edema and hinder wound healing.

6. d   Child abuse must always be considered when caring for a child with a burn. Between 10% and 20% of burns in children are intentionally inflicted, accounting for 10% of child abuse cases. Most inflicted burns are scalds. A deep wound with a geometric pattern and sharply demarcated borders suggests a contact burn. Many children with inflicted burns have a nonspecific pattern of injury and there often is not a clear history of abuse. This child is potentially a victim of child abuse because of the isolated second-degree scald burns to the buttocks without burns to the extremities. This burn pattern is suggestive of an intentional submersion injury. Fluid resuscitation is not necessary and there is no role for systemic antibiotics in the acute management of this burn. Tetanus prophylaxis is indicated, but the vast majority of 2-year-old children are up to date with their vaccinations or require only tetanus toxoid. Tetanus immunoglobulin would only be given in a child with a tetanus-prone wound and a history of two or fewer doses of tetanus toxoid. Plastic surgery consultation in the ED is not needed.

7. c   Infants and toddlers are especially at risk for electrical burns to the face and mouth from mouthing electrical cords. Deep burns at the corner of the mouth require specialized attention to prevent severe scarring and contractures. Bleeding from the labial artery 1–2 weeks after the injury, when the eschar separates, can result in significant blood loss. Most children require hospitalization for the management of these burns.

8. e   Acids cause coagulation of tissue proteins, which limit the depth of penetration. Alkali results in liquefaction of tissue and deeper injury. Caustic chemicals on the skin cause a prolonged period of burning compared with most thermal burns. Copious irrigation of chemical burns to dilute the chemical and stop the burning, whether acid or base, is the recommended treatment. Attempts to neutralize the pH are ineffective and should be avoided. Furthermore, neutralization may produce further injury because this reaction results in a thermal injury. The need for tetanus prophylaxis should be addressed in the care of all burns. Pain management is crucial in the management. Consultation and or follow-up with a plastic/hand surgeon is recommended with all burns that cross a joint.

CHAPTER **115**

Orthopedic Trauma

JOYCE SOPRANO, M.D.

QUESTIONS

1. A 5-year-old girl comes to the ED with right wrist pain after falling on an outstretched arm while rollerskating. Plain radiographs of her wrist reveal a displaced angulated fracture of the radial metaphysis. Which of the following statements is most accurate?

   a. Her bones are stronger and stiffer than an adult's; thus, they are less likely to fracture with this mechanism
   b. She is at high risk of having suffered a wrist sprain in addition to the radius fracture
   c. Fracture reduction will be difficult due to tearing of the periosteum
   d. A high degree of remodeling is expected in this patient
   e. She is at high risk of suffering a nonunion of the radius

2. A 10-year-old boy is referred to the ED after suffering an injury to his right index finger while playing basketball. His physical examination is remarkable for tenderness and swelling of the proximal interphalangeal joint. A plain radiograph of the index finger reveals a fracture line through the growth plate with extension into the metaphysis. This is classified as which type of fracture:

   a. Salter-Harris I
   b. Salter-Harris II
   c. Salter-Harris III
   d. Salter-Harris IV
   e. Salter-Harris V

3. A 4-year-old girl arrives to the ED with pain of the left forearm after falling off a swing. You note a deformity of the forearm, and plain radiographs reveal a bowing fracture of the left radius. The most appropriate management for this injury is:

   a. Sling for 14 days, then gradual return to activity
   b. Cast for 14 days, then repeat examination
   c. Closed reduction and cast placement
   d. Completion of the fracture to obtain anatomic reduction
   e. Internal fixation

4. A 3-year-old boy is brought to the ED by ambulance from the scene of a high-speed motor vehicle collision in which he was an unrestrained back-seat passenger. The only injury noted by the EMTs is an open tibial fracture. On arrival to the ED, the patient has HR 180, RR 45, and BP 70/42. You immediately notice the open left tibial fracture. After securing the airway and assessing his breathing, the most appropriate next step in management is:

   a. Apply a splint to the left lower extremity
   b. Administer IV cefazolin
   c. Obtain immediate orthopedic consultation for operative repair of the fracture
   d. Administer a normal saline (NS) bolus IV
   e. Obtain plain radiographs of the left lower extremity

5. An 11-month-old girl is brought to the ED because her parents note that she has not been using her right leg normally. On physical exam, she is afebrile and uncomfortable appearing. She has tenderness to palpation of the right lower leg. Plain radiographs reveal a spiral fracture of the right tibia. On further questioning, her parents recall that earlier in the day they found the patient crying with her right leg sticking out of the crib rails, but recall no other trauma. The most appropriate next step is:

   a. Obtain a skeletal survey
   b. Obtain a bone scan
   c. File a report with the Department of Social Services
   d. Place a posterior splint and arrange follow-up with orthopedics
   e. Place a long leg cast and discharge home

6. A 13-year-old boy is seen in the ED after falling on his left shoulder while mountain biking. On physical examination he has marked swelling and tenderness of the upper arm. He has slightly decreased sensation on the dorsum of the hand in the web space between the thumb and index finger, but normal extension of the wrist. Plain radiographs reveal a midshaft fracture of the humerus, with 15 degrees of angulation. The most appropriate management is:

   a. Sling and swathe for 3–6 weeks
   b. Sugar-tong splint and sling for 3 weeks
   c. Sling and orthopedic follow-up the following day
   d. Immediate orthopedic consultation for fracture reduction
   e. Immediate orthopedic consultation for fasciotomy

7. A 5-year-old boy is brought to the ED with severe right-arm pain several hours after falling from a rock while hiking. He has marked swelling and tenderness of the elbow and resists range of motion (ROM) testing. He has extreme tenderness of the forearm and pain when you attempt to extend his fingers. His radial pulse is present, but his arm appears pale. The most appropriate next step is:

   a. Obtain plain radiographs of the elbow
   b. Flex the elbow to 90 degrees and place a posterior splint
   c. Place a long arm cast and refer to orthopedics within 5 days
   d. Obtain an immediate orthopedic consultation
   e. Manually reduce the displacement and obtain radiographs of the elbow

8. A 3-year-old girl is referred to you after falling off a slide onto her outstretched left arm. She has been refusing to use the left arm since the injury. On physical examination, she holds her left arm slightly flexed and pronated, and she resists movement of the elbow. She has mild swelling of the elbow. Her peripheral pulses are normal, and she seems to have normal movement of the wrist and fingers. You obtain plain radiographs of the elbow that reveal faint anterior and posterior fat pads but no obvious fracture. The best management for this patient is:

   a. Supinate and flex the arm while applying pressure to the radial head
   b. Apply a long arm splint and arrange orthopedic follow-up within 5 days
   c. Apply a sling and arrange orthopedic follow-up in 3 weeks
   d. Prescribe ibuprofen and rest of the arm without immobilization
   e. Obtain immediate orthopedic consultation for internal fixation

9. A 9-year-old boy is seen in the ED for right arm pain after falling off his bicycle. Physical examination reveals a deformity of the ulna and mild swelling and tenderness of the elbow. His radial and ulnar pulses are normal. Plain radiographs of the forearm and wrist reveal a slight bowing fracture of the ulna. The most appropriate next step is:

   a. Obtain plain radiographs of the elbow
   b. Place a long arm posterior splint and refer to orthopedics the following day
   c. Perform closed reduction of the bowing fracture and cast placement
   d. Obtain immediate orthopedic consultation for internal fixation of the ulnar fracture
   e. Apply a sling and prescribe a nonsteroidal anti-inflammatory medication (NSAID)

10. A 17-year-old male patient complains of pain of the right hip that occurred acutely while he was running hurdles. He recalls feeling a "pop" at the time of the injury. On physical examination he has tenderness over the right anterior inferior iliac spine and limited ROM of the right hip. Plain radiographs reveal a minimally displaced avulsion fracture. The recommended management for this pelvic fracture is:

    a. Physical therapy with return to normal function within 3 weeks
    b. Crutches with no weight bearing for 3 weeks followed by partial weight bearing
    c. Complete bedrest for 3–4 weeks, followed by partial weight bearing
    d. Open reduction and internal fixation
    e. Closed reduction with an external fixator

11. A 13-year-old boy is referred to you with pain of his right thigh that occurred after a minor fall while playing soccer. On further questioning he also recalls intermittent mild thigh pain over the past few weeks. On physical examination he holds his right hip externally rotated and complains of increased pain when you attempt to flex or internally rotate the hip. The most likely finding on plain radiographs is:

    a. Widening of the medial clear space and detachment of the posterior labrum of the right hip joint
    b. Displaced fracture of the femoral shaft
    c. A step-off between the metaphysis and epiphysis of the femur
    d. Intertrochanteric fracture of the femur
    e. Avulsion fracture of the anterior superior iliac spine

12. A 12-year-old girl is referred to the ED with right knee pain. Her mother reports that the patient fell while playing soccer and appeared to have "bent her knee too far forward." She is unable to walk and she has significant swelling of the right knee. The most likely finding on plain radiographs of the knee is:

    a. Salter-Harris II fracture of the distal femur
    b. Elevation of the anterior tibial spine
    c. Avulsion of the tibial tuberosity
    d. Fracture of the proximal tibial growth plate
    e. Dislocation of the knee

13. A 15-year-old girl arrives to the ED complaining of left knee pain that occurred when she was hit in the leg while playing lacrosse. She reports that it felt like her knee cap "popped out." She has moderate swelling of the knee on physical exam. The most likely additional finding is:

    a. Tenderness along the lateral aspect of the patella
    b. Genu varus
    c. Laxity of the anterior cruciate ligament (ACL)
    d. Well-developed quadriceps muscle
    e. Pain and apprehension with lateral displacement of the patella

14. An 8-year-old boy is referred to you with left ankle pain following a fall down several stairs. The patient recalls twisting his ankle, and then was unable to bear weight. On physical examination he has mild swelling and tenderness over the lateral malleolus. The range of motion of the ankle appears normal. The most likely finding on plain radiographs of the ankle is:

    a. Tillaux fracture
    b. Soft tissue swelling overlying the distal fibula
    c. Triplane fracture
    d. Salter-Harris II fracture of the tibia with greenstick fracture of the fibula
    e. Jones fracture

ANSWERS

1. **d** A high degree of bone remodeling is expected in younger children, especially when the fracture occurs in the metaphysis and in the plane of motion of the adjacent joint. Nonunions are rarely seen in young children because the thick periosteum usually remains intact on one side of the fracture, aiding in anatomic reduction of the fracture and in callus formation. The epiphyseal growth plates are the weakest part of the growing skeleton, more commonly resulting in growth plate fractures than in ligamentous injuries. A wrist sprain is therefore unlikely in this scenario. Pediatric bones are more porous than are an adult's, making them pliable, but also weaker and more likely to fracture.

2. **b** A physeal fracture in which the fracture line crosses the germinal growth plate and courses into the metaphysis is classified as a Salter-Harris Type II fracture. A Salter-Harris Type I fracture involves separation of the metaphysis from the epiphysis through the growth plate and may show either a widening of the growth plate or a normal radiograph. In a Type III fracture the fracture line courses into the epiphysis; in a Type IV it involves both the epiphysis and metaphysis. A Salter-Harris Type V fracture is a crush injury of the growth plate, resulting in narrowing of the growth plate.

3. **c** A bowing fracture is a persistent deformity that has little remodeling capabilities. Fracture reduction is essential prior to immobilization. Greenstick fractures, in which one side of the cortex remains intact, often require completion of the fracture to obtain anatomic alignment. Internal fixation is rarely required for bowing fractures.

4. **d** This patient with tachycardia and hypotension is most likely in shock from acute blood loss. The mechanism of his injury puts him at risk for major organ damage as a cause for his blood loss. It is unlikely that he has had a significant amount of blood loss from a single long bone injury. Although splinting of the injured extremity is crucial to prevent further injury and for pain control, the patient's hypotension must first be treated with isotonic solution. Potential causes of life-threatening blood loss must then be evaluated and managed. IV antibiotics should be given and orthopedic consultation and radiographs should be obtained after the patient is further stabilized.

5. a   Spiral fractures of the tibia or femur in preambulatory children are suspicious for child abuse. In addition, the history of possible trauma of the leg in the crib is inconsistent with this injury. A skeletal survey is indicated in any child less than 2 years old in whom you consider child abuse. A bone scan may be indicated to detect subtle rib fractures after a skeletal survey is completed. If further workup supports a suspicion of child abuse, a report of abuse or neglect should be filed with the Department of Social Services at that time. Although the definitive treatment for the fracture is either casting or splinting, the evaluation for possible child abuse must take place prior to discharging the patient.

6. d   Most humeral shaft fractures heal without intervention because the thick periosteum limits fracture displacement and promotes healing. For incomplete fractures a sling and swathe is all that is required, and for minimally displaced fractures a sugar-tong splint is generally recommended. When there is evidence of radial nerve dysfunction, immediate orthopedic consultation is recommended for possible fracture reduction. Most radial nerve palsies resolve with proper fracture management. Compartment syndrome is not typically seen with humeral shaft fractures, and is unlikely in this scenario with only mild radial nerve dysfunction.

7. d   The most common elbow fracture in this age group is a supracondylar humeral fracture, which is associated with potentially severe complications. This clinical scenario suggests a compartment syndrome with muscle ischemia, with severe diffuse arm pain, tenderness of the forearm, and pain on passive extension of the fingers. The presence of the radial pulse does not make the diagnosis of compartment syndrome less likely. Immediate orthopedic evaluation for measurement of compartment pressures and possible fasciotomy or fracture reduction is crucial. If orthopedic consultation is unavailable, manual reduction of the fracture may then be necessary to improve neurovascular function. Flexion of the elbow beyond 20–30 degrees places increased tension on the neurovascular structures and is not advised.

8. b   The presence of a posterior fat pad indicates that there is fluid in the joint space, most likely a hemarthrosis from a subtle fracture. In this age group, a nondisplaced supracondylar fracture is the most likely fracture, although fractures of the radial neck are also relatively common. Radiographic examination of the anterior humeral line, which should intersect the middle third of the capitellum, can aide in the diagnosis of subtle supracondylar fractures. This patient most likely has a nondisplaced supracondylar fracture, which should be managed with immobilization in a long arm cast or splint with prompt orthopedic follow-up. Internal fixation is rarely required for nondisplaced fractures. The presence of swelling and the posterior fat pad are contraindications to the attempted reduction of a radial head subluxation.

9. a   Isolated ulnar fractures rarely occur in children because the force usually causes an injury to the radius as well. The presence of an ulnar fracture, including bowing fractures, should prompt a rigorous search for a radial injury. This patient has a Monteggia fracture, which is a fracture of the ulna and an associated dislocation of the radial head. The elbow swelling and tenderness are clues to the radial dislocation. It is crucial to obtain radiographs of the joints above and below the injury to look for additional fractures. A line drawn through the axis of the radius should intersect the center of the capitellum on all views. In addition, external reduction of the ulnar bowing fracture prior to immobilization is crucial because these injuries have limited ability to remodel and may result in a permanent disability if not reduced properly.

10. b   Most avulsion fractures of the pelvis can be managed conservatively with no or partial weight bearing for 4–6 weeks, followed by gradual return to function. Complete bed rest is not required. Open reduction and internal fixation is recommended only for widely displaced avulsion fractures. External fixators are used for unstable fractures of the pelvic ring.

11. c   This clinical scenario—of chronic thigh pain in an adolescent male worsening after a minor injury—is most consistent with a slipped capital femoral epiphysis (SCFE). Limited or painful internal rotation and flexion of the hip are common physical exam findings in this injury. The hip often appears normal on anteroposterior views; however, the step-off between the metaphysis and epiphysis becomes apparent on lateral hip radiograph as external rotation turns the posterior aspect of the femur medially. Widening of the medial clear space and detachment of the posterior labrum are seen with hip dislocations. Intertrochanteric and shaft fractures of the femur occur from high-energy accidents, which did

not occur in this case. An avulsion fracture of the anterior superior iliac spine would cause localized tenderness over the fracture site.

12. b Hyperflexion injuries of the knee in children with open physes are frequently associated with injuries to the anterior cruciate ligament (ACL) and an associated avulsion of the anterior tibial spine. Radiographic findings include a joint effusion and an elevation or total separation of the anterior tibial spine on plain radiographs of the knee. Salter-Harris fractures of the distal femur are extremely uncommon due to the shape of the physis and the strong perichondrial ring. They are caused by high-energy injuries. Avulsion fractures of the tibial tuberosity are most commonly seen in boys with a history of Osgood-Schlatter's disease. Fractures of the proximal tibial physis and knee dislocations occur as a result of hyperextension injuries.

13. e This patient gives a classic description of a patellar dislocation that reduced spontaneously. This occurs when a force displaces the patella laterally while the foot is planted. Lateral displacement of the patella elicits pain and apprehension as the patient feels like the patella is going to "pop out." Tenderness will be maximal along the medial aspect of the patella in the area of the medial patellar retinaculum. Risk factors include genu valgus and weak quadriceps muscles. ACL injuries are less common in this scenario.

14. b This clinical scenario is most consistent with a Salter-Harris I fracture of the distal fibula, with mild symptoms isolated to the lateral malleolus. The most-common finding on radiographs of the ankle is soft-tissue swelling overlying the fibular physis, and less frequently widening of the physis. Tillaux, triplane, and Jones fractures all occur in adolescents who are nearing skeletal maturity. The former two, along with the Salter-Harris II fracture of the tibia with greenstick fracture of the fibula, present with significant swelling, deformity, and instability of the ankle. The Jones fracture results in tenderness at the base of the fifth metatarsal.

CHAPTER **116**

Minor Trauma—Lacerations

ANDREA STRACCIOLINI, M.D.

QUESTIONS

1. A 3½-year-old girl comes into the ED with a laceration of her forehead. Her mother states that she ran into the corner of the door late last night (approximately 15 hours ago). The wound appears clean. She suffered no other injuries. Her immunizations are up to date. Your best plan of care is:

    a. Delayed primary closure
    b. Primary closure
    c. Closure by secondary intention
    d. Tertiary closure
    e. None of the above

2. A 5-year-old boy suffered a laceration of his left eyebrow when he fell from the monkey bars 4 hours ago. The wound extends to the level of the skull and is mildly gaping. There is no underlying fracture seen. The wound is clean. You decide to repair the wound primarily. The best treatment for this wound includes:

    a. A 5.0 monofilament absorbable deep layer, 6.0 nylon skin closure
    b. A 5.0 chromic gut deep layer, 6.0 nylon skin closure
    c. No deep layer, 6.0 nylon skin closure
    d. Steri-strip skin closure
    e. Tissue adhesive skin closure

3. A 13-year-old boy injured his left leg while playing lacrosse. He has a deep laceration of his left thigh just proximal to the knee. The wound is 8-cm long and 2-cm wide. The wound is clean and his neurovascular examination is normal. The most appropriate repair of this wound is closure using:

    a. Simple interrupted sutures
    b. Running or continuous sutures
    c. Vertical mattress sutures
    d. Subcuticular sutures and Steri-strips
    e. None of the above

4. A 2-year-old boy comes to the ED with a laceration of his distal right forearm from falling onto the metal edge of a rusty fence. The wound is 3-cm long. The wound appears clean and his neurovascular examination is normal. You inquire about immunizations and the mother states that she just began caring for the child and is unsure about the child's immunization status. Appropriate treatment for this wound is administration of:

    a. Td (tetanus toxoid)
    b. DPT, tetanus immune globulin (TIG)
    c. Tetanus immune globulin
    d. No tetanus prophylaxis
    e. DPT (diphtheria, pertussis, tetanus)

5. A 17-year-old male wrestler comes to the ED after sustaining blunt trauma to his left ear. On physical exam you note a smooth ecchymotic swelling that disrupts the normal contour of the auricle. There is a small adjacent laceration just medial to this area. Your next step in caring for this patient is:

    a. Local wound care
    b. Primary laceration repair
    c. Drainage of the hematoma
    d. Antibiotics
    e. Application of a pressure dressing

6. A 7-year-old girl comes to the ED with a full-thickness laceration of the upper lip extending through the vermilion border. The wound appears clean. All of her immunizations are up to date. The best choice for repair of this wound is:

    a. Skin closure with absorbable suture
    b. A three-layer repair beginning with oral mucosa
    c. Primary closure with tissue adhesive
    d. A two-layer repair beginning with skin closure
    e. Local wound care, plastic surgery follow-up

380

7. A 2½-year-old girl is in the ED with a dog bite to her left cheek. She has a 2-cm linear laceration to the left cheek. Physical exam reveals no involvement of the facial nerve, parotid duct, or facial artery. All immunizations are up to date. The best management plan for this wound is:

a. Primary closure, antibiotics
b. Closure by secondary intention, antibiotics
c. Local wound care, no antibiotics
d. Plastic surgery consult, antibiotics
e. Tape closure, no antibiotics

*[Handwritten margin notes: PROLENE → BLUE; (1) Location — cosmetic — Risk for infection; Suture — strength, inflammation/scarring; SUB Q — Vicryl/Dexon ~ absorbable; CHROMIC GUT * reactive (∅ face); Blue; vertical; parallel]*

ANSWERS

1. b   In children the infection rate is about 2% for all sutured wounds. Most wounds may thus be closed primarily, approximating the wound edges as soon after the injury as possible. As the delay in primary closure increases, the risk of subsequent infection increases. The length of time before there is a significant risk is variable. Wounds at low risk for infection can be closed 12–24 hours after the injury. Wounds of the face and scalp often heal well. Because this wound is on the face, cosmetic outcome is important. In addition, this wound is at low risk for infection. Primary closure, therefore, is appropriate. Delayed primary closure (closure after 3–5 days) is recommended for selected heavily contaminated wounds and those associated with extensive damage. Allowing the wound to heal by secondary intention would not be appropriate for this facial wound. Tertiary closure is delayed primary closure.

2. a   Suture material must have adequate strength while producing little inflammation. Monofilament nylon or polypropylene (Prolene) retain most of their tensile strength and are nonreactive. Subcuticular layers should be repaired using fine absorbable suture such as Dexon or Vicryl. Deep sutures are indicated here because the wound is deep and involves the face. Chromic gut suture is very reactive and would thus not be a good choice. The wound is too deep for Steri-strip closure or tissue adhesive alone. Prolene is preferable to Ethilon because it is blue and thus makes suture removal from the eyebrow easier.

3. c   Running sutures can be applied to close large, straight wounds that are not under significant tension. Because this wound is located in a mobile area and is gaping, a running suture would not be the best choice. Simple interrupted sutures alone will not be adequate for this high-tension wound. The vertical mattress stitch is useful for deep wounds like the one described here. It reduces tension on the wound and may close dead space within the wound. It essentially combines a deep and superficial stitch in one suture. Subcuticular sutures followed by skin closure with Steri-strips is not the best option for this large extremity wound.

4. b   If the tetanus status is unknown and the wound is significant or dirty, tetanus toxoid (Td) and tetanus immune globulin (TIG) are indicated. Wounds involving massive tissue destruction also require TIG. If the wound is clean and minor, and the patient has received three previous doses of tetanus toxoid, then a booster of tetanus toxoid is given only if 10 or more years have passed since the last dose. If the patient has received three or more previous tetanus immunizations, but the wound is a dirty, minor laceration, then tetanus toxoid is indicated if the last dose was more than 5 years prior. Thus, this child would require DPT and TIG, because his immunization status is unknown and the wound is dirty.

5. c   Blunt ear trauma can lead to a simple contusion or a significant subperichondral hematoma that can compromise the auricular cartilage. A significant perichondral hematoma is tense and appears as a smooth ecchymotic swelling that disrupts the normal contour of the auricle. This injury is particularly common among wrestlers. Auricular hematomas should be drained promptly to avoid necrosis of the cartilage and a subsequent deformed auricle or "cauliflower ear."

6. b   The lip is an important facial landmark and thus should be repaired with great care. The vermilion border should be precisely reopposed using 6.0 suture. Lip lacerations should generally be closed in layers. Full-thickness lacerations require a three-layer repair beginning with the oral mucosa, using 5.0 absorbable material, followed by the orbicularis oris muscle layer to include the inner and outer fibrofatty layers, and finishing with the skin, using 6.0 nonabsorbable interrupted suture. Plastic surgery consult is not necessary in this case. Because the wound is full thickness, a two-layered repair and local wound care with follow-up are not sufficient.

7. a   Puncture wounds resulting from animal bites should be debrided and irrigated thoroughly. Lacerations of the face from animal bites, because of the cosmetic concerns, should be closed primarily using 6.0 nonabsorbable sutures. Antibiotics should be prescribed for animal bites. Amoxicillin-clavulanic acid is recommended because it appropriately treats *Pasteurella multocida*, *Staphylococcus aureus*, and *Streptococcus* species adequately.

Surgical Emergencies

CHAPTER 117

Minor Lesions

VINCENT J. WANG, M.D.

QUESTIONS

1. A 7-year-old girl complains of pain and swelling of her left index finger. She has not had any fever and she denies trauma to her finger. On examination, she is well appearing and afebrile. She has moderate swelling and erythema of the eponychium, with scant whitish discharge from between the eponychium and the nail root. Treatment includes:

    a. Warm soaks only
    b. Incision and drainage
    c. Partial removal of the fingernail
    d. Oral griseofulvin
    e. Splinting

2. A 10-year-old boy complains of finger pain. He says he had scraped his hand when he fell off of his bicycle several days ago. He has had pain since the accident, but today his finger tip is throbbing more. On examination, the pulp of his right middle finger is tense, erythematous, and warm. Palpation suggests fluid under the skin. Your management includes:

    a. Splinting his finger
    b. Acyclovir PO
    c. Griseofulvin PO
    d. Cephalexin PO
    e. Partial removal of the fingernail

3. A 2-year-old girl is brought to the ED because she injured her finger in a car door. The mother states that she caught her finger in a car door, and has had pain since then. On examination, she has an isolated injury of her right index finger. She has a discoloration of her nailbed, under the fingernail, that involves 70% of the nailbed. Her fingernail is intact and she has no other injuries to her finger. A radiograph of the finger reveals no fractures. Treatment includes:

    a. Warm soaks
    b. Trephination of the fingernail
    c. Partial removal of the fingernail
    d. Total removal of the fingernail
    e. Cephalexin PO

4. A 3-week-old boy is brought to the ED because of persistent crying. He has been feeding well and has been afebrile, without other constitutional symptoms. The crying has been persistent since yesterday afternoon. On examination, he is well nourished and well appearing. His HEENT examination is normal, including fluoroscein staining of his eyes. His abdomen is soft and nontender, but he has mild erythema and swelling of the right fifth finger, distal to the middle of the middle phalanx. His stool test for heme is negative, as is his urinalysis. You suspect the etiology of his crying to be caused by:

    a. A hair tourniquet
    b. A corneal abrasion
    c. Intussusception
    d. Fracture of his finger
    e. Osteomyelitis of his finger

5. A 17-year-old girl comes to the ED because she is afraid she has a tumor. She complains of a painless lump on her upper back that has been getting larger. On examination, she has a dome-shaped, circumscribed, freely movable, firm, skin-colored nodule on her right shoulder. There is no drainage, erythema, or inflammation. She has not had previous trauma to the area. She has no other lesions. Your immediate treatment includes:

    a. Upper GI series
    b. Incision and drainage
    c. Biopsy of the lesion
    d. Injection of hydrocortisone into the lesion
    e. Reassurance that the lesion is not malignant

6. A 2-year-old boy is brought to the ED because of a facial lesion. The parents want a second opinion for what they were told was a hemangioma. He has a firm, noncompressible, reddish-gray nodule approximately 1 cm in diameter on the bridge of the nose. The lesion has been present since birth, and has not changed in size. Your most likely diagnosis is:

   a. Hemangioma
   b. Glioma
   c. Encephalocele
   d. Lipoma
   e. Epidermal inclusion cyst (EIC)

7. An 8-year-old girl is brought to the ED because of a neck mass. She has developed a midline neck mass over the past few days, associated with redness and fever. On examination, she has a smooth, mobile, midline mass overlying the hyoid bone. She complains of mild tenderness to palpation, and there is overlying erythema. The mass moves when she swallows. Your most likely diagnosis is:

   a. Thyroglossal duct cyst infection
   b. Submental lymphadenitis
   c. Hashimoto's thyroiditis
   d. Goiter
   e. Brachial cleft cyst infection

8. A 13-year-old girl is brought to the ED by her mother because she thinks she has neck cancer. Her maternal uncle recently passed away from esophageal cancer. The mother noticed neck swelling this afternoon, and says that she has lost 5 kg over the past few weeks, despite eating more than usual. Her vital signs are T 37°C, HR 130, RR 18, and BP 130/60. She is anxious and restless, but without signs of toxicity. She has a nontender, midline, non-erythematous neck mass below the hyoid bone. Which evaluation is likely to make the diagnosis?

   a. CBC with smear
   b. Serum glucose
   c. TSH (thyroid-stimulating hormone)
   d. Esophageal biopsy
   e. Psychiatry consult

9. A 5-year-old boy is brought to the ED by his newly adoptive parents, who know little about his past medical history. He began having left-sided tonic-clonic seizures approximately 10 minutes before arriving in the ED. He is developmentally delayed and has a mild left-sided limp, which has been chronic. He has otherwise been well, without antecedent symptoms. His vital signs are T 36.8°C, HR 140, RR 20, and BP 90/50. He continues to have left-sided tonic-clonic seizures. His pupils are reactive bilaterally, his examination is without evidence of trauma, he has a deep-red macular skin lesion involving the upper face and eyelid on the right. Which of the following tests is likely to confirm the diagnosis?

   a. Serum electrolytes
   b. Serum glucose
   c. Urine toxicologic screening
   d. Skull radiograph
   e. CSF cell count

10. A 3-week-old girl is brought to the ED by her parents because of a swelling of her umbilical stump. The umbilical cord had fallen off 10 days ago, but the stump has not healed and granulation tissue remains. The stump has had minimal, chronic clear discharge. On examination, you note excessive granulation tissue, which appears moist. There is no central lumen and the discharge on the stump appears serous. Treatment includes:

   a. Topical silver nitrate
   b. Topical isopropyl alcohol
   c. Amoxicillin PO
   d. Surgical evaluation
   e. Reassurance only

11. A 15-year-old boy is brought to the ED as a referral for resistant tinea corporis. He has had ringlike lesions on the dorsum of his right hand for many weeks. He has been treated with topical antimycotics without improvement. On examination, he is alert and well-appearing. He has two ring-shaped lesions on his right hand. The edges are raised and the center is clear. There is no scaling. You recommend:

   a. Continuing the antimycotic ointment for another 2 weeks
   b. Continuing the antimycotic ointment and beginning oral cephalexin
   c. Discontinuing the ointment and beginning oral griseofulvin
   d. Discontinuing the ointment and beginning oral ketoconazole
   e. No further treatment

ANSWERS

1. b   Treatment of a paronychia involves incision and drainage of the paronychia, under the cuticle. Once incised, warm soaks may facilitate healing. Some physicians would use oral antibiotics as well. Partial removal of the fingernail is indicated for subungual hematomas and subungual abscesses. Oral griseofulvin is indicated for onychomycosis, and splinting is appropriate for finger trauma, both of which are not indicated here. Herpetic whitlow should also be considered in the differential diagnosis, particularly if vesicles are seen.

2. d   Treatment of a felon, a deep infection of the pulp space of the fingertip, involves incision and drainage of the area, followed by a course of oral antibiotics for likely organisms. As with paronychiae, infectious agents include *Staphylococcus aureus, Streptococcus pyogenes,* and anaerobic species. There is no role for splinting the finger or removing the fingernail in the treatment of a felon. Antiviral or antifungal agents may be used for herpetic whitlow or onychomycosis, respectively.

3. d   If the subungual hematoma involves less than 50% of the nail surface and is not associated with a phalanx fracture, trephination will drain the blood and relieve pressure from the hematoma. If the subungual hematoma involves more than 50% of the nail surface and/or is associated with a phalanx fracture, the fingernail should be removed, and any nailbed lacerations should be repaired with appropriate sutures.

4. a   Hair tourniquets may be a cause of unexplained crying in an infant. The hair may encircle a digit, the penis, or the clitoris, and thereby cause strangulation of the body part. Removal may be difficult, and may require examination under magnification, such as with loupe lenses. Corneal abrasions are another cause of crying in an infant, but a negative fluoroscein staining test makes this unlikely. Intussusception may also cause crying, but the history, examination, and negative stool test make this less likely. Clinical suspicion, however, should still be the primary guide to your diagnosis of this problem.

5. e   Epidermal inclusion cysts (EICs) are keratin-filled cysts, typically occurring after puberty. Multiple large EICs may be associated with Gardner's syndrome, which is characterized by intestinal polyposis, osseous lesions, and desmoid tumors. This syndrome is important to diagnose because there is a 50% chance of malignant transformation of the intestinal polyps. In this patient, however, this is unlikely, and an imaging study is not indicated. Incision and drainage is indicated for infected EICs, which is not the case in this vignette. Biopsy and injection with hydrocortisone are not appropriate. Reassurance that the lesion is not malignant is correct, as well as outpatient referral for elective excision.

6. b   Gliomas may be confused with hemangiomas. Hemangiomas may be classified as superficial, deep, or mixed. Superficial hemangiomas are confined to the upper dermis, and are compressible, well-demarcated vascular lesions. Deep hemangiomas lie in the lower dermis and are characterized by an overlying bluish hue. Most hemangiomas are mixed, containing elements of both. Hemangiomas are not often seen at birth, but have a rapid growth phase over 6–12 months, and may be evident after several months. Most lesions will involute afterward, resolving completely by 9 years of age. Gliomas are benign growths of ectopic neural tissue. The lesions are as described in the vignette, and are usually found on the nasal bridge or intranasally. Encephaloceles are soft, compressible, and often pulsatile because these lesions have a direct communication to the central nervous system. Lipomas are compressible and are skin-colored. EICs are described previously.

7. a   Thyroglossal duct cysts result from incomplete regression of ectodermal elements after the fetal descent of the thyroid gland. Most are found intimately associated with the hyoid bone, and will therefore move with motion of the hyoid bone. The usual presentation is as a painless, smooth, midline, mobile mass overlying the hyoid bone. The initial diagnosis, however, may be made when it is infected, as it is in this case. Antibiotics are indicated for the infection, and elective excision should be made at a later time. Infection of the submental lymph nodes is typified by similar symptoms, just below the chin, but not associated with the hyoid bone. Hashimoto's thyroiditis is a disorder of the thyroid gland, which is below the hyoid bone. Hashimoto's thyroiditis does not cause erythema or tenderness. A goiter similarly causes asymptomatic enlargement of the thyroid gland. A brachial cleft cyst is usually found anterior to the sternocleidomastoid muscle.

8. c   Thyrotoxicosis may be diagnosed with an elevated T_4 level in the presence of a low TSH. This patient's symptoms are classic for Graves' disease. Neck carcinoma is unlikely, given her history and findings, and the family history is probably unrelated. Diabetes mellitus may cause weight loss, despite increased appetite, but the other findings make this less likely. Weight loss from anorexia nervosa or bulimia is diagnosed by history and examination, but her symptoms are not consistent with this diagnosis.

9. d   Sturge-Weber disease is a constellation of findings thought to be caused by anomalous development of the primordial vascular bed during the early part of cerebral development. (Haslam RHA. "Sturge-Weber Disease." In: *Nelson Textbook of Pediatrics,* fifteenth edition. Philadelphia: W.B. Saunders, 1996:1707–1708.) Associated symptoms and signs include a port-wine stain or facial nevus, seizures, intracranial calcifications, hemiparesis, and, later, mental retardation. Given the findings, this is the most likely cause; therefore, a skull radiograph will likely show intracranial calcifications.

10. a   Large umbilical granulomas should be treated with cauterization with silver nitrate. Smaller ones will resolve spontaneously, but isopropyl alcohol is often recommended to keep the area clean. In the case of pedunculated granulomas, suture ligation may be necessary. Umbilical granulomas must be differentiated from persistent embryonic remnants (e.g., a patent urachus or omphalomesenteric duct). The presence of chronic fecal or urinary discharge and or a central lumen would suggest this diagnosis. Treatment for these problems is surgical evaluation for removal of the entire remnant. There is no role for oral antibiotics.

11. e   Granuloma annulare may be confused with tinea corporis. The lesions are similar, but granuloma annulare does not have any scales. In addition, tinea corporis is rare after puberty. Most lesions will resolve within 2 years without further treatment. Corticosteroids may hasten resolution, but are not necessary.

CHAPTER **118**

Abdominal Emergencies

BARBARA M. GARCIA PEÑA, M.D., M.P.H.

QUESTIONS

1. A 5-year-old boy comes to the ED with a 3-day history of diffuse abdominal pain associated with vomiting and brown, watery diarrhea. He has had fever to 39°C since the onset of symptoms. The most likely cause for this child's findings is:

   a. Intussusception
   b. Gastroenteritis
   c. Perforated appendicitis
   d. Nonperforated appendicitis
   e. Malrotation with volvulus

2. A 2-year-old boy comes to the ED for evaluation of abdominal pain of 8-hour duration. Features of an appropriate and informative abdominal examination in this child include all of the following, EXCEPT:

   a. Spending a few minutes to gain the child's confidence
   b. Avoiding the use of narcotics
   c. Avoiding an examination when the child is sleeping
   d. Examining the child in an orderly progression
   e. Undressing and exposing the child's entire abdomen and inguinal area

3. A 9-year-old girl comes to the ED with hypogastric tenderness, low-grade fever, and a WBC count of 15,000. For these symptoms to be consistent with acute appendicitis, the inflamed appendix would most likely be lying in the:

   a. Right lateral gutter
   b. Right upper quadrant (RUQ)
   c. Right lower quadrant (RLQ)
   d. Left lower quadrant (LLQ)
   e. Lower pelvis

4. A 5 year-old boy comes to the ED with RLQ abdominal pain of 4-day duration. He has had no fever, vomiting, or diarrhea, and he is currently hungry. He is tender in the RLQ on physical examination. His WBC count is 6000. Which of the following diagnoses is the most likely explanation for this child's abdominal pain?

   a. Pneumonia
   b. Gastroenteritis
   c. Urinary tract infection (UTI)
   d. Diverticulitis
   e. Constipation

5. A 7-year-old girl comes to the ED with a 24-hour history of low-grade fever and abdominal pain that originated periumbilically and migrated to the RLQ. You suspect appendicitis. A CBC performed in this child will most likely show a WBC count in the range of:

   a. 5000–10,000
   b. 11,000–15,000
   c. 16,000–20,000
   d. 21,000–25,000
   e. 26,000–30,000

6. A 10-year-old boy comes to the ED with periumbilical pain migrating to the RLQ. The pain began 48 hours ago. His temperature is 38.4°C. He is exquisitely tender in the RLQ and has a positive Rovsing's and psoas sign. WBC count is 14,000. You are concerned about appendicitis and consider obtaining an abdominal roentgenogram (KUB). What is the likelihood that the KUB will show a fecalith?

   a. 0.01%
   b. 0.1%
   c. 1%
   d. 10%
   e. 20%

7. In addition to the presence of a fecalith, common findings on abdominal radiographs seen in children with appendicitis include all of the following, EXCEPT:

   a. Diminished air in the gastrointestinal tract
   b. Thickening of the cecal wall and mucosal folds
   c. Scoliosis concave to the right
   d. Diffuse air-fluid levels in small and large bowel
   e. Focal obliteration of the adjacent properitoneal fat pad

8. A 5-year-old girl comes to the ED with abdominal pain of 3-day duration. She is toxic appearing and febrile to 39.4°C. Her abdomen is distended and she winces in pain when you gently percuss her abdomen in any quadrant. Which of the following is the most likely diagnosis?

   a. *Salmonella* gastroenteritis
   b. Ileocolic intussusception
   c. Nonperforated appendicitis in the right lateral gutter
   d. Perforated appendicitis
   e. Nonperforated retrocecal appendicitis

9. A 10-year-old girl with history of cirrhosis comes to the ED with fever to 40.1°C, vomiting, and diffuse abdominal pain. Her WBC count is 20,000. Which of the following would be most helpful to ascertain a diagnosis?

   a. Paracentesis
   b. KUB
   c. Abdominal ultrasound (U/S)
   d. Abdominal CT scan
   e. Exploratory laparotomy

10. A 5-year-old boy comes to the ED with upper abdominal pain radiating to the back. His serum amylase level is 740 U/l. The most common cause of this condition in children is:

    a. Gallstones
    b. Trauma
    c. Congenital anomaly of the biliary tree
    d. Congenital anomaly of the pancreatic duct
    e. Choledochal cyst

11. A 6-month-old boy comes to the ED with episodes of severe crampy abdominal pain and vomiting. On rectal examination, he is hemoccult positive. He appears comfortable and quiet between the episodes. Treatment will most likely involve:

    a. Pyloromyotomy
    b. Manual reduction
    c. Detorsion
    d. Laparotomy
    e. Enema

12. An 8-month-old girl comes to the ED with episodic severe abdominal pain and currant jelly stool. Where might you expect to palpate a mass?

    a. Right upper quadrant
    b. Right lower quadrant
    c. Left upper quadrant
    d. Left lower quadrant
    e. Midepigastrum

13. Which of the following is not true regarding a child's early symptoms in the course of intussusception?

    a. There is often a history of having passed a currant jelly stool
    b. The child experiences cramping, episodic abdominal pain
    c. Between episodes of pain, the child may appear either lethargic or perfectly comfortable
    d. The child may be misdiagnosed as being in a postictal state
    e. The patient may have antecedent symptoms and signs of a viral gastroenteritis

14. A 10-month-old girl comes to the ED with cramping episodic abdominal pain of 12-hour duration. She is quiet and listless between the painful episodes. She has not passed stool in 24 hours. Based on your suspicion, you order a barium enema. Which of the following is true regarding this diagnostic modality?

    a. It is a successful therapy in more than 90% of cases
    b. It is contraindicated in the presence of free peritoneal air
    c. It should be performed with a barium column no higher than 5 feet above the abdomen
    d. It should be attempted with concomitant manual palpation of the abdomen
    e. It should not be performed with sedatives because they may mask a successful result

15. An 8-month-old boy returns to ED 3 days after barium enema reduction for intussusception. He has cramping intermittent abdominal pain similar to his symptoms when he was diagnosed with intussusception. Which of the following is true?

    a. Recurrence rate after barium enema reduction usually ranges from 8 to 10%
    b. Reduction with barium enema should not be attempted after any recurrence
    c. Reduction with barium enema should not be attempted when a child has had three episodes of intussusception in the past
    d. Recurrences are more common in younger children and are usually caused by a lead point, such as a Meckel's diverticulum
    e. Operation after the first recurrence of intussusception is not indicated in older children

16. A 20-month-old girl comes to the ED with inconsolable irritability and crying for 8-hour duration. On physical examination, a firm tender mass can be palpated at the internal inguinal ring. You suspect an incarcerated inguinal hernia. Which of the following statements is true?

    a. Incarcerated inguinal hernias occur more commonly in girls
    b. Greater than 80% of incarcerated hernias occur during the first year of life
    c. In girls, the incarceration rarely involves the ovary
    d. Strangulation usually occurs after 24 hours of a non-reduced incarcerated hernia
    e. The family and/or patient frequently know about the presence of the hernia

17. Manual reduction of an incarcerated inguinal hernia may involve all of the following, EXCEPT:

    a. Sedating the child with morphine
    b. Placing the child in the Trendelenberg position
    c. Exerting mild pressure at the internal inguinal ring
    d. Observing the child in the hospital after successful manual reduction
    e. Immediately repairing the inguinal hernia after successful manual reduction

18. A 1-month-old male infant is brought to the ED with bilious vomiting and bloody stools. On physical examination, the child is afebrile, with HR 160, RR 30, and BP 80/40. He appears toxic. Abdominal exam shows distension and rectal examination is positive for occult blood. KUB shows few dilated loops of bowel with air-fluid levels. Which of the following is the most appropriate next radiographic study?

    a. Abdominal U/S
    b. Abdominal CT
    c. Upper GI series
    d. Abdominal plain film (KUB)
    e. Barium enema

19. A 6-day-old male is brought to the ED with bile-stained vomiting since the third day of life. On physical examination, the child is afebrile, with stable vital signs. His abdomen is mildly distended. Rectal examination is negative for blood. You obtain a surgical consult and order a KUB. Which finding on KUB most suggests the diagnosis?

    a. The presence of small bowel loops overriding the splenic shadow
    b. The presence of large bowel loops overriding the liver shadow
    c. Many scattered dilated loops of bowel with air-fluid levels
    d. Scattered dilated loops of bowel distal to the lesion
    e. "Double-bubble" sign

20. A 5-week-old boy is brought to the ED with vomiting since 4 weeks of age that has been progressively worsening. The emesis is described as "curdled milk." Although the parents report he has lost 6 ounces, he appears well. You suspect pyloric stenosis. You expect all of the following, EXCEPT:

    a. Guiaic-negative stool
    b. Hypokalemia
    c. A firm, fusiform mass in the right upper abdomen
    d. Prominent gastric waves
    e. Hypochloremic acidosis

21. A 4-week-old girl is brought to the ED with nonbilious, nonbloody vomiting for 4 days. She vomits immediately after every feeding. She seems hungry when she feeds, but is unable to hold down any of her formula. She has lost 1 kg over the past week. She is afebrile, with stable vital signs. You are unable to feel any mass in the abdomen. Which of the following tests would be most helpful?

    a. KUB
    b. Abdominal U/S
    c. Upper GI series
    d. Abdominal CT
    e. Barium enema

22. A 20-month-old male is brought to the ED with abdominal pain. His parents give a history of constipation since birth. He has required frequent assistance with stooling with enemas, suppositories, and digital stimulation. He has not had vomiting. Which of the following is true in the diagnosis of this suspected disease?

    a. After a KUB has been obtained, a barium enema is the best initial diagnostic procedure
    b. There should be stimulation of the rectum for 1–2 days before radiologic examination
    c. Radiologic methods are more reliable than anorectal manometry for short, aganglionic segments
    d. Manometric studies are not dependable in infants less than 3 months of age
    e. Rectal biopsy is necessary for definitive diagnosis

23. A 4-year-old girl comes to the ED with blood in her stool of 1-day duration. She has no vomiting or fever, but is frequently constipated with hard, rocklike stools. She often strains to have a bowel movement. On examination, she has stable vital signs and looks well. Her abdomen is soft and nontender to palpation. Her rectal examination is positive for bright red blood on the examiner's finger, as well as for a small amount of blood visible at the anus. Which of the following is the most likely diagnosis?

    a. Anal fissures
    b. Juvenile polyps
    c. Meckel's diverticulum
    d. Henoch-Schönlein purpura (HSP)
    e. Omental cysts

24. A 6-year-old girl comes to the ED with painless rectal bleeding of 1-day duration. The stools are described as "currant jelly." She has no vomiting or fever. She looks well on examination. Her abdomen is nontender and rectal examination reveals grossly heme-positive stool. There are no fissures visible. Her WBC is 6.9, hct is 28%, and her ESR is 9. Which of the following is the most appropriate next step in diagnosis?

    a. Barium enema
    b. Abdominal U/S
    c. Abdominal CT
    d. Nuclear scintigraphy
    e. Abdominal MRI

25. A 2-year-old boy comes to the ED with a 4-month history of frequent urination. Urinalysis is negative. Multiple urine cultures have been sterile. Blood glucose is normal. VCUG is performed and is negative for reflux, but shows a fatty mass that arises from the ventral surface of the coccyx. Which of the following is true regarding this clinical entity?

    a. It is most commonly diagnosed at birth
    b. It is more common in males than in females
    c. It is most commonly malignant
    d. It has calcifications present in approximately 30%
    e. It is more commonly benign if it has more solid components than more cystic components

26. A 4-day-old boy is brought to the ED with an enlarged scrotal sac that he has had since birth. He is otherwise well. The scrotal sac can be transilluminated and is nontender. Treatment includes:

    a. Reassurance
    b. Aspiration
    c. Testicular U/S
    d. Immediate manual reduction
    e. Immediate exploration in OR

27. A 2-year-old boy is brought to the ED with ingestion of a bobby pin 1 hour ago. He is asymptomatic. Radiography confirms the presence of the bobby pin in the jejunum. Which of the following is the most appropriate intervention?

    a. Observation
    b. Administration of enema
    c. Administration of cathartic
    d. Endoscopic removal
    e. Exploratory laparotomy

28. A 4-year-old girl is brought to the ED for evaluation of RLQ abdominal pain. The pain started this morning. She has been otherwise well except for a cough, URI symptoms, and posttussive emesis. On physical examination she is febrile to 38.7°C, with HR 100, RR 30, and BP 90/60. The chest examination shows good aeration, with decreased breath sounds bilaterally. She has RLQ tenderness on abdominal examination without involuntary guarding or rebound. Which of the following is the most appropriate?

    a. Abdominal U/S
    b. Abdominal CT
    c. KUB
    d. CXR
    e. Fleet's enema

ANSWERS

1. b   A high fever at the onset of symptoms in a child with abdominal pain usually signifies an infectious origin (e.g., a viral gastroenteritis or urinary tract infection). The vomiting and diarrhea in this child suggest gastroenteritis. In a child with perforated appendicitis, there may be high fever, but this usually begins a few days after the onset of the abdominal pain. The child with acute nonperforated appendicitis usually has a low-grade fever that develops after the onset of the vague midepigastric pain. Children with intussusception and malrotation with volvulus usually do not have high fever at the onset of their symptoms.

2. c   Many children find it difficult to cooperate during the abdominal examination. Spending a few minutes gaining the child's confidence is important to the child and helpful to the physician. Once the child is relaxed, the physical examination should follow an orderly progression. It is helpful to let the distressed, crying child go to sleep. A second examination while the child is sleeping may help to determine whether or not there is true tenderness. The use of narcotics in such a young child should be avoided because they may mask findings of peritonitis on subsequent examinations. All children should have an examination that is not hindered by his/her clothes.

3. d Because the position of the appendix varies in children, the localization of the pain and tenderness may also vary. An appendix pointed toward the left lower quadrant will usually cause hypogastric tenderness. An appendix located in the lateral gutter may produce flank pain and lateral abdominal tenderness. An inflamed appendix in the lower pelvis may cause diarrhea from direct irritation of the sigmoid colon.

4. e One needs to consider other causes of abdominal pain that may resemble appendicitis, but are non-surgical. Gastroenteritis, constipation, urinary tract disease, emotional disturbance, and pneumonia are common explanations for the cause of the abdominal pain. The boy in this scenario is afebrile and does not have vomiting or diarrhea. This makes the diagnoses of pneumonia, gastroenteritis, and urinary tract infection less likely. Diverticulitis, a common cause of left lower quadrant pain in adults, is extremely rare in childhood. Constipation is a common childhood cause of abdominal pain.

5. b A CBC in a child with appendicitis usually shows an elevated WBC count in the range of 11,000–15,000 in the first 12–24 hours of the illness. As the appendix becomes more gangrenous, the WBC count rises further and the differential demonstrates more neutrophils and bands.

6. d Abdominal roentgenograms are normal in the majority of cases of acute appendicitis. In 8–10% of cases, however, a calcified appendiceal fecalith can be identified.

7. d Most children with acute nonperforated appendicitis show diminished air in the gastrointestinal tract. This is due to the symptoms of anorexia, vomiting, and diarrhea. Other roentgenographic signs of appendicitis are: thickening of the cecal wall and mucosal folds, indistinct psoas margins with scoliosis concave toward the right, focal obliteration of the adjacent preperitoneal fat pad. The presence of air in the appendix may be a sign of appendicitis; however, a retrocecal appendix may be filled with gas in the normal person. Diffuse air-fluid levels in small and large intestines are usually seen with gastroenteritis.

8. d Young children with perforated appendicitis usually show signs of toxicity. The abdomen may be rigid with extreme tenderness. There is marked elevation of the WBC count, usually above 15,000/mm³, high-grade fever, and hypoactive or absent bowel sounds. The clinical findings may initially be confused with those of pneumonia because the abdominal pain may cause shallow respirations and decreased air entry, or with meningitis, as any movement of the child will produce pain and irritability. In this scenario, however, the child had a distended abdomen and peritoneal signs.

9. a Primary peritonitis is a bacterial infection of the peritoneal cavity usually secondary to a lymph- or blood-borne infection. It occurs in children with nephrosis and cirrhosis, and it may often mimic appendicitis. Primary peritonitis is usually caused by pneumococcus, group *A Streptococcus,* or Gram-negative organisms. Once the diagnosis is suspected, the patient should undergo prompt paracentesis for Gram stain and culture. KUB, abdominal ultrasound and abdominal CT scan are unnecessary if the diagnosis of bacterial peritonitis is suspected. Laparotomy is not indicated.

10. b The most common cause of acute pancreatitis in children is abdominal trauma. When pancreatitis occurs in a child without a history of trauma, the patient should be evaluated for possible congenital abnormalities of the biliary tree or pancreatic ducts (e.g., the presence of a choledochal cyst). Gallstones, a common cause of pancreatitis in adults, are rarely a cause for pancreatitis in children.

11. e The child in this vignette comes with the classic symptoms of intussusception. The presentation of episodic crampy pain with periods of lethargy or listlessness between episodes is characteristic of intussusception. The most common intussusception is ileocolic and an air contrast or barium enema would be indicated for diagnosis and treatment. Pyloromyotomy would be indicated for pyloric stenosis, manual reduction for an incarcerated inguinal hernia, detorsion for testicular torsion, and laparotomy for malrotation with volvulus.

12. a If the abdomen is not too distended, the intussuscepted bowel can most often be palpated as an ill-defined, sausage-shaped mass in the right upper quadrant of the abdomen. The localized portion of the intussusception leads to either partial or complete obstruction and general abdominal distension.

13. a Children who present to the ED early in the course of intussusception often have no history of having passed a "currant jelly" stool. Thus, the absence of bloody stools should not preclude making the diagnosis of intussusception. As the bowel becomes more tightly intussuscepted, the mesenteric veins be-

come compressed, leading to the production of the characteristic bloody stool. The main manifestation of intussusception is crampy abdominal pain. This pain may be preceded by the symptoms and signs of a viral gastroenteritis or upper respiratory infection (URI). During the painful episodes, the child may scream out, but then appears to be perfectly comfortable or only slightly cranky between the episodes. Lethargy is a typical sign that occurs between the episodes of pain. The child may become still and pale and exhibit a shocklike state because of the intense pain. Because of this, children with intussusception have been misdiagnosed as being in the postictal state.

14. b   A barium enema reduction is contraindicated if there is free peritoneal air. Hydrostatically controlled barium enema reduction has been a successful therapy in more than 50% of cases. The barium column should be no higher than 3 feet above the abdomen and manual palpation of the abdomen during the study is contraindicated. A dose of morphine or the use of another sedative is often helpful to relax the child during the study or if there is difficulty with the reduction.

15. c   The recurrence rate after barium enema reduction is 1–3%. When there is recurrence, a second attempt at reduction may be performed by barium enema. With a third episode of intussusception, however, an exploratory laparotomy should be performed. Recurrences are more common in older children and may be caused by a lead point such as a Meckel's diverticulum, polyp, or intraluminal tumor. It may be wise, therefore, to operate with the first recurrence in an older child.

16. a   Incarcerated inguinal hernias occur more frequently in boys. In girls, they usually involve the ovary rather than the intestine. Approximately 60% of incarcerated hernias occur during the first year of life. The patient or family commonly has no previous knowledge of the presence of a congenital hernia. Strangulation can occur within 24 hours of a nonreduced incarcerated hernia, because of progressive edema of the bowel due to lymphatic and venous obstruction.

17. e   Unless the child is very ill with signs of obstruction or toxic from gangrenous bowel, a manual reduction of the incarcerated hernia should be attempted. The child may be sedated with IV morphine. The mother should hold the child until he/she falls asleep. An older child may be placed in the Trendelenberg position in order to allow gravity to facilitate the reduction. When the child is asleep, gentle manipulation of the incarcerated hernia should be attempted. Mild steady pressure should be exerted at the inguinal ring with one hand, while the other attempts to squeeze fluid or gas out of the incarcerated bowel back into the abdominal cavity. If the reduction is unsuccessful, the child should be taken immediately to the operating room. After the hernia has been reduced manually, the child may be admitted for observation, but not for immediate repair. The hernia sac is quite edematous after a reduction and this makes the repair difficult. It is usually done 24 hours after admission.

18. c   The child in this vignette demonstrates concerning signs and symptoms for malrotation with volvulus. The study of choice when assessing a child for malrotation is the upper GI series. The ligament of Treitz is absent in malrotation, so the C-loop of the duodenum is not present. The duodenum lies to the right of the spine and the jejunum presents a coiled spring appearance in the right upper quadrant. The cecum is not fixed and is usually situated in the right upper quadrant; however, because it is mobile, the cecum on barium enema may be visualized in the right lower quadrant. Hence, barium enema is not the most reliable study to rule out malrotation.

19. e   A "double-bubble" sign is often present on an upright film in a child with malrotation and volvulus because of partial obstruction of the duodenum which causes distension of the stomach and first part of the duodenum. The presence of loops of small bowel overriding the liver shadow is also suggestive of an underlying malrotation. When complete volvulus has occurred, there may be only a few dilated loops of bowel with air–fluid levels. Distal to the volvulus there may be little or no gas in the GI tract.

20. e   The vomitus in a child with pyloric stenosis usually does not contain bile or blood. Infants with pyloric stenosis may also become jaundiced. The hyperbilirubinemia usually improves postoperatively for unknown reasons. On physical examination, palpating under the edge of the liver, one may feel a firm, fusiform mass in the shape of an olive. There may also be prominent peristaltic waves that course from left to right across the abdomen. Serum electrolytes may be abnormal due to gastric losses. The potassium and chloride will be low and serum bicarbonate high, thus producing a hypochloremic alkalosis.

21. b   This infant has historical findings of hypertrophic pyloric stenosis. If a classic history of vomiting is not elicited and a mass cannot be felt, real-time ultrasound is the study of choice to confirm the diagno-

sis. The hypertrophic pyloric muscle can be seen as a thick hypoechoic ring surrounding a central echogenic mucosal and submucosal region. If the ultrasonography does not show a hypertrophic pylorus, an upper GI series should then be done to eliminate gastroesophageal reflux, malrotation, and antral web as possible diagnoses.

22. a   After flat and upright abdominal roentgenograms have been obtained, a barium enema is the best initial diagnostic procedure. There should be no bowel preparation and no rectal stimulation (e.g., enemas or digital examinations) for 1–2 days before the procedure. Anorectal manometry to determine the presence or absence of internal anal sphincter relaxation can help establish the neurogenic dysfunction of the bowel. Rectal manometric studies are more reliable than radiologic methods for short, aganglionic segments. Manometric studies are not dependable in infants less than 3 weeks of age. If the barium enema and anal manometry studies indicate Hirshsprung's disease, rectal biopsy is not necessary to confirm the diagnosis.

23. a   The child in this vignette has a history of constipation with hard, rocklike stools. There is bright red blood on rectal examination that is visible at the anus. An anal fissure is the most likely cause of the blood. Juvenile polyps and Meckel's diverticulum may cause rectal bleeding, but there is usually no history of constipation. HSP is unlikely in this scenario, because the patient does not have abdominal pain, rash, or joint pain. Omental cysts are rare, usually asymptomatic, and can reach gigantic size. They usually present as an intra-abdominal mass.

24. d   This patient's symptoms are consistent with a Meckel's diverticulum. Clinical problems are seen in only 2% of patients with a Meckel's diverticulum. The most common presentation is a bleeding ulcer due to ectopic gastric mucosa that produces the characteristic "currant jelly" appearance. Barium studies will usually fail to identify a Meckel's diverticulum. The imaging modality of choice for detection of ectopic gastric mucosa in a bleeding Meckel's diverticulum is nuclear scintigraphy. The accuracy of scintigraphy in detecting ectopic gastric mucosa is 95%. Ultrasound and MRI are of no use in identifying a Meckel's diverticulum.

25. a   The presacral sacrococcygeal teratoma is the most frequent tumor of the caudal region in childhood, and is more common in females than in males. Most tumors are benign and are noted at birth. Tumors in patients beyond neonatal age have a higher incidence of malignancy. Calcifications are present in 60% of presacral sacrococcygeal teratoma and are more frequent in benign tumors. Those tumors with more solid components are more malignant than are those with more cystic components. Frequently, children (like the child in this vignette) may present with polyuria, as the teratoma presses on the bladder.

26. a   A physiologic hydrocele is trapped fluid around the testicle in the tunica vaginalis at the time of embryologic closure of the processus vaginalis. This is a normal newborn finding. The fluid will generally be absorbed in the first 12 months of life. Physiologic hydroceles should not be surgically repaired as soon as they are diagnosed.

27. a   Foreign bodies that reach the stomach, whether pointed or sharp-edged, usually pass completely through the intestinal tract and will be evacuated. Cathartics and other efforts to increase transit-time should not be used. Coins may remain in the child's stomach for a considerable time and will eventually pass, even after a month or more. A foreign body will occasionally lodge in the esophagus, necessitating removal. Once an esophageal foreign body has been identified, it should be promptly removed to prevent complications such as edema, ulceration, aspiration, pneumonia, or perforation. A long, thin foreign body (e.g., a bobby pin) sometimes may not be able to traverse the turn where the duodenum joins the jejunum at the ligament of Treitz.

28. d   The symptoms and physical examination findings (fever and tachypnea) in this child are consistent with right lower lobe pneumonia. Right lower quadrant pain is sometimes found in children with right lower lobe pneumonia, which can mimic appendicitis.

CHAPTER 119

Thoracic Emergencies

VINCENT J. WANG, M.D.

QUESTIONS

1. A 1-month-old girl is brought to the ED because of respiratory distress. She was born at 29 weeks gestation, but never required mechanical ventilation. She has had noisy breathing since birth, but over the last 2 days, she has had a cough and rhinorrhea. She developed respiratory distress today, with noisier than normal breathing. Her vital signs are: T 38°C, HR 130, RR 48, and BP 90/50. O_2 saturation is 95% on room air. She has moderate intercostal retractions and inspiratory stridor at rest. She does not have wheezing or rales. Treatment includes:

   a. Endotracheal intubation
   b. Albuterol nebulizer treatments
   c. Dexamethasone IM
   d. Racemic epinephrine nebulizer treatments
   e. Admission and observation

2. A 2-week-old boy is brought to the ED because of noisy breathing. He was born full term, after a normal spontaneous vaginal delivery without complications. The parents believe that his breathing has always been noisy, and that he has been a slow feeder. His vital signs are: T 37°C, HR 140, RR 44, and BP 85/55. He has coarse upper airway sounds with expiratory wheezing. When he is arching his back and extending his neck, the symptoms improve. His CXR reveals a midline trachea at the level of the carina. Which of the following is most likely to confirm the diagnosis?

   a. Echocardiography
   b. Barium esophagram
   c. Bronchoscopy
   d. Gastric pH probe
   e. Trial of nebulized dexamethasone

3. A 15-year-old boy is brought to the ED after being assaulted by another adolescent. Witnesses report that he was hit in the right eye, and punched several times in the chest and abdomen. He complains of pain at these sites, but also complains of shortness of breath. His vital signs are: T 37°C, HR 150, RR 44, and BP 110/70, with an O_2 saturation of 94% on room air. On examination, he has moderate swelling around his right eye. He is unable to look upward and outward. He has moderate tenderness over his right chest, with significant contusions over the lower right chest. He is dyspneic and has decreased breath sounds over the right side of his chest. He has moderate left upper quadrant (LUQ) tenderness and pain of his shoulder. His extremities are well perfused and his neurological examination is normal. Immediate management includes:

   a. Obtaining an abdominal CT scan
   b. Ophthalmologic consultation
   c. IV methylprednisolone 30 mg/kg
   d. Needle thoracostomy
   e. Obtaining a CXR

4. A 9-year-old girl is brought to the ED because of cough and fever. She has had cough for 1 week and fever for 5 days. She was evaluated at another medical center 3 days ago and was told that she had a right-sided pneumonia. She has been taking amoxicillin for 3 days. Since then, she developed right-sided chest pain when she breathes deeply. Her vital signs are: T 38.3°C, HR 110, RR 26, and BP 110/70, with an O_2 saturation of 94% on room air. She is somewhat ill appearing, but awake and alert. Her cardiovascular examination is normal, but she has decreased breath sounds at the right base. Her abdomen is soft and nontender. Your management would be:

   a. Obtain a CXR
   b. Chest CT scan
   c. Needle thoracostomy
   d. Oral amoxicillin-clavulanate
   e. Oral azithromycin

5. A 2-month-old girl is brought to the ED for cough and respiratory distress. She was born without complications. She has had an occasional cough for the past 3 weeks, and the parents think that she is breathing faster. Her vital signs are T 36.8°C, HR 130, RR 64, and BP 85/50. She is tachypneic, with mild intercostal retractions, and has decreased aeration over her right upper chest. Her physical examination is otherwise normal. A CXR reveals a radiolucency of the right upper lobe, with faint pulmonary markings throughout the lucency. You suspect the following diagnosis:

   a. Tension pneumothorax
   b. Congenital lobar emphysema
   c. Vascular sling
   d. Cystic fibrosis
   e. Congenital diaphragmatic hernia

6. A 12-year-old boy is brought to the ED for cough and wheezing. He has had multiple episodes of cough and wheezing over the past few months. He was diagnosed with asthma, and treated with bronchodilators and corticosteroids with good effect. His symptoms, however, appear to be more frequent now. His vital signs are: T 37.2°C, HR 110, RR 28, and BP 110/70, with an O_2 saturation of 98% on room air. He is comfortable, in no acute distress. He has mild wheezing and minimal tachypnea, but his examination is otherwise normal. His CXR reveals a density, shaped like a sail on the AP view, and in the anterior mediastinum on the lateral view. Your management is:

   a. Outpatient management with albuterol and prednisone over 5 days
   b. Admission for albuterol and methylprednisolone
   c. Admission for cefuroxime
   d. Obtain a CT scan of the chest
   e. Obtain a gastric aspirate for acid fast bacilli

7. A 5-year-old girl is diagnosed with non-Hodgkin's lymphoma and is transferred to your ED for admission and chemotherapy. Upon arrival by ambulance, you notice that she is in mild distress. Upon your examination, she has a dark red/blue complexion to her face and she has distended neck veins. Her face and neck also appear edematous. You suspect that the etiology of her symptoms is:

   a. Superior vena cava syndrome
   b. Hyperleukocystosis
   c. Thrombocytopenia
   d. Graft versus host disease
   e. Hyperkalemia

8. A 3-month-old boy is brought to the ED because of vomiting. He has been vomiting for the past 2 days and has not been able to feed. He has not had a bowel movement in 2 days as well. His vital signs are: T 37.2°C, HR 170, RR 68, and BP 90/50. His lungs are clear, but he is tachypneic. His breath sounds seem diminished at the left base. His abdomen is distended and he has diffuse tenderness. He has blood in his stool. On chest and abdominal radiographs, he has several cystic lesions in the left lower lobe, and multiple loops of distended bowel in the upper abdomen. The diagnosis may be confirmed by:

   a. Air contrast enema
   b. Rectal biopsy
   c. Upper GI series
   d. Sweat testing
   e. Needle aspiration of the lesions

9. A 14-year-old boy complains of lower chest pain. He had been wrestling with a friend and complains of right lateral chest pain. He does not remember significant trauma. On examination, he has point tenderness over the lower right ribs. He has no abdominal tenderness. His CXR reveals a lytic lucency of his right tenth rib, on the lateral aspect. You suspect:

   a. Rib fracture
   b. Ewing's sarcoma
   c. Chondrosarcoma
   d. Anaplastic sarcoma
   e. Osteosarcoma

ANSWERS

1. e This patient has tracheomalacia or laryngomalacia, which is complicated by a concurrent URI. Treatment for this condition is supportive, but if the patient develops significant respiratory distress, assisted ventilation may be necessary. In this vignette, supportive care and observation are all that are necessary. The other three treatment choices are not indicated: albuterol for bronchiolitis or asthma, dexamethasone for croup, and racemic epinephrine for croup or bronchiolitis.

2. a Vascular rings may cause tracheal and esophageal compression, resulting in both respiratory and feeding difficulty. Patients are usually diagnosed early in infancy, but may occasionally be misdiagnosed and present later with more severe symptoms. A CXR may reveal a right aortic arch, but this may be difficult to determine because of the size of the thymus. Another radiographic sign is a midline trachea (normally the trachea is displaced slightly to the right at the level of the carina). A double aortic arch and a right aortic arch may cause this radiographic finding. Even though a barium esophagogram will determine the presence of either one of these, only echocardiography or angiography will distinguish between these two. Bronchoscopy might detect the presence of compression on the trachea, but will not be able to determine the etiology of extrinsic causes. (Mandell VS, and Braverman RM. Vascular Rings and Slings. In *Nadas' Pediatric Cardiology*. St. Louis: Mosby-Yearbook, Inc. 1992:719–726.)

3. d The most emergent problem this patient has is a pneumothorax, which must be decompressed immediately. Obtaining a CXR would confirm this diagnosis, but would delay the definitive treatment unnecessarily. The patient also appears to have a blowout fracture of his orbit, and will require ophthalmological consultation and potentially surgery. His abdominal findings suggest a splenic injury, with referred pain to the shoulder (Kehr's sign). Both of these emergencies must be addressed after decompressing the pneumothorax, however. There is no evidence of a spinal injury; therefore, the use of methylprednisolone is not indicated.

4. a This patient has failed outpatient therapy and warrants admission; changing to more broad-spectrum oral antibiotics as an outpatient should not be an option. A follow-up CXR is warranted to determine the presence of a pleural effusion, which may complicate pneumonia. The presence of an effusion might warrant needle thoracentesis, or even chest tube placement, depending on the size and persistence of the effusion. Decision of appropriate inpatient antibiotics can be made once a repeat CXR has been done. She has no clinical signs of tension pneumothorax, which would require thoracostomy. A chest CT scan is not indicated at this time.

5. b Congenital lobar emphysema accounts for approximately 50% of all congenital lung malformations. Infants may be normal at birth, but develop symptoms gradually over the next few weeks to months. The upper lobes are the most commonly involved. Pneumothorax may be suspected, but this is less likely with faint pulmonary markings and a more chronic history of symptoms. A vascular sling should not produce a radiolucency on radiograph; cystic fibrosis would produce multiple cystic lucencies late in the course of the disease, but not at the infant age; and congenital diaphragmatic hernia would be seen as bowel-shaped lucencies, as the bowel herniates through the diaphragm. This will usually be evident in the left lower lung, rather than the right upper lung.

6. d The most common causes of mediastinal masses are neurogenic tumors, lymphomas, and germ-cell tumors. This patient should have a chest CT scan to define the mass further and to evaluate tracheal compression. Further treatment for asthma is inappropriate, and the patient's symptoms may have been masked with corticosteroid treatment in the past. Pneumonia is a diagnostic possibility, but this radioopacity should be further evaluated. Thymus enlargement is also a possibility, but this would be extremely rare in this age group. The radiographic findings are not consistent with tuberculosis.

7. a Each of the choices are oncologic emergencies, and the consequence of a primary oncologic process. (Crist WM, and Heslop H. Table 448–2: Oncologic Emergencies. In: *Nelson Textbook of Pediatrics*, fifteenth edition. Philadelphia: W.B. Saunders, 1996:1451.) Her symptoms and oncologic process support the diagnosis of superior vena cava syndrome. Even though hyperleukocytosis may cause vascular occlusion, it would be unlikely to occur in the head and neck area alone. Thrombocytopenia may cause petechiae and purpura, but this would be unlikely to cause distended neck veins or facial and neck

edema. Graft versus host disease is a complication of bone marrow transplantation. Hyperkalemia may be a complication of lymphoma, but would not present with these symptoms.

8. c   Diaphragmatic hernias that become symptomatic after the neonatal period often cause gastrointestinal complaints, especially if the bowel is strangulated within the diaphragm. The cystic lucencies in the left lower lobe represent loops of bowel. An upper gastrointestinal series or an abdominal and chest CT scan would confirm the diagnosis. Intussusception should be suspected in a child with abdominal pain, vomiting, and heme-positive stool, but this diagnosis is unlikely given the radiologic findings; therefore, an air contrast enema is not helpful. Rectal biopsy would be indicated to diagnose Hirschprung's disease, which may cause distended loops of bowel, but not bloody stools or cystic lesions in the lung. Cystic fibrosis would produce multiple cystic lucencies late in the course of the disease, but not at the infant age; therefore, sweat testing is not indicated. Needle biopsy would be indicated for abscesses of the lung, but this diagnosis is less likely given the signs and symptoms.

9. b   Childhood chest wall tumors are likely to be malignant. Ewing's sarcoma typically involves the lateral aspects of the ribs, whereas chondrosarcoma usually involves the costal cartilages between the distal rib end and the sternum and anaplastic sarcomas involve the sternum. A rib fracture will not be radiolucent on x-ray. Osteosarcoma is usually a sclerotic lesion, rather than a lytic lesion.

CHAPTER **120**

Ophthalmic Emergencies

CYNTHIA JOHNSON MOLLEN, M.D.

QUESTIONS

1. A 4-year-old boy is brought to the ED for a 2-day history of severe right eye swelling and tactile fevers. His vital signs are: T 37.5°C, HR 100, RR 20, and BP 100/60. There is no discharge noted from the eye. Extraocular muscles are intact and there is no proptosis. There is facial tenderness to palpation below the right eye. Treatment should include:

   a. Mupiricin only
   b. Cool compresses and discharge to home
   c. IV cefuroxime
   d. Amoxicillin PO
   e. Percutaneous aspiration of the area of cellulitis

2. A patient has periorbital cellulitis. Which of the following conditions requires inpatient treatment for the patient?

   a. A bug bite is visible at the edge of the cellulitis
   b. The patient is 3 years old
   c. The patient's temperature is 38.7°C
   d. The periorbital swelling involves the upper and lower lids
   e. The patient does not have a primary care provider (PCP)

3. A 6-year-old boy is brought to the ED because of tenderness, localized swelling, and drainage near the lid margin of his left eye. He has not had fever and he has no other medical problems. The conjunctiva appears pink. His physical examination is otherwise normal. The most likely diagnosis is:

   a. Infectious conjunctivitis
   b. Allergic conjunctivitis
   c. Periorbital cellulitis
   d. Bug bite
   e. Stye (external hordeolum)

4. A 2-year-old girl arrives in the ED in distress after pulling an open bottle of hair relaxer off a shelf. Her mother is holding a wet washcloth over the patient's left eye. On physical examination, the conjunctiva is pale. Immediate management is:

   a. Application of a topical anesthetic
   b. Ocular lavage with 2 l of normal saline (NS)
   c. Sedation prior to intervention
   d. Aggressive mechanical debridement
   e. No treatment is necessary

5. An 18-month-old boy who attends day care has had 3 days of drainage from his eyes. The mother reports that his eyes are crusted shut each morning, and it takes her several minutes to clean them off with a washcloth. Bacterial conjunctivitis is the most likely diagnosis if:

   a. There are multiple infected contacts
   b. It is bilateral
   c. There is purulent drainage
   d. There is itching
   e. There is chemosis

6. A 2-day-old infant girl, just discharged from the nursery, is brought to the ED by her father because of eye drainage. The eye is swollen and there is a thick discharge. Initial treatment should include all of the following, EXCEPT:

   a. Topical erythromycin ointment
   b. Parenteral cephalosporin
   c. Hourly saline ocular lavage
   d. Topical gentamicin ointment
   e. Oral erythromycin

7. A 15-month-old boy is brought to the ED because of eye redness and swelling. He rubs his eye many times while you are in the examining room with him. You note that he has a vesicular rash on his trunk and face, with some lesions near his eyes. The mother states he has had the rash recurrently over the last 12 months two or three times. He has also had fever and vomiting. Therapy should include:

a. Gentamicin drops
b. Ophthalmology consult
c. Anesthetic drops
d. Ophthalmologic follow-up within 24 hours
e. Steroid drops for the swelling

ANSWERS

1. c Treatment for periorbital cellulitis should include IV antibiotics, or an oral antibiotic that would provide appropriate coverage for the likely organisms. Close follow-up is essential if oral antibiotics are chosen. Amoxicillin is not appropriate, nor are topical antibiotics or cool compresses. It is not essential to aspirate the area because this will rarely provide an organism and is painful. The differential diagnosis of eye swelling includes infectious and allergic conjunctivitis, both of which can be treated topically; however, there is no discharge or injection of the eye in this patient. This cellulitis is most likely due to a sinusitis, given the facial tenderness over the maxillary sinus area. A CT should be considered to evaluate the extent of disease.

2. c If systemic signs or symptoms exist, including fever, a patient with periorbital cellulitis should be treated with IV antibiotics. A patient who shows no improvement in 24–48 hours should also be treated with IV antibiotics, as should all infants. If there is suspicion of severe sinusitis, IV therapy should be strongly considered because this complication has the potential to spread to the meninges. Periorbital cellulitis in a well-appearing older child, especially if it is thought to be due to an insect bite, can be treated with oral or IM antibiotics and careful follow-up. The lack of a PCP is not a contraindication to outpatient therapy, as long as follow-up can be guaranteed.

3. e The localization of symptoms to the lid margin helps make the diagnosis of a stye, which is a blocked gland within the eyelid. A more generalized swelling and drainage can exist in conjunctivitis, but the hallmark is an injected conjunctiva, which is not the case in this patient. A periorbital cellulitis rarely has eye drainage, and a bug bite is usually visible on close inspection.

4. b This is a true ocular emergency. When a patient has a potentially severe chemical burn to the eye, irrigation should be performed immediately, even before sedation or anesthesia of the eye. Alkali burns are extremely dangerous, and can cause blanching rather than injection of the eye, as in this patient. This can indicate a poor prognosis. With any history of an ocular chemical burn, irrigation should be performed, regardless of whether the eye appears irritated. The patient can be discharged home (without treatment) only if the substance was clearly not alkali or strongly acidic, and if there is no injection. Debridement is required only if there are visible particles.

5. c Clear serous drainage is more often seen with conjunctivitis due to a viral etiology, whereas bacterial etiologies often cause more purulent discharge. Multiple contacts and bilateral infection are more often associated with viral conjunctivitis, although these can occur with bacterial infection. Pruritis and chemosis are more often associated with allergic conjunctivitis. One viral infection that can be severe enough to mimic bacterial infection is epidemic keratoconjunctivitis due to adenovirus. The hallmarks of this infection are dramatic lid swelling, a sandy foreign body sensation, and preauricular lymphadenopathy. The symptoms usually start in one eye and quickly spread to the other.

6. d Neonatal purulent conjunctivitis, which is assumed to be a gonococcal infection until cultures are negative, must be treated with an IV cephalosporin (ceftriaxone or cefotaxime). Co-infection with

chlamydia should be assumed, so therapy with both topical and oral erythromycin should be started empirically. Oral erythromycin is necessary to eradicate the carriage state, which can lead to pneumonia. Saline lavage may decrease the number of organisms in contact with the cornea. Topical gentamicin has no role in this infection.

7. **b** This patient may have a herpetic ocular infection, which may rapidly progress to corneal destruction. Ophthalmologic consultation should therefore be obtained immediately, in addition to the commencement of IV antivirals. Steroid and anesthetic drops should only be prescribed by an ophthalmologist. Inappropriate use of steroids can lead to glaucoma, cataracts, increased severity of a corneal viral infection, or rebound symptoms. Even though ocular anesthetics are safe for use in the ED, prolonged use can lead to corneal ulceration; therefore, they should not be prescribed for outpatient use.

CHAPTER **121**

Otolaryngologic Emergencies

JEFFREY P. LOUIE, M.D.

QUESTIONS

1. A 3-year-old comes to the ED with a chief complaint of right-sided ear pain for 12 hours. His mother reports that this would be his second ear infection in 3 years. He is otherwise well appearing and is diagnosed with an acute otitis media. For this patient, which of the following is NOT a likely etiology of acute otitis media?

   a. *Streptococcus pneumoniae influenzae*
   b. *Haemophilus influenzae*
   c. *Moraxella catarrhalis*
   d. Adenovirus
   e. *Pseudomonas* species

2. A 16-year-old is brought to ED with a chief complaint of left ear pain. He swims daily in the public pool. He denies fevers or headache. On examination, the external canal is slightly swollen and very tender. A foul smell is noted. Which statement best describes the management of this condition?

   a. The ear canal should be flushed with iodine
   b. The ear canal should be drained using a number eleven surgical blade
   c. Oral antibiotics should be prescribed
   d. Antibiotic ear drops should be prescribed
   e. A wick should be placed and topical antibiotics prescribed

3. A 10-year-old boy is brought to the ED for acute onset of dizziness that he describes as a spinning sensation. He denies any medical problems other than a cold last week. He is afebrile, with a normal neurologic exam and tympanic membranes that appear normal. Which of the following is the best treatment option?

   a. Oral steroids
   b. Amoxicillin
   c. Azithromycin
   d. No treatment
   e. Diphenhydramine

4. A 9-year-old girl comes to the ED with recurrent nasal drainage. The mother states that her daughter has been on antibiotics with some relief, but the drainage always returns. Of the etiologies given, which is a possible cause of chronic or recurrent nasal discharge?

   a. Asthma
   b. Septal deviation
   c. Chronic pharyngitis
   d. Septal hematoma
   e. Herpangina

5. A 5-year-old child is brought to the ED for epistaxis. The mother reports that her son has had recurrent nosebleeds for a whole month. He is otherwise a healthy child, with no recent head trauma or significant past medical history. All of the following are possible causes of his symptoms, EXCEPT:

   a. Nose picking
   b. Septal hematoma
   c. Rendu-Osler-Weber disease
   d. Sinusitis
   e. Leukemia

6. A 3-week-old infant boy is brought to the ED with a 2-day history of noisy breathing. The history reveals a possible tactile temperature and an exposure to an older sibling with a cold. The vital signs are: T 37.6°C, HR 160, and RR 60; pulse oximetry reveals an O_2 saturation of 90% on room air. On physical examination, inspiratory stridor is noted. In addition, there is a small (1 cm × 1 cm) raised red lesion on his left cheek that does not blanch with pressure. The patient responds to supplemental oxygen, nebulized racemic epinephrine, and dexamethasone. Two hours after his last treatment the patient is resting comfortably on room air. Which of the following should be done for this patient?

   a. Start oral steroids as an outpatient
   b. CXR
   c. AP and lateral neck radiographs
   d. No further treatment
   e. Direct laryngoscopy

7. A 5-year-old boy is brought to the ED with a 1.5 cm × 1.5 cm lump on his neck for 1 week. The lump became red and painful 3 days ago and he was placed on oral amoxicillin (40 mg/kg/day) by his pediatrician. A PPD placed at that time shows 5 mm of erythema (mumps control positive). The lump is still red and tender to palpation. He is afebrile and otherwise well appearing. Which of the following should be done?

   a. Surgical excision
   b. Amoxicillin 75 mg/kg/day
   c. Cephalexin 50 mg/kg/day
   d. Start isoniazid
   e. Admit for IV antibiotics

8. A 16-year-old mother brings her 5-day-old baby into the ED because of a "mass" on her baby's face. The mother is upset and would like the "mass" removed. On exam, the baby is well appearing, but has a 3 ×3 cm hemangioma on the left cheek. Which of the following would you recommend?

   a. No treatment
   b. Topical steroids
   c. Lasar therapy
   d. Surgical removal
   e. Oral steroids

9. A 3-day-old infant is brought to the ED for evaluation of a neck mass. The parents are not sure if the mass has been present since birth. The parents report no fevers, changes in feeding, or in number of wet diapers. On examination, the baby is well appearing. When the neck is turned to the left, a 1-cm mass is noted on the right side of the neck. The mass is firm and nontender. What is the most likely diagnosis?

   a. Rhabdomyosarcoma
   b. Wry neck
   c. Lymphoma
   d. Retropharyngeal abscess
   e. Histiocytoma

ANSWERS

1. **e**   *Streptococcus pneumoniae, Haemophilus influenzae, Moraxella catarrhalis,* and adenovirus are common causes of acute otitis media. *Pseudomonas* species is generally found in chronic otitis media and mastoiditis. It is not a usual cause of acute otitis media.

2. **d**   Most otitis externa can be managed by debridement (i.e., suction or curette) and otic antibiotics (e.g., neomycin, bacitracin, and hydrocortisone). If the external canal is swollen, which would impede the topical otic drops, a wick can be placed into the canal to open it and allow topical exposure of the medication to the walls of the external canal. Oral antibiotics are generally not recommended for simple external otitis unless there is a cellulitis, cervical adenitis, or an abscess.

3. **d**   This patient is describing vertigo. It is most often caused by a self-limited labyrinthitis, often associated with a recent URI. No specific therapy is usually required in uncomplicated cases. In cases where the vertigo is disabling or recurrent, treatment with meclizine or dimenhydrinate should be considered.

4. **b**   Chronic pharyngitis, asthma, minor trauma, or a septal hematoma do not result in persistent nasal discharge. Any obstruction of a nasal passage may result in chronic nasal discharge; thus, a neoplasm, a foreign body, septal deviation, adenoid hypertrophy, choanal atresia, and allergic polyps are all potential causes of persistent nasal discharge. Other possible causes are dental disease and immunodeficiency syndromes.

5. **b**   Nose picking is the most common cause of nose bleeding. Any bleeding abnormalities (e.g., idiopathic thrombocytopenia purpura, leukemia (thrombocytopenia), Rendu-Osler-Weber disease, hemophilia, or von Willebrand's disease) may also present with recurrent nosebleeds. Infectious etiologies such as sinusitis can also cause nosebleeds. Tumors (benign or malignant) are also included in the differential diagnosis, as are foreign bodies. Dental pathology or recurrent tonsillitis are not causes of nosebleeds. A septal hematoma is caused by nasal trauma and is a true emergency requiring drainage, but it is not a cause of recurrent epistaxis.

6. e Any patient with a cutaneous hemangioma and stridor should be evaluated by an otolaryngologist to rule out a subglottic hemangioma (50% of infants with subglottic hemangiomas will have a cutaneous lesion). Thus, this patient requires laryngoscopy to exclude the diagnosis of subglottic hemangioma prior to discharge.

7. c Adenitis is commonly seen in children and is usually caused by *Streptococcus* species or *S. aureus*. Failure of treatment with amoxicillin points to *Staphylococcus* as the cause in this case. As this patient is afebrile and well appearing, outpatient treatment with an oral antibiotic with better *Staphylococcus* coverage (e.g., cephalexin) is appropriate. Tuberculosis and atypical mycobacteria can also cause an isolated neck lesion, but they are unlikely in this scenario.

8. a Indication for hemangioma removal include airway obstruction, thrombocytopenia, skin necrosis, and bleeding. Neutropenia, chronic pain, or thrombocytosis are not usually associated with hemangiomas. Cosmesis is rarely an indication for hemangioma removal. Most lesions will slowly resolve in 1–2 years; thus, observation is the preferred treatment modality. If the hemangioma causes heart failure or airway obstruction, it can be removed with several methods: systemic steroids, cryotherapy, CO_2 laser excision, interferon, sclerosing agents, and surgical excision.

9. b Wry neck is a very common cause of torticollis in newborn infants and range of motion exercises are the treatment modality. The mass is fibrous tissue. Rhabdomyosarcoma is the most common soft tissue sarcoma of the head and neck in children, but it is rare in infants, as are lymphomas and histiocytomas. All three of these do not cause torticollis. A retropharyngeal abscess can present as torticollis, and may be associated with a palpable mass (adenopathy), but these patients are usually febrile and toxic appearing.

CHAPTER **122**

Urologic Emergencies

VINCENT J. WANG, M.D.

QUESTIONS

1. A 4-month-old boy has had a fever for 2 days. His foreskin is nonretractable. A urine specimen obtained by suprapubic aspiration is negative. Concerning the foreskin, you recommend:

    a. No further therapy
    b. Surgical correction
    c. Manual reduction
    d. Mupirocin ointment
    e. Hydrocortisone ointment

2. A 4-year-old uncircumcised boy is brought to the ED for swelling of his penis. His foreskin is retracted behind the glans penis, and he has swelling of the glans. He has mild erythema of the site. Appropriate initial treatment includes:

    a. Wrapping suture material around the glans
    b. Application of ice to the penis
    c. Administration of furosemide
    d. Placing the patient in the supine position
    e. Surgical division of the foreskin

3. A 3-year-old boy is brought to the ED for swelling and erythema of his foreskin. He is afebrile, and his examination reveals swelling and erythema of the foreskin only. His examination is otherwise normal. Your treatment includes:

    a. Incision and drainage
    b. IV antibiotics
    c. Manual reduction
    d. Oral antibiotics
    e. Circumcision

4. A 3-year-old white boy is brought to the ED because of priapism. There is no history of trauma. He is otherwise healthy, but appears pale to you. His examination is normal except for the priapism. The most useful diagnostic test is a:

    a. Toxicology screen
    b. Psychiatric referral
    c. Hemoglobin electrophoresis
    d. Rectal palpation of the prostate
    e. Peripheral blood smear

5. A 6-year-old boy is brought to the ED because part of his foreskin is trapped in his zipper. Treatment involves:

    a. Dissecting the foreskin free
    b. Application of ice to the penis
    c. Cutting the median bar of the zipper
    d. Gently retracting the zipper
    e. Gently advancing the zipper

6. In which of the following patients is a urine culture NOT indicated?

    a. Well-appearing 4-month-old boy with a temperature of 39.8°C
    b. An 18-month-old girl with vomiting and a temperature of 38.3°C
    c. A 12-month-old boy with cough and a temperature of 38.3°C
    d. A 5-year-old girl with dysuria and a temperature of 37°C
    e. A 3-year-old girl with hematuria and a temperature of 37.8°C

7. A 6-year-old girl complains of fever and dysuria. Her abdomen is soft and nontender, and she has no costovertebral angle (CVA) tenderness. Her urethral and perineal examinations are normal. A urinalysis reveals 20–50 WBCs/hpf and Gram-negative rods. Empiric treatment with which of the following would be appropriate:

a. Trimethoprim-sulfamethoxazole
b. Nitrofurantoin
c. Methenamine mandelate
d. Tetracycline
e. Cranberry juice

ANSWERS

1. a   Adhesions between the glans and the foreskin are normal in infants, and the foreskin should not be retracted. Retraction may be painful for the child, and may also lead to inflammation and scarring. Between the ages of 2 and 4 years, 90% of children will have spontaneous lysis of these adhesions.

2. b   The initial step is to apply ice and steady local manual compression. An injection of lidocaine to block the dorsal penile nerve will help reduce discomfort. If manual reduction fails, surgical division of the foreskin is indicated. Wrapping silk suture material has been used for ring removal from the fingers. The other techniques are not recommended.

3. d   Balanoposthitis is a form of cellulitis of the foreskin, which may extend to the glans. The acute infection should be treated with warm soaks and oral antibiotics. Voiding into a tub of warm water may make voiding easier for the child. Incision and drainage, IV antibiotics, and manual reduction are not indicated. Circumcision may be considered if the patient has multiple episodes of infection.

4. e   Priapism is rare in children. The most common etiology of priapism is a vaso-occlusive crisis involving the corporal bodies. Sickle-cell disease, however, is unlikely in this scenario. Other etiologies of priapism include trauma and leukemic infiltration. Given the lack of trauma, therefore, a peripheral blood smear would be the most useful. Toxic ingestions are unlikely to cause priapism. A 3-year-old boy may have normal exploratory behavior, but this will not cause priapism. Prostatitis is a common cause of priapism in adults, but not in children; thus, palpation of the prostate is unlikely to be helpful.

5. c   You suspect there is something about Mary to this story. Cutting the median bar of the zipper will release the two halves of the zipper from engagement, and the zipper will fall apart. Dissecting the foreskin is not indicated. Application of ice will reduce edema, but not enough to solve this problem. Advancing or retracting the zipper will be painful for the patient, and will lacerate the tissue.

6. c   A urinary tract infection (UTI) may produce nonspecific findings. In an infant, there may be unexplained fevers, irritability, failure to thrive, or gastrointestinal symptoms. The urine may be cloudy or foul-smelling. In an older child, he/she may complain of frequency, urgency, dysuria, secondary enuresis, and fever. Hematuria may also be seen in older girls. Cough and fever in an infant would suggest a URI rather than a UTI.

7. a   Trimethoprim-sulfamethoxazole is the most frequently used antibiotic for UTIs in children. Nitrofurantoin is effective, but may produce gastrointestinal upset in children. Methenamine mandelate has no role in childhood UTIs. Tetracycline should not be used routinely in children under 8–10 years of age because it can cause discoloration of teeth. Drinking cranberry juice and other foods that may acidify the urine are helpful adjuncts, but will not definitively treat the UTI. The choice of antibiotic will be influenced by the spectrum of organisms isolated in the bacterial community and the antibiotic susceptibility pattern of these organisms.

CHAPTER 123

Orthopedic Emergencies

JOYCE SOPRANO, M.D.

QUESTIONS

1. A 10-day-old girl is referred to you with a fever of 38.5°C. On physical examination you note that she is not moving her right leg and becomes irritable when you examine her. Plain radiographs of the hip and lower extremity are normal. A bone scan shows increased uptake in the proximal femur. The most appropriate antibiotic choice is:

   a. IV ampicillin
   b. IV gentamicin
   c. IV nafcillin and gentamicin
   d. IV ampicillin and gentamicin
   e. IV cefazolin

2. A 12-year-old girl complains of redness and swelling of the right foot that has been worsening over the past 2 days. On physical exam, she has a low-grade fever, marked swelling, and erythema of the right foot, and a small healing puncture wound on the sole of the foot. She recalls having stepped on a nail several days ago. Plain radiographs show soft-tissue swelling of the foot. The most appropriate initial management is:

   a. Cephalexin PO for 5 days
   b. Cephalexin PO for 14 days
   c. Repeat plain radiographs in 10 days
   d. Obtain a bone scan
   e. IV gentamicin for 14 days

3. A 2-year-old boy comes to the ED refusing to walk. On arrival, his temperature is 38.7°C. He has no obvious erythema or swelling of the lower extremities, but he holds his left leg externally rotated and flexed at the hip. Internal rotation of the femur elicits pain. His WBC count is 13,000, ESR is 42 mm/hr, and plain radiographs of his left hip appear normal. The most appropriate next step is:

   a. Discharge on ibuprofen and bedrest
   b. Hip ultrasound
   c. Bone scan
   d. Plain radiographs of the left knee
   e. MRI of the left hip

4. A 3-year-old boy comes to the ED complaining of right leg pain. On physical exam he is afebrile, has a slight limp, and has mild pain when you attempt to internally rotate his right hip fully. His CBC reveals a WBC count of 10,000 and his ESR is 16. Plain radiographs of the hip suggest a right hip effusion. A sample of the joint fluid is obtained by ultrasound-guided aspiration and shows 1000 WBCs/mm³ and a negative Gram stain. The most appropriate management is:

   a. Immediate orthopedic consultation for joint irrigation
   b. Broad-spectrum IV antibiotics
   c. Cephalexin PO for 10 days
   d. Bone scan
   e. Nonsteroidal anti-inflammatory medications and rest

5. A 13-month-old girl is brought to the ED refusing to move her left arm after falling while running at home. On physical exam she appears to be in no discomfort but holds her left arm slightly flexed at the elbow. You observe no swelling, deformity, or tenderness of the arm, but she cries when you flex her left elbow. The most appropriate management is:

   a. Supinate and flex the patient's elbow
   b. Obtain a plain radiograph of the right shoulder and arm
   c. Place a posterior splint and refer the patient to an orthopedist
   d. Obtain a social services consult
   e. Obtain a CBC and ESR

6. A 13-year-old obese boy complains of a 3-week history of left thigh pain that increased after falling while playing soccer. On physical exam he is afebrile and well appearing. He holds the left leg flexed and externally rotated at the hip. An AP plain radiograph of the left hip is normal. The most appropriate next step in management is:

    a. Obtain a WBC count
    b. Obtain a lateral radiograph of the left hip
    c. Obtain immediate orthopedic consultation
    d. Obtain plain radiographs of the left knee
    e. Obtain an ultrasound of the left hip

7. You are most likely to diagnose a slipped capital femoral epiphysis (SCFE) in which of the following patients?

    a. A 15-year-old female gymnast who has doubled her practice time in the past month
    b. A 16-year-old male defensive end who complains of left hip pain after a tackle
    c. A 12-year-old obese boy who fell out of a tree
    d. A 14-year-old boy with a 3-week history of worsening right hip pain but no known injury
    e. An 11-year-old girl who is being followed by an endocrinologist for short stature and delayed bone age

8. All of the following contribute to the increased incidence of SCFE in adolescence, EXCEPT:

    a. Increased body weight
    b. Thinning of the perichondrial ring with decreased support of the physis
    c. Decreased height of the physis
    d. Vector of body weight more perpendicular to the femur
    e. Increased activity in sports

9. A 7-year-old boy is referred to you with worsening right hip pain after falling off his bicycle. His mother reports that he has had "growing pains" of his right hip and thigh for the past 3 months. He is afebrile on arrival to the ED. You note decreased range of motion (ROM) of the right hip, but otherwise a normal physical exam. The most likely abnormal finding is:

    a. An ESR of 60
    b. 80% lymphoblasts on a peripheral blood smear
    c. A right hip effusion on a hip ultrasound
    d. Periosteal reaction of the proximal femoral metaphysis on plain radiograph
    e. Irregularity and flattening of the femoral epiphysis on plain radiograph

10. A 6-year-old girl complains of a 9-day history of nonspecific back pain. Her mother reports no traumatic injury. She has a temperature of 39°C and is lying still on the examination table. The most likely finding on physical examination is:

    a. A left foot drop
    b. Tenderness of the lower lumbar spine
    c. Decreased ROM of the left hip
    d. Decreased left patellar reflex and sensation of the left foot
    e. Normal straight-leg raise bilaterally

11. A 15-year-old boy who recently joined the crew team at his school is seen with a several-month history of low back pain that is exacerbated when he rows. He recalls no traumatic injury to his back. On physical examination you find mild tenderness to the lumbar spine and tight hamstrings on straight-leg raise. His reflexes and sensory examination are normal. You obtain lumbar spine radiographs that reveal a lucency of the pars interarticularis of L-5 on oblique view but no abnormality on lateral view. The appropriate management for this patient is:

    a. No change in current level of activity
    b. Avoidance of activity that causes pain until evaluated by an orthopedist
    c. Complete bedrest for 1 month, then slow return to normal activities
    d. Immediate orthopedic consultation for surgical intervention
    e. Complete spinal immobilization with brace

12. Overuse syndromes are particularly common during adolescence for all of the following reasons, EXCEPT:

    a. Growth of muscle-tendon units exceeds skeletal growth
    b. Cartilage is more susceptible to injury from repetitive forces
    c. Tendons have not yet fused to bone
    d. Increased participation in sports
    e. Rapid growth spurt

13. A 10-year-old boy complains of right elbow pain 1 month after starting baseball. He tells you that the pain is worse when he throws the baseball. On physical exam you find tenderness over the medial aspect of the elbow. Plain radiographs of the elbow are normal. The most appropriate management is:

    a. Decrease activity by 50% for 2 weeks, then increase gradually over 2 weeks
    b. Splinting with the elbow in 90 degrees flexion for 2 weeks
    c. Immediate orthopedic referral for possible pinning
    d. Rest for 1 month, then slowly return to activity after pain has resolved
    e. Strength training of the upper extremity muscles

14. A child is seen for a 1-month history of knee pain. On physical exam, you find tenderness and slight prominence of the upper tibia bilaterally. When you flex the child's knees fully you illicit pain. The patient most likely is:

a. A 17-year-old boy who is the kicker for the football team
b. A 13-year-old female gymnast
c. A 14-year-old male who participates in multiple track and field events
d. An 11-year-old boy who recently began riding his new bicycle
e. A 13-year-old obese girl who spends most of her free time sitting at her computer

15. A 14-year-old female ballet dancer complains of right knee pain for 4 months. She reports that the pain is worse after she dances but improves with rest. She felt like her knee "locked" when she was walking down stairs several times. Your evaluation is most likely to reveal:

a. Completely normal physical examination and plain radiographs
b. A large joint effusion and laxity of the anterior cruciate ligament
c. Tenderness of the medial femoral condyle and a radiodense object in the joint space
d. Lytic lesions of the distal femoral metaphysis with periosteal reaction
e. Limited internal rotation and flexion of the right hip

16. A 13-year-old girl is referred to you with a 2-month history of anterior left knee pain that is especially severe when she is climbing stairs. She has recently joined the track team at school. Your evaluation of the knee is most likely to reveal:

a. Tenderness along the patellar margins and normal plain radiographs
b. A moderate sized joint effusion and lateral joint line tenderness
c. Normal magnetic resonance imaging
d. Q angle less than 15%
e. A relatively weak lateral quadriceps muscle

ANSWERS

1. c   This newborn infant has osteomyelitis of the femur. The most likely organisms in this age group are *Staphylococcus aureus,* group B *Streptococcus,* and Gram-negative bacilli, especially *E. coli.* Although both nafcillin and first-generation cephalosporins cover *S. aureus,* cefazolin would not cover the Gram-negative organisms. Gentamicin and nafcillin together would cover all these organisms. Ampicillin would not cover *S. aureus* and many Gram-negative organisms, and gentamicin alone would be insufficient to cover the Gram-positive organisms.

2. d   This clinical scenario is worrisome for osteomyelitis of the foot, caused by a puncture wound. Bone scan is the definitive test to make the diagnosis in this case. A repeat radiograph in 10 days may show lytic changes seen with osteomyelitis, but diagnosis should not be delayed. Although the patient may have a simple cellulitis that could be treated with oral antibiotics, osteomyelitis must first be ruled out. After the diagnosis of osteomyelitis is made, the antibiotic of choice in this patient with the puncture wound would be an IV antibiotic effective against *Pseudomonas.*

3. b   This clinical scenario is suggestive of septic arthritis of the hip. The WBC count and plain radiographs may be normal early in the disease process. The ESR may be elevated in 90% of cases of septic arthritis, but can be elevated in other disease processes as well, so it can not confirm the diagnosis. An ultrasound of the hip is the most sensitive means of identifying an effusion. Bone scan and MRI may be helpful in determining the site of infection if a hip ultrasound is normal, and would be the next diagnostic tests if your suspicion was high and the ultrasound was negative. Although young children are often unable to localize pain, the physical exam findings identify the hip as the site of pain; thus, knee radiographs are likely to be normal.

4. e   This patient's clinical picture suggests that he has toxic synovitis of the hip and not a septic arthritis. The treatment for this condition is nonsteroidal anti-inflammatory medications and rest, with close follow-up. Antibiotics are not indicated for this inflammatory condition. Joint irrigation is indicated for septic arthritis. Bone scan is not necessary to make this diagnosis.

5. a   This clinical picture is most consistent with a subluxation of the radial head. The mechanism of injury is mild, and the patient is holding her arm in the characteristic position. Because no swelling or deformity is noted on physical examination, radiographs are not required prior to reduction maneuvers. Splinting is not required as long as the reduction is successful. Because the injury is common and the mechanism is consistent with the injury, a social services consultation is not necessary. There are no signs of infection in this patient; thus, WBC count and ESR are likely to be normal.

6. b   This patient likely has a chronic SCFE with acute slippage after a minor injury. Anteroposterior (AP) hip radiographs are often normal, and alone cannot rule out an SCFE. Lateral radiographs of the hip are more likely to reveal a step-off between the metaphysis and the epiphysis. Because his symptoms are focused on the hip, knee radiographs are likely to be normal. Ultrasound is not used in the diagnosis of SCFE. Orthopedic consultation would be required once the appropriate diagnosis is made.

7. d   SCFE is thought to be caused by weakening of the physeal-epiphyseal complex seen in adolescence. Acute slippage is uncommon due to the convexity of the physis toward the epiphysis and the strong collagenous bridges that traverse the physis. A gradual slippage with chronic symptoms is more commonly seen. Although obese children are predisposed to SCFE, weight alone does not predict slippage. The 16-year-old football player is likely to have closed physes and not be at risk for SCFE. Girls tend to have a SCFE earlier than boys, at age 11–13 years versus 13–15 years, so the gymnast is less likely to have this condition. Increases in exogenous or endogenous growth factor are risk factors for SCFE, but short stature alone is not.

8. c   The increased incidence of SCFE in adolescence is thought to be due to weakening of the physeal-epiphysis complex and changes in geometry and weight that are seen in this age group. Increased, not decreased, height of the physis lengthens the lever arm and increases the shearing forces on the growth plate.

9. e   This boy has had chronic hip pain with an acute exacerbation after an injury. The most likely diagnosis is Legg-Calvé-Perthes disease. With more advanced cases, irregularity and flattening of the femoral epiphysis are seen on radiographs of the hip. This clinical scenario is not consistent with an acute infection; thus, the ESR is likely to be normal, and no signs of osteomyelitis or septic arthritis should be seen. Because the patient has an otherwise normal examination, acute lymphoblastic leukemia is unlikely.

10. b   This girl has symptoms most consistent with diskitis. The most common finding on physical examination is tenderness over the involved portion of the spine. Due to spasm of the paravertebral and hamstring muscles, the straight-leg raise maneuver often causes pain. Range of motion of the hip is usually normal in diskitis. It is uncommon to have neurologic deficits of the lower extremities.

11. b   This patient has spondylolysis but no signs of spondylolisthesis on plain radiographs. Although this injury is exacerbated with repeated stress to the spine, cases without displacement of the vertebral body are unlikely to progress. The patient should avoid the activities that are exacerbating the pain until evaluated by an orthopedist or sports medicine physician; however, complete bedrest or spinal immobilization is not recommended. Surgical intervention is rarely required in mild cases.

12. a   Overuse syndromes are primarily due to rapid growth spurt in adolescence that leads to skeletal growth exceeding growth of the muscle-tendon unit. This causes repeated stress at the apophysis, leading to inflammation and weakening of the bone. In adults, the tendon fuses to the bone, resulting in tendonitis rather than apophysitis.

13. d   This patient has a clinical picture consistent with little-leaguer's elbow, a medial humeral epicondylitis caused by repetitive valgus stress on the elbow. Recommended treatment includes a 1-month period of rest of the affected arm, with gradual return to activity after pain has resolved. Routine stretching and ROM exercises improve outcome, so splinting would not be recommended. Surgical intervention is only indicated for displaced avulsion fractures.

14. c   This clinical scenario describes a patient with Osgood-Schlatter's disease, an apophysitis of the tibial tubercle. This overuse syndrome is seen most commonly in boys ages 11–15 years who are involved in running and jumping sports. It is seen less commonly in children who are not involved in sports and in older adolescents.

15. c   This young ballet dancer has osteochondritis dissecans of the medial femoral condyle. Her symptoms suggest that she has advanced disease with a free body in the joint space, so you are likely to find tenderness of the medial femoral condyle and a radiodense object in the joint space on plain radiographs. Anterior cruciate ligamentous injuries are uncommon in this age group. The symptoms are not consistent with osteomyelitis, so lytic lesions and periosteal reaction should not be seen. The patient has no symptoms referable to the hip, so she should have a normal hip exam.

16. a   This clinical scenario is consistent with chondromalacia patellae. The typical findings are tenderness along the patellar margins and crepitus. Radiographs are generally normal. Magnetic resonance imaging is at least 80% sensitive in diagnosing the condition. Joint effusions are rare and should lead you to alternative diagnoses. The cause of this condition is thought to be malalignment of the patella and abnormal tracking over the femoral condyles, exacerbated by weak medial quadriceps muscles and Q angles greater than 20 degrees (the Q angle is between a line from the center of the tibial tubercle to the center of the patella and a line from the center of the patella to the anterior superior iliac spine).

CHAPTER 124

Dental Emergencies

VINCENT J. WANG, M.D.

QUESTIONS

1. A 12-year-old boy complains of bleeding from the site of an extracted tooth. The procedure was performed approximately 48 hours ago and the site has continued to bleed despite applying pressure to it. Appropriate management at this time would be:

   a. Reassurance and continued application of pressure
   b. Oral saline rinses
   c. Suturing the extraction site
   d. Pain medication and oral antibiotic therapy
   e. Application of a tea bag to the site

2. A 16-year-old girl complains of pain at a mandibular extraction site. She had a tooth extracted approximately 4 days ago. On examination, she has no swelling, bleeding, or edema of the site. Appropriate management would include:

   a. Oral saline rinses
   b. Application of moist heat
   c. Suturing the extraction site
   d. Pain medication and oral antibiotic therapy
   e. Application of a tea bag to the site

3. A 6-year-old boy presents with a soft, raised, fluid-filled nodule on the floor of the mouth. The borders are well-delineated and the lesion appears translucent. Initial treatment includes:

   a. Excision
   b. Application of moist heat
   c. Further evaluation with MRI
   d. Observation
   e. Penicillin PO

4. A 7-year-old boy complains of pain in his upper incisor, mobility of the tooth, and soft-tissue swelling of the gingiva. Which of the following signs or symptoms would lead you to suspect an etiology other than a dentoalveolar abscess?

   a. Fever
   b. Bleeding
   c. Fistulous tracts
   d. Extrusion of the tooth
   e. Lymphadenopathy

5. In which of the following scenarios must the patient with a dentoalveolar abscess be admitted for treatment?

   a. A 7-year-old boy whose abscess culture has grown anaerobic organisms
   b. An 8-year-old boy with eye pain and tenderness over the orbits
   c. A 9-year-old girl who has a temperature of 38.6°C
   d. A 6-year-old girl with a penicillin allergy
   e. A 4-year-old boy with erythema and swelling around the tooth

6. A 6-year-old girl complains of pain distal to her molars. She has edema and erythema of the surrounding soft tissues. She also has lymphadenopathy, trismus, and dysphagia. Management includes:

   a. Tooth extraction
   b. Oral rinses and heat
   c. Application of local pressure
   d. Application of viscous lidocaine
   e. Incision and drainage

7. A 3-year-old boy complains of "mouth sores." He has had high fevers and fussiness for the past 2–3 days. On the day of the visit, the mother noticed lesions in his mouth. His vital signs are: T 39°C, HR 110, and RR 20. On your examination, you note ulcers with surrounding erythema on the tongue and lips. Treatment includes:

a. Penicillin PO for 7 days
b. Half-strength hydrogen peroxide mouth rinses
c. Debridement of the affected areas
d. Salt-water rinses
e. Pain relief

8. An infant presents with an oral lesion in his mouth. Which of the following requires excision for treatment?

a. Pyogenic granuloma
b. Epstein's pearls
c. Bohn's nodules
d. Dental lamina cysts
e. Epidermolysis bullosa

ANSWERS

1. c   An extraction site may continue to ooze for 8–12 hours after extraction, and somewhat longer for a permanent tooth. Bleeding for 48 hours after extraction requires treatment. The patient should be assessed for complications of bleeding, and appropriate tests should be done to determine if the patient has an underlying bleeding disorder. Oral saline rinses, antibiotics, and pain medication are helpful for infections, but are unlikely to be helpful in a bleeding patient. Application of a moistened tea bag releases tannic acid, which may accelerate or initiate coagulation; however, this is a temporizing home remedy, and not definitive treatment. The site should be closed with sutures to stop the bleeding.

2. d   This patient has an alveolar osteitis, caused by a disintegration of the clot in the tooth socket. This usually occurs approximately 3 days after a mandibular extraction, and is typically painful. Treatment includes debridement of the socket, followed by packing with iodoform gauze or Bipp's paste. Oral analgesics and antibiotic therapy are part of the treatment. Oral saline rinses and application of moist heat are helpful for postextraction infections, but not for an alveolar osteitis. Suturing the extraction site and application of a tea bag to the site are treatments for postextraction bleeding.

3. a   The patient has a mucocele, or, more specifically, a ranula, because the lesion is on the floor of the mouth. Mucoceles should be excised, and ranulas should be marsupialized. Further evaluation is not indicated, and the other treatments are not helpful.

4. b   Etiologic factors for a dentoalveolar abscess include gross or recurrent caries and trauma. Fistulous tracts may be present if the abscess is long standing. Because of the presence of fluid in the periradicular space, the tooth may become extruded. Lymphadenopathy and fever are nonspecific signs of infection, and may occur at any time during the development of the abscess. Bleeding is not a typical characteristic of a dentoalveolar abscess.

5. b   Each of the patients may be treated as an outpatient except the patient with eye pain and tenderness over the orbits. Complications of a dentoalveolar abscess include airway compromise, brain abscess, septicemia, and cavernous sinus thrombosis. Eye pain and tenderness over the orbits may be early signs of cavernous sinus thrombosis.

6. b   Management of a pericoronitis includes local curettage, oral rinses, heat, and scrupulous oral hygiene. Penicillin may also be indicated. Tooth extraction and incision and drainage may be indicated with carious teeth causing a dentoalveolar abscess. Application of local pressure is helpful for bleeding extraction sites. Application of viscous lidocaine has been advocated for herpetic gingivostomatitis, but this medication must be used sparingly.

7. e   Primary herpetic gingivostomatitis (HG) is a common cause of ED visits. The typical case is an infant or toddler who presents with poor oral intake, high fever, and irritability. The gingivae may be erythematous with areas of spontaneous hemorrhage. Vesicles develop and then rupture, causing painful ulcers. Secondary infection is rare. Treatment is supportive for hydration, analgesics, and fever control. Pain may be relieved by kaopectate/diphenydramine orally, viscous lidocaine topically, or aceta-

minophen with codeine orally. Acute necrotizing ulcerative gingivitis (ANUG) is typically seen in adolescents or young adults, and may be misdiagnosed with HG. Treatment includes improving oral hygiene with mouth rinses, an oral course of penicillin, and debridement of affected areas.

8. a   Pyogenic granulomas develop as a response to trauma or an irritant. Treatment consists of excision of the granuloma and removal of the causative agent. Epstein's pearls and Bohn's nodules are often present in newborns and disappear within weeks of birth. Dental lamina cysts appear in newborns or young infants. These disappear with time or with the eruption of teeth. Epidermolysis bullosa is a hereditary vesicobullous condition that affects the teeth and mucous membranes. Treatment consists of pain relief and nutritional support.

CHAPTER **125**

Neurosurgical Emergencies, Nontraumatic

DAVID GREENES, M.D.

QUESTIONS

1. A 12-year-old boy with sickle-cell disease was noted 2 hours ago to be slurring his words and to have difficulty walking. There is no history of trauma, drug use, toxin exposure, or fever. On physical examination, he has dysarthria and weakness of the right upper and lower extremity. Head CT scan, performed without contrast, is normal. Which of the following would be the most appropriate next step?

   a. Initiation of an IV heparin infusion
   b. Observation in the ICU with no intervention
   c. Initiation of an IV infusion of tissue plasminogen activator (TPA)
   d. Preparation for immediate exchange transfusion
   e. Preparation for immediate cerebral angiography

2. A 3-year-old boy with a history of aqueductal stenosis had a ventriculoperitoneal shunt placed 2 years ago. He comes to the ED with a complaint of 2 days of fever to as high as 39.3°C. There is no history of runny nose, cough, sore throat, vomiting, or diarrhea. He has been less active than usual, but playful when his fever is brought down with antipyretics. On physical examination, he appears well, with no erythema, swelling, or tenderness overlying the shunt, no meningismus, a normal abdominal examination, and a normal neurologic status. What is the most appropriate course of action at this time?

   a. Tapping of the shunt
   b. Radiographic shunt series, with tapping of shunt only if abnormal
   c. Careful clinical observation and follow-up
   d. Lumbar puncture
   e. Head CT, with tapping of the shunt only if the CT is abnormal

3. A 5-year-old boy has a ventriculoperitoneal shunt for hydrocephalus associated with a Dandy-Walker malformation. The shunt was revised 4 months ago. His mother reports that he has been less active than usual for several days, with intermittent complaints of headache, and that he vomited in the morning yesterday and today. There has been no fever. Physical examination is entirely normal. The most appropriate next step is:

   a. A radiographic "shunt series" and head CT
   b. Pumping of the shunt reservoir, with head imaging only if the shunt fills abnormally
   c. Tapping of the shunt
   d. Discharge to home with instructions to return if symptoms worsen
   e. Radiographic "shunt series," with follow-up head CT if shunt series is abnormal

4. A 9-year-old girl has recently been diagnosed with a brainstem glioma. She arrives at the ED with a complaint of increasing somnolence. On physical examination, her HR is 52, BP is 140/90, and she is breathing irregularly. She is unresponsive to painful stimuli. Her left pupil is 6 mm and nonreactive; the right pupil is 4 mm and reactive. Her right arm and leg are stiff and extended. You perform endotracheal intubation, obtain IV access, begin hyperventilation, and initiate therapy with IV mannitol. On repeat physical examination, both pupils are dilated and nonreactive. What is the most appropriate next step?

   a. Emergent ventriculostomy
   b. Transfer to the OR for resection of the tumor
   c. IV dexamethasone and admission to the ICU
   d. Immediate MRI scan of the head
   e. Administration of IV atropine and hydralazine

5. A 6-year-old boy complains of recurrent frontal head-aches over the past 2 weeks. Which of the following his-torical features would be LEAST consistent with a diag-nosis of brain tumor?

   a. The headaches wake him from sleep
   b. He feels better after vomiting
   c. The headaches improve with a brief nap
   d. He feels better after getting up in the morning
   e. He has never had headaches in the past

6. A 4-year-old girl complains of back pain, fever, and re-fusal to walk. Physical examination reveals moderate ten-derness over the lower thoracic spine and weakness and decreased reflexes in both lower extremities. Plain radi-ographs of the thoracic and lumbar spine are normal. The most appropriate next step is:

   a. IV antibiotic therapy
   b. Lumbar puncture
   c. Radionuclide bone scan
   d. MRI scan of the spine
   e. High dose IV methylprednisolone therapy

ANSWERS

1. d   Patients with sickle-cell disease are at risk for ischemic stroke caused by sickling crises in the cerebral vasculature. This patient's history and physical examination findings are consistent with a stroke. Nor-mal findings on a head CT do not exclude the possibility of a recent ischemic stroke. Stroke in patients with sickle-cell disease is treated with simple or exchange transfusion to reduce the fraction of hemo-globin S in the circulation, and to prevent further sickling. It would be inappropriate to observe this pa-tient without some effort to reduce the likelihood of further sickling. IV heparin and TPA are used for patients with thrombotic or embolic strokes, which are less likely diagnoses in this scenario. Cerebral angiography is helpful for diagnosing vascular anomalies, but it has little utility as an emergency proce-dure in patients with ischemic stroke.

2. c   Shunt infection is always a consideration when evaluating febrile children with ventriculoperitoneal shunts. Shunt infection occurs predominantly in the first several weeks to months after the shunt is placed, and it is an uncommon infection thereafter. Shunt infections are often indolent and may present with nonspecific signs of illness; fever, meningeal signs, and leukocytosis are frequently absent. Con-comitant shunt malfunction is sometimes, but not always, evident. Shunt infection is diagnosed by tap-ping the shunt to obtain CSF. The decision to tap the shunt must be weighed carefully, because there is a risk of introducing bacteria and causing shunt infection by performing the tap. In this scenario, with a shunt placed 2 years ago and a patient who appears well, it is most appropriate not to tap the shunt at this time. Because hydrocephalus is sometimes, but not always, present in shunt infection, it does not make sense to decide about tapping the shunt on the basis of a head CT. In this patient with noncom-municating hydrocephalus, lumbar puncture would not yield information about the ventricular (or shunt) fluid. A radiographic shunt series will seldom be abnormal in cases of shunt infection and is not indicated in this case.

3. a   Shunt malfunction causes symptoms and signs as intracranial pressure begins to increase. Head-ache, lethargy, vomiting, abnormalities of gaze, dilation of the pupils, and focal neurologic findings may all be present as intracranial pressure increases. Early signs of shunt malfunction, however, may be quite subtle. Parental report of minor alterations in the child's behavior is often the first indication of shunt malfunction. In this scenario, with headache, morning vomiting, and decreased activity, the most ap-propriate course of action is to perform a shunt series and head CT. Many shunt malfunctions are asso-ciated with no radiographic abnormality of the shunt itself, so it is not appropriate to perform only a shunt series. Pumping of the shunt, to assess for obstructed flow, has been found to be an unreliable means of diagnosing shunt malfunction. Tapping of the shunt raises the possibility of introducing bac-teria into the shunt and is not often necessary in evaluations for shunt malfunction. Although the pa-tient may do well even if the malfunctioning shunt is not replaced for hours or days, there is a chance of rapid neurologic deterioration, so it is appropriate to make the diagnosis and institute therapy as soon as concerns for shunt malfunction arise.

4. a   The patient is showing signs of impending tentorial herniation, with Cushing's triad of bradycardia, hypertension, and irregular respirations, as well as pupillary dysfunction and posturing. In the context

of a known brainstem tumor, the most likely reason for this acute deterioration is obstructive hydro-cephalus. With such rapid deterioration, the patient will likely suffer irreversible brain injury in the next several minutes. The most appropriate course of action is immediate reduction of intracranial pressure (ICP). Along with hyperventilation and mannitol therapy, the most effective means of reducing ICP is to relieve the hydrocephalus by placement of a ventriculostomy catheter. IV dexamethasone therapy may shrink edema associated with the brain tumor, but it would not rapidly relieve the hydrocephalus. Resection of a brainstem tumor would be technically difficult, if not impossible, and would not be fast enough to provide relief of the intracranial hypertension. IV atropine and hydralazine would treat the bradycardia and hypertension but would not relieve the underlying problem of increased ICP. MRI scan would require too much time and should not be considered until the patient is stabilized. If the patient can be stabilized, it would be reasonable to perform emergent head CT to assess for acute bleeding or other surgical lesions. With impending herniation, however, the neurosurgeon may need to perform ventriculostomy even before head CT can be performed.

5. c   Headache is a common complaint in pediatrics, and the vast majority of patients with headache do not have intracranial mass lesions. The clinician should consider a diagnosis of intracranial masses, however, in cases associated with neurologic abnormalities, or if the history or physical examination suggests increased intracranial pressure. Headaches associated with ICP are usually worse when patients are sleeping, probably because their supine positioning leads to increased intracranial CSF volume, and perhaps because the hypoventilation during sleep leads to intracranial vasodilation. Histories of night-time or morning headaches, especially if they get better upon arising, are worrisome for possible intracranial mass lesions. Patients with intracranial masses often report feeling better after vomiting, perhaps because they hyperventilate when vomiting, thereby decreasing intracranial volume. Patients with chronic histories of headaches are less likely to have an intracranial mass lesion than are patients with the acute development of new symptoms. Patients with migraines often feel better after a nap. In contrast, patients with intracranial masses may actually feel worse if they lie down for a nap.

6. d   The scenario of back pain, fever, refusal to walk, and decreased lower extremity reflexes suggests an epidural abscess. Other causes of spinal cord compression (e.g., tumors or hemorrhage) should also be considered. Many such lesions, including abscesses and tumors, will require immediate surgical intervention to relieve the compression. Neurologic prognosis after spinal cord compression is directly related to the duration of the compression, so decompression must occur without delay. MRI is the best imaging modality to visualize the spinal cord and surrounding tissues, and it should be performed emergently to look for operative lesions. Although IV methylprednisolone may improve the prognosis with spinal cord compression, it is not definitive therapy and does not replace the need for surgical decompression. Bone scan may show bony abnormalities not seen on the plain x-rays, but it would not yield information about the spinal cord, which is the priority here. Lumbar puncture is not indicated in the workup for spinal cord compressive lesions.

CHAPTER **126**

Transplantation Emergencies

DOMINIC CHALUT, M.D.

QUESTIONS

1. A 2-year-old child newly transplanted with a living donor kidney complains of abdominal pain and high fever. The child was transplanted 2 weeks ago. What is the most likely type of infection?

   a. Cytomegalovirus (CMV) infection
   b. Herpes simplex virus (HSV) reactivation
   c. *Pneumocystis carinii* pneumonitis
   d. Fungal infection
   e. UTI

2. A 6-year-old boy is 6 months post–liver transplant. He complains of dysphagia, odynophagia, and fever. Which diagnosis should be suspected?

   a. *Candida* esophagitis
   b. CMV esophagitis
   c. HSV esophagitis
   d. *Aspergillus* esophagitis
   e. Peritonsillar abscess

3. A 16-year-old girl is now 4 months post–liver transplant. She complains of a 6-week history of persistent and progressive headache. Her daily activities are limited by those headaches. She is reporting occasional low-grade fever. She has never had headaches before. Which diagnosis should be suspected?

   a. Organ rejection
   b. *Candida* meningitis
   c. *Pneumocystis carinii* pneumonitis
   d. Migraine
   e. HSV reactivation

4. A patient 4 weeks post–liver transplant is referred to you because of abnormal laboratory values. She had routine postoperative blood tests done earlier today, and is called back because of elevated liver aminotransferase levels. On exam the wound is healing nicely and the liver seems enlarged. You confirm that her liver aminotransferases are elevated. Which initial study will you request for this patient?

   a. Hepatitis B serology
   b. Liver biopsy
   c. Renal function
   d. Abdominal x-ray
   e. Ultrasound examination

5. A 12-year-old girl post–renal transplant is on immunosuppressive therapy. Her compliance is good. She complains of abdominal pain, and laboratory evaluation shows increased amylase and lipase levels. Which therapy may explain these symptoms?

   a. Azathioprine
   b. OKT3
   c. Mycophenolate mofetil
   d. Cyclosporine
   e. Tacrolimus

6. A 4-year-old boy, now 2 years post–renal transplant, is diagnosed with a UTI. His current medication includes prednisone, tacrolimus, and azathioprine. Which antibiotic should you use to treat his infection?

   a. Eythromycin
   b. Trimethoprim-sulfamethoxazole
   c. Amoxicillin
   d. Gentamicin
   e. Cefixime

ANSWERS

1. e   In the first few weeks after transplantation, the most common infections are UTI and wound infection with bacterial pathogens. *Pneumocystis carinii* pneumonitis is becoming increasingly uncommon in transplant patients because of routine prophylaxis. CMV, HSV, and fungal infections will usually present later.

2. a   A common fungal infection is *Candida esophagitis* between 1 and 6 months post-transplant. The patient usually presents with dysphagia or odynophagia. Although CMV, HSV, and *Aspergillus* can cause esophagitis, they are less common. *Aspergillus* infection is associated with the highest mortality.

3. b   Fungal infections generally do not occur in the first month after transplant, but they appear in the subsequent months. Between the first and sixth months, *Candida* species are the major fungal pathogens. Fungal infection of the CNS may be difficult to assess because the classic signs of CNS infection (e.g., meningismus and fever) may be absent in immunosuppressed patients. The common presentation of headache, often without fever, may be the only indication that there is a CNS infection. These cases warrant a thorough neurological evaluation, lumbar puncture with fungal stains and cultures, and possibly an imaging study of the brain. Acute or subacute meningitis is most commonly caused by *Listeria monocytogenes,* whereas chronic meningitis is most often caused by *Cryptococcus neoformans,* and focal brain abscess is often caused by *Aspergillus* species.

4. e   Elevated liver aminotransferases may be a sign of rejection, arterial or venous thrombosis of the graft, or even biliary stricture and obstruction, with resultant cholangitis. An ultrasound examination with Doppler study would visualize arterial or venous blood flow to the graft and assess the biliary tree for evidence of dilation, which suggests obstruction. A liver biopsy would be required to assess the possibility of rejection, but it is usually not the first study done.

5. a   Pancreatitis is seen as a complication of taking azathioprine. OKT3 predisposes patients to opportunistic infections. The most common side effects of mycophenolate mofetil are gastrointestinal complaints including esophagitis, gastritis, diarrhea and emesis; bone marrow suppression, including leukopenia, anemia, and thrombocytopenia, is dose related and may necessitate a decrease in dose. Cyclosporine and tacrolimus mainly cause nephrotoxicity and neurotoxicity.

6. e   Erythromycin decreases the tacrolimus metabolism, causing increased levels. Trimethoprim-sulfamethoxazole and aminoglycosides can cause synergistic nephrotoxicity with tacrolimus. Cefixime offers a better coverage against the coliform bacteria compared with amoxicillin.

CHAPTER 127

Approach to the Care of the Technology-Dependent Child

JILL C. POSNER, M.D.

QUESTIONS

1. A 2-year-old boy with a tracheostomy has had fever, increased tracheal secretions, and mild respiratory distress at home. En route to the ED, the paramedics performed a cannula change and started the patient on 0.25 cc of nebulized albuterol. On arrival to the ED, the patient has developed severe respiratory distress. He is tachypneic and has significant accessory muscle use. His vital signs are: T 37.2°C, HR 180, RR 66, and BP 126/60. Pulse oximetry reveals an O_2 saturation of 85% despite 100% supplemental oxygen and suctioning. You immediately:

   a. Perform an arterial blood gas (ABG) analysis
   b. Increase the dose of albuterol to 1 cc
   c. Obtain a portable CXR
   d. Perform a tracheostomy tube change
   e. Begin manual ventilation

2. A 15-year-old boy with Down syndrome and a tracheostomy for obstructive apnea is brought to the ED for bleeding from the tracheostomy tube. The management involves all of the following, EXCEPT:

   a. Administer humidified air through the tracheostomy tube
   b. Inspect the peristomal skin for the site of bleeding
   c. Perform a cannula change
   d. Send tracheal secretions for bacterial and viral studies
   e. Apply direct pressure to a visualized site of bleeding

3. A 4-year-old girl has a tracheostomy for bronchopulmonary dysplasia (BPD). She no longer requires mechanical ventilation and is in the process of weaning from nighttime CPAP (continuous positive airway pressure). She becomes decannulated while playing with her siblings and has not developed respiratory distress. Her mother reports that she is unable to insert a replacement tube through the stoma. Your management is to:

   a. Apply lubrication, and with firm pressure gently force the tube into the stoma
   b. Call an otorhinolaryngologist to perform an emergent surgical augmentation of the stoma
   c. Place a Foley catheter in the stoma and inflate the balloon
   d. Begin a trial of permanent decannulation, because the patient has demonstrated the ability to tolerate it
   e. Insert an endotracheal tube of smaller diameter through the tracheal stoma and initiate successive dilatation

4. The feature that correlates best with CSF shunt failure is:

   a. A history of persistent vomiting
   b. A history of headache
   c. A history of lethargy
   d. A history of irritability
   e. A history of activity patterns resembling a previous episode

5. An 18-month-old girl is brought to the ED by ambulance. Her vital signs are: T 37.1°C, HR 40, BP 138/70, and RR 26 and irregular. Pupils are 5 mm and sluggishly reactive bilaterally. She is unresponsive to all stimuli. A dextrostick shows a blood glucose of 132 mg/dl. A "double bubble" CSF shunt reservoir is palpable in the right parietal region. There is no neurosurgeon available at your hospital. You immediately:

   a. Obtain a noncontrast head CT scan and radiographic "shunt series"
   b. Administer atropine
   c. Administer epinephrine
   d. Aspirate CSF from the proximal shunt "bubble"
   e. Aspirate CSF from the burr hole

6. A 6-year-old boy with a ventriculoperitoneal shunt (VPS) for congenital aqueductal stenosis has fever, vomiting, and diarrhea. He has not had any surgery since the initial placement of the shunt at 2 months of age. On physical examination, the vital signs are normal and he appears well. You should:

   a. Send a blood specimen for CBC and culture
   b. Tap the shunt for a CSF specimen for cell counts and culture
   c. Recommend antipyresis, a bland diet, and close follow-up with the primary care physician (PCP)
   d. Obtain a head CT and radiographic shunt series
   e. Administer a single dose of IM ceftriaxone and ensure close follow-up with the PCP

7. A 16-year-old boy with spina bifida and a history of multiple VPS revisions complains of daily headaches for the last 2 weeks. He awakes in the morning asymptomatic, but the headache becomes so intense that by the early afternoon he has been going to the school nurse's office daily. Lying down for a few hours improves his symptoms. The most likely cause of this patient's headache is:

   a. Migraine headaches
   b. Slit ventricle syndrome
   c. Malingering
   d. Tension headaches
   e. Shunt infection

8. A 4-year-old boy with newly diagnosed acute lymphoblastic leukemia (ALL) is brought to the ED after he inadvertently pulled on the externalized portion of his indwelling central venous catheter (CVC). You are unable to draw back free-flowing blood from the device. The management includes:

   a. Use a 20-cc syringe of saline to dislodge the obstructing clot
   b. Infuse urokinase through the line
   c. Remove the device completely and apply pressure
   d. Obtain a contrast dye study
   e. Advance the catheter with gentle pressure

9. A 6-year-old girl with cerebral palsy and mental retardation pulls out her gastrostomy tube. Her mother brings a replacement tube along with her to the ED. You are unable to insert the new tube. Your next step in management is:

   a. Dilate the stoma with progressively larger Foley catheters
   b. Ask the surgeons to perform an immediate surgical augmentation
   c. Using lubricant and gentle pressure, force the tube into the stoma
   d. Cover the stoma with sterile, saline-soaked gauze
   e. Place an IV for hydration and admit the patient for surgery

10. A 10-year-old boy with cystic fibrosis and a gastrostomy tube for supplemental nutrition complains of sudden onset of nonbilious vomiting. He has no fever or diarrhea. He denies ingesting medications or toxins, and denies abdominal trauma. On physical examination he appears quite uncomfortable. Vital signs are: T37.2°C, HR 130, RR 18, and BP 122/62. He continues to retch and vomit throughout your exam. Your immediate management is to:

    a. Administer an antiemetic agent
    b. Pull back on the gastrostomy tube (g-tube)
    c. Vent the g-tube
    d. Place a nasogastric (NG) tube
    e. Obtain abdominal radiographs

11. A 4-month-old girl with a colostomy secondary to Hirschsprung's disease is brought to the ED for irritability and absent stool output. Physical exam reveals T 37.8°C, HR 140, RR 20, and BP 88/50. Her abdomen is distended and tender. There is bowel prolapsing through a dusky-colored stoma. Your immediate management is to:

    a. Obtain an obstruction series
    b. Perform a digital dilation of the stoma
    c. Decompress the stomach with an NG tube
    d. Prepare the patient for immediate surgical intervention
    e. Ease the prolapsed contents back into the stoma

12. A 14-year-old girl with Crohn's disease and an ileostomy complains of the sudden onset of colicky abdominal pain. She has had no fever, weight loss, rash, or joint complaints. She denies emesis or change in her ostomy output. Vital signs are: T 37.4°C, HR 104, RR 16, and BP 108/65. In between episodes of pain, her abdomen is soft, with normal bowel sounds. The most likely diagnosis is:

    a. Bowel perforation
    b. Small bowel obstruction
    c. Nephrolithiasis
    d. Flare of inflammatory bowel disease (IBD)
    e. Viral gastroenteritis

ANSWERS

1. d   The most life-threatening complication in a patient with an artificial airway is cannula obstruction or decannulation. A patient with a tracheostomy and respiratory distress should be assumed to have one of these complications until proven otherwise. The patient should be assessed for proper placement of the tracheostomy tube. The physician should recognize that a tube in the stoma does not necessarily indicate a tube in the trachea. A false passage into the paratracheal soft tissues may occur, especially if the tube change is performed in a highly pressured situation or with inexperienced personnel. In the vignette, although the history of increased tracheal secretions and fever suggest an infection, the recent cannula change, followed by a decline in the patient's respiratory status, indicates malpositioning of the replacement cannula.

2. c   The most common cause of light bleeding from a tracheostomy tube is friability and irritation of the tracheal mucosa due to inadequate humidification. The bleeding may also be due to granuloma formation, peristomal irritation, or infection. If the site of bleeding is visualized, direct pressure should be applied. Peristomal granulomas can be treated with topical antibiotics, or with cauterization in refractory cases. Large amounts of bleeding may indicate erosion of the tracheostomy tube into a major vessel, most commonly the innominate artery. In this surgical emergency, vascular access and volume replacement should be initiated immediately. Frequent suctioning to clear the airway and to prevent aspiration is appropriate. The cannula should not be removed, however, because this may be the best way to ensure an airway. The surgeons and OR staff should be notified immediately if erosion is suspected.

3. e   A stoma that is maintained patent with a technologic device is likely to constrict if that device is removed. Replacement of a dislodged tracheostomy tube or gastrostomy tube may become more difficult if there is a delay. A tube should never be forced into the stoma, because this will not only traumatize the stoma but the child as well, and it may result in a false passage of the tube into the paratracheal soft tissues. When faced with a constricted tracheostomy stoma, options include: 1) attempting to recannulate with a tracheostomy tube one-half size smaller than the patient's usual size; 2) using a smaller-sized endotracheal tube and progressively "dilating up"; and 3) using a small-sized oxygen catheter as an obturator to guide the tube through the stoma. Any plan to alter the patient's long-term airway management should be made in conjunction with the primary care physician, pulmonologist, and/or intensive care physician, and should not be determined solely by the ED physician.

4. e   Patients with mechanical malfunction of a CSF shunt may present with a variety of nonspecific signs and symptoms. A history of headache, lethargy, irritability, vomiting, or visual changes should be sought. The history provided by the parent that the child "just isn't acting right" or that "this is exactly how he acted the last time his shunt was obstructed" should be taken very seriously because this may be the most reliable indicator of shunt malfunction.

5. d   Cushing's triad (hypertension, bradycardia, and an abnormal respiratory pattern) occurs late in the course of patients with elevated intracranial pressure (ICP) and indicates impending herniation. Patients with any component of the triad require emergent maneuvers to decrease the ICP while arranging for definitive operative repair of the shunt. Hyperventilation will decrease ICP by reducing the blood volume within the cranial vault through hypocarbia-induced cerebral vasoconstriction. Medications such as dexamethasone and acetazolamide may reduce tissue inflammation and decrease CSF production, respectively; however, the therapeutic effect is not immediate. The removal of CSF from the proximal portion of the shunt may serve as a temporizing means, resulting in a sufficient reduction in ICP until a surgical shunt revision can be performed. "Tapping the shunt" will not be effective if a complete proximal shunt obstruction is present. In these rarer cases, the only nonsurgical approach is to aspirate fluid through a needle placed directly into the ventricle via the burr hole. This procedure tears the shunt and disrupts brain parenchyma. It should therefore be used only in the patient in extremis in whom an attempt at a shunt tap has failed to remove fluid, and when emergent surgical revision is not possible.

6. c   Technology-dependent children are afflicted with the same pediatric illnesses as other children. Even though one must consider that the presence of an indwelling device predisposes the patient to infection, it is also important to remember that "common things are common." For example, a patient with a CSF shunt, fever, vomiting, and diarrhea is more likely to have gastroenteritis than a shunt malfunction. The

possibility of a shunt infection or malfunction should be considered in the differential diagnosis; however, obtaining a head CT and shunt series should not be reflexive. Given that the child in the vignette has not had the shunt manipulated in 6 years, a shunt infection as the cause of his fevers is not likely. For this patient, further evaluation beyond that what is done for the usual child with viral gastroenteritis in not necessary. As with most children seen in an ED setting, close follow-up with the primary care physicians should be encouraged.

7. b   Overdrainage of the CSF system is an occasional complication experienced by children with CSF shunts. In these cases, the shunt works "too well" and results in collapse of the ventricles around the proximal shunt tip. The drainage of CSF shunts increases when the patient is upright, and decreases in the supine position. Patients with slit ventricle syndrome, therefore, are more symptomatic when they have been upright for a few hours, and may find some relief when they lie supine. Symptoms include headache, nausea, vomiting, and lethargy. The diagnosis is generally made based on historical features because many patients with CSF shunts will have small ventricles on CT scan, yet only a small proportion have slit ventricle syndrome. The CT scan is best used to aid in eliminating shunt obstruction with resultant hydrocephalus as the cause of the symptoms, rather than to diagnose slit ventricle syndrome.

8. d   The inability to draw blood or infuse fluid through a CVC can be due to either catheter occlusion or malposition. There may be a fibrin or blood clotted in the lumen, or there may be a precipitate of parenteral nutrition or medication solutions. Maneuvers to increase venous pressure (e.g., having the patient hold his arms above his head, cough, or Valsalva) or placing the patient in reverse Trendelenburg position may help. Gentle irrigation of the clot with 2–3 ml of saline in a back and forth motion may loosen the clot without forcing it into the venous circulation. If blood still cannot be withdrawn, specific agents such as 70% ethanol, 0.1 normal hydrochloric acid, or urokinase may dissolve the precipitate or clot. In the vignette, however, the patient recently placed traction on the line. The difficulty in drawing blood is more likely due to catheter malposition or dislodgment. It the catheter is positioned against a vessel wall, the maneuvers to increase venous pressure may allow for the withdrawal of free-flowing blood. If dislodgment is suspected, the catheter should not be used. Clamp the catheter (use a clamp without "teeth," which can destroy the catheter, or cushion a hemostat with multiple layers of gauze), secure it close to the chest, and obtain a contrast dye study to locate the catheter tip.

9. a   The interval of time since the dislodgment of the gastrostomy tube is an important historical feature. If the tube has been dislodged for hours, it is likely that the stoma will have constricted. The constricted stoma will be unable to accommodate the same-sized tube. Forcing an oversized tube into the stoma will traumatize the stoma (and the child), and may result in the passage of the tube into the peritoneal cavity through a false track. The management of a constricted stoma is to either insert a smaller-sized gastrostomy tube, or to dilate the stoma using progressively larger Foley catheters.

10. b   Gastric outlet obstruction is a rare complication of gastrostomy tubes. It occurs when the tube migrates into the pyloric channel. Patients present with sudden onset of wretching and emesis. Treatment is to pull the g-tube back into its proper location against the abdominal wall. This should relieve the symptoms. If it is unsuccessful, the tube may need to be removed completely.

11. e   Prolapse of the stoma occurs in greater than 20% of patients with stomas and usually is not an emergency. Rarely, the prolapse can be associated with circulatory compromise, in which case the situation becomes more emergent. Patients with incarceration of the bowel usually present with pain, decreased output, and a dusky color of the stoma. This is managed by easing the prolapsed contents back into the stoma using gentle pressure and both hands. Prolapse may recur, so this procedure may need to be done repetitively.

12. c   Patients with ileostomies are prone to developing urinary stones, most commonly comprised of uric acid (60%) or calcium oxalate (40%). The initial management is the same as for other patients with calculi: analgesia and hydration. Treatment and prevention of further stone development is aimed at decreasing ileostomy output and increasing urine output.

SECTION VI Psychosocial Emergencies

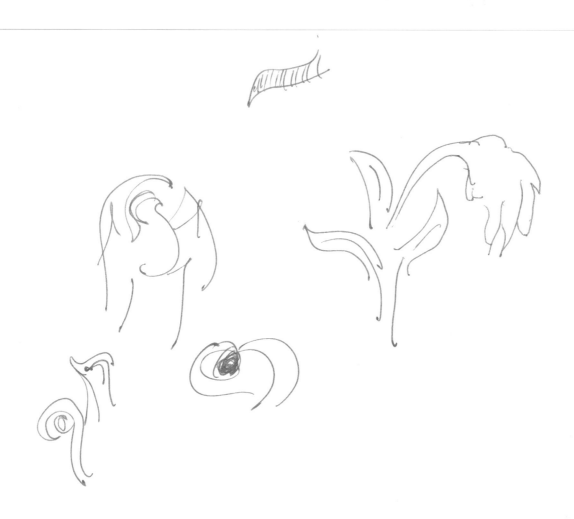

CHAPTER 128

Child Abuse

KATHY BOUTIS, M.D.

QUESTIONS

1. A 4-year-old girl is brought to the ED because of a new rash. On exam, you notice looped-shaped contusions on the skin. You suspect that the child has been injured by a:

   a. Cord
   b. Belt
   c. Rope
   d. Hand
   e. Paddle

2. A 9-month-old boy is brought to the ED by his parents because they noticed that he is not moving his left leg. The father reports that the problem began after the baby fell off the couch and landed on a hardwood floor. Exam reveals swelling over the left distal femur. A skeletal survey is done. Which of the following findings most supports your diagnosis?

   a. Transverse fracture of the femur
   b. Spiral fracture of the femur
   c. Comminuted fracture of the femur
   d. Multiple acute fractures
   e. "Bucket handle" fracture of the femur

3. Two weeks ago, a 5-month-old girl had been diagnosed with a humerus fracture that she sustained after a reported fall from her mother's arms. She was brought to the ED today because she was found by her father not moving or breathing. On examination her vital signs were absent and after a lengthy resuscitation, she was pronounced dead. The most likely cause of death is:

   a. Dehydration
   b. Brain hemorrhage
   c. Gastrointestinal bleeding
   d. SIDS (sudden infant death syndrome)
   e. Central apnea

4. For which of the following children would you be most likely to order a skeletal survey:

   a. An 18-month-old who tripped and fell and has a spiral fracture of the tibia
   b. A 6-month-old female who rolled off a parent's lap and has a midshaft humerus fracture
   c. A 3-year-old fell off of monkey bars and has a supracondylar fracture
   d. A 4-year-old who fell on an outstretched hand and has radius and ulna fractures
   e. A 1-week-old, delivered vaginally, with a fractured clavicle

5. An 8-month-old is brought to the ED because of a "rash." You notice that the rash appears to be several healing small circular burns. You suspect these to be cigarette burns. You:

   a. Tell the parents nothing but immediately call the police
   b. Discharge the child for follow-up with the pediatrician
   c. Report the case but do not tell parents you suspect abuse
   d. Report the case and speak with the child protection agency about disposition
   e. Report the case and then discharge patient to home

6. A 16-year-old boy and a 13-year-old girl were found to be engaging in mutual, consensual sexual exploration. The mother of the girl brings her daughter into the ED and wants to file sexual abuse charges against the boy. On physical exam there are no abnormal findings. Which of the following would be the most appropriate course of action:

   a. Report this as a case of child sexual abuse in which the boy is the perpetrator
   b. Report this as a case of child sexual abuse in which the girl is the perpetrator
   c. Reassure parents that this is not sexual abuse and send the family home
   d. Discuss with a child protection agency and file for an investigation
   e. Encourage the family to obtain a restraining order for the boy involved

7. A 4-year-old girl is brought to the ED with complaints of itching and pain in the vaginal area in association with urinary frequency. The genital exam does not reveal any vaginal erythema or bleeding. In addition to obtaining a urine culture, you would do which of the following?

   a. Obtain a vaginal culture
   b. Obtain a culture if any vaginal discharge
   c. Call the child protection team
   d. Get a social services consult
   e. Perform a pelvic examination

8. A 6-year-old girl complains of dysuria and is found to have obvious vaginal discharge. You send vaginal and urine cultures as well as an RPR. The urine culture is negative, but one of the tests is positive. Which of the following is true?

   a. If the test shows herpes simplex, do not file a report of abuse
   b. Positive cultures (except group A strep) or positive RPR mandate a report of abuse
   c. If RPR is positive, this is unlikely to be a case of abuse
   d. If it is positive for group A *Streptococcus,* file an abuse report
   e. Even if all tests are negative, file a report of abuse

9. A 15-year-old girl is brought to the ED because of a 3-month history of chronic abdominal pain. She has been to see her pediatrician about it several times. The family feels the pain is getting worse would like some more definitive answers as to the cause of the pain. She has missed several days of school in the past 2 weeks. She was healthy prior to the onset of the pain. Social history reveals that the parents are recently divorced and mother's new boyfriend is now living in the home. Her exam is unremarkable. Her pediatrician has done an extensive workup. No abnormalities were found. The best course of action would be the following:

   a. Arrange for the gastroenterologist to see her now
   b. Immediately repeat most of the tests that were done by the pediatrician
   c. Recommend patient/family counseling
   d. Tell the parent to call pediatrician in the morning
   e. Interview the patient privately

10. A mother and father with very high expectations believe that the best way to encourage their 11-year-old child is to tell him constantly that he should be doing better. In addition, after he has performed a chore, they insist he repeat it until it is perfect. Which of the following statements regarding children who suffer emotional abuse is true?

   a. The rate of drug/alcohol abuse in these children is the same as the general population
   b. They are usually developmentally ahead of their peers
   c. The may present to ED for asylum due to fear
   d. They are at high risk for developing frequent illnesses
   e. Other forms of abuse are rare in these scenarios

11. A 5-month-old infant is brought to the ED because by his mother because he is "not growing and the pediatrician is not able figure out why." The mother states that the baby was born healthy and his height, weight, and length were all in the fiftieth percentile. In the last 3 months, the baby has dropped his weight to the twenty-fifth percentile, but his length and head circumference have relatively been preserved, with length at 40% and head circumference at 50%. No other symptoms are reported except for frequent upper respiratory tract infections (URIs) since he started attending day care at 4 months of age. His physical exam is significant for dull, apathetic facies, poor hygiene, and a lack of interest in surroundings. The mother, who is young and single, also shows a lack of concern when the baby cries. Which of the following is the most appropriate course of action?

    a. Report suspicion of neglect and recommend outpatient services
    b. Admit the child and defer reporting until nonorganic failure to thrive is confirmed
    c. Report your suspicion of neglect and admit the child
    d. Discharge home if serum electrolytes and glucose are normal
    e. None of the above

12. A 16-year-old boy has sex with a 16-year-old girl who is mentally handicapped. The parents of the girl consider this rape and are seeking legal action. Which of the following statements is true?

    a. The boy did not commit a criminal offense
    b. This is not likely to be considered rape
    c. This is likely to be considered as rape and the boy will likely face criminal charges
    d. It has to be determined whether or not the girl is intellectually capable of giving consent
    e. Regardless of the circumstances, the boy has committed a felony

13. A 2-month-old boy is brought to the ED after a fall from a changing table. He reportedly rolled off when the mother went to answer the phone. He cried immediately. His mother now notices a contusion on the occiput and reports that the baby has vomited twice. Exam is otherwise significant for some drowsiness in the infant. Skull x-rays reveal a fracture. The most appropriate next step in management is:

    a. Obtain a head CT and if negative and clinical improvement send home
    b. Contact child protection services and obtain a skeletal survey and head CT
    c. Observe the baby in the ED for 4 hours; with improvement, send home
    d. Obtain a head CT and admit the child for observation
    e. Admit the child for observation

ANSWERS

1. a Specific skin injuries associated with child abuse are those that clearly reflect the method or object used to inflict the trauma. Loop-shaped marks are readily visualized following a beating with an electric cord or wire. Linear marks may be seen from a belt or paddle injury. Rope burns result in circumferential marks on the wrists, ankles, or around the neck when a child has been bound. Another common specific integument lesion is a hand print on the side of the face or symmetrically on the upper arms.

2. e Metaphyseal chip fractures occur when the extremity is pulled or yanked; the periosteum is most tightly adherent at the metaphysis, causing small bone fragments to avulse. Metaphyseal chip fractures are almost exclusively caused by abuse. Subperiosteal hematomas produce a characteristic radiograph. The elevation of the periosteum is visualized as a linear opacification running parallel to the bone surface. Subperiosteal hematomas are produced by direct trauma to the bone. It is often difficult to differentiate the true etiology of the other fractures. Although multiple fractures in different stages of healing are also highly suggestive of abuse, there is a broader differential for multiple fractures in different stages of healing than there is for metaphyseal fractures (e.g., abuse, osteogenesis imperfecta, infantile

cortical hyperostosis, scurvy, syphilis, osteoid osteoma, neoplasms, rickets, hypophosphatasia, and osteomyelitis).

Subdural Bleed. of Bridging Veins

3. b   Injuries to the central nervous system (CNS) are the main cause of child abuse deaths. These injuries may be subdivided into two categories—direct trauma and shaking injuries. Shaking injuries characteristically cause serious CNS damage without evidence of external trauma. The infant's relatively large head size and weak neck muscles are predisposing factors for whiplash injury.

4. b   Humerus fractures in children less than 3 years of age (except for supracondylar) are highly likely to be associated with abuse. The remaining injuries are all common forms of accidental injury. Clavicular fractures are common following birth, which would be a reasonable explanation in this 1-week-old infant.

5. d   It is the obligation of the physician to report suspected, not only confirmed, child abuse. The emergency physician should become familiar with her or his state law. The definition of abuse is central to each of the reporting laws. A stated age will define a child. The laws will also specify who must report and who may report. For most mandated reporters there is both a specific penalty for failure to report, and protection from liability if the report of suspected abuse turns out to be unfounded once investigated. Reports are made to child protective services, to police departments, or to some combination of law enforcement and social services personnel. Notification of parents is important. The overall approach to the parents must be based on concern for the child. It is important to use the words "child abuse report."

6. c   The sexual exploration that occurs between children of the same age is not sexual abuse, although on occasions an uninformed parent may consider it as such.

7. b   Parents may bring their child to the ED for the complaint of vaginal discharge. Gonorrhea may also appear in cases where there are a number of less well-defined symptoms, such as vaginal pain, itching, urinary frequency, or enuresis. Recent studies indicate that only children with vaginal discharge have a sufficiently high rate of positive results as to make cultures clinically indicated.

8. b   The Centers for Disease Control (CDC) indicate in their treatment guidelines that "any sexually transmitted infection in a child should be considered as evidence of sexual abuse until proven otherwise." Some infections are virtually always transmitted through sexual contact (e.g., gonococcal and syphilis infections); other infections are usually transmitted sexually (e.g., HSV or HPV). Dysuria is a common complaint in prepubertal children and more often indicates a urinary tract infection or pinworms; only occasionally does it indicate sexual abuse.

9. e   Nonspecific physical complaints often occur in children who are victims of physical or sexual abuse. In this case, repeating a medical workup is unlikely to yield any more useful information. Given the social history, the age of the girl, and the nature of the complaint, which has escalated to school avoidance, you should speak to the patient privately to inquire about sexual activity, including the possibility of a nonconsensual relationship with the mother's boyfriend.

10. c   Emotional abuse manifests in many forms. Some children may seek hospital asylum because of excessive fear of their parents. Adolescent "runaways" may include a subset of children who are emotionally abused. Developmental delay may be recognized in the ED, but the cause of the delay can rarely be identified. Children with drug or alcohol abuse may be high-risk group for prior emotional abuse. Children who are emotionally abused are at risk for other forms of abuse; however, they are not known to have an increased risk of developing frequent illnesses.

11. c   In this case, there are several features suggesting nonorganic failure to thrive, likely secondary to neglect. Historical features include isolated low infant weight and young single mother. Physical exam suggested an understimulated child with the dull, apathetic facies and a lack of interest in surroundings. In addition, the child has noted poor hygiene. If you are suspicious of neglect it is your responsibility to report. In addition, organic failure to thrive is still a possibility and an admission to hospital would help to confirm your initial suspicion and rule out organic causes.

12. d   A person commits a felony when he engages in sexual intercourse with another person not his spouse: 1) by forcible compulsion; 2) by threat of forcible compulsion that would prevent resistance by

a person of reasonable resolution; 3) when the person is unconscious; or 4) when the person is so mentally deranged or deficient that such person is incapable of consent. In this case, there is no mention of how handicapped the girl is and it is important to determine her ability to give consent before deciding whether or not this is rape.

13. b   In this case, a child reportedly rolled off a changing table. This is a developmental stage beyond the capability of a normal 2-month-old; therefore, suspicion should be cast on the reliability of the history to explain the mechanism. At a minimum, in addition to the head CT, one should perform a skeletal survey and contact the child protection team for further advice.

* Sexual Abuse - Vaginal / urine / Rectal !!

DDx/
Osteogenesis Imperfecta (Blue sclera)
Rickets
Hypo PO4
Osteomyelitis
neoplasm

* Suggestive of Abuse:
- Metaphyseal chip Frx (yanked ext)
- Humerus Frx (< 3yr)

CHAPTER 129

Psychiatric Emergencies

THOMAS H. CHUN, M.D.

QUESTIONS

1. A father brings his 16-year-old daughter to the ED for evaluation of depression. He states that there is a strong family history of mood disorders and observes that she has been more irritable than usual. The patient does not openly exhibit any symptoms of depression, but does note multiple vague somatic complaints. She and her father both agree that her psychosocial functioning is normal. She is not suicidal and her physical examination is unremarkable. Your advice to the patient and her father should be:

   a. She is exhibiting normal adolescent behavior and no follow-up is needed
   b. She has no evidence of depression, but they should follow up with her primary care provider for somatic complaints
   c. Depression is rare in adolescents, and they should follow her symptoms over time
   d. Depression is common in adolescents, and they should seek timely mental health evaluation
   e. She should be admitted for an evaluation of depression and suicidality

2. A 7-year-old otherwise healthy boy is brought to the ED with concerns of depression and suicidality. His vital signs and physical examination are unremarkable. ED evaluation of this patient should also include:

   a. T_3, T_4, and TSH (thyroid function tests)
   b. Serum toxicology screen
   c. Psychological testing
   d. Emergent consultation with his pediatrician
   e. Family evaluation

3. A mental status examination (MSE) includes orientation, appearance, memory, cognition, behavior, relating ability, speech, affect, and thought content and process. In evaluating children with psychiatric complaints, the most correct statement is:

   a. A formal MSE should performed on all patients
   b. A full battery of psychological tests should done
   c. Relevant MSE data usually can be gathered in the course of interviewing the child
   d. Only a mental health clinician should perform the MSE
   e. None of the above

4. Symptoms of depression in children and adolescents:

   a. Vary with the age of the patient
   b. Always include a sad or forlorn mood
   c. Are usually easily recognized by parents, caregivers, and physicians
   d. Are less common in children with disabilities
   e. Rarely includes suicidal ideation

5. A 16-year-old boy with a known history of bipolar disorder, substance abuse, and previous suicide attempts is brought to the ED for evaluation by his mother. She unexpectedly discovered a suicide note by the patient and found him attempting to hang himself. He admits to also having taken an entire bottle of "aspirin" 3 hours ago. There is a strong family history of depression. On examination he is sullen, unengaging, and says he "doesn't want to talk about it." His vital signs and physical examination are unremarkable. This patient will most likely benefit from:

   a. Inpatient admission, without further ED evaluation
   b. Inpatient admission, after further ED evaluation
   c. Discharge, if he makes a "no-suicide commitment" (i.e., "contracts for safety")
   d. Discharge, if he makes a "no-suicide commitment" and promises to see his psychiatrist
   e. Discharge, if your mental health clinician via phone consultation says discharge is "OK"

6. The single most useful piece of information in assessing the severity of a child's or adolescent's suicidal attempt is:

   a. The patient's stated intent
   b. How strongly the patient denies being "seriously" suicidal
   c. The medical lethality of their attempt
   d. The patient's stated perception of the lethality of their attempt
   e. There is no single predictor of the lethality of a patient's suicide attempt

7. A 9-year-old girl, with no past history of medical, psychiatric, or behavioral problems, is brought to the ED by her parents for evaluation. After arguing with her parents, she stated she was going to jump out of the window. There is no family history of psychiatric problems or suicide. She is doing well in school. She and her parents are engaging and cooperative. Her medical examination and mental status examination are unremarkable. She denies any suicidal ideation at the present time, and states that says that she threatened to hurt herself "because I was mad" and had no intention of harming herself. A mental health clinician assesses the patient and feels that she is a low suicide risk and that the family can adequately care for the child. Appropriate management for this patient would be:

   a. Inpatient admission, without further ED evaluation
   b. Inpatient admission, after further ED evaluation
   c. Discharge, without further ED evaluation or intervention
   d. Discharge, if she makes a "no-suicide commitment"
   e. Discharge, if she makes a "no-suicide commitment" and will see a mental health clinician the next day

8. A 15-year-old girl with no past history or medical, psychiatric, or behavioral problems and no history of any prodromal symptoms, is brought to the ED because of an acute change in behavior and mental status. There is no family history of psychiatric problems. On evaluation she is agitated, confused, and disoriented to time and place. She is tachycardic and diaphoretic. Her neurologic examination is unremarkable. On MSE, there is evidence of bizarre, incoherent thought process and visual and tactile hallucinations. The most likely cause of this patient's psychotic symptoms and most appropriate disposition are:

   a. Organic; inpatient medical admission
   b. Organic; inpatient psychiatric admission
   c. Psychiatrically based; inpatient medical admission
   d. Psychiatrically based; inpatient psychiatric admission
   e. Psychiatrically based; discharge with appropriate mental health follow-up

9. A 17-year-old boy is brought to the ED for agitation. He believes that the "neighbors" want to hurt him and says that a voice in his head is telling him to kill himself before the "neighbors" do. His mother says that over the past 2 months he has become more socially withdrawn and isolated, bathing and changing his clothes only when prompted, frequently muttering to himself, and has made failing grades at school. There is a family history of mental illness, but she is reluctant to talk about it. On examination, he is disheveled and agitated. His vital signs and physical exam are unremarkable. In speaking, he jumps from one topic to the next, without any apparent relationship between topics. He is unable to complete three simple, sequential instructions. His affect ranges from sad and crying to angry and hostile. This patient's most likely diagnosis is:

   a. Depression
   b. Schizophrenia
   c. Asperger's disorder
   d. Drug-induced psychosis
   e. Adjustment disorder

10. After being psychiatrically hospitalized and discharged on medications, the patient in Question 9 presents to the ED 6 months later, with confusion and agitation. His mother is unsure if he is taking his medication. On examination, his temperature is 39°C and HR is 110. He is diaphoretic, agitated, confused, and complains that his muscles feel "tight." Possible etiologies for this presentation include:

    a. Meningoencephalitis
    b. Exacerbation of underlying condition secondary to noncompliance
    c. Neuroleptic Malignant Syndrome (NMS)
    d. Posttraumatic Stress Disorder (PTSD)
    e. Any of the above

11. A 16-year-old girl with a known diagnosis of bipolar (manic-depressive) disorder is brought to the ED for evaluation of a 2-week history of hyperactivity, distractibility, pressured speech, irritable and labile mood, and decreased need for sleep. Her mother states that the girl has not been taking her medication. On evaluation, she is agitated, provocative, and unable to control herself. For acute relief of symptoms, the most appropriate medication is:

    a. Lithium carbonate
    b. Valproic acid
    c. Carbamazepine
    d. Haloperidol
    e. Fluoxetine

12. A 7-year-old girl is brought to the ED for evaluation, be-cause "she's sick all the time and she's missing a lot of school." The girl's complaints are varied, ranging from stomachaches, to headaches, to "just not feeling good." She is the only child of an older couple, and she has com-pletely recovered from leukemia diagnosed at age 2 years. Her physical and intellectual development is appropriate for her age. Vital signs and physical exam are unremark-able. ED management should include:

a. Mental health consultation
b. Comprehensive laboratory workup
c. Discussion of possible school refusal
d. Psychiatric hospitalization
e. Medical hospitalization

13. A 12-year-old boy is brought to the ED for disruptive and aggressive behavior, with irritable mood and poor frustration tolerance. Thorough medical evaluation is not suggestive of an organic cause for his symptoms. In the ED management of this patient, the most important goal is:

a. Obtaining appropriate mental health consultation and/or follow-up
b. Ensuring the safety of the patient, with himself, his family, and in his environment
c. Arriving at a psychiatric diagnosis (e.g., ADHD, con-duct disorder, substance abuse, psychosis, etc.)
d. Starting psychotropic medications
e. Psychiatric hospitalization

14. A 10-year-old boy, recently diagnosed with a motor tic (Tourette's) disorder and treated with oral pimozide (Orap, a neuroleptic), is brought to the ED with his head and neck stiffly tilted to one side for the past several hours. His vital signs, physical examination, and MSE are otherwise normal. The most appropriate first-line med-ication is:

a. Pimozide
b. Diazepam
c. Dantrolene
d. Diphenhydramine
e. Bromocriptine

ANSWERS

1. d Estimates of the prevalence of depression in children and adolescents vary widely. A 20% lifetime prevalence is a conservative, and the most frequently agreed upon, estimate. Depression is a common problem in children and adolescents, who frequently present to EDs with vague complaints. All children and adolescents with vague or recurrent somatic or behavioral complaints should be screened for de-pression. Depression is more common in children and adolescents with school problems, learning dis-abilities, attention-deficit hyperactivity disorder (ADHD), chronic medical problems, female gender, and family histories of mood disorders. Symptoms of depression include mood disturbance (e.g., de-pressed or irritable mood, crying easily); changes in sleep, appetite, or energy level; anhedonia; poor self-esteem; social isolation or withdrawal; feelings of hopelessness, helplessness, or worthlessness; poor school performance; psychomotor retardation or agitation; and poor concentration. Other symptoms may include pervasive thoughts of death or guilt, substance abuse, or antisocial behavior. Patients with-out suicidality and adequate psychosocial functioning can be safely managed as outpatients.

2. e Necessary data for evaluating a psychiatric emergency include orienting data, relevant history, med-ical evaluation and physical examination, mental status examination, and family evaluation (see Table 129.2 of *Textbook of Pediatric Emergency Medicine,* fourth edition). Integrating all of these sources of in-formation is essential in understanding the crisis that precipitated the psychiatric emergency and in de-ciding among possible treatment options. "Medical clearance" of psychiatric patients entails a careful assessment for possible medical etiologies of the psychiatric symptoms. It does not necessarily include laboratory investigation. Laboratory investigations should be obtained on the basis of clinical suspicion for a medical etiology (see Chap. 18 of text). Formal psychological testing is not indicated in the ED set-ting. Emergent consultation with a primary care provider should be obtained on a case-by-case basis.

3. c   In the ED setting, interviewing the child and observing his or her interaction with his or her family and the examiner is usually sufficient to assess the child's mental status. Formal psychological testing has no routine utility in the ED setting. Anyone is capable of performing an MSE. All ED physicians should be familiar with how to perform an MSE.

4. a   Symptoms of depression vary widely with age. Infants usually manifest apathy, listlessness, staring, hypoactivity, poor feeding, weight loss, and increased susceptibility to illness. Preschool and school-age children may exhibit mood changes (e.g., sadness, "moodiness," anger, or irritability), crying easily, self-deprecatory thoughts, multiple or vague somatic complaints, poor school performance, runaway behavior, phobias, or firesetting. Depressive symptomatology in adolescents is similar to that of school-age children, but it may also include substance abuse, promiscuity, aggressive behavior, and stealing. Appearing irritable or angry, without appearing "sad," is a common presentation of depression in children and adolescents. Symptoms of depression are protean and are often mistaken for other causes. Children with medical or psychological disabilities have an increased incidence of depression. Depression is a major risk factor for suicide.

5. b   This patient manifests multiple factors that put him at high risk for suicide, including a past history of psychiatric problems and suicide attempts, substance abuse, multiple and lethal suicide methods, evidence of premeditation and secrecy, and unwillingness to establish rapport with caregivers. Tables 129.8–129.16 in *Textbook of Pediatric Emergency Medicine* (fourth edition) list factors associated with suicide that should be evaluated in suicidal patients. This patient clearly needs further toxicological evaluation/treatment, as well as a comprehensive mental health evaluation. A "no suicide" commitment (also known as "contracting for safety")—a convincing promise by a patient not to hurt himself or herself and to seek help if he or she should feel suicidal again—is not sufficient for avoiding hospitalization in this vignette. Given this patient's high risk for suicide, discharge should not be considered. After medical stabilization in the ED, appropriate dispositions for this patient would include medical admission with suicide precautions, or psychiatric hospitalization, if available.

6. e   No single factor is predictive of a patient's suicidal intent. Children and adolescents in the ED setting are often embarrassed, scared, or are unwilling or untrusting to discuss their suicide attempt. They may want to appease their parents or the examiner. As a result, they frequently deny or minimize their suicidal intent. They also frequently misjudge the lethality (either under- or overestimate) of their attempt. Perceived or actual degree of medical lethality of their attempt is thus an unreliable measure of suicidal intent. The impulsivity of the act and the strengths and support of the family are also important in this assessment. All suicide attempts, regardless of severity or lethality, should be taken seriously and need to be assessed carefully.

7. e   This patient meets criteria for low suicide risk, and has been adequately evaluated. Outpatient management of a suicidal patient may be considered if the child and family are cooperative and engageable, the attempt was not "serious" (re: intent, medical lethality), the child is not actively suicidal or psychotic, the child provides an earnest "no suicide" commitment, the family is willing and able to assume responsibility for the child, and timely outpatient follow-up is arranged. Families should be discharged with guidelines for the prevention of suicide and early-warning signs of suicide (see Tables 129.18–129.19 in *Textbook of Pediatric Emergency Medicine*, fourth edition).

8. a   Differentiating between organic and psychiatrically based etiologies is critical in the appropriate ED management of psychotic patients. Misdiagnosis can result in delay of appropriate treatment, inappropriate treatment, and psychological trauma. Acute onset of symptoms, lack of prodromal symptoms or previous psychiatric problems, and evidence of medical instability, impaired cognition, and visual hallucinations raise suspicion for an organic etiology of this patient's psychosis. Table 129.20 in the text summarizes the common findings of organic versus psychiatrically based psychosis. Tables 129.21–22 list some of the many etiologies of organic psychosis. Acute management should include a thorough evaluation for potentially unstable medical conditions. Patients in whom an organic psychosis is suspected should be medically admitted for diagnostic evaluation and treatment.

9. b   This patient's presentation of acute psychosis, auditory hallucinations, and persecutory ideation, preceded by a prodrome of cognitive, behavioral, and social impairment, is a textbook presentation of schizophrenia. These patients frequently have "loose associations" of speech; blunted, flat, or inappropriate affect; and agitated, withdrawn, or labile mood. There is a wealth of evidence of a strong genetic

basis for schizophrenia. Even though some depressed patients may have psychotic features, they do not have this full complement of symptoms. Organic psychoses usually have an acute onset of symptoms. Asperger's disorder, one of the pervasive developmental disorders, may present with bizarre but not frankly psychotic behavior.

10. e   Any of these conditions may account for this presentation. Careful evaluation for possible medical causes of abnormal behavior is critical in all patients, including those with known or suspected psychiatric disorders. Noncompliance with medication is a common reason for an exacerbation of symptoms. NMS occurs in between 0.1 and 1% of patients on antipsychotics. Patients develop hyperthermia and muscle rigidity, frequently associated with mental status changes and signs of autonomic instability. Distinguishing between NMS and other causes of these symptoms can be quite vexing. These patients' symptoms are frequently treated with repeated doses of antipsychotics, which worsen the condition. Young, muscular boys are particularly at risk for NMS. Dystonic reactions to antipsychotics are common in children and adolescents. PTSD typically manifests as some form of disturbing recollection of traumatic events or as a generalized "numbing" to events or people, but in some cases can manifest as agitation, confusion, or frank psychosis.

11. d   This patient has an acute manic episode. Although lithium, valproic acid, and carbamazepine are excellent mood-stabilizing medications, they are not efficacious in the acute setting. These medications must be given for at least 2 weeks for effect. The acute management of mania involves antipsychotics such as haloperidol. There are newer, atypical neuroleptics, such as risperidone (Risperdal), clozapine (Clozaril), and olanzapine (Zyprexa), which have more advantageous side-effect profiles. They have not been widely studied in children or adolescents, but are probably efficacious and safe. Low-dose benzodiazepines may be effective adjunctive medications. Antidepressants such as fluoxetine (Prozac) may exacerbate or trigger manic symptoms.

12. c   School refusal is a common problem that the ED may face. It is commonly seen in chronically ill children, "vulnerable" children (i.e., those that have survived serious illness), "special" children (i.e., children who are especially "wanted" particularly by older parents or parents who had difficulty with conception), and in children from overprotective families. The classic triad is vague physical complaints, normal medical evaluation, and poor school attention. ED management priorities are detection of school refusal and evaluation for significant medical illness. Extensive laboratory testing is not required. Mental health referral may be warranted, but it is rarely required emergently. Hospitalization is not necessary.

13. b   The goals for evaluating psychiatric patients in the ED setting are threefold. First and foremost is ensuring the safety of the child. Keep in mind that behavior may be situation dependent (i.e., the child may look "safe" and "in control" in the ED, but his or her behavior may be very unsafe when returned to the home environment). The second goal is to rule out possible medical causes and severe psychiatric conditions. The third aim is to gather sufficient information to decide on a disposition for the patient. A definitive psychiatric diagnosis is much less important. Need for consultation, disposition, and treatment depends most on assessing the patient for safety and less on psychiatric diagnosis. Patients with conduct or attention-deficit disorder are at high risk for other problems (e.g., depression and suicidality).

14. d   This patient has an acute dystonic reaction. Dystonic reactions are a common adverse effect of neuroleptics. Such a reaction is best treated with diphenhydramine IM, IV, or PO. His presentation is not consistent with a motor tic; thus, more pimozide is not indicated. His presentation is also not consistent with neuroleptic malignant syndrome, obviating the use of dantrolene (a skeletal muscle relaxant) or bromocriptine (a direct CNS dopamine agonist). Although benzodiazepines may be helpful, they are not considered first-line medications for acute dystonic reactions.

CHAPTER 130

Adolescent Emergencies

CHRISTINA FONG, M.B.B.S., M.P.H.

QUESTIONS

1. A 17-year-old girl is brought to the ED because of a syncopal episode. She has been light-headed and amenorrheic for the last 2 months. Physical examination and evaluation should include all of the following, EXCEPT:

   a. Weight and height
   b. Urine HCG test
   c. Blood sugar
   d. Streptococcal throat swab
   e. Orthostatic vital signs

2. Which of the following patients, with a previously known diagnosis of anorexia nervosa, can be discharged for outpatient management of anorexia?

   a. A 17-year-old girl who presents with syncope. Her K^+ = 2.8 meq/l and on ECG her QTc interval is 0.5 msec
   b. An 18-year-old boy who weighs 70% of ideal body weight; has HR 53, BP 90/60; and a blood glucose level of 48 mg/dl
   c. A 14-year-old girl who has a fear of becoming fat, has missed a period last month, and has a body mass index of 19 kg/m²
   d. A 16-year-old girl who has been amenorrheic for the last 3 months and has lanugo; HR 55, BP 85/60, and T 35.6°C; and K^+ = 3.0 meq/l
   e. A 14-year-old boy who has been vomiting up to eight times per day, a body mass index of 19 kg/m²; HR 160 and a BP 60/45; and has cool, clammy hands and feet

3. A 13-year-old asthmatic boy on albuterol inhalers comes to the ED with shortness of breath and carpopedal spasm. Examination reveals: RR 32, HR 99, O_2 saturation 100%, and good air entry, with no wheezes on auscultation. Treatment should include:

   a. Performing an ABG analysis
   b. Giving him a nebulized albuterol treatment
   c. Giving him IM midazolam to sedate him
   d. Slapping him on the face to stop his panic attack
   e. Having him breathe into a paper bag

4. A 15-year-old girl with a past history of pelvic inflammatory disease (PID) complains of right lower quadrant abdominal pain. She has guarding and rebound tenderness. Her HR is 110 and her BP is 70/44. She is cool, clammy, and sweaty. The next step in her management after IV fluid resuscitation includes:

   a. Pelvic ultrasound (U/S)
   b. Abdominal CT scan with rectal contrast
   c. Urine microscopy
   d. Operative intervention
   e. CBC

5. A 16-year-old prima gravida whose last normal menstrual period was 7 weeks ago complains of mild vaginal bleeding and lower abdominal cramps for 1 day. An ultrasound last week showed a single intrauterine pregnancy. She is afebrile, with HR 82, and BP 115/70. On pelvic examination she has an open internal cervical os with a gray, membrane covered tissue in the vaginal vault. The likely diagnosis in this patient is:

   a. Threatened spontaneous abortion
   b. Inevitable spontaneous abortion
   c. Incomplete abortion
   d. Placenta previa
   e. Placental abruption

6. An intern on his first day in the ED is assessing a 15-year-old girl who ingested an overdose of a 1-month packet of an oral contraceptive pill and 20 amoxicillin tablets. Risk factors for suicide include each of the following, EXCEPT:

   a. Marijuana use
   b. Previous suicide attempts
   c. Previous mental health care
   d. Poor school performance
   e. Smoking

7. A 16-year-old boy with a past history of depression comes to the ED after taking an overdose of 25 20-mg fluoxetine (Prozac) tablets. He was brought in last week because he was complaining of auditory and visual hallucinations after smoking a joint. He was discharged to the care of his father, a police officer, and he was advised not to smoke marijuana. Management in the ED should include:

   a. Discharging him to the care of his father, but advising the father to empty and conceal or lock up the bullets from his gun
   b. Increasing the fluoxetine dose to 20 mg twice a day
   c. Stopping fluoxetine and starting him on chlorpromazine
   d. Assessing suicidal ideation and signs of underlying mental disorder
   e. Advising him to start smoking marijuana again, because this may be a withdrawal effect

8. A 14-year-old boy is brought into the ED following a motor vehicle collision. He was found alone, agitated, screaming, and walking around the crash site. On arrival, he was restrained on the stretcher by handcuffs behind his back and was held down by two police officers and two paramedics, who were unable to obtain IV access. He smelled of alcohol, and empty beer cans and a gram of cocaine were visible on the front car seat. Treatment includes:

   a. Putting the patient in a protected room and calling for a psychiatric consult
   b. Putting the patient in the resuscitation bay, applying four-point leather restraints, administering oxygen, and obtaining IV access
   c. Injecting 5 mg IM midazolam and waiting until the patient calms down
   d. Placing the patient in hog-tie restraints and waiting until the effects of alcohol and cocaine diminish
   e. Putting the patient in a cervical collar, requesting the security guards to hold each limb down, and returning at a later time

9. The police finally locate the parents of the patient in Question 8 in an Amnesty International protest march. They arrive and insist that their son be removed from the restraints despite his agitated state. You should:

   a. Apologize and release the patient to the care of his parents
   b. Inform the parents of his cocaine and alcohol use
   c. Reassure the parents that the restraints are applied for his safety
   d. Demonstrate to the parents how violent he is by removing the restraints
   e. Sedate the parents

10. A 16-year-old obese girl comes to the ED with a 2-week history of sharp left-sided chest pain. She has T 37.6°C, HR 92, and saturated O_2 100% on room air. Auscultation of the chest is normal. She has otherwise been well. She takes the oral contraceptive pill regularly, and she smokes cigarettes. Initial ED investigation should include:

    a. CXR, ECG and ABG
    b. CXR, ECG and CBC
    c. CXR, ESR, and PEFR (peak expiratory flow rate)
    d. CXR, ECG, and PEFR
    e. No diagnostic testing

11. A 17-year-old boy complains of an acute onset of fatigue, malaise, myalgia, and mental exhaustion. You think he has chronic fatigue syndrome. Some of the factors on history that are NOT consistent with chronic fatigue syndrome include:

    a. Increasing fatigue at the end of the day, relieved by rest
    b. Low-grade fever
    c. Painful lymphadenopathy
    d. Persistent fatigue
    e. Recent history of a viral infection

12. A 12-year-old girl is referred by her primary care physician with a suspicion of anorexia nervosa. Which of the following features is NOT consistent with an eating disorder?

    a. Delayed puberty
    b. Dependent edema
    c. Lanugo
    d. Enlarged parotids
    e. Gum hypertrophy

13. You are the director of an ED where six of the seriously injured adolescents from the local high school massacre were treated last week. One of the victims died in the ED, and the rest are still in the ICU. The adolescent responsible for the shootings is one of the patients in the ICU. The following should be part of the disaster planning after the acute phase:

    a. Appear on television talk shows to share your experience with the rest of the nation
    b. Run debriefing sessions for the staff and families involved and increase security in the hospital
    c. Refuse to give press releases, stating that patient confidentiality should be maintained
    d. Take your vacation early, as you are too distressed by the incident
    e. Write up the incident as a case study for publication

14. A 15-year-old girl comes to the ED with complaints of dysuria and frequency. Urinalysis shows evidence of a UTI. During the examination, you notice a lower abdominal fullness and you suspect a 16-week gravid uterus midway between the pubic symphysis and the umbilicus. The patient denies being sexually active and claims to be a virgin. Management of this patient, apart from treating the UTI, should include the following:

   a. Confirming the pregnancy with a β-HCG urine test without informing the patient

   b. Explaining to the patient that a pregnancy test, as well as other tests (e.g., a pelvic ultrasound), is important as part of the investigation of an abdominal mass

   c. Contacting her parents and to ask if they want their grandchild aborted

   d. Explaining to the patient while waiting for the urine β-HCG test her options, including keeping the baby, putting up the baby for adoption, or terminating the pregnancy

   e. Advising the patient to return to her primary care physician to diagnose her abdominal mass

ANSWERS

1. d   It is important to document the patient's body mass index as part of the evaluation for anorexia. The vignette does not describe any weight gain, but she may be in the first trimester of pregnancy and may be experiencing morning sickness. Weight loss, lethargy, and changes in the menstrual cycle can be an insidious presentation of diabetes without overt ketoacidosis, and she should be screened for with a simple finger-stick glucose test or a urinalysis for ketones and glucose. A throat swab has no relevance in any of the likely differential diagnoses entertained in this case scenario, which includes anorexia nervosa, diabetes mellitus, pregnancy, occult malignancy, chronic infection, inflammatory bowel disease, hyperthyroidism, or Addison's disease. Vital signs are vital, as the name suggests! They should be part of all examinations; however, an orthostatic BP will be useful in helping in the diagnosis of this case.

2. c   Patient (a) has hypokalemia, which has caused a cardiac arrhythmia (probably ventricular tachycardia [VT]) that has precipitated her syncope. A prolonged QT_c is a harbinger of VT. Patients (b) and (d) may not be acutely ill but their symptoms fulfill the criteria for admission (see Table 130.8 in *Textbook of Pediatric Emergency Medicine,* fourth edition). Patient (c) has no medical complications. Patient (e) needs resuscitation!

3. e CO_2 rebreathing is the most effective way of treating hyperventilation. This scenario can be difficult because this boy is an asthmatic patient; however, the clue to suggest the diagnosis is the carpopedal spasm. Respiratory alkalosis causes Ca^{2+} to be bound by the negatively charged protein anions, so that there is a relative hypocalcemia leading to tetany and muscular spasm. In asthma, there is a retention of CO_2 so that there is a respiratory acidosis. ABGs will not help and in fact drawing blood may cause more pain and hyperventilation. Albuterol will heighten his anxiety state and exacerbate tachycardia. Sedation is unnecessary and dangerous in this scenario. Slapping the patient is not suggested.

4. d   This patient is in shock. Several etiologies are possible: She may have a ruptured ectopic pregnancy (PID is a risk factor, especially if she had salpingitis and damaged fallopian tubes), perforated appendicitis, or acute PID. Regardless of the etiology, she is hypotensive and has peritonitis requiring surgical intervention. Diagnostic imaging such as ultrasound and CT will only delay the treatment. Urine microscopy and a CBC would not aid in the diagnosis and would delay definitive treatment.

5. c   Threatened spontaneous abortion has a closed internal cervical os with no products of conception expelled. Inevitable abortion has an open cervical os but no tissue or products of conception are expelled. This girl has an open os and tissue has been expelled, which is diagnostic of an incomplete abortion. Placenta previa and placental abruption are third-trimester obstetrical emergencies.

6. e   Smoking per se is not a suicidal risk factor. Five risk factors as reported by Slap and Vorters (Slap GB, Vorters DF, et al. Risk factors for attempted suicide during adolescence. Pediatrics 1989; 84:762–772.) include (a)–(d) and dependence on the ED for primary care.

7. d   The ED evaluation should focus on assessing his risk of suicidality and underlying mental disorders, because both need to be addressed. These are crucial to the evaluation because this determines whether the patient should be admitted or discharged for outpatient care. This patient has multiple risk factors for suicide: He has a premorbid history of depression and is already on antidepressants; he has had auditory and visual hallucinations, which are not usual effects of marijuana, but are likely his first presentation of schizophrenia, precipitated by cannabis; he has a history of substance abuse; and he may have easy access to a firearm. He should NOT be discharged. There is no evidence to suggest that increasing the fluoxetine dose has an increased antidepressant effect. Moreover, he just took an overdose of it! The half-life of Prozac (fluoxetine) is also up to 1–2 weeks. It is not a treatment emergency physicians should initiate because it needs follow-up. Leave it to the psychiatrists. This patient is not psychotic and does not need chlorpromazine, even though there is a suggestion of schizophrenia in the history. As with option (c), this is not acute management. Answer (e) is just ridiculous.

8. b   This cause of this patient's excited delirium can be from alcohol intoxication, head injury, hypoxia, cocaine, or even a premorbid paranoia state. We do not know. In any case, the patient is not suitable for a psychiatric assessment just yet, but requires acute resuscitation. The patient should be put in an environment where airway and monitoring equipment are available (e.g., the resuscitation bay). He needs to be restrained initially for the staff to assess and treat him safely. After that, the priorities are airway, breathing, and circulation. (This patient is obviously protecting his airway, because he is probably spitting at you at this stage.) Administer O_2 for breathing while you assess his ventilation, then obtain IV access for circulation and pharmacological sedation. Answer (c) is incorrect because it is unsafe to sedate a patient immediately, before assessing his airway or monitoring him. Hog-tie restraints are NOT recommended in the United States. This form of restraint has been shown to cause positional asphyxia in excited delirium states. (Chan TC, Vilke GM, Neuman T, Clausen JL. Restraint position and positional asphyxia. Ann Emerg Med 1997; 30(5):578–586.) Putting a violent patient in a cervical collar can be a challenge and should be attempted after ABCs have been attended to; pragmatically, this will probably be possible after sedation. Ideally, there should be five, not four, people to hold this patient down—one for each limb and one to secure the head and neck.

9. c   This question is designed to highlight two important points: 1) The patient is a minor and consent for treatment is still a legal requirement. However, in cases where the parent is not available or their wishes against proper medical care may endanger the life of the patient, the physician can be the patient's advocate if it is deemed that removing the restraints will seriously endanger the patient's life. Other examples are blood transfusions in Jehovah's witnesses or emergency surgery. 2) In response (b), patient confidentiality should be respected. The physician should try not to disclose information regarding the patient's substance abuse until the adolescent is well enough to consent or if the patient's outcome is fatal or near fatal.

10. a   Even though the most likely diagnosis in this patient is musculoskeletal anterior chest wall pain, other important causes should be excluded, including pulmonary emboli, myocarditis, pericarditis, pneumonia, and pneumothorax. A CXR will help to exclude pneumonia and pnuemothorax; ECG may demonstrate PR depression or widespread concave ST elevation indicative of pericarditis or ST elevation, T-wave inversion, or arrhythmia consistent with myocarditis; and an ABG may show a widened alveolar–arterial (A–a) gradient despite a 100% O_2 saturation, which is suggestive of a pulmonary emboli. Answers (b)–(e) do not include obtaining an ABG in the responses and will be unable to exclude a pulmonary emboli with any confidence. Risk factors in this girl are that she smokes and is on the oral contraceptive pill.

11. a   "Increasing fatigue at the end of the day, relieved by rest" will often have an underlying medical cause for the fatigue. On the other hand, chronic fatigue syndrome patients have fatigue that is present

upon awakening and is not relieved by rest or sleep. The other responses are true of chronic fatigue syndrome.

12. e   Gum hypertrophy is a manifestation of chronic phenytoin use, and not anorexia nervosa or bulimia. The other responses are true of eating disorders.

13. b   Deaths from violent homicide among adolescents are on the rise in the United States, and emergency physicians should be aware of this and be prepared for this epidemiological trend. One of the less frequently addressed areas of disaster planning is the aftermath or postacute phase, because this phase is often overlooked. It is vital for both staff and the families to be debriefed and counseled. For the staff, apart from assisting them in dealing with their emotional stress, debriefing is also a form of quality assurance. An appraisal of how well the department coped with the disaster can help identify whether any improvements should be made. Security should be increased to protect not only the perpetrator but also the staff looking after him, because family and friends of victims may be vengeful toward the shooter and the staff looking after him. It is important to talk to the press without divulging too much medical information and still maintain patient confidentiality. Answers (a), (d), and (e) are just plain silly!

14. b   The patient should have adequate explanation of and be informed of any test that the physician is going to perform on her. This includes pregnancy testing, which should be done privately. The decision to act on those results will be that of the adolescent, her partner, and/or a support person whom she has identified. Thus, answers (a) and (c) are wrong, and (d) is too presumptive because the patient may not be pregnant. If she is pregnant, discussing options regarding a pregnancy will probably scare her away. She already shows signs of denial and/or ignorance. Answer (e) is wrong because this is a high-risk pregnancy and the adolescent is likely not to make the appointment and therefore will not have appropriate prenatal care. She may not want to see her primary care physician for fear that the physician will notify her parents of the pregnancy. It is important to keep the patient within the health care system by first obtaining a diagnosis, and then referring her to adolescent health services.

CHAPTER **131**

Behavioral Emergencies

VINCENT J. WANG, M.D.

QUESTIONS

1. An 18-month-old boy has had a syncopal episode. He was in his usual state of health when he became upset and began crying. He stopped breathing, became cyanotic, limp, and then has opisthotonic posturing. He returned to normal within 45 seconds. On examination he is afebrile and well appearing. His physical examination is normal. Appropriate treatment/management includes:

    a. Obtaining a serum glucose level
    b. Obtaining a toxicological screen
    c. Obtaining serum electrolyte levels
    d. Performing a head CT scan
    e. Reassurance and discharge

2. A 10-year-old boy has had twitching movements for the past 3 months. He has had right-sided blinking occurring several times a minute. The activity seems to be worse when he is in a stressful situation. On examination, he is well appearing, but you note intermittent blinking on the right. He is able to suppress the activity with encouragement. The rest of his examination is normal. Diagnostic testing should include:

    a. Head CT scan
    b. Head MRI scan
    c. EEG
    d. Antistreptolysin O titer
    e. No further testing

3. A 12-year-old girl with a history of anxiety complains of dizziness and numbness in her hands bilaterally. These symptoms have occurred intermittently for 4 months. She appears well and her physical examination is normal. While in the ED she complains of shortness of breath and begins to hyperventilate. Immediate treatment includes:

    a. Albuterol via nebulization
    b. Oxygen
    c. Rebreathing into a bag
    d. Needle decompression of her chest
    e. Propranolol

4. A 4-year-old boy awakens 30 minutes after he has fallen asleep. He is screaming as if in pain. He is extremely anxious, sweating, hyperpneic, and tachycardic. The patient comes to the ED after this event. He is now sleeping and your physical examination is normal. You suspect that he has:

    a. Somnambulism
    b. Pavor nocturnus
    c. Somniloquy
    d. Narcolepsy
    e. Obstructive sleep apnea

5. A 16-year-old girl has had a syncopal episode and is brought by the teacher to your ED. She says she was at school when she felt limp, but she remembered the entire event. She is normally a good student, but has had difficulty recently because she often falls asleep in the classroom. She also reports an inability to move as she awakes from sleep. Treatment includes:

    a. Phenytoin
    b. DDAVP (desmopressin acetate)
    c. Social services evaluation
    d. Dextroamphetamine
    e. Sumatriptan succinate

ANSWERS

1. e   Breath-holding spells are a common cause of syncope in children. Breath-holding spells may be cyanotic, pallid, or indeterminate. This patient demonstrates characteristics of a cyanotic spell. Diagnosis of breath-holding spells is based on the history and a normal physical examination. Some experts have suggested obtaining a hemoglobin level because this has been associated with breath-holding spells, but the other tests are not necessary. Other causes in the differential diagnosis include seizures, structural heart disease, and apnea from a secondary cause (e.g., infection, brain tumor, or injury). The history and exam do not suggest these etiologies.

2. e   Tics are stereotypical, involuntary, repetitive movements or vocalizations that usually involve the muscles of the head and neck. Unlike seizures, they are nonrhythmic and partially suppressible. Males are more commonly affected than are females, and tics tend to increase during times of fatigue, stress, or anxiety. Given that this boy's movement is suppressible, seizures are unlikely. Dystonic reactions to medications may mimic tics, but there is no history of medication use in this child. Sydenham's chorea may also mimic tics, but this would be unlikely without other stigmata of acute rheumatic fever.

3. c   Hyperventilation occurs in males and females equally, with a typical age of onset between 6 and 18 years of age. Patients may have tachypnea, anxiety, lightheadedness, paresthesias, chest pain, palpitations, blurred vision, syncope, and seizure activity. The history and observation often make the diagnosis. Rebreathing into a bag is the classic remedy for this syndrome. If the patient had an asthma exacerbation, albuterol via nebulization and oxygen would be indicated. Needle decompression of the chest is indicated for patients with pneumothorax. Migraine headaches may present similarly, but this is not the case here, and propranolol is not indicated.

4. b   Night terrors, or pavor nocturnus, characteristically occur in preschool-aged children. Shortly after falling asleep, the child awakens in terror, as if in pain. The patient may seem extremely anxious and may have tachycardia, tachypnea, sweating, and flushing. The child may be inconsolable afterward. Somnambulism is otherwise known as "sleepwalking." Somniloquy is talking while sleeping. Narcolepsy is manifested by extreme tiredness, daytime sleep attacks, sleep paralysis, hypnagogic hallucinations, and disturbed nighttime sleep. Obstructive sleep apnea results from upper airway obstruction, which may manifest with apneic spells during sleep.

5. d   This patient demonstrates cataplexy (a sudden loss of muscle tone, while remaining conscious), daytime sleepiness, and sleep paralysis (inability to move during awakening or onset of sleep). Her condition, therefore, is consistent with narcolepsy. Treatment includes regularly scheduled naps, stimulant drugs for daytime sleepiness, and tricyclic antidepressants for cataplexy, sleep paralysis, or hypnagogic hallucinations. Phenytoin would be indicated for seizures (partial absence) but this is not the case. DDAVP may be used for nocturnal enuresis. Social services evaluation is not necessary, and sumatriptan succinate would be used for migraine headaches, which is also not the case here.

CHAPTER 132

The ED Response to Incidents of Biologic and Chemical Terrorism

VINCENT J. WANG, M.D.

QUESTIONS

1. General characteristics of chemical terrorism regarding weapons of mass destruction (WMD) include:

   a. The patient's clinical presentation usually defines the agent
   b. Decontamination of patients exposed to chemical agents is less important than for biological agents
   c. Most facilities are well equipped to triage patients
   d. ED physicians do not require the same personal protective equipment (PPE) as rescue workers
   e. Chemical weapons are more difficult to deploy than nuclear weapons

2. General characteristics of biological terrorism regarding WMD include:

   a. Patients usually complain of symptoms within hours of the exposure
   b. Most biological agents are lethal
   c. Pets of patients are rarely affected
   d. No agents are endemic to parts of the world
   e. ED physicians are at relatively low risk from secondary exposure

3. Recommendations for universal decontamination include all of the following, EXCEPT:

   a. Utilization of an outdoor facility
   b. Complete disrobement
   c. Containment of clothes in impervious bags
   d. Copious rinse with warm 10% hydrogen peroxide solution
   e. Washing with brushes or sponges

4. Twenty children being evaluated in your ED have high fever, difficulty breathing, and poor perfusion. They report having fever, cough, chest tightness, and headaches for the preceding 2 days. Multiple other EDs in the area report an overwhelming number of children and adults with similar symptoms. All patients attended a circus event 3 days ago. You suspect the etiologic agent to be:

   a. Sarin nerve gas
   b. Cyanide gas
   c. *Bacillus anthracis*
   d. Smallpox
   e. Influenza type B

5. You and your colleagues have noticed a number of patients who have fever, malaise, and cough, and are particularly ill. They have been brought to local EDs over the past 2 weeks and many have required admission and ICU care. You perform a Gram stain of the sputum of one patient and note bipolar-staining safety-pin–like bacilli. You call the Centers for Disease Control (CDC) and begin treatment with:

   a. Trimethoprim-sulfamethoxazole PO
   b. IV penicillin
   c. IV gentamicin
   d. Acyclovir PO
   e. IM ceftriaxone

6. A 16-year-old boy is brought to the ED for fever and malaise, followed by vesicular lesions beginning on the trunk and spreading to the arms and legs. Over the past 24 hours, several children from his neighborhood have presented to your ED and other local hospitals with similar symptoms. He is otherwise well appearing. Treatment includes:

   a. Administration of acyclovir
   b. Administration of atropine
   c. Vaccination with smallpox vaccine
   d. Administration of vaccinia immune globulin
   e. Administration of amoxicillin-clavulanate

7. Three siblings are brought to the ED with ptosis, photophobia, blurry vision, and a bulbar palsy. Two other children presented similarly earlier in the day. On examination, they have varying degrees of dysphagia, dysarthria, and dysphonia. All children attended a picnic hosted by a political party 2 days ago. You begin treatment with:

   a. Clindamycin
   b. Vancomycin
   c. Ceftriaxone
   d. Chloramphenicol
   e. No antibiotics

8. A terrorist organization claims responsibility for releasing anthrax via aerosol at a basketball game 1–2 days ago. A number of school-aged children who attended the game are brought to your ED without complaints, but with fear from exposure at the game. The local health authorities confirm that anthrax was indeed aerosolized at the game. Their physical examinations are normal. Cultures are sent. Treatment includes:

   a. Ciprofloxacin
   b. Penicillin
   c. Trimethoprim-sulfamethoxazole
   d. Anthrax vaccine
   e. Admission and observation

9. A terrorist organization releases aerosolized *Yersinia pestis* at a wrestling match. A number of school-aged children are brought to your ED because they had attended the match and are concerned about contracting the disease. They are currently asymptomatic 1 day after the exposure. Treatment includes:

   a. Acyclovir
   b. Penicillin
   c. Trimethoprim-sulfamethoxazole
   d. Plague vaccine
   e. Observation until symptomatic

10. A 7-year-old boy is brought to the ED because of blurry vision, nausea, and weakness. He had apparently been playing in a farmhouse, near an abandoned military base just 1 hour earlier. The mother says that she saw a number of canisters with the label "GC" on them. The local military officials confirm that canisters labeled GC are on the base, but they do not believe any chemical or biological weapons are on the base. His vital signs are T 37.2°C, HR 50, RR 36, and BP 80/40. He is in mild respiratory distress. His eyes have excessive tearing and miosis, his lungs have diffuse wheezing, and his skin is flushed. You suspect that he had been exposed to:

    a. Mustard gas
    b. Nerve agents
    c. Malathion
    d. Cyanide
    e. Anthrax

11. A 2-year-old boy is brought to the ED after inhalational exposure to Sarin nerve gas. The patient was one of many children exposed to Sarin at a daycare center. He is pulseless and apneic. As you prepare to intubate him with rapid-sequence intubation, the best combination of medications is:

    a. Succinylcholine, atropine, midazolam, fentanyl
    b. Succinylcholine, midazolam, fentanyl
    c. Succinylcholine, atropine, ketamine
    d. Rocuronium, atropine, midazolam
    e. Vecuronium, midazolam, fentanyl

12. A 16-year-old girl is brought to the ED because she developed blisters on her hands. She had been unpacking and organizing old military hardware and munitions. One of boxes had a dark-brown residue seeping through the edges. She says that it had a garlic odor. After she had touched the residue, she complained of burning at the site. She also complains of coughing and shortness of breath. On physical examination, she has mild conjunctival injection and lid edema. The sites of contact are erythematous with blisters in the center. Because of this exposure, you immediately treat by:

    a. Administering atropine
    b. Administering thiosulfate
    c. Debriding the areas of blistering
    d. Dermal spray with 1-chloroacetophenone
    e. Administering acetaminophen

13. A 15-year-old boy is one of many school children brought to the ED because of a possible chemical exposure. The local police department reports that a terrorist group left a message claiming responsibility for "poisoning the school." The boy says that he has a history of allergies, and noticed that he had developed eye itching and nasal irritation earlier, associated with cough and chest tightness. He had attributed this to his allergies, but he does admit this is worse than before. The schoolteacher says that the air has smelled like new-mown hay since the beginning of school that day. Treatment may include any of the following, EXCEPT:

   a. Oxygen
   b. Copious saline irrigation
   c. Bedrest
   d. Ibuprofen
   e. N-acetylcysteine

14. Twenty school-aged children are brought to the ED after a threatened terrorist attack. Many of the children have complained of difficulty breathing. Other children complain of headache, dizziness, and flushing. One of the patients has begun seizing. On examination of the children, you notice a cherry-red color to many of the children's faces and a bitter almond odor to their breaths. You immediately begin treatment with:

   a. Pralidoxime
   b. British anti-lewisite (BAL)
   c. Methylene blue
   d. Thiosulfate
   e. Doxycycline

15. A 14-year-old girl is one of many children brought to the ED after an unknown exposure at a high school auditorium A local terrorist group is claiming responsibility for the act, which occurred 2 hours ago. She says that she initially felt twitching of her muscles, and then she felt weak. She also complains of eye pain, excessive tearing, shortness of breath, and nausea. On physical examination, you note wheezing and diaphoresis. You immediately begin treatment with:

   a. Pralidoxime
   b. BAL
   c. N-acetylcysteine
   d. Thiosulfate
   e. Doxycycline

16. A distraught father of a recently deceased child comes to your ED saying that he wants to join his daughter. He says he is a military chemist in the antichemical warfare division. He is waving a canister and says that he hopes to bring a few others with him to join his daughter. Shortly after he detonates the device in front of him, he begins hyperventilating. He then begins to seize, and then becomes comatose. He dies shortly thereafter. He has no evidence of cyanosis, oral or nasal secretions, or miosis. The most likely agent is:

   a. Nerve gas
   b. Cyanide
   c. Phosgene
   d. Capsaicin
   e. Mustard

ANSWERS

1. d   ED physicians are not required to wear the same PPE as rescue workers. Patients transported to medical centers should be decontaminated to a degree and screened appropriately. Rescue workers are required to wear Level A or B PPE, but hospital-based health-care workers routinely wear Level C PPE. The clinical presentation may be confusing, and there may have been multiple agents used. Biological agents are unlikely to reaerosolize, and with the exception of mycotic agents, are not dermally active. Decontamination of biological exposures, therefore, is less critical than chemical exposures, which may be dermally active and may be readily aerosolized. Most medical centers are not well equipped to triage a WMD disaster. Chemical and biological WMD are easier to deploy than nuclear weapons, and have been used by countries that do not have nuclear weapons.

2. e   ED physicians are at relatively low risk from secondary exposure for multiple reasons: 1) biological agents do not aerosolize readily from the patient's clothes; 2) if aerosolized, the ideal particle size is 1–5 μm, which is unlikely to result from a patient's cough or from aerosolization from his clothes; 3) only mycotic agents are dermally active; 4) biological agents are not volatile; 5) patients often present in the ED days after the exposure and are therefore unlikely to have the agents on their clothes. Most agents are not lethal, and pets are often affected with similar illnesses. Many agents (e.g., anthrax) are endemic to parts of the world.

3. d   Each of the previous statements is true except for (d). All patients should undergo a copious warm water rinse, rather than a warm 10% hydrogen peroxide solution rinse.

4. c   *Bacillus anthracis,* the etiologic agent of anthrax, represents the greatest biological threat. After an incubation period of 1–6 days, a flulike illness begins, characterized by fever, cough, headache, myalgia, and chest tightness. After a brief intervening period of improvement, a rapid deterioration then ensues, characterized by high fever, cyanosis, dyspnea, and shock. Death is universal in untreated cases. Sarin nerve gas and cyanide gas would produce symptoms within minutes of exposure. The incubation period of smallpox is 7–17 days and a vesicular rash is characteristic. Influenza type B is not known as a biologic WMD, and infection would be unlikely to present so acutely.

5. c   *Yersinia pestis* (plague) may be treated with streptomycin, gentamicin, or doxycycline. Chloramphenicol may be used for cases of meningitis. For prophylaxis oral tetracycline, doxycycline, or trimethoprim-sulfamethoxazole are recommended. Trimethoprim-sulfamethoxazole is not recommended for primary treatment. Penicillin, acyclovir, and ceftriaxone are ineffective.

6. a   Chickenpox is the primary differential diagnostic consideration for smallpox. In contrast to smallpox, which begins in the periphery and spreads to the trunk, chickenpox spreads from the trunk to the arms and legs. Smallpox has been eradicated, but research stockpiles are kept at the CDC in Atlanta and at a Russian institute in Koltsovo. Some experts fear stockpiles exist elsewhere. Nevertheless, this vignette is consistent with chickenpox, which may be treated with acyclovir.

7. e   Botulism is characterized by cranial nerve dysfunction such as ptosis, photophobia, bulbar palsy, and blurred vision. This progresses to include dysphonia, dysphagia, and dysarthria, and then a descending, symmetric, flaccid paralysis. Antibiotic treatment is not indicated unless the patient develops a secondary infection. Supportive care, including ventilatory support, is the primary means of treatment. Antitoxin may prevent progression of symptoms, but it is unlikely to reverse the disease.

8. a   In cases of known exposure, prophylaxis with ciprofloxacin or doxycycline are recommended. Even in children, these antibiotics should be given because of the risk imposed by this agent. *Bacillus anthracis* is susceptible to penicillin, but resistant strains are easily produced in vitro; therefore, penicillin is not recommended prophylactically. Anthrax vaccine is approved for adults only. Admission and observation is not indicated in asymptomatic children.

9. c   Prophylaxis for *Yersinia pestis* exposure includes tetracycline, doxycycline, or trimethoprim-sulfamethoxazole. In the absence of symptoms, prophylaxis is reasonable, but if suspicion were high, the patient should be admitted and treated with parenteral gentamicin or doxycycline.

10. c   This patient exhibits symptoms of organophosphate poisoning, with cardiovascular, ocular, respiratory, and dermatologic muscarinic effects, but neurologic nicotinic effects. Malathion is a common organophosphate found in pesticides. Nerve agents are organophosphorus compounds, which may produce similar findings. However, nerve agents are unlikely to be found in abandoned military barracks. In addition, the nerve agents are designated GA (tabun), GB (sarin), GD (soman), and VX (Venom X). There is no GC designation, and it is believed that GC was deliberately not used to avoid confusion with the common designation for gonorrheal infections. Mustard gas is a vesicant and would produce symptoms later; it would be unlikely to cause miosis or skin flushing. Cyanide may cause similar respiratory, gastrointestinal, and dermatologic findings, but the cardiovascular findings are tachycardia rather than bradycardia. Anthrax does not cause immediate symptoms.

11. d   Succinylcholine is contraindicated because its effect will be markedly prolonged, as the effects of acetylcholinesterase are inhibited. Atropine is an antidote and should be administered immediately. In addition, it would be a useful adjunct for rapid-sequence intubation. Choice (e) is acceptable, but choice (d) is better.

12. e   Mustard is a vesicant that produces symptoms as noted in this vignette. Treatment is supportive, but does include removing all clothes and decontaminating the eyes and skin with copious saline irrigation. Atropine is an antidote for nerve agent poisoning. Thiosulfate may be used for cyanide poisoning. Debriding the blisters is not indicated. 1-chloroacetophenone is the chemical name for the riot control agent "Mace," and would not be indicated here.

13. b   Phosgene is a toxic inhalant agent that causes injury via multiple mechanisms: 1) asphyxia by displacing oxygen; 2) topical damage to alveoli; 3) allergic hypersensitivity reactions; and 4) systemic absorption through the pulmonary vasculature. Phosgene is considered to have very low solubility and re-

quires prolonged exposure to be toxic. However, because it smells like new-mown hay, and may initially produce no symptoms, exposure may be prolonged before the victim realizes the problem. The most important method of decontamination is removing the patient from the exposure, and administering oxygen if necessary. Bedrest may lessen phosgene-induced pulmonary edema. The use of anti-inflammatory agents (e.g., ibuprofen and N-acetylcysteine) have improved pulmonary edema in animal models.

14. d   Cyanide poisoning will classically present as described in this vignette. Treatment is supportive initially, including provision of 100% O_2 and dermal decontamination. Symptomatic patients should receive antidotal therapy, which is a two-step process. Sodium nitrite is administered to form methemoglobin, which has a high affinity for cyanide and will disassociate it from cytochrome oxidase. The second step is provision of a sulfur donor, typically sodium thiosulfate, which is combined with the cyanide and enzymatically converted to thiocyanate. The second step may be used alone, if the exposure is uncertain. Pralidoxime is indicated for nerve agent poisonings. BAL may be used for lewisite exposures. Methylene blue is used to treat methemoglobinemia. Doxycycline may be used to treat anthrax cases.

15. a   This patient exhibits findings of organophosphate toxicity, secondary to a nerve agent poisoning. If given in time before a stable covalent bond is formed, pralidoxime (2-PAM) splits the organophosphate away from the cholinesterase and regenerates the enzyme. BAL was developed by British scientists as an antidote to lewisite, a vesicant. The choices are treatment for phosgene, cyanide, and anthrax, respectively.

16. b   In a chemical attack, symptoms of convulsions and death within minutes of exposure implies that the weapon is either a nerve agent or cyanide. The course for nerve agent toxicity, however, is typically somewhat longer than that of cyanide toxicity. Patients with lethal nerve agent exposures typically have copious nasal and oral secretions, muscle fasciculations, miotic pupils, and preterminal cyanosis. Phosgene requires much longer exposures to produce symptoms. Capsaicin is also known as pepper spray, and usually manifests as ocular and pulmonary symptoms. Mustard exposure is also unlikely to present so acutely.

Index

A
Abdominal distension
    diagnosis/management, 353, 356
    differential diagnosis, 29–31
Abdominal pain
    diagnosis/management, 303, 304
        differential, 389–395
    symptoms, 136–138
Abdominal trauma, 353–357
    decompression, 354, 356
    diagnostic peritoneal lavage, 354, 356
    imaging in, 354, 356
    laboratory diagnosis, 353, 356
    laparotomy in, indications for, 354,
        356
    mortality in, 353, 356
    penetrating, 355, 357
Abscesses
    Bartholin's gland, 293, 296
    dentoalveolar, 413, 414
    epidural, 417, 418
    pharyngeal, 229, 236
    retroorbital, 150, 151
    retropharyngeal, 76, 82, 126, 127, 144,
        145, 188–191, 229, 236
    tubo-ovarian, 293, 296
Accidents. See also entries under Trauma
    environmental, diagnosis/management,
        264–268
    motor vehicle, 335–340, 355, 357
    radiation, diagnosis/management,
        269–273
ACL injuries, 109, 110–111
ACL tear, 109, 110
Acoustic neuromas, bilateral, 93, 94
Acoustic trauma, 93, 94
Acrocyanosis, 329, 331
Acrodermatitis enteropathica, 172, 173
Acute life-threatening event, 32, 33
Acute lymphoblastic leukemia, 153, 154
Acute poststreptococcal
        glomerulonephritis, 97, 99
Acute radiation syndrome, 270, 271
Acute rheumatic fever
    diagnosis/management, 219, 221
    symptoms, 152, 154
Addison's disease, 212, 213
Adenitis

cervical, diagnosis/management, 229,
        236
    diagnosis/management, 404, 405
Adenomatous polyps, 286, 288
ADH deficiency, and polydipsia, 161, 162
Adhesions
    foreskin/glans, 406, 407
    labial, 292, 294
Adolescent emergencies, 437–441
Adrenal hyperplasia, congenital
    salt-losing form of, 307, 308
    symptoms, 184, 185, 199, 200
Adrenal insufficiency, 306, 308
Advanced life support providers, 19, 20
Airway, artificial, complications, 421, 423
Airway assessment, 3, 5
Airway management, 16–18. See also
        Endotracheal intubation; Rapid-
        sequence intubation
Airway rupture, 349, 351
Allergic colitis, 286, 288
Allergic reactions
    bites/stings, 176, 177, 274–279
        anaphylactic reaction to, 275, 278
    diagnosis/management, 59, 60, 280–284
    to dietary protein, 280–284, 286, 288
    urticaria in, 176
Allergic rhinitis, 282, 284
Alport's syndrome, 92, 93
Alveolar osteitis, 413, 414
Anal fissures, 286, 288
Analgesia, 13–15
Anaphylaxis
    diagnosis/management, 281, 284
    stings/bites, 275, 278
    symptoms, 210, 211
Anemia
    aplastic, 158, 159
    autoimmune hemolytic, 248, 251
    differential diagnosis, 158, 160
    hypoplastic, 158, 159
    iron-deficiency, 158, 160
    microangiopathic, 159, 160
    nonimmune hemolytic, 248, 251
    nutritional, 158, 159
    sickle-cell, 95, 96
    sideroblastic, 158, 159
Angioedema, hereditary, 190, 191

Anion gap, 254, 255, 258, 259
Anisocoria, physiologic, 69, 70
Ankle injuries, 104, 105
Anterior uveitis, acute, 71, 72
Antihistamines, as cardiac toxins, 255, 260
Antipsychotic drugs, and syncope, 193, 194
Aorta, traumatic rupture of thoracic, 349,
        352
Aphthous ulcers, 134, 135
Apley compression test, 111
Apnea
    breath-holding events, 32, 33
    choking events, 32, 34
    diagnosis/management, 32, 33
    differential diagnosis, 33, 34
    in infants, 32, 33
    obstructive sleep, 300, 302
Apophysitis, 409, 411
    of calcaneus, 119, 120
Appendicitis, 136, 137, 389, 393
    pelvic, 198, 199
Arrest of labor, with beta-
        sympathomimetics, 8, 9
Arthritis
    complications of, 324, 326
    gonococcal, 152, 153
    pauciarticular-onset juvenile
        rheumatoid, 102, 103
    septic
        diagnosis/management, 231, 232, 238,
            408, 410
        symptoms, 152, 153
Artificial airway, complications, 421, 423
Asphyxia, traumatic, 349, 351
Aspiration, diagnosis/management
    fluids, 298, 301
    foreign bodies, 47, 48, 85, 86, 190, 191,
        210, 211, 280, 282
    pulmonary, 210, 211
Aspiration pneumonia, 299, 301
Aspirin toxicity, 181, 182.
Asthma
    cough-variant, 143, 280, 282
    diagnosis/management, 280–281, 283
    pneumothorax with, 280, 283
    ventilation in, 297, 300
    wheezing in, 211
Ataxia, 35–36

Atlanto-axial subluxation, 126, 127
    differential diagnosis, 127, 128
Atopic dermatitis
    diagnosis/management, 312, 314
    symptoms, 163, 164, 165
Atrial contractions, premature, 196, 197
Atrial fibrillation, 218, 220
Auricular hematomas, 380, 381
Autoimmune hemolytic anemia, 248, 251

B
Back pain, 139–140
Bacteremia
    meningococcal, 76, 81
        purpura in, 174, 175
    risk for, 227, 234, See also Sepsis
Balanoposthitis, 406, 407
Bartholin's gland abscess, 293, 296
Basilar skull fracture, and hearing loss, 92,
    93
Battle's sign, 106, 107, 342, 345
Bedwetting, 139, 140
Bee stings, 275, 277
    reaction to, 177
Behavioral changes, 55–56
Behavioral emergencies, 442–443
Benign fibrous cortical defects, 102, 103
Beta-blocker overdose, 256, 261
Beta-sympathomimetics, 8, 9
Bicycle accident trauma, 335, 336, 355, 357
Biguanide overdose, 256, 261
Bites/stings, 274–279
    diagnosis/management, 274–279, 275,
        278, 313, 316
    symptoms, 176, 177
Bladder injuries, 359, 360
Bleeding. See also Epistaxis; Ulcers
    dysfunctional uterine, 201, 202, 292, 295
    gastrointestinal, 87–89
    tooth extraction site, 413, 414
    of unclear etiology, 299, 301
    upper gastrointestinal, 285, 288
    vaginal, 201–202
Blepharitis, 63, 65
Blood, swallowed maternal, 286, 288
Blood disorders
    anemia
        aplastic, 158, 159
        autoimmune hemolytic, 248, 251
        differential diagnosis, 158, 160
        hypoplastic, 158, 159
        iron-deficiency, 158, 160
        microangiopathic, 159, 160
        nonimmune hemolytic, 248, 251
        nutritional, 158, 159
        sickle-cell, 95, 96
        sideroblastic, 158, 159
    clotting, 61, 62, 250, 253
Blow-out fracture, diagnosis/management,
    66, 67, 364, 365, 396, 398
Blunt trauma, 338, 339
Bone tumor, 319, 321
Botulism
    diagnosis/management, 224, 226, 233,
        239
    symptoms, 144, 145, 181, 182, 208, 209
Bowel disease, inflammatory, 212, 213
Bowel obstruction, 29–31

Bowel perforation/transection, 355, 357
Brachial plexus, congenital, 330, 332
Brain injuries, child abuse, 427, 430
Brain tumor, 319, 321
Branch-chain ketoacid decarboxylase
    defect, 129, 130
Breast lesions, 37–38
Breast-feeding, jaundice and, 114, 115
Breath-holding spells, 32, 33
    cyanotic symptoms, 47, 48, 186, 187
    and syncope, 192, 193, 442, 443
    vs. seizures, 222, 224
Bronchiolitis, 210, 211
    dehydration in, 230, 237
    diagnosis/management, 230, 237, 280,
        282
Bullous impetigo, diagnosis/management,
    231, 238
Bupivacaine, 13, 14
Burn injuries
    acidic, 373, 374
    diagnosis/management, 265–268
    electrical, 373, 374
    intentionally inflicted, 373, 374
    major, 372, 373
    minor, 372, 373
    ocular, 400, 401
    oral, 370, 371
    second-degree, 372, 373
    symptoms, 178, 179
    thermal, 372, 374

C
Calcium channel blocker overdose, 256,
    261
Cancer. See Malignancies; Oncologic
    symptoms/processes
Candidiasis, in infants, 134, 135
Carbon dioxide monitoring, end-tidal, 3, 6
Carbon monoxide poisoning,
        diagnosis/management, 72, 73, 265,
        267
Cardiac. See also entries under Heart
Cardiac contusion, 350, 352
Cardiac disease, and syncope, 192, 193
Cardiac symptoms,
        diagnosis/management, 217–221
Cardiogenic shock, infant, 217, 220
Cardioversion, synchronized, 5, 7
Cat bites, 276, 279
Catheter placement
    intraosseous, 10, 12
    saphenous vein, 4, 6
Cat-scratch disease, 233, 239
Cellulitis, diagnosis/management
    bacterially induced, 231, 238
    of foreskin, 406, 407
    periorbital, 59, 60, 400, 401
    retroorbital, 150, 151
Central anticholinergic poisoning, 75, 80
Central cord syndrome, 341, 343
Central nervous system injuries, child
        abuse, 427, 430
Central venous catheter, complications,
        422, 423
Cephalohematomas, 328, 331
Cerebellar ataxia, acute, 224, 226
Cerebellitis, postinfection, 224, 226

Cerebrovascular event, 223, 225
Cervical adenitis, 229, 236
Cervical fractures, 126, 127. See also Neck
        trauma
Cervical subluxations, 126, 127
    differential diagnosis, 127, 128
Chance fractures, 355, 357
Chancroid, 90, 91
Chest pain, 141–143. See also Myocardial
        infarction
    cardiac, 24, 25, 141, 142
    in cystic fibrosis, 303, 305
    differential diagnosis, 141, 142, 143, 438,
        440
    drug induced, 141, 142
    etiology of, adult, 24, 25
    myocardial ischemic, 24, 25
Chickenpox. See Varicella infection
Child abuse, 427–431
    reporting responsibilities, 427, 430
Chlamydia pneumonitis, 44, 45
Chlamydia trachomatis infection
    neonatal, diagnosis/management, 329,
        331
    symptoms, 71, 72
Chloral hydrate, 14, 15
Chloramphenicol (IV), for RMSF, 77, 82
Choanal atresia, 144, 145, 180, 182
Choking episodes
    and cough, 45, 46
    in infants, 32, 34
Cholangitis, acute, 287, 289
Cholecystitis, acute, 287, 289
Cholesteatoma, 92, 93
Chondromalacia patellae, 410, 412
Clostridium difficile infection, 231, 237
Clotting factor deficiencies, 61, 62. See also
        Hematologic symptoms
Coarctation of aorta, hypertension and,
        100, 101
Colic, 49–50
Colitis, allergic or ulcerative, 286, 288
Coma, 39–40
Commotio retinae, 71, 72
Community-acquired pneumonia, 45, 46
Concussion, 106, 107, 341, 343. See also
        under Head trauma
Condyloma acuminata, 293, 296
Congenital adrenal hyperplasia, 184, 185,
        199, 200
    salt-losing form of, 307, 308
Congenital heart block, 217, 220
Congenital heart disease, 8, 9, 47, 48
    heart murmur in, 95, 96
Congenital lobar emphysema, 397, 398
Congestive heart failure, 59, 60, 210, 211
    diagnosis/management, 217, 220
    differential diagnosis/management, 217,
        219
    in infants, 30, 31
Conjunctivitis
    allergic, 63, 65
    differential diagnosis, 400, 401
    viral, 121, 122
Consciousness, altered levels of, 39–40
Consent, parental, in emergencies, 438, 440
Constipation
    acute, 41, 43

differential diagnosis, 41, 42, 43, 391, 395
functional, 42, 54
and urinary frequency, 199, 200
Contact lenses, 63, 64
Corectopia, 69, 70
Corneal abrasions, 49, 50
diagnosis/management, 364, 366
Cortical blindness, 72, 73
Cortical defects, benign fibrous, 102, 103
Cough, diagnosis/management, 281, 283
differential diagnosis, 44, 45, 46
Cough syrup overdose, 4, 7
Cough-variant asthma, 142
Coxsackie A16 infection, 167, 169
Coxsackie virus infection, 188, 189
Crohn's disease, 134, 135
Croup, 45, 46
differential diagnosis, 180, 181, 190, 191
treatment of, 229, 236
Crying
and colic, 49–50
diagnosis/management, 329, 331
differential diagnosis, 385, 387
Cryptorchidism, 90, 91
CSF shunt. *See* Shunts
Cushing's triad, 344
Cyanosis, diagnosis/management, 217, 219
differential diagnosis, 47, 48, 186, 187
heart murmur and, 48, 95, 96
Cyanotic spells, 219, 221
Cystic fibrosis, 184, 185, 210, 211
diagnosis/management, 303–305
Cystic hygroma, 124, 125
Cysts
differential diagnosis, 385–388
oral, neonatal, 329, 332

D
Darier's sign, 170, 171
DDAVP, for trauma in von Willebrand's
disease, 250, 253
Defibrillation, 5, 7
Dehydration, 51–52
in bronchiolitis, 230, 237
diagnosis/management, 243–244,
245–246
indications for IV antibiotics in, 51, 52
Dental emergencies, 413–415
Dental infection, 150, 151
Dental trauma, 369–371
Dentoalveolar abscess, 413, 414
Depression, 432, 434, 435, 438, 440
Dermatitis. *See also* Dermatologic
symptoms; Rash
atopic, 163, 164, 165, 312, 314
diagnosis/management, 312–317
perianal, 286, 288
poison ivy, 313, 316
Rhus, 164, 165
seborrheic, 163, 164
Dermatitis/erythroderma, exfoliative, 163,
165
Dermatologic symptoms,
diagnosis/management, 312–317
Diabetes, and polydipsia, 161, 162
Diabetes insipidus, 307, 308
Diabetic ketoacidosis, 136, 137
odor in, 129, 131

Diagnostic peritoneal lavage, 354, 356
Diaper rash, 312, 315
Diaphragmatic injury, 349, 351
Diarrhea, 53, 54
Discitis, 409, 411
Diskitis, 409, 411
Dislocations. *See*
Subluxations/dislocations; Trauma
Disseminated intravascular coagulation,
11, 12
Disturbed children, 55–56
Diving event, 264, 266
Dizziness, 57–58
Dobutamine (IV fluid replacement),
indications for, in shock, 10, 11
Dog bites, 276, 279
Doll's-eyes maneuver, 66
Dopamine (IV fluid replacement),
indications for, in shock, 11, 12
Double-bubble sign, 391, 394
Doxycycline (IV), for RMSF, 77, 82
Drowning event, 264, 267
Duodenal hematomas, 355, 357
Dyscoria, 69, 70
Dysfunctional uterine bleeding, 201, 202
diagnosis/management, 292, 295
Dysmenorrhea, 292, 294, 295
Dysphagia, 144–145
Dystonic reaction, acute, 434, 436
Dysuria, 146–147

E
Ear, innervation of, 148, 149
Ear infection, 148, 149
Ear pain, 148–149
Ear trauma, middle, 367, 368
Earache, 148–149
Ecchymoses
mastoid, 106, 107
periorbital, 106, 107
Eczema, 163–166
Edema, 59–60
of scrotum, 156, 157
Electrical injuries, 266, 268
Electrocardiograms, in tachycardia,
195–197
Electrolyte imbalance, 10–12. *See also*
specific electrolyte or electrolyte
disorder
diagnosis/management, 243–247
Emergency medical technicians, 19, 20
Emergency Treatment and Active Labor
Act, 21, 22
Emotional abuse, 428, 430
Emphysema, congenital lobar, 397, 398
Encephalitis, symptoms, 223, 225
Encephalopathy, differential
diagnosis/management, 241, 242
Endocarditis, infective, 219, 221
Endocrine symptoms,
diagnosis/management, 306–309
Endotracheal intubation, 3, 5. *See also*
Rapid-sequence intubation
rapid-sequence, tube size, 16, 18
tube placement, 3, 6
tube size, 3, 4, 6
Enteritis, viral, 53, 54
Enterobius vermicularis infestation, 146, 147

Enterotoxins, 255, 259
Environmental accidents, 264–268
Epicondylitis, 409, 411
Epidemic keratoconjunctivitis, 63, 65
Epidermal inclusion cysts, 385, 387
Epididymitis, 155, 157
Epidural abscess, 417, 418
Epidural hematoma, 342, 345
Epiglottitis
diagnosis/management, 229, 236
differential diagnosis, 180, 181, 188, 189
endotracheal intubation in, 3, 5
Epinephrine, indications and dosages, 4, 6
Episcleritis, 63, 64
Epistaxis, 61–62
recurrent, differential diagnosis, 403, 404
Epstein-Barr viral infection, 233, 239
Erythema, 313, 315
Erythema infectiosum, 168, 169
Erythema multiforme, 146, 147, 167, 168
Esophageal compression, 396, 398
Esophageal injury, 349, 351
Esophageal varices, 285, 288
Esophagitis, 285, 287
Examination, of children
sexual abuse, 293, 295
sexual history-taking, 291, 294
in trauma, 112, 113, 335–336
Eye(s). *See also* Ophthalmic emergencies
injuries of, 364–367
innervation of, 67
red, 63–65
strabismus, 66–68
unequal pupils, 69–70
visual disturbances, 71–73
Eyelid lacerations, 364, 365

F
Facial fractures, 361–363
and injury to deeper structures, 362, 363
Facial trauma, 361–363
Factor VIII deficiency, hemorrhage in, 250,
253
Failure to thrive, 429, 430
Falling injuries, suspicious, 429, 431
Fatigue, increasing, 438, 440
Felon, 385, 387
Femoral head, aseptic necrosis, 118, 119
Fentanyl, 13, 15, 17, 18
Fever
asymptomatic, 75, 80
diagnosis/management, 74, 78, 79
differential diagnosis/management
in infant urinary tract infection, 227,
234
infants, 232, 238
in seizures, 228, 235
measurement of, 75, 80
persistent, 227, 234
after antibiotics, 77, 83
symptomatic
bacterial infections, 75, 76, 77, 79, 80,
81, 83
heat-related illness, 76, 82
herpetic gingivostomatitis, 77, 83
Kawasaki's disease, 76, 82
malaria, 78, 84
malignant hyperthermia, 77, 84

Fever, symptomatic (*continued*)
    neck pain, 126, 128
    petechiae, 76, 81
    retropharyngeal abscess, 76, 82
    Rocky Mountain spotted fever, 77, 82
    rubeola, 77, 82
    seizures, 74, 79
    toxic ingestion, 75, 80
    toxic shock syndrome, 77, 83
    vesicular eruption, 76, 81
    viral infections, 75, 77, 79, 82
First responders, training and
    responsibilities, 19, 20
Flaccid paralysis, 207–209
Flail chest, 349, 351
Fluid replacement, 10–12. *See also*
    Electrolyte imbalance;
    Resuscitation; and specific
    electrolyte or electrolyte disorder
Foreign body(ies)
    aspiration, 47, 48, 85, 86, 190, 191, 210,
      211
      diagnosis/management, 280, 282, 367,
        368
    esophageal, 144, 145
    ingested, 85, 86, 392, 395
    ocular, 364, 366
    unusual odors, 129, 130
    vaginal, 203, 204, 291, 294
Foreskin, cellulitis, 406, 407
Foreskin/glans adhesions, 406, 407
Fracture(s)
    blow-out, 66, 67, 364, 365
    bone growth and, 375, 377
    bowing, 375, 377
    cervical, 126, 127
    Chance, 355, 357
    clavicular, 112, 113
    elbow, 376, 378
    facial, 361, 362, 367, 368
    fibula, 377, 379
    humeral, 376, 378, 427, 430
    juvenile Tillaux, 104, 105
    mandibular, 361, 362
    metaphyseal chip, 427, 429
    nasal bone, 361, 362, 363, 367, 368, *See
      also* Facial fractures
    orbital, 361, 362
    pars interarticularis, 139, 140
    pelvic, avulsed, 376, 378
    physeal, 375, 377
    Salter-Harris
      diagnosis/management, 377, 379
      physeal symptoms, 102, 103, 104, 105,
        109, 110
    severe, management, 375, 377
    skull, 341, 342, 343, 344, 345
    spinal, 375, 378
    supracondylar, nondisplaced, 376, 378
    supracondylar humeral, 102, 103
    tooth, 369, 370
    triplanar, 104, 105
    ulnar, 376, 378
    vertebral compression, 139, 140
    zygomatic, 361, 362
Fungal infection, of skin, 313, 316
Furosemide, and nephrolithiasis, 97, 98

G
Galactorrhea, antidepressant-induced, 133
Gardner's syndrome, 385, 387
Gastroenteritis, viral, 230, 237
Gastroesophageal balloon tamponade, 285,
    288
Gastrointestinal bleeding, 87–89
Gastrointestinal symptoms,
    diagnosis/management, 285–291
Gastronomy tubes, complications, 422,
    424
Genitourinary trauma, 358–360
Gilbert's syndrome, 116
Gingival hypertrophy, 438, 441
Gingivostomatitis, primary herpetic, 77, 83,
    414
Glasgow Coma Scale, 39, 40, 106, 107
Glaucoma, juvenile, 63, 65
Glenohumeral joint dislocations, 112, 113
Gliomas, differential diagnosis, 386, 387
Glomerulonephritis, acute
    poststreptococcal, 97, 99
Glucose-6-dehydrogenase deficiency, 248,
    251
    syndrome of, 114, 115
Gonadal dysgenesis, 292, 294
Granulomas, 386, 388
    granuloma annulare *vs.* tinea corporis,
      170, 171, 386, 388
    pyogenic, 414, 415
Graves' disease, 386, 388
Groin masses, 90–91
Group A beta-hemolytic streptococci, 75,
    80
Growing skull fracture, 341, 343
Guillain-Barré syndrome, 207, 208
Gum hypertrophy, 438, 441
Gunshot wounds, 336, 342, 344, 355, 357
    to abdomen, 355, 357
Gynecologic symptoms,
    diagnosis/management, 291–296

H
Hair tourniquets, surgical management,
    385, 387
Hamartomatous polyps, 286, 288
Hand-foot-mouth disease, 167, 169
Head tilt, differential diagnosis, 127, 128
Head trauma
    diagnosis/management, 335, 336, 337,
      339, 341, 342, 343, 344
    symptoms/diagnosis, 106–108, *See also*
      entries under Trauma
Headaches, 150–151
    intracranial masses and, 417, 418
Hearing loss, 92–94
    sensorineural, 92, 94
Heart block, congenital, 217, 220
Heart disease, congenital, 8, 9, 47, 48
    heart murmur in, 95, 96
Heart failure, 217, 220
    congestive, 59, 60, 210, 211
      differential diagnosis/management,
        217, 219, 220
    in infants, 30, 31
Heart lesion, congenital, 184, 185
Heart murmurs, 95–96

Heart rate
    infant, increasing, 8, 9
    in shock, 10, 11
Heat-related illness, 76, 82
    cramps, 265, 267
    exhaustion, 265, 267
    stroke, 265, 267
Hemangiomas
    differential diagnosis, 386, 387
    removal, indications for, 404, 405
    subglottic, 403, 405
Hematemesis, 285, 287
Hematobilia, 355, 357
Hematocolpos, 30, 31
Hematologic symptoms,
    diagnosis/management, 248–253
Hematomas
    auricular, 380, 381
    duodenal, 355, 357
    epidural, 342, 345
    septal, 367, 368
    subdural, 342, 345
    subungual, 385, 387
Hematometrocolpos, 30, 31
Hematuria, 97–99, 358, 359
    absence of, 358, 360
Hemoglobinopathies, 158, 159
Hemolytic anemia
    autoimmune, 248, 251
    nonimmune, 248, 251
Hemolytic uremic syndrome, 245, 247, 286,
    289
Hemophilia, 61, 62
    purpura in, 174, 175
    trauma management in, 250, 252
Hemoptysis, in cystic fibrosis, 303, 305
Hemorrhagic diatheses, 61, 62
Hemorrhagic disease, of newborn, 87, 88
Hemorrhagic shock, 87, 88
    in abdominal trauma, 353, 356
Hemorrhagic symptoms,
    diagnosis/management, 248–253
Hemothorax, 350, 352
Hemotympanum, 148, 149
Henoch-Schönlein purpura, 137, 138, 174,
    175
    electrolyte imbalance in, 245, 247
Hepatitis
    toxic, 116, 117
    viral, 116, 117
Hepatitis B infection, urticaria in, 176, 177
Herpes simplex infection
    congenital, 317
    corneal, 64, 401, 402
    neonatal, 77, 83, 184
      diagnosis/management, 330
    oral, 77, 135
Herpes zoster lesions, 178, 179
Herpes zoster oticus, 148, 149
Herpetic gingivostomatitis, primary, 77, 83,
    414
High-risk births, 8, 9
High-voltage injuries, 266, 268
Hip, transient synovitis of, 118, 119
Hirschsprung's disease, 42, 43
Histiocytosis, Langerhans' cell, 163, 165,
    199, 200

Hodgkin's lymphoma, 122, 123
Homicide, 438, 441
Horner's syndrome, 69, 70
Hornet stings, 275, 277
Human bites, 276, 279
Human immunodeficiency virus infection, diagnosis/management, 240–242
Hyaline membrane disease, 8, 9
Hydrocele, testicular, 156, 157, 392, 395
Hydrometrocolpos, 42, 43
Hymenoptera stings, 275, 277
Hyperbilirubinemia
conjugated, 116–117
unconjugated, 114–115
Hyperdynamic flow murmur, 95
Hyperkalemia
arrhythmia and, 218, 221
in renal failure, 245, 247
Hypersensitivity reactions. See Allergic reactions
Hypertension, 100–101
and coarctation of aorta, 100, 101
complications of therapy, 101
pheochromocytoma and, 100, 101
Hyperthermia, malignant, 17, 18
succinylcholine and, 77, 84
Hyperventilation
diagnosis/management, 437, 439, 442, 443
and syncope, 193, 194
therapeutic, 341, 343
Hyphema, 365, 366
Hypocalcemic seizure, 244, 246
Hypoglycemia
diagnosis/management, 306, 308
toxicologic symptoms, 254, 257
Hypokalemia, 29, 31, 437, 439
paralysis in, 208, 209
Hyponatremia, 186, 187
diagnosis/management, 243, 246
in neonatal seizures, 330, 332
Hypotension, 10, 11
traumatic, diagnosis/management, 342, 344
Hypothermia, 267, 268
Hypothyroidism, 42
Hypoxemic spells, 219, 221
Hysterical reaction, 71, 72

I
Idiopathic thrombocytopenic purpura, 174, 175
intracranial hemorrhage, 150, 252
Ileostomy patients, urinary stone development, 422, 424
Immobile arm, 102–103
Immunizations, reaction to, 49, 50
Impetigo, bullous, 231, 238
Inborn errors of metabolism, 129, 130
diagnosis/management, 310–311
neonatal, 330, 332
Incontinence, 139, 140
Indomethacin, 8, 9
Indwelling devices, complications with, 421–424
Infectious diseases, 227–239
odors in, 130, 131
vomiting and, 205, 206

Infective endocarditis, 219, 221
Inflammatory bowel disease, 212, 213
diagnosis/management, 286, 289
Inguinal hernia, incarcerated, 90, 91, 391, 394
Inhalant toxins, 255, 256, 260, 263
Injuries. See Accidents; Fracture(s); Subluxations/dislocations; Trauma
Insect sting, reaction to, 176
Insulin replacement, in endocrine events, 306, 307
Interstitial pneumonia, 298, 301
Intracranial pressure
brain tumor, 319, 321
hemorrhage, in idiopathic thrombocytopenic purpura, 250, 252
masses, 417, 418
and shunt malfunction/infection, 416, 417
therapeutic hyperventilation in, 341, 343
trauma, 342, 344
trauma symptoms, 106, 107
Intraosseous needle infusions, in shock, 10, 12
Intravenous fluids/infusions, 10–12. See also Electrolyte imbalance; specific solution or electrolyte
Intrusion injuries, 369, 370
Intubation, fluid requirements, 298, 300
Intussusception
in children, 87, 88, 205, 206, 390–391, 393–394
in infants, 49, 50
Iritis, traumatic, 365, 366
Ischemia
myocardial, chest pain, 24, 25
stroke, in sickle-cell disease, 416, 417
Ischemic stroke, in sickle-cell disease, 416, 417

J
Jaundice
breast-feeding and, 114, 115
conjugated hyperbilirubinemia, 116–117
unconjugated hyperbilirubinemia, 114–115
Jaw-thrust maneuver, 3, 5
Jellyfish stings, 274, 276
Jervell-Lange-Nielsen syndrome, 92, 94
Joint, septic, 118, 119
Joint pain, 152–154. See also Fracture(s); Rheumatologic symptoms; Trauma
Juvenile rheumatoid arthritis
complications, 323–326
diagnosis/management, 323, 325
pauciarticular-onset symptoms, 102, 103

K
Kasabach-Merritt syndrome, 329, 331
Kawasaki disease, 76, 82, 121, 122, 167, 168
diagnosis/management, 325, 326, 327
Kehr's sign, 112, 113, 398
Kernicterus, 114, 115
Ketamine, 13, 14, 16, 18
adverse reactions, 14, 15
Kidneys. See entries under Renal

Knee injuries, 109–111
hyperflexion, 377, 379
patellar dislocation, 109, 110
diagnosis/management, 377, 379
patellar menisci injury, 109, 111
Knife wounds, 335, 336

L
Labial adhesions, 292, 294
Labor, beta-sympathomimetic arrest of, 8, 9
Labyrinthitis, viral, 93, 94
Lacerations, 380–382
eyelid, 364, 365, 380–384
infection rate for sutured, 380, 381
lip, 380, 382
puncture, 381, 382
ungual, 369, 370
vaginal, 359, 360
Laparotomy, indications for, in abdominal trauma, 354, 355, 356, 357
Laryngomalacia, 191, 396, 398
Lead poisoning, 256, 261
Legg-Calvé-Perthes disease, 118, 119, 152, 153, 409, 411
Leptomeningeal cyst, 341, 343
Lesions
differential diagnosis/management, See also under specific lesion
pityriasis rosea vs. secondary syphilis, 172, 173
tinea corporis vs. granuloma annulare, 170, 171, 386, 388
Lesions, differential diagnosis/ management. See also Rash; specific lesion
breast, 37–38
coin-shaped, 312, 314
cysts, 385–388
gastric mucosal, 285, 288
hyperpigmented, 313, 317
oral, 134–135
papular, 170–171
papulosquamous, 172–173
tinea capitis, 164, 165
tinea versicolor, 168, 169
vaginal, 233, 239
varicella-zoster, 178, 179
vesiculopustular, 313, 317
Letterer-Siwe disease, 163, 165
Leukemia, 318, 320
infection in, 318, 320
risk for sepsis, 227, 234
Leukorrhea, physiologic, 203, 204
Lichen sclerosus, 203, 204
Lichen striatus, 170, 171
Lidocaine, toxic effects of, 14, 15
Life-threatening event, acute, 32, 33
Ligament injury, anterior talofibular, 104, 105
Limping, 118–120, 139, 140
Liver disease, 287, 290
Liver trauma, 355, 357
blunt, 354, 357
Lobar emphysema, congenital, 397, 398
Lung disease, restrictive, 297, 300
Lyme disease, 325, 327
Lymphadenitis, 121, 122, 124, 125

Lymphadenopathy, 121, 122
  bacterial, symptoms, 121, 122, 124, 125
  cervical, 121, 122
  Hodgkin's, 122, 123
  mediastinal mass and, 122, 123
  persistent regional, 121, 122
  viral causes, 121, 122
Lymphocytic interstitial pneumonitis, 240, 242

M
Maculopapular rash, 167–169
Malaria, 78, 84
Malignancies, 407. *See also* Oncologic
      symptoms/processes
  cholesteatoma, 92, 93
  gliomas, differential diagnosis, 386, 387
  hemangiomas
    differential diagnosis, 386, 387
    removal, indications for, 404, 405
    subglottic, 403, 405
  Hodgkin's lymphoma, 122, 123
  infections in, 318, 319, 320, 321
  neuromas, acoustic, 93, 94
  pheochromocytomas, 100, 101
  presacral sacrococcygeal teratoma, 392, 395
Malignant hyperthermia, 17, 18
  succinylcholine and, 77, 84
Mallory-Weiss tear, 88, 89
Malnutrition, and oligomenorrhea, 132, 133
Malrotation, 136, 137, 391, 394
Mandibular dislocation, 370, 371
Manic episodes, 433, 436
Mantoux reaction, 230, 237
Marcus Gunn 'jaw-winking' phenomenon, 69, 70
Marcus Gunn pupil sign, 69, 70
Marfan's syndrome, 139, 140
Mastitis, 37–38
  neonatal, 77, 83, 329, 332, 414
McKusick-Kaufman syndrome, 292, 294
Measles, 77, 82, 167, 168
Measles encephalopathy, 233, 239
Meckel's diverticulum, 87, 89, 392, 395
Mediastinal mass
  differential diagnosis of, 397, 398
  and lymphadenopathy, 122, 123
  and respiratory distress, 318, 321
Meningitis
  antibiotic management, 228, 235
  bacterial
    fever complications, 228, 235
    pathogens causing, 228, 235
  differential diagnosis/management, 223, 225, 227, 235
Meningococcemia, 76, 81
  purpura in, 174, 175
Menstruation, vicarious, 61, 62
Mental status examination, 56
Metabolic symptoms,
      diagnosis/management, 310–311
Metabolism, inborn errors of
  diagnosis/management, 310–311
Metabolism, inborn errors of,
  diagnosis/management, 129, 130
Metaphyseal chip fractures, 427, 429
Metastatic oncologic disease, 319, 321

Methanol poisoning, 72, 73
Methemoglobinemia, 47, 48
  diagnosis/management, 249, 252
Midgut volvulus, 87, 88, 136, 137, 391, 394
Migraine, 57, 58
  diagnosis/management, 223, 225
Möbius' syndrome, 67, 68
Molluscum contagiosum, 313, 317
Mongolian spots, 328, 330
Motor vehicle accident trauma, 335–340, 355, 357
Muciprocin, 231, 238
Mucocele, 413, 414
Mumps orchitis, 155, 157
Muscle stress, 265, 267
Myocardial infarction, 25–26. *See also*
      Chest pain
  ECG, 24, 25
Myocardial ischemia, 24, 25

N
Narcolepsy, 442, 443
Narcotic withdrawal, neonatal, 330, 332
Nasal discharge, persistent, 403, 404
Near-drowning event, 264, 266
Neck, soft tissue injury, 367, 368
Neck mass, 124–125
Neck pain, fever and, 126, 128
Neck stiffness, 126–128
  differential diagnosis/management, 228, 235, 236
Neck trauma, 338, 339, 341, 343, 346–347
Necrotizing fasciitis, in varicella infection, 231, 238
Neonatal symptoms,
      diagnosis/management
  acrocyanosis, 329, 331
  brachial plexus, congenital, 330, 332
  cephalohematomas, 328, 331
  Chlamydia trachomatis infection, 329, 331
  congenital muscular torticollis, 329, 331
  crying, 329, 331
  herpes simplex viral infection, 328, 330
  inborn errors of metabolism, 330, 331, 332
  Kasabach-Merritt syndrome, 329, 331
  mastitis, 329, 332
  Mongolian spots, 328, 330
  narcotic withdrawal, 330, 332
  oral cysts, 329, 332
  pupillary reflex, 331
  seizures, 330, 332
  spina bifida occulta, 330, 332
  transient tachypnea, 328, 330
Nephrolithiasis, furosemide and, 97, 98
Nephrosis, electrolyte imbalance, 244, 246
Nephrotic syndrome, 59, 60
  electrolyte imbalance management, 244, 246
Neuritis, optic, 224, 226
Neurologic symptoms,
      diagnosis/management, 222–226
Neurologic trauma, 341–346
Neuromas, bilateral acoustic, 93, 94
Neuronitis, vestibular, 57, 58
Neuropathy, peripheral, 224, 226
Neurosurgical emergencies, 416–418
Night terrors, 442, 443

Nitrous oxide, effects of, 13, 14
Nonimmune hemolytic anemia, 248, 251
Normal saline (IV fluid replacement)
  indications for, in dehydration, 51, 52
  indications for, in shock, 10, 11
Nose bleeds, 61, 62
  recurrent, differential diagnosis, 403, 404
Nuchal rigidity. *See* Neck stiffness

O
O$_2$. *See* Oxygen
Obstipation, 29, 31
Obstruction
  diagnosis/management
    intestinal, in cystic fibrosis, 303, 304
    sleep apnea, 300, 302
  symptoms
    hematuria, 97, 98
    mechanical, 29, 30, 87, 88
    uropathic, in newborn, 30, 31
Ocular. *See* Eye(s); Ophthalmic
      emergencies
Odors
  body, 129, 130
  detection of human, 129, 130
  in infectious diseases, 130, 131
  of toxins, 130, 131
  unusual, 129–131
    in infants, 129, 131
Oligomenorrhea, 132–133
Oncologic symptoms/processes, 397, 398.
      See also Malignancies
  diagnosis/management, 318–322
  metastatic, 319, 321
Ophthalmic emergencies, 400–402
Opioid toxicity, 254, 257, 258
Optic neuritis, 224, 226
Oral lesions, 134–135
Oral trauma, 369–371
Orchitis, mumps, 155, 157
Organophosphate poisoning
  diagnosis/management, 256, 261
  symptoms, 208, 209
Orthopedic emergencies, 408–412
Orthopedic trauma, 375–379. *See also*
      Fracture(s);
      Subluxations/dislocations
Osgood-Schlatter disease, 110, 111, 410, 412
Osmolar gap, 254, 255, 258, 259
Osteitis, alveolar, 413, 414
Osteochondritis dissecans, 110, 111, 410, 412
Osteomyelitis, 105
  diagnosis/management, 232, 238, 408, 410
Otitis externa, 148, 149
  diagnosis/management, 229, 236, 403, 404
Otitis media, 148, 149
  diagnosis/management, 228, 229, 236
  organisms causing, 403, 404
Otolaryngologic emergencies, 403–405
Otolaryngologic trauma, 367–368
Ovarian cyst, torsed, 30, 31
Overdoses
  beta-blocker, 256, 261
  biguanide, 256, 261
  calcium channel blocker, 256, 261

phenothiazine, 256, 262
sulfonylurea, 256, 261
theophylline, 256, 262
tricyclic antidepressants, 256, 262
Oxygen
delivery methods for, 3–6
indications for, 8, 9

P
Pain
abdominal, 136–138
back, 139–140
chest, 141–143
dysphagic, 144–145
dysurial, 146–147
ear, 148–149
head, 150–151
joint, 152–154
scrotal, 155–157
Pain pills, ingestion of
diagnosis/management, 255, 259, 260
symptoms, 181, 182
Pallor, 158–160
Palpitations, 195–197
Pancreatic pseudocyst formation, 35, 357
Pancreatitis, 287, 289
traumatic, 390, 393
Papular lesions, 170–171
Papulosquamous lesions, 172–173
Paralysis
descending, 144, 145
flaccid, 207–209
Parental consent, 438, 440
Parinaud's syndrome, 66, 67
Paronychia, 385, 387
Patellar dislocation, 109, 110
diagnosis/management, 377, 379
Patellar menisci, injury to, 109, 111
Patellofemoral pain syndrome, 109, 110,
111
Pavor nocturnus, 442, 443
Pelvic appendicitis, 198, 199
Pelvic examination, 291, 294
Pelvic inflammatory disease, 137, 138
diagnosis/management, 293, 296
Penile trauma, 359, 360, 406, 407
Pentobarbital, 13, 14, 15
Peptic ulcer disease, 286, 289
Perianal dermatitis, 286, 288
Pericardial tamponade, 348, 350
Pericarditis, acute, 219, 221
Pericoronitis, 413, 414
Perilymphatic fistula, 93, 94
Periodontal injuries, 369, 370
Periorbital cellulitis, 59, 60, 400, 401
Periorbital ecchymoses, 106, 107
Peripheral neuropathy, 224, 226
Peritoneal lavage, diagnostic, 354, 356
Peritonitis, primary, 390, 393
Peritonsillar cellulitis/abscess, 188, 189
diagnosis/management, 229, 236
Pertussis, 44, 46, 183, 185
management/complications, 230, 237
Pertussis vaccinations, 49, 50
Pharyngeal abscess, 229, 236
Pharyngitis, 188–189
diagnosis/management, 228, 236
streptococcal, 134, 135
Phenothiazine overdose, 256, 262

Phenytoin
chronic use, 438, 441
for seizures, 186, 187
Pheochromocytoma, hypertension and,
100, 101
Photosensitivity reaction *vs.* sunburn, 164,
165
Pityriasis rosea, 172, 173
Pityriasis rubra pilaris, 172, 173
Plant toxins, ingestion of, 255, 260
Plasma (IV fluid replacement), indications
for, in shock, 11, 12
Pleural effusion, 299, 301–302
Pneumocystis carinii pneumonia, 240, 241
Pneumomediastinum, 124, 125
Pneumonia
abdominal pain in, 136, 137
aspiration, 299, 301
community-acquired, 45, 46
complications in, 229, 236
diagnosis/management, 230, 237, 396,
398
differential, 229, 236
interstitial, 298, 301
organisms causing, 229, 230, 236, 237
Pneumocystis carinii, 240, 241
right-lower lobe, 392, 395
Pneumonitis
Chlamydia, 44, 45
lymphocytic interstitial, 240, 242
Pneumothorax, 124, 125
with asthma, 280, 283
diagnosis/management, 350, 352, 396,
398
open, 348, 350
small, 348, 350
tension, 180, 181
diagnosis/management, 348, 350
Poison ivy dermatitis, 313, 316
Poisoning. *See* Toxins
Polyarthritis, hepatitis B–induced, 153, 154
Polydipsia, 161–162
Polyps, hamartomatous and adenomatous,
286, 288
Positive-end expiratory pressure, 298, 300
Posttraumatic seizures, 106, 107
Precordial catch syndrome, benign, 141,
142
Pregnancy
adolescent, 30, 31, 132, 133, 198, 199,
339, 441
bleeding management, 201, 202
Prehospital care, 19–20
Premature atrial contractions, 196, 197
Premature ventricular contractions, 195,
197
Presacral sacrococcygeal teratoma, 392,
395
Priapism, 406, 407
Prostaglandins, for shock, 10, 11
Protein C deficiency, 250, 253
Protein S deficiency, 250, 253
Pseudomembranous colitis, 53, 54
Pseudostrabismus, 66, 67
Pseudovertigo, 57, 58
Psoriasis, 168, 169, 172, 173
Psychiatric emergencies, 432–436
evaluation goals, 434, 436
Psychiatric symptoms, 55–56

Psychotic emergencies, organic *vs.*
psychiatric-based, 433, 435, 436
Pulmonary aspiration, 210, 211
Pulmonary edema, 299, 301
Pulmonary hypertension, in cystic fibrosis,
304, 305
Pulmonary symptoms,
diagnosis/management, 297–302
Pulmonic stenosis, peripheral, 95
Puncture wounds, 381, 382
Pupillary reflex, neonatal, 329, 331
Pupils, unequal, 69–70
Purpura rash, 174–175
Pyelonephritis, 146, 147
Pyloric stenosis, 205, 206, 391, 394
Pyogenic granuloma, 414, 415

Q
QT syndrome, prolonged, 192, 193
diagnosis/management, 219, 221
QTc (corrected QT interval), 255, 260

R
Rabies, 276, 279
Raccoon's eyes. *See* Ecchymoses
Radiation accidents
decontamination procedures, 270, 272,
273
diagnosis/management, 269–273
estimating, 270, 272
Ramsay Hunt syndrome, 148, 149
Ranula, 413, 414
Rape, determination of, 429, 430
Rapid-sequence intubation, 16–18
in brain tumor, 17, 18
fentanyl use and effects, 17, 18
ketamine use and effects, 16, 18
in multiple injuries, 17, 18
sedatives/anesthetics, 16, 17, 18
in status asthmaticus, 16, 17, 18
in status epilepticus, 17, 18
tube size, 16, 18
Rash. *See also* Lesions
atopic, 163, 164, 165, 312, 314
B. burgdorferi, 233
diagnosis/management, 312–317
diaper, 312, 315
eczematous, 163–166
in Kawasaki disease, 325, 327
maculopapular, 167–169
perianal, 286, 288
petechial, 233, 239
poison ivy, 313, 316
purpura, 174–175
Rhus, 164, 165
rubella and, 233, 239
seborrheic, 163, 164
skin, in drug reactions, 312, 314
urticaria, 176–177
vesicobullous, 178–179
Rectal prolapse, 303, 304
Red eyes, 63–65
Reflux, gastroesophageal, 205, 206
Renal failure
acute, hypertension, 244, 246
hyperkalemia in, 245, 247
Renal functioning determination, 358, 359
Renal symptoms, diagnosis/management,
243–247

Renal trauma, 358–360
Respiratory distress, 180–182
  differential diagnosis/management, 281, 283
  mediastinal mass and, 318, 321
Respiratory events/disease mortality, 297, 300
Respiratory muscle fatigue, 181, 182
Respiratory stabilization, 8, 9
  in abdominal distension, 30, 31
Respiratory syncytial virus infection, 298, 301
Restraint, of patient, 438, 440
Restrictive lung disease, 297, 300
Resuscitation
  agitated/uncooperative patient, 438, 440
  basic and advanced, 3–7
  inadequate, 8, 9
  neonatal, 8–9
Resuscitation lines, ideal, 4, 6
Retinal artery occlusion, 71, 73
Retinal hemorrhage, 106, 107
Retinal neovascularization, 71, 72
Retrograde urethrography, 359, 360
Retropharyngeal abscess, 76, 82, 126, 127, 144, 145
  diagnosis/management, 229, 236
  differential diagnosis, 188, 189, 190, 191
Reye's syndrome, 287, 289
Rheumatic fever, acute, 152, 154
  diagnosis/management, 219, 221
Rheumatologic symptoms,
      diagnosis/management, 323–327
Rhus dermatitis, 164, 165
Rickets, 307, 308
Rocky Mountain spotted fever, 77, 82, 167, 169
  diagnosis/management, 233, 239
Rotavirus infection, 230, 237
Rubella, 233, 239
Rubeola, 77, 82, 167, 168
Ruptured globe, 364, 365

S
Salmonella enterocolitis, 76, 80
Salmonella infection, 231, 237
Salter-Harris fractures
  diagnosis/management, 377, 379
  physeal symptoms, 102, 103, 104, 105, 109, 110
Scabies infection, rash of, 164, 166
Scarlet fever, 168, 169
School refusal, 434, 436
Scleritis, 63, 64
Scorpion stings, 274, 277
Scrotal injuries, 359, 360
Scrotum. *See also* Testes
  diagnosis pathology, 155, 156
  pain, 155–157
Seborrheic dermatitis, 163, 164
Sedation, 13–15
Seizures, 186–187
  as complications
      of bacterial meningitis, 228, 235
      of pertussis, 230, 237
  differential diagnosis/management
      breath-holding spells, 222, 224
      febrile, 228, 235

febrile, 74, 79, 222, 224
  with focal features, 222, 225
  hypocalcemic, 244, 246
  neonatal, 330, 332
  posttraumatic, 106, 107
  status epilepticus, 222, 225
Sensorineural hearing loss, 92, 94
Sepsis, diagnosis/management, 227, 234
  in abdominal distension, 29, 30
  in leukemia, 227, 234
  neonatal, 183, 184
  in Wiskott-Aldrich syndrome, 250, 253
Septal hematoma, 367, 368
Septic-appearing infant, 183–185
Serum sickness, 282, 284
Severe combined immunodeficiency, 318, 320
Sever's disease, 119, 120
Sexual abuse, examination in, 293, 295
Sexual exploration, 428, 430
Sexual history-taking, 291, 294
Sexually transmitted diseases, 90, 91
  in child abuse, 428, 430
  diagnosis/management, 232, 238
Shark bites, 274, 277
Shigella infection, 231, 237
Shock, diagnosis/management, 10–12, 437, 439. *See also* Electrolyte imbalance
  hemorrhagic, 87, 88, 353, 356
  indications for IV antibiotics, 11, 12
  septic, 227, 235, 244, 246
  spinal, 342, 344
  in supraventricular tachycardia, 218, 220
Shoulder injuries, 112–113
Shunts, complications, 416, 417, 421, 422, 423
Sickle-cell anemia, 95, 96
Sickle-cell disease, 102, 103
  diagnosis/management, 249, 251–252
  and ischemic stroke, 416, 417
Sinusitis, acute, 229, 236
Skin
  fungal infection of, 313, 316
  injuries, child abuse, 427, 429
  rash, in drug reactions, 312, 314
Sleep apnea, obstructive, 300, 302, 442, 443
Slipped capital femoral epiphysis, 110, 111, 118, 120
  diagnosis/management, 376, 378, 409, 411
Smoke inhalation, 265, 267. *See also* Burn injuries
Smoking, maternal history of, 8, 9
Snake bites, 275, 278, 279
Sodium bicarbonate (IV fluid replacement)
  for aspirin toxicity, 181, 182
  indications for, 4, 6
Somnambulism, 442, 443
Somniloquy, 442, 443
Sore throat, 188–189
  streptococcal, 134, 135
Spider bites, 274, 277
Spina bifida occulta, 330, 332
Spinal cord disorder, 223, 225
Spinal cord infection, 223, 225
Spinal cord injury. *See also* entries under Fracture(s); Trauma
  without radiographic abnormality, 126, 127
  diagnosis/management, 342, 344

Spinal cord trauma, 341, 342, 343, 344
Spinal shock, 342, 344
Splenic sequestration crisis, 249, 252
Spondylolysis, 139, 140, 409, 411
Stab wounds, 335, 336, 355, 357
Staphylococcal scalded-skin syndrome, 313, 315
Status epilepticus, 222, 225
Steeple sign, 191
Stevens-Johnson syndrome, 146, 147
  diagnosis/management, 313, 315
Stiff neck. *See* Neck stiffness
Stingray stings, 274, 276
Stings/bites
  anaphylactic reaction, 275, 278
  dermatologic reaction to insect, 313, 316
  diagnosis/management, 274–279
  symptoms, 176, 177
Stomas, complications, 421, 422, 423, 424
Stomatitis, herpes, 134, 135
STORCH, 92, 94, 116, 117
Strabismus, 66–68
Stridor, 190–191
Stroke, sickle-cell disease and ischemic, 416, 417
Sturge-Weber disease, 386, 388
Stye, 400, 401
Subdural hematoma, 342, 345
Subluxations/dislocations
  atlanto-axial, 126, 127, 128
  cervical, 126, 127, 128
  hyperflexion of knee, 377, 379
  patellar dislocation, 109, 110, 377, 379
  radial head, 102, 103, 408, 411
  slipped capital femoral epiphysis, 110, 111, 118, 120, 376, 378
Subungual hematoma, 385, 387
Succinylcholine
  effects of, 17, 18
  and malignant hyperthermia, 77, 84
Suicide, 432, 433, 435
  risk factors, 437, 438, 440
Sulfonylurea overdose, 256, 261
Sunburn *vs.* photosensitivity reaction, 164, 165
Superior vena cava syndrome, 122, 123
Supraventricular tachycardia, 5, 7
  febrile, 184, 185
  OTC cold preparations and, 218, 220
  shock in, 218, 220
Sutured wounds
  infection rate for, 380, 381
  tetanus immune globulin, 380, 381
Sutures, 380, 381
SVC syndrome, 122, 123
Swelling, 59–60. *See also* Edema
Swimmer's ear, 148, 149
Sydenham's chorea, 224, 226
Synchronized cardioversion, 5, 7
Syncope, 192–194, 442, 443
Syndrome of inappropriate antidiuretic hormone, 307, 308
Synovitis
  toxic, 41, 153, 154, 408
  transient, of hip, 118, 119
Syphilis, congenital, 183, 185
Systemic illness, and unusual odors, 129, 131

Systemic lupus erythematosus, 153, 154
   management/ complications of, 324, 326

T
Tachycardia, 195–197
Tamponade
   diagnosis/management, 219, 221
   gastroesophageal balloon, 285, 288
   pericardial, 348, 350
Teeth. *See also* entries under Dental
   avulsed primary, 369, 370
   extraction complications, 413, 414
Tension pneumothorax, 180, 181
   diagnosis/management, 348, 350
Tentorial herniation, 416, 417
Teratoma, presacral sacrococcygeal, 392, 395
Terrorism, biological and chemical, 444–448
Testes. *See also* Scrotum
   hydrocele, physiologic, 156, 157, 392, 395
   injuries, 359, 360
   retractile or undescended, 90, 91
   torsed, 137, 138, 155, 156, 157
Testicular appendage, torsion of, 155, 156
Testicular feminization syndrome, 292, 294
Tetanus immune globulin, 380, 381
Tetracaine/epinephrine/cocaine, 14, 15
Tetralogy of Fallot, 47, 48
   heart murmur in, 95, 96
Thalassemia
   diagnosis/management, 249, 252
   syndromes of, 158, 159, 160
Theophylline overdose, 256, 262
Therapeutic hyperventilation, 341, 343
Thoracentesis, 299, 301–302
Thoracic emergencies, 396–399
Thoracic trauma, 348–353
Thoracic tumors, 397, 399
Thyroglossal duct cysts, 124, 125
   diagnosis/management, 386, 387
Thyroid storm, 307, 309
Tics, 442, 443
Tinea capitis, 312, 314
Tinea versicolor, 168, 169
Tongue lacerations, 369, 370
Tonsillar hypertrophy, 188, 189
Tooth. *See* Teeth
TORCH, 92, 94, 116, 117
Torticollis
   acute, drugs causing, 126, 127
   brain tumor causing, 127, 128
   congenital muscular, 329, 331
   differential diagnosis, 126, 127, 404, 405
Tourette's syndrome, 44, 46
Toxic child, and abdominal distension, 29, 30
Toxic epidermal necrolysis, 163, 165
   diagnosis/management, 313, 315
Toxic megacolon, 286, 289
Toxic shock syndrome, 61, 62
   fever in, 77, 83
Toxicologic symptoms,
      diagnosis/management, 254–263
Toxins. *See also* Terrorism, biological and
      chemical
   antihistamines as cardiac, 255, 260
   carbon monoxide, 72, 73, 265, 267
   central anticholinergic, 75, 80

chemical, 256, 263
diagnosis/management
   anion gap, 254, 255, 258, 259
   gastrointestinal decontamination, 254, 258
   hypoglycemia signs, 254, 257
   osmolar gap, 254, 255, 258, 259
   whole bowel irrigation, 255, 258
ingestion of
   aliphatic hydrocarbons, 255, 259
   caustic agents, 255, 259
   enterotoxins, 255, 259
   lead, 256, 261
   methanol, 72, 73
   organophosphate, 208, 209
   organophosphates, 256, 261
   pain pills, 181, 182, 255, 260
   plant, 255, 260
   purpura in, 175
   tricyclic antidepressants, 256, 262
   vomiting and, 205, 206
inhalant, 255, 256, 260, 263
odors of, 130, 131
overdoses
   beta-blocker, 256, 261
   biguanide, 256, 261
   calcium channel blocker, 256, 261
   phenothiazine, 256, 262
   sulfonylurea, 256, 261
   theophylline, 256, 262
paralysis by, 208, 209
profiling patients, 254, 257
Tracheal compression, 396, 398
Tracheomalacia, 396, 398
Transient tachypnea, of newborn, 328, 330
Transplantation emergencies, 419–420
Transport
   air vs. ground, 21–23
   contraindications, 21, 22
   patient management, 21, 22
Transverse myelitis, 207, 208
Trauma. *See also* Accidents
   abdominal, 353–357
   acoustic, 93, 94
   ankle, 104–105
   bicycle accident, 335, 336, 355, 357
   blunt, 338, 339
   burn, 178, 179, 265–268, 370, 371, 372–374
   dental, 369–371
   diagnosis/management, 248–253, *See also* entries under specific trauma
   examination of children, 112, 113, 335–336
   eye, 364–367
   facial, 361–363
   genitourinary, 358–360
   gunshot wounds, 336, 342, 344, 355, 357
   head, 106–108, 335, 336, 337, 339, 341, 342, 343, 344
   knee, 109–111
   knife wounds, 335, 336
   lacerations, 380–382
   major, 337–340
   motor vehicle accident, 335–340, 355, 357
   neck, 338, 339, 341, 343, 346–347
   neurologic, 341–346
   oral, 369–371

orthopedic, 375–379, *See also* Fracture(s)
   otolaryngologic, 367–368
   renal, 358–360
   shoulder, 112–113
   spinal cord, 341, 342, 343, 344
   stab wounds, 335, 336, 355, 357
   thoracic, 348–353
   urethral, 338, 339
Traumatic asphyxia, 349, 351
Traumatic iritis, 365, 366
Trichomonal vaginitis, 203, 204
   diagnosis/management, 293, 295
Tricyclic antidepressants overdose, 256, 262
Tuberculosis
   diagnosis/management, 230, 237
   hematuria in, 98, 99
Tubo-ovarian abscess, 293, 296
Tumor lysis syndrome, 318, 320
Tumors
   bone, 319, 321
   brain, 17, 18, 319, 321
      torticollis and, 127, 128
   thoracic, 397, 399
   Wilm's, 319, 321
Typhlitis, 319, 321

U
Ulcerative colitis, 286, 289
Ulcers. *See also* Lesions
   aphthous, 134, 135
   peptic, 286, 289
Uncal herniation syndrome, 69, 70
Ureteral trauma, 358, 360
Urethral disruption, 353, 356
Urethral prolapse
   diagnosis/management, 292, 294
   and hematuria, 97, 98
   vaginal bleeding in, 201, 202
Urethral trauma, 338, 339, 359, 360. *See also* Genitourinary trauma
Urethritis
   chemically induced, 146, 147
   STD diagnostic testing, 146, 147
Urethrography, retrograde, 359, 360
Urinary frequency, childhood, 198–200
Urinary obstruction, 198, 199
   in newborn, 30, 31
Urinary tract infections, 198, 199
   diagnosis/management, 232, 238, 406, 407
   infants, 227, 234
   laboratory analysis, 232, 238
   risk factors, 232, 238
   hematuria in, 97, 98
   vomiting, 285, 288
Urologic emergencies, 406–407
Urticaria, 176–177, 313, 317
Uveitis, acute anterior, 71, 72

V
Vaginal bleeding, 201–202
Vaginal discharge, 203–204, 428, 430
Vaginal laceration, 359, 360
Vaginal lesions, diagnosis, 233, 239
Vaginal secretions/odors, 129, 130
Vaginitis, trichomonal, 203, 204
   diagnosis/management, 293, 295
Vaginosis, bacterial, 203, 204
   diagnosis/management, 293, 295

Varicella infection, 75, 80
  diagnosis/management
    in asthmatic patient, 233, 239
    complications, 231, 238
Varicella-zoster infection
  lesions of, 178, 179
  and remission in ALL, 320, 322
Vascular event, intracranial, 150, 151
Vascular rings, 396, 398
Vasodilation, cerebral, 150, 151
Vasovagal syncope, 192, 193
Venereal disease. *See* Sexually transmitted
    diseases
Ventilation. *See also* Respiratory
    stabilization
  airway assessment, 3, 5
  airway management, 16–18
  artificial airway, complications, 421, 423
  of asthmatic patient, 297, 300
  endotracheal intubation, 3, 5
    rapid-sequence, tube size, 16, 18
    tube placement, 3, 6
    tube size, 3, 4, 6
  rapid-sequence intubation, 16–18
    in brain tumor, 17, 18
    fentanyl use and effects, 17, 18

ketamine use and effects, 16, 18
    in multiple injuries, 17, 18
    sedatives/anesthetics, 16, 17, 18
    in status asthmaticus, 16, 17, 18
    in status epilepticus, 17, 18
    tube size, 16, 18
  in resuscitation
    agitated/uncooperative patient, 438,
      440
    basic and advanced, 3–7
    inadequate, 8, 9
    neonatal, 8–9
Ventricular contractions, premature, 195,
    197
Ventricular fibrillation, bretylium for, 4, 7
Ventricular septal defect, 30, 31
Ventricular tachycardia, 218, 221
Vertebral compression fractures, 139, 140
Vertigo, 57, 58, 403, 404
Vesicobullous rash, 178–179
Vestibular neuronitis, 57, 58
Vicarious menstruation, 61, 62
Visual disturbances, 71–73
Visual loss, diagnosis, 365, 366
Vitreous hemorrhage, 72, 73
Vomiting, 205–206

and urinary tract infection, 285, 288
von Willebrand's disease, trauma
    management in, 250, 253

W
Warts, genital, 293, 296
Wasp stings, 275, 277
Weakness, 207–209
Weber's test, 92, 93
Weight loss, 212–213
Weight loss, neonatal, 328, 331
Werdnig-Hoffman disease, 43, 207, 208
Wheezing, 281, 283
  differential diagnosis, 210–211
Wilm's tumor, 319, 321
Wilson's disease, 69, 70
  diagnosis/management, 287, 290
Wiskott-Aldrich syndrome, 318, 320
  sepsis in, 250, 253

X
X-linked hypogammaglobulinemia, 318,
    320

Y
Yellow jacket stings, 275, 277